ESSENTIALS OF
PATHOPHYSIOLOGY
FOR NURSING PRACTICE

Sara Miller McCune founded SAGE Publishing in 1965 to support the dissemination of usable knowledge and educate a global community. SAGE publishes more than 1000 journals and over 800 new books each year, spanning a wide range of subject areas. Our growing selection of library products includes archives, data, case studies and video. SAGE remains majority owned by our founder and after her lifetime will become owned by a charitable trust that secures the company's continued independence.

Los Angeles | London | New Delhi | Singapore | Washington DC | Melbourne

NEAL COOK
ANDREA SHEPHERD
JENNIFER BOORE
STEPHANIE DUNLEAVY

FOREWORD BY
BRENDAN MCCORMACK
AND TANYA MCCANCE

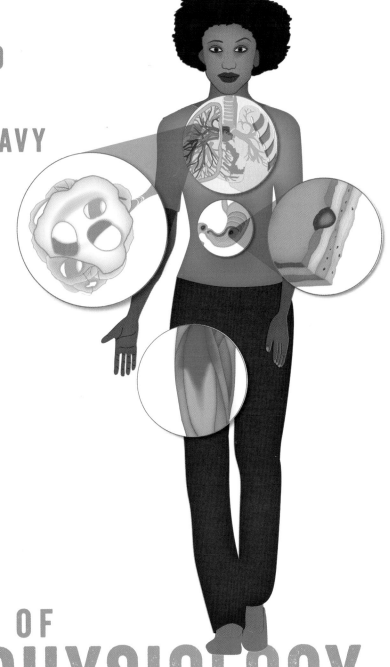

ESSENTIALS OF
PATHOPHYSIOLOGY
FOR NURSING PRACTICE

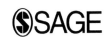

Los Angeles | London | New Delhi
Singapore | Washington DC | Melbourne

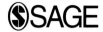

Los Angeles | London | New Delhi
Singapore | Washington DC | Melbourne

SAGE Publications Ltd
1 Oliver's Yard
55 City Road
London EC1Y 1SP

SAGE Publications Inc.
2455 Teller Road
Thousand Oaks, California 91320

SAGE Publications India Pvt Ltd
B 1/I 1 Mohan Cooperative Industrial Area
Mathura Road
New Delhi 110 044

SAGE Publications Asia-Pacific Pte Ltd
3 Church Street
#10-04 Samsung Hub
Singapore 049483

Editor: Alex Clabburn
Development editor: Laura Walmsley
Editorial assistant: Jade Grogan
Assistant editor, digital: Sunita Patel
Production editor: Tanya Szwarnowska
Copyeditor: Elaine Leek
Proofreader: Sharon Cawood
Marketing manager: George Kimble
Cover design: Shaun Mercier
Typeset by: C&M Digitals (P) Ltd, Chennai, India
Printed in the UK

Library of Congress Control Number: 2018960418

British Library Cataloguing in Publication data

A catalogue record for this book is available from the British Library

ISBN 978-1-4739-8022-8
ISBN 978-1-4739-8023-5 (pbk)
ISBN 978-1-5264-9481-8 (pbk & Interactive eBook)

At SAGE we take sustainability seriously. Most of our products are printed in the UK using responsibly sourced papers and boards. When we print overseas we ensure sustainable papers are used as measured by the PREPS grading system. We undertake an annual audit to monitor our sustainability.

CONTENTS

How to Use Your Book   viii

Overview of Your Book   xi

The Bodie Family   xv

About the Authors   xxv

Foreword   xxvii

Preface: Pathophysiology in the Context of Person-Centred Nursing   xxix

Acknowledgements   xxxiii

Terminology   xxxvii

Abbreviations   xli

Section 1 Health and Disease   **1**

1   Variation and Disease   3

2   Health and Disease in Society   23

3   Integrated Health Care   45

4   Principles of Pharmacology   83

5   Genetic Disorders   103

6   Mental Ill-Health   131

Section 2 Key Causes of Disease   **147**

7   Disorders of Immunity and Defence   149

8   Disorders of Blood and Blood Supply   189

9   Cellular Adaptation and Neoplastic Disorders   223

10   Disorders of Support and Protection   259

Section 3 Disorders of Homeostasis   **301**

11   Disorders of Renal Function and Fluid Balance   303

12   Disorders of Nutrient Supply and Faecal Elimination   335

13   Disorders of Metabolism   371

14   Disorders of Oxygenation and Carbon Dioxide Elimination   411

15   Disorders of the Cardiovascular System   447

Section 4 Disorders of Control and Coordination   479

16   Disorders of Neurological Control   481
17   Disorders of Endocrine Regulation   533
18   Disorders of the Female Reproductive System   553
19   Disorders of the Male Reproductive System   595

Appendix 1: American English Spelling Guide   617
Glossary   619
Index   673

HOW TO USE YOUR BOOK

Essentials of Pathophysiology for Nursing Practice has been developed with a number of features and online resources to help you succeed in your study.

FOUR STAGE LEARNING JOURNEY

Each chapter guides you through your learning journey in four stages, using video, activities, key concepts and examples to support you along the way.

2. APPLY: Put your knowledge and understanding into practice

1. UNDERSTAND: Get to grips with the 'need to know' essentials

3. REVISE: Test your knowledge, understanding and application

4. GO DEEPER: Engage with more advanced concepts

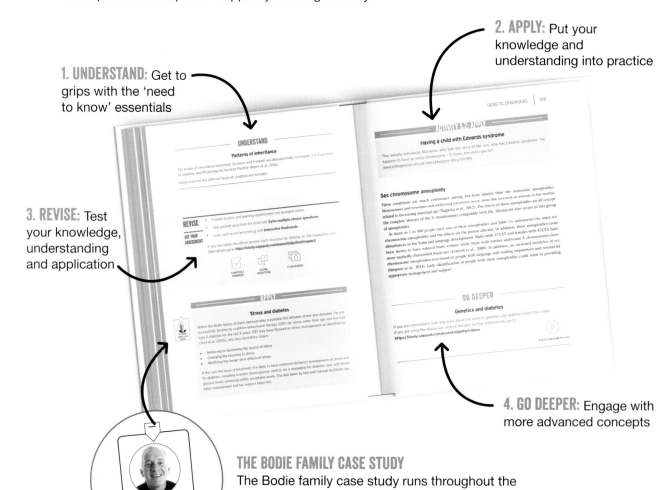

RICHARD JONES CASE NOTES

THE BODIE FAMILY CASE STUDY

The Bodie family case study runs throughout the book, helping you to place person-centredness at the heart of your learning. Meet the family on p. xv.

CURATED ONLINE RESOURCES

Online resources help to consolidate your knowledge and understanding and bring each chapter to life.

 Visualise essential concepts, theory and practice with curated video links.

 Test and refresh your knowledge with quizzes and assessment questions.

 Check your understanding of new vocabulary with flashcards for each chapter and an audio glossary.

 Advance your knowledge and build your bibliography with further reading.

HOW TO ACCESS THE ONLINE RESOURCES

An interactive eBook version of the text has been created so that you can easily navigate through the online resources while reading. Simply click on the icons throughout the book to be taken directly to each resource. **Download the free interactive eBook using your access code on the inside front cover.**

Alternatively, you can access the online resources by visiting https://study.sagepub.com/essentialpatho

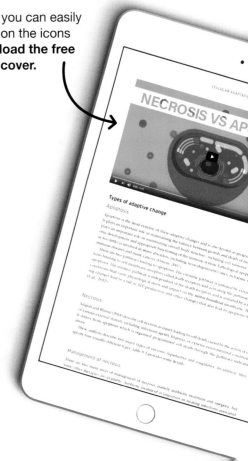

FOR LECTURERS

A wealth of accompanying digital resources, including a video teaching guide, testbank and image bank, is available to upload to your VLE/LMS and use in your teaching. To access the resources, visit

https://study.sagepub.com/essentialpatho

OVERVIEW OF YOUR BOOK

Before reading this book, it is important to recognise that this text is primarily a pathophysiology text; while we may recap on anatomy and physiology in places, this text is not a substitute for learning anatomy and physiology thoroughly before attempting to understand pathophysiology. We therefore strongly recommend that you are fresh and up to date with anatomy and physiology before delving into the complexities of pathophysiology. This book is structured to follow on from *Essentials of Anatomy and Physiology for Nursing Practice* (Boore et al., 2016) and our recommendation is to use the Revise sections in that book to check your anatomy and physiology knowledge and understanding. We will refer you to key chapters and sections in Boore et al. (2016) throughout this text.

In recognising that this is a pathophysiology text, we do make links to practice to assist you in applying the content you are learning. However, this text is not a treatment/intervention text; the knowledge you will learn in this book will help you to understand the physiological principles upon which interventions are based and will enable you to understand your practice and what is occurring with the people in your care. A thorough understanding of pathophysiology is central to being able to think critically and analyse signs and symptoms.

STRUCTURE

This book is laid out in four sections to provide a logical structure for the content. The sections are structured in a manner that shows you how they interrelate. Additionally, person-centredness spans all sections:

Section 1: Health and Disease (Chapters 1–6)

This section of the book examines some of the core issues that influence health and disease in society; the subject areas of this section span across the chapters and influence health in a wide context, such as genetics, epidemiology, interprofessional practice and social factors.

Section 2: Key Causes of Disease (Chapters 7–10)

This section starts to narrow down some of the key concepts in Section 1 to look more specifically at the key physiological disturbances which can influence the presentation of disease in various systems of the body. Later sections look at the different systems of the body and their disorders, but this section focuses on the way these disturbances occur and affect body tissues. For example, this section deals with disorders of blood and blood supply, which affects all systems, as does cellular adaptation and change, disorders of infection and immune response and disorders of support and protection. Together with Section 1, core concepts across systems are addressed.

Section 3: Disorders of Homeostasis (Chapters 11-15)

The concepts and issues addressed in Sections 1 and 2 will impact on homeostasis across systems. In this section, we examine disorders of systems of the body and in doing so apply wider concepts in a more focused, systematic way. This section includes looking at disorders of the renal, cardiovascular and respiratory systems, alongside disorders of metabolism and nutrient supply and elimination.

Section 4: Disorders of Control and Coordination (Chapters 16-19)

Finally, Section 4 recognises that life begins and continues through reproduction and that physiological and homeostatic processes are regulated by the nervous and endocrine systems. In this respect, disorders in these processes will have a systemic impact and therefore these systems are at the core.

Figure 0.1 illustrates how the sections of this book interrelate. Sections 1 (outer white segment) and 2 (blue segment) have a widespread impact across all systems, represented in the outer circles of the model

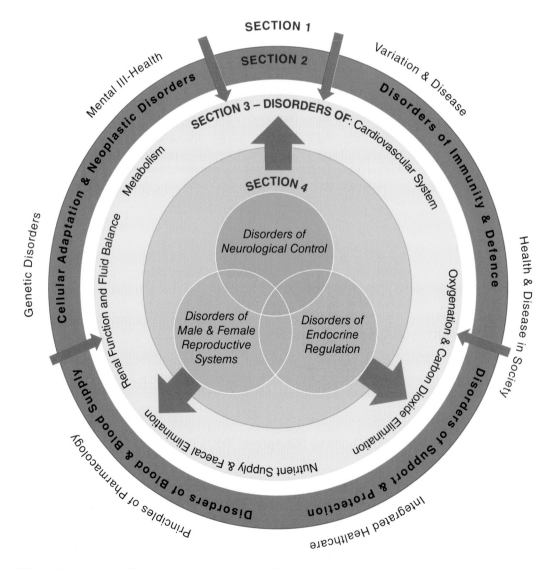

Figure 0.1 Interrelationship between the four different sections of the book

that have an inward influence. At the core, with influence radiating out, is Section 4 (grey segment), as it represents the control and coordination systems (including reproduction). Directly influenced by Section 4 below it and Sections 1 and 2 above, Section 3 (the yellow segment representing the disorders of systems) is positioned between these influencing factors.

We have endeavoured to write this book so that each chapter can be studied alone and make sense on its own, thus allowing chapters to be studied in the order of individual preference or to match your order of study. However, as can be seen, each section influences or is influenced by another and so we cross-reference between chapters in recognising that each chapter does not sit in isolation but is integral to the others. We advocate that you read the chapters in Sections 1 and 2 first, considering their widespread influence across all chapters of the book.

This book is further supported by a range of online resources for both students and lecturers to aid learning and teaching. These can be accessed via the interactive eBook version of the text, or via the companion website: **https://study.sagepub.com/essentialpatho**. For students, using these online resources alongside the book will help you during your initial learning and as you consolidate your knowledge and prepare for tests and exams.

1 Understand	• Learners are often unsure as to how much or how little they need to know. This book will identify the material that is fundamental to understand each particular system or component of the human body in order that you know that this is what you really need to learn. There will be some activities to support this process. Guidance to specific materials, including animations, will be provided which will aid understanding of certain body actions.
2 Apply	• Understanding pathophysiology is not enough as a nurse caring for people. Being effective as a nurse requires you to be able to apply the knowledge and understanding that you have gained. In this book, content that enables you to apply what you are learning to the care of people in society is highlighted.
3 Go Deeper	• For some of you, curiosity and only knowing the fundamentals of pathophysiology will not be enough for your personal needs. You may also want to improve and advance your knowledge for professional reasons. This section will highlight content that goes deeper than the essential knowledge you need to have. Some of you will find this helpful or just interesting, while others may choose not to study these areas.
4 Revise	• At this stage, you have learned the essential knowledge, applied it to practice and gone deeper if you wanted or needed to. You may have had a gap in your learning, or you may wish to refresh your knowledge or prepare for an exam. This stage will guide you on how you can revise through key points, and direct you to interactive activities to test your knowledge, understanding and application.

Figure 0.2 Four stages of learning

THE FOUR STAGES OF LEARNING

This book is set out in a staged process that takes you through your learning journey, using a colour-coded sequence. Four main approaches are used within each of the different topic areas covered: see Figure 0.2.

Throughout these four stages, this book will relate the content to a fictional family living in society: the Bodie family. Those of you who have read *Essentials of Anatomy and Physiology for Nursing Practice* (Boore et al., 2016) will be familiar with this family. Changes to our health are multifactorial, and it is within this context that nursing care is provided. Through relating to the Bodie family throughout this book, we aim to keep you focused on placing people at the centre of your nursing practice.

REFERENCE

Boore, J.R.P., Cook, N.F. and Shepherd, A. (2016) *Essentials of Anatomy and Physiology for Nursing Practice.* London: Sage.

THE BODIE FAMILY

In order to develop your application of pathophysiology to person-centredness you need to be able to reflect on how the experience of ill-health in society relates to a multi-generational family. Through this book we will develop your understanding of how pathophysiological processes result in illness and disease through applying the content to a variety of situations and conditions that can impact on what we do as nurses. Thinking about caring in the context of a family will help you to do this effectively. You may also be able to relate these situations to people you have met in practice or indeed your own family. In order to achieve this, we have created the fictional Bodie family and you will come across different members of the family in the various chapters of this book. Look out for the Bodie family icon, which will remind you to refer back to the Bodie family tree (Figure 0.3) and individual profiles. So now it is time to meet the family.

The grandparents are:

- George Bodie, an 84-year-old retired engineer, worked for a major rail company network for around 50 years. He remains very active and has a strong interest in cars. George met his wife, Maud, now 77 years of age, at the Young People's Guild at their local church. Maud was a dinner lady at a primary school before her marriage. They have been married for 59 years and have three children, four grandchildren and one great-grandchild and a Jack Russell dog, which they take for walks together. They now live in a bungalow in a small housing development on the outskirts of a small town. Their children all live within a 20-mile radius.

The three children and their families are:

- Edward Bodie, a 57-year-old accountant who is married to Sarah, a 55-year-old community midwife. Their 30-year-old son, Thomas, is a pilot with an international airline. He lives primarily in New York with his partner, Jack Garcia.
- Hannah Jones, a 54-year-old social worker who is married to Richard Jones, the 54-year-old vice-principal of a primary school. They have three children. The eldest, Derek, is a 29-year-old anaesthetist in a regional hospital, and they also have 27-year-old identical twin daughters, Michelle and Margaret. Michelle is a linguist who works as a translator for the EU in Brussels where she met her husband, Kwame Zuma, a 28-year-old South African civil servant. They have a 2-month-old baby girl, Danielle. Margaret is in Australia undertaking post-graduate research in marine biology of the Barrier Reef.
- Matthew Bodie is a 45-year-old unemployed electrician with a keen interest in competing in triathlons.

More information about each family member can be found in their individual profiles that follow.

Now that you know how this book works and you have met the Bodie family, it is time to start your learning journey.

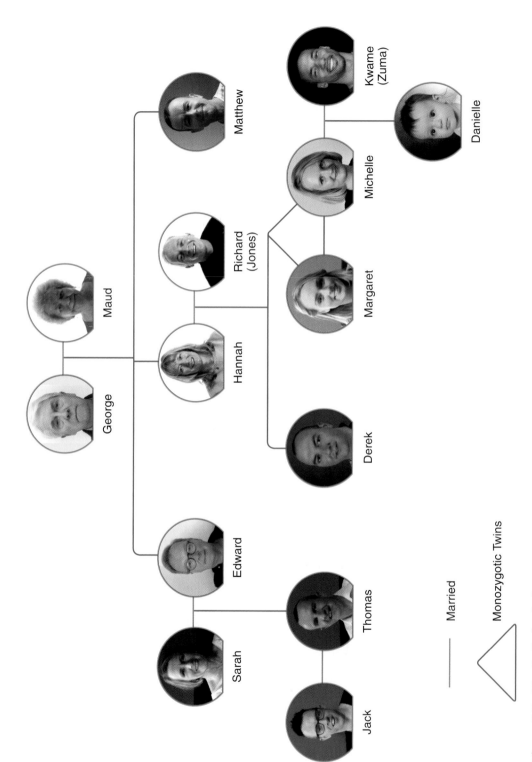

Figure 0.3 The Bodie family tree

Married

Monozygotic Twins

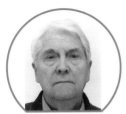

George Bodie

Social:

Marital Status: Married to Maud Bodie for 59 years.

Children: Father to Edward, Hannah and Matthew.

Occupation: Retired engineer, having worked for a major rail network for 50 years.

Hobbies: George is very active, having a strong interest in cars, walking their dog and spending time with the children, grandchildren and great-grandchild.

Housing: Lives in a bungalow in a small housing development with Maud. Their children live within a 20 mile radius.

Health

Age:	84	**Weight:**	84 kg
Height:	1.8 m (5'11")	**Eye Colour:**	Brown

BMI: 25.9 (overweight category (lower end))

History: Appendix removed at the age of 15. Has had raised cholesterol (hypercholesterolaemia) since he was 75, since when he has taken statins to lower it successfully. George gets the flu vaccine every year from his GP. George is not consciously aware of being thirsty.

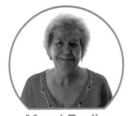

Maud Bodie

Social:

Marital Status: Married to George Bodie for 59 years

Children: Mother to Edward, Hannah and Matthew.

Occupation: Dinner lady until she married George.

Hobbies: Maud likes to walk their dog and spend time with the children, grandchildren and great-grandchild.

Housing: Lives in a bungalow in a small housing development with George. Their children live within a 20 mile radius.

Health

Age:	77	**Weight:**	73 kg
Height:	1.68 m (5'6")	**Eye Colour:**	Blue

BMI: 25.8 (overweight category (lower end))

History: Maud was diagnosed with heart failure three years ago (right ventricular failure) following a heart attack (myocardial infarction). She is prescribed digoxin and warfarin to improve the contractility of her heart and to thin her blood for better perfusion. She also was diagnosed with hypothyroidism at the age of 53, for which she takes thyroxine. Maud gets the flu vaccine every year from her GP.

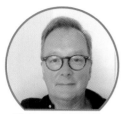

Edward Bodie

Marital Status:	Married to Sarah Bodie for 30 years.
Children:	Father to Thomas Bodie.
Occupation:	Accountant.
Hobbies:	Edward enjoys wine, and likes to make homemade wine in his spare time. He also likes to read modern fiction and is close to his son, Thomas.
Housing:	Lives in semi-detached house with a garden, located down a country lane.

Health

Age:	57	Weight:	90 kg
Height:	1.8 m (5'11")	Eye Colour:	Brown

BMI:	27.7 (overweight category)
History:	Edward suffers from chronic lower back pain.

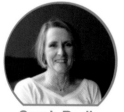

Sarah Bodie

Social:

Marital Status:	Married to Edward Bodie for 30 years.
Children:	Mother to Thomas Bodie.
Occupation:	Community Midwife.
Hobbies:	Sarah is an active painter, favouring watercolours. She also loves to play the guitar, having learned it as a child.
Housing:	Lives in semi-detached house with a garden, located down a country lane.

Health

Age:	55	Weight:	65 kg
Height:	1.73 m (5'8")	Eye Colour:	Brown

BMI:	21 (healthy weight category)
History:	Sarah had childhood chickenpox. Sarah is currently going through the menopause. She has recently stopped taking hormone replacement therapy after doing so for 2½ years.

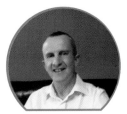

Thomas Bodie

Social:

Marital Status:	Partner to Jack Garcia for six years.
Children:	None, although he and Jack are keen to adopt in the future.
Occupation:	Pilot for an international airline.
Hobbies:	Thomas loves to ski and snowboard. He is very passionate about music, having learned to play the guitar from his mother. Thomas also loves to sing. Thomas attends the gym three times weekly to stay fit.
Housing:	His primary home is with Jack in New York, although he often stays with his parents when his work brings him in their direction. He and Jack live in a city-centre apartment.

Health

Age:	30	**Weight:**	72 kg
Height:	1.83 m (6′)	**Eye Colour:**	Brown

BMI:	21.4 (healthy weight category)
History:	Thomas is very healthy, eating a balanced diet. He has regular health checks as part of his occupation. Because of irregular hours of work, he has to ensure adequate sleep to maintain circadian rhythm.

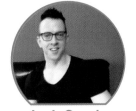

Jack Garcia

Social:

Marital Status:	Partner to Thomas Bodie for six years.
Children:	None, although he and Thomas are keen to adopt in the future.
Occupation:	Self-employed sculptor with his own studio in New York.
Hobbies:	Jack is very active in the gym, attending most mornings. He also collects art and is a volunteer at a local pet rescue centre.
Housing:	Jack lives in a city-centre apartment with Thomas.

Health

Age:	28	**Weight:**	73 kg
Height:	1.85 m (6′1″)	**Eye Colour:**	Blue

BMI:	21.3 (healthy weight category)
History:	Jack is very healthy, eating a balanced diet. His father has a history of testicular cancer and so Jack has been vigilant in performing Testicular Self-Examination (TSE) monthly since he was a teenager.

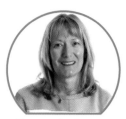

Hannah Jones

Social:

Marital Status:	Married to Richard Jones for 28 years.
Children:	Mother to Derek, and Michelle and Margaret (identical twins).
Occupation:	Social worker.
Hobbies:	Hannah likes to read and has an interest in hobby crafts.
Housing:	Hannah lives with her husband in a detached Victorian home in the countryside.

Health

Age:	54	**Weight:**	57 kg
Height:	1.7 m (5'7")	**Eye Colour:**	Brown

BMI:	19.7 (healthy weight category)
History:	Hannah likes to eat healthily, being fond of wholemeal bread and plenty of fruit and vegetables (five-a-day). Hannah smoked in her early 20s, but has successfully given up. She is currently going through the menopause. Hannah currently takes hormone replacement therapy using patches which are reportedly effective.

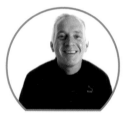

Richard Jones

Social:

Marital Status:	Married to Hannah Jones for 28 years.
Children:	Father to Derek, and Michelle and Margaret (identical twins).
Occupation:	Primary school teacher.
Hobbies:	Richard is a keen cyclist.
Housing:	He lives with his wife in a detached Victorian home in the countryside.

Health

Age:	54	**Weight:**	64 kg
Height:	1.78 m (5'10")	**Eye Colour:**	Brown

BMI:	20.1 (healthy weight category)
History:	Richard, like his wife, is fond of wholemeal bread and plenty of fruit and vegetables (five-a-day). He has suffered from stress in the past that was successfully managed through six weeks of cognitive behavioural therapy. Richard was diagnosed with type 2 diabetes five years ago.

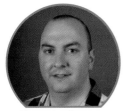

Derek Jones

Social:

Marital Status:	Single.
Children:	None.
Occupation:	Anaesthetist in a regional hospital.
Hobbies:	Derek is a keen chef and often takes cooking course holidays in different countries to widen his culinary skills and knowledge.
Housing:	Lives alone in a new build riverside apartment.

Health

Age:	29	**Weight:**	69 kg
Height:	1.85 m (6'1")	**Eye Colour:**	Blue

BMI: 20.1 (healthy weight category)

History: Derek has had mild persistent asthma since childhood for which he has been prescribed a β_2 agonist and a low-dose corticosteroid inhaler to reduce inflammation and dilate his airways. He is particular about having spare inhalers.

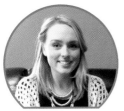

Margaret Jones

Social:

Marital Status:	Single.
Children:	None.
Occupation:	Post-graduate researcher in marine biology in Australia.
Hobbies:	Margaret likes to go horse-riding and goes running four times weekly.
Housing:	Lives with friends in a shared city-centre home.

Health

Age:	27	**Weight:**	69 kg
Height:	1.73 m (5'8")	**Eye Colour:**	Brown

BMI: 23 (healthy weight category)

History: Margaret has hay fever, which she manages well with antihistamines when it flares up.

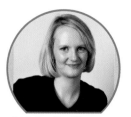

Michelle Zuma

Social:

Marital Status:	Married to Kwame Zuma for three years.
Children:	Mother to Danielle.
Occupation:	Linguist, working as a translator for the EU in Brussels.
Hobbies:	Michelle has a love for the theatre and has pursued both dance and acting interests.
Housing:	Lives with Kwame and Danielle in their house in Brussels.

Health

Age:	27	**Weight:**	64 kg
Height:	1.68 m (5′6″)	**Eye Colour:**	Brown

BMI:	21.3 (healthy weight category)
History:	Michelle broke (fractured) her right ankle during dance classes when she was 22. This healed uneventfully. She was severely ill when she was 10 and her growth was slowed: she is still slightly shorter than her twin sister. Michelle is currently breast-feeding Danielle after some initial difficulties.

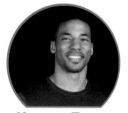

Kwame Zuma

Social:

Marital Status:	Married to Michelle Zuma for three years.
Children:	Father to Danielle.
Occupation:	South African civil servant working in Brussels.
Hobbies:	Kwame loves growing plants and vegetables. He is also a keen chess player.
Housing:	Lives with Michelle and Danielle in their house in Brussels.

Health

Age:	28	**Weight:**	85 kg
Height:	1.90 m (6′3″)	**Eye Colour:**	Brown

BMI:	23.5 (healthy weight category)
History:	Kwame has no significant medical history.

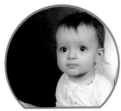

Danielle Zuma

Social:

Marital Status:	Single.
Children:	None.
Occupation:	Sleeping, eating and developing.
Hobbies:	Bath toys, plastic keys and being read stories.
Housing:	Lives with her parents in their house in Brussels.

Health

Age:	2 months	**Weight:**	5 kg (11 lb)
Height:	0.58 m (23″)	**Eye Colour:**	Brown

History: Danielle is a healthy baby and is still being breast-fed by her mother. She is undergoing routine vaccinations.

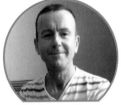

Matthew Bodie

Social:

Marital Status:	Single.
Children:	None.
Occupation:	Electrician (currently unemployed).
Hobbies:	Matthew has a keen interest in undertaking triathlons. He also likes to restore vintage cars, which his father enjoys helping with. Matthew also enjoys DIY activities.
Housing:	Lives alone in a cottage.

Health

Age:	45	**Weight:**	82 kg
Height:	1.83 m (6′)	**Eye Colour:**	Brown

BMI: 24.4 (healthy weight category)

History: Matthew has suffered from depression since his early 30s. This is successfully treated with antidepressant therapy.

REFERENCES

AACN (American Association of Colleges of Nursing) (2008) *The Essentials of Baccalaureate Education for Professional Nursing Practice*. Washington: AACN.

EU (2005) Directive 2005/36/EC of the European Parliament and of the Council of 7 September 2005 on the recognition of professional qualifications, Article 31. Available at: http://eur-lex.europa.eu/LexUriServ/LexUriServ.do?uri=OJ:L:2005:255:0022:0142:EN:PDF (accessed 5 January 2015).

McCormack, B. and McCance, T. (2010) *Person-centred Nursing: Theory and Practice*. Oxford: Wiley-Blackwell.

NMC (Nursing and Midwifery Council) (2010) *Standards for Pre-registration Nursing Education*. London: NMC.

ABOUT THE AUTHORS

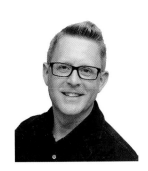

Dr Neal Cook is a Reader and the Associate Head of School at the School of Nursing, Ulster University and a Fellow of the Higher Education Academy. He is the Athena SWAN Champion for the School. He is also President of the European Association of Neuroscience Nurses and an Executive Board Member of the British Association of Neuroscience Nurses. Neal has taught anatomy, physiology and pathophysiology to undergraduate and postgraduate nursing students across a number of courses since he commenced working in higher education. Neal is also an Advanced Life Support Instructor, teaching life support courses in Health and Social Care Trusts and in the University. He has worked in the fields of neurosciences and critical care since registering as a nurse, becoming a specialist practitioner and subsequently moving into education and research. Neal has published clinical, research and education papers in the fields of education and neurosciences and remains very active in these endeavours. He remains clinically active in neurosciences and is still a registered nurse with the Nursing and Midwifery Council (UK).

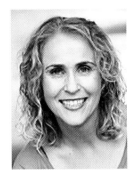

Andrea Shepherd is a Lecturer in Nursing at the School of Nursing, Ulster University and a Fellow of the Higher Education Academy. She has taught anatomy, physiology and pathophysiology to undergraduate and postgraduate nursing students across a number of courses since she commenced working in higher education. Andrea is also an Advanced Life Support Instructor, teaching life support courses in Health and Social Care Trusts and in the University. She has worked in the fields of critical care and orthopaedics since registering as a nurse, becoming a specialist practitioner and subsequently moving into education. She currently takes a lead role in adult pre-registration nursing, is clinically active in critical care and remains a registered nurse with the Nursing and Midwifery Council (UK).

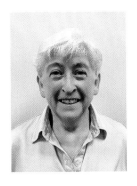

Professor Jennifer Boore is Emeritus Professor of Nursing at the School of Nursing, Ulster University. Jenny started her career as a registered nurse, followed by becoming a midwife. She practised as a nurse and midwife in the UK and Australia for some years before returning and beginning her first degree in human biology. After working as a clinical teacher with the degree students, she obtained a Research Fellowship at the University of Manchester and completed her PhD on preoperative preparation of patients. From 1977 to 1984 Jenny worked as a Lecturer in Nursing at the Universities of Edinburgh and Hull and was then appointed as Professor of Nursing at the University of Ulster in 1984 (the first Professor of Nursing in Ireland). Jenny has an extensive background in education, research and professional regulation. She has taught anatomy, physiology and pathophysiology to undergraduate and postgraduate nursing students across a number of courses throughout her career. Her contributions to nursing have been recognised in achieving the honours of Fellow of the Royal College of Nursing in 1993 and Officer of the Order of the British Empire in 1996. Jenny continues to be active in nursing education and writing.

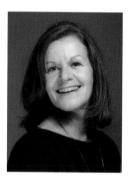

Stephanie Dunleavy is a Lecturer in Nursing and academic lead for pre-registration Nursing programmes at the School of Nursing, Ulster University and a Fellow of the Higher Education Academy. She has taught anatomy, physiology and pathophysiology to undergraduate and postgraduate nursing students across a number of courses since she commenced working in higher education. Stephanie is also an Immediate Life Support Instructor, teaching life support courses in the School. She has worked in the fields of critical care and neurosciences and has completed a BSc (Hons) in Life Sciences and a Masters of Business Administration since registering as a nurse, subsequently moving into education. She currently takes a lead role in adult pre-registration nursing and curriculum design, and remains a registered nurse with the Nursing and Midwifery Council (UK).

ULSTER UNIVERSITY

The School of Nursing at Ulster provides pre-registration and post-registration nursing education across two campuses in Northern Ireland and internationally. The Person-Centred Nursing Framework (McCormack and McCance, 2010, 2019) informs the curricular framework for pre-registration nursing courses at the School and influence a wide variety of programmes and research activity within the School and the Institute of Nursing and Health Research. Both the School and the Institute of Nursing and Health Research are recognised as excellent and leading in their field nationally and internationally.

REFERENCES

McCormack, B. and McCance, T. (2010) *Person-Centred Nursing: Theory and Practice*. Chichester: Wiley–Blackwell.

McCormack, B. and McCance, T. (eds) (2017) *Person-Centred Practice in Nursing and Health Care: Theory and Practice*, 2nd edn. Chichester: Wiley–Blackwell.

FOREWORD

It is a pleasure to write this foreword for the book *Essentials of Pathophysiology for Nursing Practice* by Neal Cook, Andrea Shepherd, Jennifer Boore, and Stephanie Dunleavy. We commend the authors for the approach they have adopted in this book and in their previous publication, *Essentials of Anatomy and Physiology for Nursing Practice*, i.e. a person-centred one! That might seem like a strange statement to make in a pathophysiology textbook for nurses, which of course is going to be about persons, i.e. human beings. However, as the history of science has shown us, the development of knowledge has a sketchy track record when it comes to adopting holistic approaches. Whilst few contemporary scientists would endorse Cartesian Dualism as a valid way of looking at persons, it is still the case that much of our knowledge development, testing and validation processes divide the person into individual (or, at best, grouped) parts. This is a significant challenge when trying to teach the science of nursing, where curricula often make a (false) distinction between the science and art of nursing or, at best, show connections between the two.

A person-centred approach holds the holistic uniqueness of all persons as central. The biological and pathophysiological make-up of persons is critical to this perspective of course, acting as the container and carrier for the ontological positioning of the person in their world. A person-centred perspective holds that our physical make-up integrates with our existential make-up and together make us a person. The approach taken in this book makes this approach explicit in its teaching of pathophysiology. It enables the student and educator to engage in a holistic conversation about persons (the whole), whilst at the same time paying attention to individual parts, systems and processes. We believe that this approach to the teaching of pathophysiology will enable future nurses to hold a holistic worldview from the start and to take that knowledge into their chosen field of practice. The need for nurses to stand firm with this approach has never been greater, in a world that is obsessed with safety, control and regulation.

Professor Brendan McCormack, Queen Margaret University, Edinburgh
Professor Tanya McCance, Ulster University, Northern Ireland

PREFACE

PATHOPHYSIOLOGY IN THE CONTEXT OF PERSON-CENTRED NURSING

This textbook is designed to be synergistic with your preparation to become a nurse or to enhance your knowledge as a registered nurse. While the content is very biological at its core, the intention is that you will learn about pathophysiology within the context of person-centredness. In writing this text, we have ensured the content is synergistic with the Person-Centred Nursing Framework (PCNF) (McCormack and McCance, 2019) (Figure 0.4) in that we believe that your development and knowledge cannot be separated from your ethos of practice and the values of the nursing profession. Ultimately, nurses need to be able to deliver safe, compassionate and effective nursing care and this requires that any new knowledge you develop is not isolated from how you practise, your philosophical approach to care and the impact you can have on people and society.

In caring for people, families and communities, nurses need to remember to be relational, rather than process-driven, in order to make those human connections and develop therapeutic relationships with people that enable care to be compassionate and aligned with their fundamental values, wishes and rights. Understanding health and disease in society is central to the public and population health agenda globally; the World Health Organisation (WHO) monitors its member countries' achievements in terms of their Sustainable Development Goals (SDGs) (WHO, 2018). SDGs each have specific targets for achievement within 15 years through one health goal and 50 health-related targets. These are universal across all countries involved. This book starts with a section on health and disease in order to equip you with some key knowledge that is necessary in building your knowledge for practice that is fundamental to understanding and delivering on this public and population health agenda. Being politically aware in terms of health and social care policy, both nationally and globally, is an essential component of professional practice and therefore we have given some focus to epidemiology; nurses of the future are expected to be strategic leaders while also being able to deliver on effective **health promotion, health protection** and in preventing ill-health (Nursing and Midwifery Council [NMC], 2018). As a result, learning pathophysiology is not just intended to give you the knowledge to provide care to people who are ill, but also to understand what causes ill-health in order that you can contribute to keeping the population healthy. Delivering on this requires strategic direction and a knowledgeable workforce; understanding the factors that contribute to health and disease enables nurses to contribute to developing and delivering on such strategies and we are part of that workforce and must be able to work with a range of professionals and interdisciplinary teams to achieve this (McCormack and McCance, 2017; NMC, 2018).

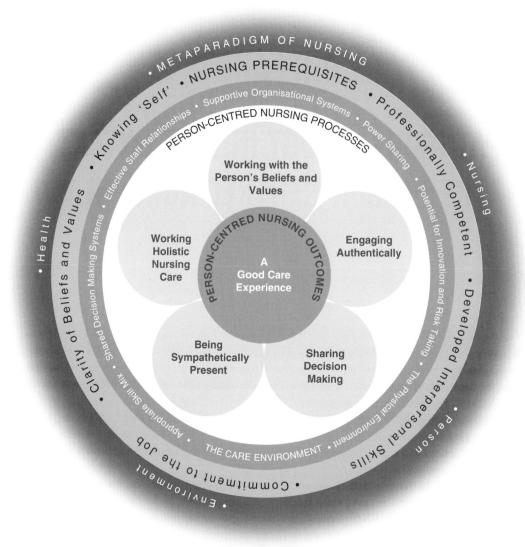

Figure 0.4 Person-Centred Nursing Framework

Source: © McCormack and McCance, 2019. Reproduced with permission.

When nurses lack compassion, the people they care for are no longer at the centre of their practice. This devalues the person and can leave them feeling unsupported (Bramley and Matiti, 2014). Being compassionate requires us to have sympathetic presence (McCormack and McCance, 2017), whereby we understand the experience of the person not purely from a biological perspective but how that illness affects them across all components of their life – socially, emotionally, spiritually, physically. In having a strong understanding of pathophysiology, you will be able to make the connections with the person's presenting signs and symptoms as well as the necessary medical interventions to restore, where possible, homeostasis. However, this cannot be at the expense of understanding the wider impact on the person. Nurses therefore need to be relational and reflective; this requires authentic engagement if care is to be person-centred.

Emotional intelligence is recognised as a key attribute of a registered nurse (NMC, 2018) and is central to bringing together knowledge and skills into nursing practice that is compassionate and person-centred. In this book we have provided opportunities for you to reflect and to apply your knowledge to caring within a person-centred context; how much you do this is down to you and we encourage you to take those opportunities so that you can be holistic and compassionate in your approach to care.

Finally, when reading this book, it is important to focus on understanding; the danger always lies in trying to memorise content for the purpose of assessment when instead it is much more important that you understand what is happening physiologically in a person. This knowledge is central to you being a confident practitioner who can think critically; understanding is central to applying your knowledge in order that your practice as a nurse is expert, informed and safeguards the welfare of the people in your care. There are interactive elements within the text to help develop that understanding alongside the revision sections and other study aids. Unless you have a confident understanding of anatomy and physiology, you will find it very challenging to understand pathophysiology. We therefore also recommend that you reconnect with the anatomy and physiology that you have learned, and in places we refer you to Boore et al. (2016) in order to help direct you to relevant content.

So now we invite you to engage with this book in anticipation that you gain an understanding of pathophysiology that enables you to practise through a compassionate, person-centred approach.

REFERENCES

Boore, J.R.P., Cook, N.F. and Shepherd, A. (2016) *Essentials of Anatomy and Physiology for Nursing Practice.* London: Sage.

Bramley, L. and Matiti, M. (2014) How does it really feel to be in my shoes? Patients' experiences of compassion within nursing care and their perceptions of developing compassionate nurses. *Journal of Clinical Nursing, 23* (19–20): 2790–9.

McCormack, B. and McCance, T. (eds) (2017) *Person-centred Practice in Nursing and Health Care: Theory and Practice,* 2nd edn. Chichester: Wiley–Blackwell.

McCormack, B. and McCance, T. (2019) The Person-Centred Nursing Framework 2010 Revised. Belfast: Ulster University. Available at: https://www.ulster.ac.uk/nursingframework (accessed 15 April 2019).

Nursing and Midwifery Council (NMC) (2018) *Future Nurse: Standards of Proficiency for Registered Nurses.* London: NMC.

World Health Organisation (WHO) (2018) *World Health Statistics 2018 – Monitoring Health for the SDGs.* Geneva: WHO.

ACKNOWLEDGEMENTS

AUTHOR ACKNOWLEDGEMENTS

The authors would like to thank all who have provided support, direction and inspiration in the development of this book. The book was inspired by student nurses in anticipation that it will support them in their learning and development. In particular, we would like to thank:

- Our partners, families, friends and colleagues, who have supported, encouraged and motivated us throughout. This is our third book on this theme and was yet another great undertaking for us and this support is invaluable.
- The team at SAGE, who continue to be supportive, enthusiastic and professional critical friends throughout. We are fortunate to be able to continue to work with you all.
- Professor Brendan McCormack and Professor Tanya McCance. Thank you for the inspiration and drive for person-centred nursing and for the eloquent Foreword. We are delighted with your continued support for this theme of work and to be able to integrate your pioneering body of work with ours.

The Bodie family have enabled us to make connections between people and physiological processes; this is central to remaining focused on the care of people and aims to promote compassion, dignity and empathy. The Bodie family are made more real by those who kindly provided their photographs; you continue to make a lovely family! Thank you to:

- Annalee Cook
- David Freeman
- Deirdre Ward
- Derek Shepherd
- Ian Munnerley
- Joseph Friel
- Kevin Holly
- Leslie Smith
- Maureen Smith
- Niamh O'Doherty
- Peter Monaghan
- Stephanie Cook
- Tracy Munnerley
- Trevor Adams

To Professor Owen Barr for your expertise in reviewing, and guiding us in revising our chapter on genetic disorders. We appreciate the time you took to support us.

To Marie O'Neill for your expertise in reviewing our chapter on mental ill-health. Your passionate and significant contributions to the field of mental health helped us identify the need for a chapter of this type in a pathophysiology text and so we are forging forward with a new trend.

We have had so much support and encouragement to write this text from nursing students. Our goal is to support you in your learning and we are proud of all of your contributions to the care of people in society.

PUBLISHER'S ACKNOWLEDGEMENTS

The publishers would like to thank all of the academic reviewers who contributed thoughtful and helpful feedback on various parts of the book at draft stage, shaping the present book for the better. Special thanks also to Tom Walvin, Plymouth University, for writing the Multiple Choice Questions for the book.

Didy Button, Flinders University
Denise Cheung, University of Hong Kong School of Nursing
David Gallimore, Swansea University
Alison Grant, Glasgow Caledonian University
Natalie Hay, Robert Gordon University
John Knight, Swansea University
Richard Leece, Robert Gordon University
Andrew Powell, Birmingham City University
Mark Ranson, University of Suffolk
Mari Salminen-Tuomaala, Seinäjoki University of Applied Sciences
Sheila Sobrany, Middlesex University
David Tait, Edinburgh Napier University
Donald Todd, Robert Gordon University
Anne Williams, Queen Margaret University
Marjorie Wilson, Teeside University
Deborah Willson, Stellenbosch University

Student reviewers

Grant Byrne, Queen Margaret University
Maria Lynass, Queen Margaret University

THIRD-PARTY MATERIAL

The publishers are grateful to all third parties for permission to reproduce the following material:

Figure 0.4 McCormack, B. and McCance, T. (2019) The Person-Centred Nursing Framework 2010 Revised. Belfast: Ulster University. Available at: https://www.ulster.ac.uk/nursingframework (accessed 15 April 2019).

Table 1.1 Variation in Biological Characteristics (Overfield, 1995). Overfield, T. (1995) *Biologic Variation in Health and Illness: Race, Age and Sex Differences*, 2nd edn. Menlo Park, CA: Addison-Wesley.

Figure 2.1 Illustration of Global Charter for the Public's Health (Lomazzi, M. 2016). A Global Charter for the Public's Health – the public health system: role, functions, competencies and education requirements. *European Journal of Public Health*, 26(2): 210–212. Available at: https:// www.ncbi.nlm. nih.gov/pmc/articles/PMC4804738/ (accessed 13 June 2018).

Table 2.3 Ten Essential Public Health Operations (EPHOs) (WHO Europe, 2012). *European Action Plan for Strengthening Public Health Capacities and Services*. Copenhagen: World Health Organisation Regional Office for Europe. Available at: www.euro.who.int/__data/assets/pdf_ file/0005/171770/RC62wd12rev1-Eng.pdf (accessed 9 March 2018).

Figure 2.3 Global Strategic Directions for Strengthening Nursing and Midwifery 2016–2020. WHO (2016b) Global strategic directions for strengthening nursing and midwifery 2016–2020. Geneva: World Health Organisation. Available at: www.who.int/hrh/nursing_midwifery/global-strategic-midwifery2016-2020.pdf (accessed 6 October 2018).

Table 3.3 Classification of Surgery. Meeker, M.H. and Rothrock, J.C. (1999) *Alexander's Care of the Patient in Surgery*, 11th edn. St. Louis, MO: Mosby.

Table 3.4 Side Effects of Chemotherapy (NHS Choices, 2015b). Chemotherapy – Side effects. NHS Online. Available at: www.nhs.uk/Conditions/Chemotherapy/Pages/Definition.aspx (accessed 20 March 2016).

Table 3.8 Connect's core values (Anderson and Van Der Gaag, 2005, p18). Anderson, C. and Van Der Gaag, A. (2005) *Speech and Language Therapy: Issues in Professional Practice*. London: Whurr Publishers.

Table 3.13 Interprofessional Education Approaches (Barr and Low, 2011). Barr, H. and Low, H. (2011) *Principles of Interprofessional Education*. Fareham, England: Centre for the Advancement of Interprofessional Education (CAIPE) Available at: https://www.caipe.org/resources/publications/barr-low- 2011-principles-interprofessional-education (accessed 22 July 2017).

Table 3.14 Characteristics of a good interdisciplinary team (Nancarrow et al., 2013, Table 5, page 9 of 11). Nancarrow, S.A., Booth, A., Ariss, S., Smith, T., Enderby, P. and Roots, A. (2013) Ten principles of good interdisciplinary team work. *Human Resources for Health*, 11:19. doi: 10.1186/1478-4491-11-19. Available at: http://human-resources-health.biomedcentral.com/ articles/10.1186/1478-4491-11-19 (accessed 21 March 2016).

Table 4.4 Pharmacokinetics in Young and Old (from Lilley et al., 1917)]. Lilley, L.L., Collins, S.R. and Snyder, J.S. (2017) *Pharmacology and the Nursing Process*, 8th edn. St. Louis, MO: Mosby.

Table 5.5 Autosomal Chromosomal Aneuploidies (from Jorde et al., 2016). Jorde, L.B., Carey, J.C. and Bamshad, M.J. (2016) *Medical Genetics*. Philadelphia, PA: Elsevier.

Table 5.6 Sex Chromosomal Aneuploidies (from Jorde et al., 2016). Jorde, L.B., Carey, J.C. and Bamshad, M.J. (2016) *Medical Genetics*. Philadelphia, PA: Elsevier.

Table 5.8 Examples of Mitochondrial Diseases (Jorde et al., 2016). Jorde, L.B., Carey, J.C. and Bamshad, M.J. (2016) *Medical Genetics*. Philadelphia, PA: Elsevier.

Table 5.9 Preparing Family Trees (Skirton et al., 2005, pp. 37–39). Skirton, H., Patch, C. and Williams, J. (2005) *Applied Genetics in Healthcare: A Handbook for Specialist Practitioners*. New York/Abingdon: Taylor and Francis/T & F Informa.

Table 8.6 Types of Anaemia (Mayo Clinic, 2017). Mayo Clinic (2017) Anemia. Mayo Foundation for Medical Education and Research. Available at: https://www.mayoclinic.org/diseases-conditions/anemia/symptoms-causes/syc-20351360 (accessed 9 May 2018).

Figure 9.4 Mechanism by which tumour cells evade the immune system. Abbas et al. (2015): *Cellular and Molecular Immunology*, 8th edn. Philadelphia, PA: Elsevier Saunders. p. 390.

Figure 9.7 Estimated world cancer incidence and mortality in 2012 for both sexes combined in the major world regions (IARC World Cancer Report 2014). International Agency for Research on Cancer (2014) World Cancer Report 2014. Lyon, France: IARC.

Figure 9.8 Estimated European cancer 5-year prevalence proportions by major sites, in both sexes combined, 2012. (IARC, World Cancer Report 2014). International Agency for Research on Cancer (2014) World Cancer Report 2014. Lyon, France: IARC.

Table 9.9 Evidence based screening methods. (2018) Cancer Staging System. Chicago: American Joint Committee on Cancer. Available at: https://cancerstaging.org/references-tools/Pages/ What-is-Cancer-Staging.aspx (accessed 1 August 2018).

Table 13.8 Causes and Risk Factors in Diabetes Mellitus Type 2 (NHS Choices, 2016b). NHS Choices (2016b) Type 2 diabetes. Available at: www.nhs.uk/conditions/Diabetes-type2/ Pages/Introduction. aspx?url=Pages/what-is-it.aspx (accessed 17 September 2017).

Table 13.11 Examples of Liver Disorders (NHS Choices, 2014). NHS Choices (2014) Liver Disease. Available at: www.nhs.uk/conditions/liver-disease/Pages/Introduction.aspx (accessed 31 August 2017).

Table 13.12 Types of Hepatitis (NHS Choices, 2016c). NHS Choices (2016c) Hepatitis. Available at: www.nhs.uk/Conditions/Hepatitis/Pages/Introduction.aspx (accessed 1 September 2017).

Table 15.1 NICE (2011) Definitions of Hypertension. NICE (National Institute for Health and Care Excellence) (2011) Hypertension in adults: diagnosis and management. London: NICE.

TERMINOLOGY

Table T.1 Prefixes

Prefix	Meaning
adip/o-	fat
ab-	away from
ad-	toward, near to
aer-/o	air
af-	toward
all/o-	other
a/an-	without
ana-	up, apart, backward, again, anew
ante-	before, forward
angi/o-	vessel (blood)
anti-	against
apo-	off, away
ather/o-	plaque (fatty substance)
aut/auto-	self, own
bar/o-	pressure, weight
bas/o-	base, opposite of acid
bi-	two, twice, double
brady-	slow
cata-	down, lower
chrom/o-	colour
chondr/o-	cartilage
circum-	around
contra-	against, counter
cost/o	pertaining to a rib
cyt/o	pertaining or referring to a cell
de-	lack of, down, less, removal of
dia-	through, completely, across, apart
dipl/o-	double

Prefix	Meaning
dis-	apart, to separate
dys-	bad, painful, difficult, abnormal
ecto-	out, outside
eff-	out, out of, from
em/en-	in, on
end/o-	in, within
eosin/o-	red, rosy, dawn-coloured
epi-	above, upon, on
erg/o	work
erythr/o-	red
eu-	good, normal
ex-	out, away from
extra-	outside
glyc/o-, glycos/o-	glucose, sugar
haem-	blood
hapl/o-	simple, single
hemi-	half
hepat/o-	liver
homeo-	sameness, unchanging, constant
hydr/o-	water
hyper-	above, excessive
hypo-	deficient, below, under, less than normal
infra-	beneath
inter-	between
intra-	within, into
intro-	into, within
is/o-	same, equal
juxta-	near

Prefix	Meaning	Prefix	Meaning
kary/o-	nucleus	pneum/o-, pneumon/o-	lung, air, gas
kerat/o-	hard, horny tissue	poly-	many, much
kines/o-, kinesi/o-	movement	post-	after, behind
leuk/o-	white	pre-	before, in front of
lip/o-	fat, lipid	pro-	before, forward
ly/o-	to dissolve, loosen	proxim/o-	near
macro-	large	pseud/pseudo-	false
mal-	bad	quadri-	four
mega-	large, enlarged	retro-	backward, located behind
meso-	middle	sarc/o-	flesh (connective tissue)
meta-	change, beyond	semi-	half, partly
micro-	small	somat/o-	body
multi-	many	steno-	narrow, contracted
my/o-	muscle	sub-	under, below
neo-	new	super-	above
necro-	death	supra-	above, upper
neur/o-	nerve	syn- / sym-	together, with
neutr/o-	neutral	tachy-	fast, rapid
noci-	to cause harm, injury or pain	tel/o-	complete
oligo-	few, less than	thromb/o-	clot
oste/o-	bone	trans-	across, through
para-	near, beside, abnormal, apart from, along the side of	tri-	three, triple
patho-	disease	ultra-	beyond, in excess
per-	through	viscer/o-	internal organs
peri-	surrounding, around		

Table T.2   Suffixes

Suffix	Meaning	Suffix	Meaning
-able, -ible	ability to, capable of	-crine	to secrete, separate
-aemia, -aemic	pertaining or referring to blood	-cyte	pertaining or referring to a cell
-aesthesia	condition of sensation	-ectasis	dilation, distension
-al, -ar	pertaining to	-ectomy	removal, cutting out
-algia	referring to pain	-emesis	vomiting
-ary	pertaining to, connected with	-flux	flow
-ase	enzyme	-form	shape, structure
-ate	action or state	-fugal	movement away from
-blast	embryonic, immature cell	-genesis, -gen, -genic	producing, forming
-centesis	a piercing		
-cle, -cula, -cule, -culum, -culus	diminutive	-gram	record, recording, writing
		-ia	state, condition

Suffix	Meaning
-ic	pertaining to
-ile	pertaining to, characteristic of
-ion	process, action
-ism	process, condition
-itis	inflammation
-ity	state
-kinesis	movement
-lith	stone
-logy	study of, branch of
-lysis	breakdown, separation, destruction, loosening
-metry	process of measuring
-oid	resembling, derived from
-ole	little, small
-oma	tumour
-oxia	condition of oxygenation
-penia	deficiency of
-phage, -phagia	eat, swallow, ingestion of, consumption

Suffix	Meaning
-philia	like, love, attraction to
-phobia	fear
-plasia	growth, formation
-plegia	paralysis of
-poiesis	formation
-rrhagia	bleeding from, flow of
-rrhoea	flow
-sclerosis	hardening
-sis	state or process
-stasis	to stop, control, place
-tax/o	order, coordination
-tomy	cut/incise
-ton/o	tension
-trophy	nourishment, development (condition of)
-uria	refers to urine condition
-zyme	enzyme

ABBREVIATIONS

Abbreviation	Expansion
ABPM	ambulatory blood pressure monitoring
ACE	angiotensin-converting enzyme
acetyl CoA	acetyl coenzyme A
ACh	acetylcholine
AChE	acetylcholinesterase
ACSM	American College of Sports Medicine
ACTH	adrenocorticotrophic hormone
ADA	adenosine deaminase
ADH	anti-diuretic hormone
ADP	adenosine diphosphate
ADRs	adverse drug reactions
AF	atrial fibrillation
AGCT	adult granulosa cell tumour
AGNC	Association of Genetic Nurses and Counsellors
AIDS	acquired immune deficiency syndrome
AIET	autologous immune enhancement therapy
AKD	acute kidney diseases and disorders
AKI	acute kidney injury
ALD	assistive listening devices
ALI	acute lung injury
ALS	amyotrophic lateral sclerosis
AMI	acute myocardial infarction
ANA	antinuclear antibodies
ANP	atrial natriuretic peptide
ANS	autonomic nervous system

Abbreviation	Expansion
ANTT	aseptic non-touch technique
APA	American Psychiatric Association
APA	anti-pituitary antibodies
APC	antigen-presenting cells
APP	acute phase proteins
APPs	amyloid precursor proteins
APR	acute phase response
ARDS	acute respiratory distress syndrome
ART	anti-retroviral treatment
ASD	autism spectrum disorder
ASHG	American Society for Human Genetics
AT	atrial tachycardia
ATN	acute tubular necrosis
ATP	adenosine triphosphate
AV	atrioventricular
AVNRT	atrioventricular nodal reentrant tachycardia
AVRT	atrioventricular reciprocating tachycardia
AVSD	atrioventricular septal defect
B/P	blood pressure
BAcC	British Acupuncture Council
BBB	blood-brain barrier
BCG	Bacillus Calmette-Guérin (vaccine)
BCOP	blood colloid osmotic pressure
BMD	bone mineral density
BMD	Becker muscular dystrophy
BMI	body mass index

Abbreviation	Expansion
BMR	basal metabolic rate
BNF	British National Formulary
BNP	B-type natriuretic peptide
BPH	benign prostatic hyperplasia
bpm	beats per minute
BRCA1	Breast Cancer gene 1
BRCA2	Breast Cancer gene 2
BSA	body surface area
Ca	cancer
CAA	cerebral amyloid angiopathy
CAC	citric acid cycle
CAD	coronary artery disease
CAG	cytosine, adenine and guanine
CAM	complementary and alternative medicine
CAP	community-acquired pneumonia
CARS	counter anti-inflammatory response syndrome
CBT	cognitive behavioural therapy
CDC	Centers for Disease Control and Prevention (USA)
CF	cystic fibrosis
CFTCR	cystic fibrosis transmembrane conductance regulator
CHCs	combined hormonal contraceptives
CHD	coronary heart disease
CHH	congenital hypogonadotropic hypogonadism
CHP	capsular hydrostatic pressure
CHT	congenital hypothyroidism
CIPD	chronic inflammatory demyelinating polyneuropathy
CKD	chronic kidney disease
CK-MB	creatinine-kinase myocardial band
CLA	cutaneous lymphocyte antigen
CMV	cytomegalovirus
CNBP	cellular nucleic acid-binding protein
CNDI	central neurogenic diabetes insipidus
CNHC	Complementary and Natural Healthcare Council
CNO	chronic non-bacterial osteomyelitis

Abbreviation	Expansion
CNS	central nervous system
CO	cardiac output
CO_2	carbon dioxide
CoA	coarctation of the aorta
COAD	chronic obstructive airway disease
COPD	chronic obstructive pulmonary disease
COX-1	cyclo-oxygenase 1
COX-2	cyclo-oxygenase 2
CPP	cerebral perfusion pressure
CRH	corticotrophin-releasing hormone
CRMO	chronic recurrent multifocal osteomyelitis
CRP	C-reactive protein
CS	caesarean section
CSF	cerebrospinal fluid
CSWS	cerebral salt-wasting syndrome
CT	computed tomography (scan)
CVD	cardiovascular disease
CVP	central venous pressure
CVS	cardiovascular system
D&C	dilation and curettage (of the uterus)
DAI	diffuse axonal injury
DALYs	disability-adjusted life years
DCIS	ductile carcinoma in situ
DCT	distal convoluted tube
DDAVP	1-deamino-8-d-arginine vasopressin (desmopressin)
DES	diethylstilboestrol
DHA	omega-3 docosahexaenoic acid
DHT	dihydrotestosterone
DI	diabetes insipidus
DIC	disseminated intravascular coagulation
DIT	diiodotyrosine
DKA	diabetic ketoacidosis
DM	diabetes mellitus
DMD	Duchenne muscular dystrophy
DMPK	dystrophia myotonica protein kinase or myotonic dystrophy protein kinase

Abbreviation	Expansion
DNA	deoxyribonucleic acid
DOCs	disorders of consciousness
DTH	delayed-type mediated hypersensitivity
DVT	deep vein thrombosis
EBA	epidermolysis bullosa acquisita
EBV	Epstein–Barr virus
ECDC	European Centre for Disease Prevention and Control
ECF	extracellular fluid
ECG	electrocardiogram
ECLS	extracorporeal life support
ED	erectile dysfunction
EDs	endocrine disruptors
EDSS	expanded disability status scale
EEG	electroencephalograph
eGFR	estimated glomerular filtration rate
EGFR	epidermal growth factor receptor
EIM	extraintestinal manifestations
EPHOs	essential public health operations
EPI	epirubicin
EPO	erythropoietin
ER	endoplasmic reticulum
ER	oestrogen/estrogen receptor
ESBL	extended spectrum beta-lactamase
ESC	European Society of Cardiology
ESH	European Society of Hypertension
ESR	erythrocyte sedimentation rate
ESRD	end stage renal disease
ETC	electron transport chain
EU	European Union
EV	enteroviruses
EWAS	epigenome-wide association studies
FAST	Face Arms Speech Time
FEV	forced expiratory volume
FFAs	free fatty acids
FG	fast glycolytic
FiO$_2$	fraction of inspired oxygen
FISH	fluorescence in situ hybridisation
FM	fibromyalgia

Abbreviation	Expansion
FOG	fast oxidative-glycolytic
FP	filtration pressure
FRAX	fracture risk assessment tool
FRG	familial renal glucosuria
FSH	follicle-stimulating hormone
FSHD	facioscapulohumeral muscular dystrophy
FVC	forced vital capacity
G	gap (phase)
GA	general anaesthetic
GA1	glutaric acidaemia type 1
GABA	gamma-aminobutyric acid
GBS	Guillain–Barré syndrome
GCC	General Chiropractic Council
GCPH	Global Charter for the Public Health
GCRB	Genetic Counsellor Registration Board
GCS	Glasgow Coma Scale
GCT	granulosa cell tumour
GDC	General Dental Council
GDM	gestational diabetes
GERD	See GORD
GFR	glomerular filtration rate
GH	growth hormone
GHD	growth hormone deficiency
GHP	glomerular hydrostatic pressure
GHRH	growth hormone-releasing hormone
GI	gastrointestinal
GINA	Global Initiative for Asthma
GIT	gastrointestinal tract
GLUT	glucose transporter
GMC	General Medical Council
GnRH	gonadotropin-releasing hormone
GOC	General Optical Council
GORD	gastroesophageal reflux disease
GOsC	General Osteopathic Council
GP	General Practitioner
GRCCT	General Regulatory Council for Complementary Therapies

Abbreviation	Expansion
GSD	glycogen storage disease
GSL	General Sales List
GVHD	graft-versus-host disease
HAP	hospital-acquired pneumonia
HAT	histone acetyltransferase
HbA1c	glycated haemoglobin
HBPM	home blood pressure monitoring
HCAP	health care-associated pneumonia
hCG	human chorionic gonadotrophin
HCPC	Health and Care Professions Council
HCU	homocystinuria
HD	Huntington's disease
HDAC	histone deacetylase
HDL	high density lipoprotein
HER-2	human epidermal growth factor receptor-2
HFEA	Human Fertilisation and Embryology Authority
hGH	human growth hormone
HHNKS	hyperosmolar hyperglycaemic non-ketotic syndrome
HHV-6	human herpesvirus 6
HIF-1	hypoxic inducible factor-1
HIV	human immunodeficiency virus
HLA	human leucocyte antigen
HMP	Human Microbiome Project
HPA	hypothalamic-pituitary-adrenal
hPL	human placental lactogen
HPV	human papilloma virus
HR_{max}	maximal heart rate
HRT	hormone replacement therapy
HSC	health and social care
HSV	herpes simplex virus
HTM	high threshold mechanoreceptors
HTT	Huntingtin (Huntington) gene
IASSW	International Association of Schools of Social Work
IBD	inflammatory bowel disease
IBS	irritable bowel syndrome
IBS-d	IBS with diarrhoea

Abbreviation	Expansion
ICE	In Case of Emergency
ICF	intracellular fluid
ICH	intracerebral haemorrhage/haematoma
ICP	intracranial pressure
ICS	International Continence Society
ICSH	interstitial cell-stimulating hormone
IFG	impaired fasting glucose
IFSW	International Federation of Social Workers
Ig	immunoglobulin
IGF-1	insulin-like growth factor-1
IGT	impaired glucose tolerance
IL	interleukin
ILD	interstitial lung disease
iNPH	idiopathic normal pressure hydrocephalus
IPF	idiopathic pulmonary fibrosis
IQ	Intelligence Quotient
IRT	immunoreactive trypsinogen
IU	International Unit
IVA	isovaleric acidaemia
IVF	in vitro fertilisation
IVP	intravenous pyelogram
JGA	juxtaglomerular apparatus
JGCT	junior granulosa cell tumour
KS	Kaposi sarcoma
KS	Kallmann syndrome
KSHV	Kaposi sarcoma herpes virus
LCFA	long-chain fatty acids
LCIS	lobar carcinoma in situ
LCPUFA	long-chain polyunsaturated fatty acids
LDLs	low density lipoproteins
LH	luteinising hormone
LMN	lower motor neuron
LOS	lower oesophageal sphincter
LPS	lipopolysaccharides
LRT	lower respiratory tract
LRTIs	lower respiratory tract infections
LTV	left testicular vein

Abbreviation	Expansion
MAP	mean arterial pressure
MCADD	medium-chain acyl-CoA dehydrogenase deficiency
MCP	metacarpophalangeal (joint)
MCS	minimally conscious state
MCV	molluscum contagiosum virus
MDR	multidrug resistant
MDT	maggot debridement therapy
MHC	major histocompatibility complex
MI	myocardial infarction
MIF	Müllerian-inhibiting factor
miRNA	Micro RNA
MIT	monoiodotyrosine
MMD	myotonic muscular dystrophy
MMR	measles, mumps and rubella
MND	motor neurone disease
MODS	multiple organ dysfunction
MRI	magnetic resonance imaging
mRNA	messenger RNA
MRSA	methicillin-resistant Staphylococcus aureus
MS	multiple sclerosis
MSUD	maple syrup urine disease
MTB	Mycobacterium tuberculosis
MTP	metatarsophalangeal (joint)
MV	minute volume
NAFLD	non-alcoholic fatty liver disease
NAPQI	N-acetyl-p-benzoquinoneimine
NASH	non-alcoholic steatohepatitis
NDI	nephrogenic diabetes insipidus
NEC	necrotising enterocolitis
NF	nuclear factor
NFP	net filtration pressure
NHP	net hydrostatic pressure
NHS	National Health Service (UK)
NICE	National Institute for Health and Care Excellence
NIH	National Institutes of Health (USA)
NK	natural killer (cells)
NMC	Nursing and Midwifery Council
NMDA	N-methyl-D-aspartate

Abbreviation	Expansion
NMJ	neuromuscular junction
NO	nitric oxide
NREM	non-rapid eye movement
NRT	nicotine replacement therapy
NS	nociceptive specific
NSAIDs	non-steroidal anti-inflammatory drugs
NST	no special type
NSTEMI	Non ST segment elevation MI
NTDs	neural tube defects
NT-proBNP	N-terminal pro b-type natriuretic peptide
O_2	oxygen
OA	osteoarthritis
OGTT	oral glucose tolerance test
OTC	over the counter
OTs	occupational therapists
PAF	platelet activating factor
PAMPs	pathogen-associated molecular patterns
PaO_2	partial pressure of oxygen
Pap	Papanicolaou
$pBtO_2$	brain tissue oxygenation
PCa	prostate cancer
PCA	primary cicatricial alopecia
PCOS	polycystic ovary syndrome
PCNF	Person-Centred Nursing Framework
PCR	polymerase chain reaction
PCT	proximal convoluted tube
PCV	pneumococcal conjugate vaccine
PDA	patent ductus arteriosus
PDB	Paget disease of bone
PDGF	platelet-derived growth factor
PE	pulmonary embolism
PEFR	peak expiratory flow rate
PEH	paraoesophageal hernia
PF_3	Platelet Factor 3
PFC	prefrontal cortex
PHE	Public Health England
PID	pelvic inflammatory disease
PIN	prostate intraepithelial neoplasia

Abbreviation	Expansion
PIP	proximal interphalangeal (joint)
PKU	phenylketonuria
PMN	polymodal nociceptors
PNS	peripheral nervous system
POM	prescription-only medicines
PPH	postpartum haemorrhage
PPI	proton pump inhibitor
PPMS	primary-progressive MS
PPV	pneumococcal polysaccharide vaccine
PrEP	pre-exposure prophylaxis
PRMS	progressive-relapsing MS
PSA	Professional Standards Authority for Health and Social Care
PSA	prostate-specific antigen
PsA	psoriatic arthritis
PSMA	prostate-specific membrane antigen
PSNI	Pharmaceutical Society of Northern Ireland
PTE	post-traumatic epilepsy
PTH	parathyroid hormone
PUBS	percutaneous umbilical cord blood sampling
RA	rheumatoid arthritis
RAAS	renin-angiotensin-aldosterone system
RAS	reticular activating system
Rb	retinoblastoma
RBC	red blood cell
RBCs	red blood cells (erythrocytes)
RCPCH	Royal College of Paediatrics and Child Health
REM	rapid eye movement
RFs	rheumatoid factors
RFS	refeeding syndrome
RICE	Rest, Ice, Compression and Elevation
RIFLE	Risk, Injury, Failure, Loss and End-stage
RNA	ribonucleic acid
ROS	reactive oxygen species
RRMS	relapsing-remitting MS

Abbreviation	Expansion
RRT	renal replacement therapy
RTA	renal tubular acidosis
RTIs	respiratory tract infections
SA	sinoatrial
SADS	sudden arrhythmic death syndrome
SBP	spontaneous bacterial peritonitis
SCD	sickle cell disease
SCFA	short-chain fatty acids
SCIDs	severe combined immunodeficiencies
SDGs	Sustainable Development Goals
SFs	synovial fibroblasts
SG	specific gravity
SIADH	syndrome of inappropriate secretion of antidiuretic hormone
SIGN	Scottish Intercollegiate Guidelines Network
SIRS	systemic inflammatory response syndrome
SJS	Stevens-Johnson syndrome
SLE	systemic lupus erythematous
SLTs	speech and language therapists
SNRIs	serotonin and norepinephrine reuptake inhibitors
SO	slow oxidative
SOD1	superoxide dismutase
SPF	Sun Protection Factor
SPMS	secondary-progressive MS
SR	sarcoplasmic reticulum
SRY	sex-determining region of the Y
SSRIs	selective serotonin reuptake inhibitors
STD	sexually transmitted disease
STEMI	ST segment elevation MI
STI	sexually transmitted infection
T_3	triiodothyronine
T_4	thyroxine
TB	tuberculosis
TCFA	thin cap fibroatheroma
TDF	Testis-Determining Factor
TEF	thermic effect of food
TEN	toxic epidermal necrolysis

Abbreviation	Expansion
TENS	transcutaneous electrical nerve stimulation
TFT	thyroid function test
TGA	transposition of the great arteries
T_h	T-helper (cells)
TIA	transient ischaemic attack
TLRs	toll-like receptors
TMJ	temporomandibular (joint)
TN	trigeminal neuralgia
TNF	tumour necrosis factor
TNM	tumour nodes metastasis
TRH	thyrotrophin-releasing hormone
TSE	testicular self-examination
TSG	tumour suppressor genes
TSH	thyroid-stimulating hormone
TTH	tension-type headache
U3A	University of the Third Age
UC	ulcerative colitis
UHC	Universal Health Coverage
UKPHR	UK Public Health Register
UMN	upper motor neuron
URT	upper respiratory tract
URTIs	upper respiratory tract infections
USPSTF	US Preventive Services Task Force

Abbreviation	Expansion
UTI	urinary tract infection
UV	ultraviolet
UVA	ultraviolet A
UVB	ultraviolet B
UWS	unresponsive wakefulness syndrome
V/Q	ventilation–perfusion ratio
VacA	vacuolating cytotoxin A
VAP	ventilator-associated pneumonia
VDLD	very low density lipoprotein
VEGF	vascular endothelial growth factor
VF	ventricular fibrillation
VIPS	Vitiligo Impact Patient Scale
VRE	vancomycin-resistant enterococcus
VS	vegetative state
VSDs	ventricular septal defects
VT	ventricular tachycardia
VTE	venous thromboembolism
WBC	white blood cell
WCC	white cell count
WDR	wide dynamic range
WHO	World Health Organisation
WHR	waist–hip ratio
ZIP1	zinc transport protein

SECTION 1
HEALTH AND DISEASE

This section of the book examines some of the generic issues that are relevant in most of the different chapters in the book. It consists of six chapters as follows:

Chapter 1: Variation and Disease. While emotional, social and spiritual aspects of health and illness are recognised, it is also important to understand physiological variation and how individuals differ in structure, function and presentation of disease, including mental health and learning disabilities. Types and causes of variation are presented in this chapter along with factors that can cause or modify disease. In addition, the main categories of disease (acute, sub-acute and chronic) are reviewed.

Chapter 2: Health and Disease in Society. Studying illness in groups of people is important in identifying relationships between environmental factors, behaviours and illness or injury. The value of epidemiological methods in nursing is considered, including in infection control, community and occupational health nursing.

Chapter 3: Integrated Health Care. This chapter introduces the major approaches to the management of physiological disorders including: surgery, radiotherapy, chemotherapy, microbial therapy, immunotherapy, physiotherapy, occupational therapy, speech and language therapy, nutrition and psychological therapies. To provide high-quality person-centred care, it is important to understand the contribution and be able to collaborate with the range of health care professionals involved.

Chapter 4: Principles of Pharmacology. This chapter introduces the other major type of medical intervention – the use of drugs. Understanding the main principles of drug therapy in treating common disorders enables safe person-centred care in relation to drugs. This introduction is designed to support student nurses in preparing to be 'prescribing ready' (not prescribers), but is not all the content they will need to learn.

Chapter 5: Genetic Disorders. This chapter examines the role of genetics in disease causation and how such disorders are diagnosed and treated. Growing understanding of genetics has enhanced the ways in which these conditions can be managed and, in many instances, has increased life expectancy. It considers the different modes of inheritance and the implications for treatment and care.

Chapter 6: Mental Ill-Health. While disorders of anatomy and physiology are the major focus of pathophysiology, disorders of mental health are just as important in considering quality of life and well-being. Thus, this chapter aims to integrate mental and physical health in preparing you for providing person-centred care.

VARIATION AND DISEASE

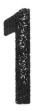

LEARNING OUTCOMES

When you have finished studying this chapter you will be able to:

1. Discuss causes of biological and behavioural variation in health and disease.
2. Differentiate between acute, sub-acute, chronic and acute on chronic disease conditions.
3. Identify a range of different causes of disease.
4. Explain factors influencing disease presentation.
5. Understand the importance of diagnosis and identify how signs, symptoms and a range of haematological, biochemical and radiological tests facilitate diagnosis.

INTRODUCTION

When we consider people with the same medical condition, they rarely exhibit exactly the same signs and symptoms at the same stage of their disorder; each journey through illness is largely unique in how it manifests and progresses. This chapter examines how and why individuals differ in health and **disease**. Disease patterns (i.e. **acute**, **sub-acute** and **chronic**), causes and diagnosis of disease are also reviewed.

This chapter builds on the study of anatomy and physiology (e.g. Boore et al., 2016) and aims to develop your understanding of disease through the examination of a number of different factors that influence the development, presentation and progress of ill-health. The focus on person-centred nursing (McCormack and McCance, 2019) throughout this book means that the variation between individuals and how this influences disease must be taken into account in order that we can individualise the provision of care. From your previous and varied areas of study, you will understand how people can differ both biologically and behaviourally, and that these can influence the presentation of disease and how individuals respond.

Within this chapter the categories and causes of disease will be examined. We will discuss how signs, symptoms and a range of haematological, biochemical and radiological tests are used to achieve a diagnosis and guide treatment.

———— PERSON-CENTRED CONTEXT: THE BODIE FAMILY ————

BODIE FAMILY
CASE NOTES

Think back to the Bodie family introduced at the start of the book and you will quickly see that there are a number of issues in relation to health that are relevant to this chapter. In general, as a family they are well adapted to any variations in their health and have learned to live fulfilling lives in spite of any illness or disorder. However, there are a number of issues which individuals have to cope with in order to achieve this balance.

Several members of the family have chronic physical disorders which they manage successfully. Following a **myocardial infarction** (heart attack), Maud was diagnosed with **heart failure**, now under good control. She also has **hypothyroidism** successfully managed with medication. Richard has type 2 **diabetes mellitus**, Derek has **asthma** and Margaret has hay fever. However, all of them are managing their conditions effectively.

Richard and Matthew have both suffered from mental health problems. Richard had an acute **stress** response in the past treated effectively with cognitive behavioural therapy. Matthew has had **depression** for 15 years (i.e. a chronic condition), although it is being managed successfully with medication and support from the community mental health team.

Within this family, several of them have undertaken approaches to maintain their health or prevent disease. For example, Hannah and Richard Jones eat a diet containing plenty of wholemeal bread and at least five portions a day of fruit and vegetables. Hannah smoked in her early 20s but gave up a number of years ago.

Still considering prevention, they ensure that they have appropriate **immunisations**: early in life for Danielle (the youngest member of the family); before holidays abroad as appropriate; annually against flu for the two older people and Derek who, as an asthmatic, is at increased risk of respiratory infections.

HUMAN VARIATION

Individuals vary in the ways in which they behave, develop, function and respond to their environment. All of these can influence health, the development of disease and how they respond. There are a number of terms used in describing health status and they need to be clearly understood, as follows:

- *Health*: the WHO (1948) definition is 'Health is a state of complete physical, mental and social well-being and not merely the absence of disease or infirmity'.
- *Disease*: 'any impairment of normal physiological function affecting all or part of an organism, especially a specific pathological change caused by infection, stress, etc., producing characteristic symptoms; illness or sickness in general' (Collins English Dictionary, 2012).
- *Illness*: 'poor health resulting from disease of body or mind; sickness' (American Heritage, 2016).
- *Disability*: an umbrella term, covering impairments, activity limitations and participation restrictions. An impairment is a problem in body function or structure; an activity limitation is a difficulty encountered by an individual in executing a task or an action; while a participation restriction is a problem experienced by an individual in involvement in life situations (WHO, 2018).

Altered health status can be considered as a disturbance from normal. But we need to ask *what is normal?* The use of the term 'normal' is controversial in health care and largely relates to factors being within healthy, homeostatic parameters. Various aspects of variation are considered and help to clarify what is 'normal'.

Physical variation

Physiologically, normality and abnormality are defined in relation to certain limits. Measurements of anatomical, physiological and biochemical characteristics are interpreted by comparison with standards; standard norms (i.e. the range of normal) are obtained by measuring the specific characteristic in large numbers of readily available subjects, if possible representative of the population (e.g. Sanders and Duncan, 2006). However, it is important to take into account that variation in such measurements can occur between ages and ethnic background. Some results which indicate disorder in some groups may be within normal limits for others and, in judging the implication of such results, knowledge and clinical expertise must be applied.

Variation can occur in all aspects of bodily makeup, anatomy, physiology, biochemistry, and growth and development. In essence, such variation is determined by nature (i.e. genetic composition) or nurture (i.e. environmental factors) but is largely a combination of both. The factors involved can be related to such circumstances as: age, gender, ethnic background, or environmental conditions, including **nutrition**, during development or later in life. A number of examples of such variations are presented in Table 1.1 based on work by Overfield (2017), which is a useful text with wide coverage of human variation.

Susceptibility to disease is another issue that varies across individuals and will be indicated as relevant in this book.

Behavioural variation

We have considered a range of factors that cause variation in the biological parameters shown in Table 1.1 and which need to be taken into account in understanding the presentation of disease. However, human behaviour is also important in causation of and response to disease and merits some consideration here: it is based on a mix of nature and nurture.

Behaviours associated with lifestyle, and often with an element of choice, can play an important role in the development of disease. Many diseases, particularly chronic ones, are a result of lifestyle factors, including diet, exercise, smoking, and use of drugs or alcohol. Whilst some of these occur through choice, some do not; for example, poverty can limit the ability to purchase adequate healthy food. These issues receive further attention in Chapter 2 (Health and Disease in Society) which considers **epidemiology** and **health promotion**.

Management of stressful events is also important in promoting or damaging health. The way in which individuals respond to illness can influence their physiological functioning, as discussed in the section on Stress later in this chapter.

Table 1.1 Variation in biological characteristics

Characteristic	Variation
ANATOMICAL VARIATION	
Height/weight	1. Less than genetically programmed height: inadequate nutrition during period of growth, or insufficient production of hormones affecting growth
	2. Long limbs and digits: occurs when growing up in a hot climate (enhances heat loss); also in **Marfan syndrome** – a genetic disorder of **connective tissue**
Chest size	Enlarged thorax: growing up at high altitudes; low oxygen levels stimulate growth of enhanced chest capacity for respiration
Bones	Density increased and muscle attachments on bone are larger when exposed to strong forces (e.g. from heavy work)
	Bone density may be reduced when inadequate **vitamin D** production occurs due to limited exposure to sun
PHYSIOLOGICAL VARIATION	
Adult lactose tolerance (Deng et al., 2015)	Varies with areas of historic cattle domestication: 90% N. European; ≈ 50% in Spain, Italy, pastoralist Arabian populations; low in Asia and most of Africa.
	Intolerance causes bloating, flatulence and cramps
Heat tolerance (Daanen and Lichtenbelt, 2016; Foster and Collard, 2013)	1. Body size increases as temperature decreases. Bodies of people living in colder climates tend to be larger than those in warmer climates, and more suited to the cold. This applies with considerable differences in latitude and temperature between groups
	2. Children and older people tolerate heat less well
BIOCHEMICAL VARIATION	
Malaria susceptibility	Several variations in the structure of **haemoglobin** or of red blood cell enzymes in heterozygotes (i.e. only one gene carried) protect individuals against malaria to some extent. Examples of such conditions include:
	Sickle cell **anaemia**, thalassaemia, glucose-6-phosphate dehydrogenase (G6PD) deficiency, Duffy blood group
Drug metabolism	1. Atypical form of pseudocholinesterase (enzyme which degrades succinylcholine – a muscle relaxant used in **surgery**) – results in prolonged paralysis and an inability to breath
	2. Slow or fast inactivation of isoniazid (used in treatment of TB) will alter level of drug in body and efficacy of treatment and susceptibility to side-effects
VARIATION IN GROWTH AND DEVELOPMENT	
Pelvic size and fetal maturity	African women: smaller pelvis and smaller baby than Caucasian (white) women, but babies are more mature for same weight than Caucasian babies
Growth curves	Growth curves are similar shape for different racial groups, but growth spurts in Asians occur later than in Caucasian children

Source: Adapted from Overfield, 2017

DISEASE PRESENTATIONS

Disease is a state of disordered functioning and in this book we are focused mainly on disordered physiological function as defined by the medical practitioner. However, understanding of physiological disturbances resulting in mental ill-health is increasing and will receive some attention. Differing from this is the illness suffered by the person affected: this consists of the subjective experience of their symptoms.

There are three broad groups of disease presentations used in medicine: acute, sub-acute and chronic, with differing implications for the individual concerned, for their family and for the relevant health care team. The following sections clarify these different groups of conditions.

Acute

An *acute illness* is one in which signs and symptoms develop suddenly; the condition is usually severe and lasts for a relatively short period of time or becomes sub-acute or chronic if it persists but becomes controlled. It is important to differentiate acute from severe as the terms are sometimes, but incorrectly, used interchangeably. An acute condition can be minor, such as a cut finger, or severe such as a myocardial infarction or fractured femur. In other words, the severity of the condition does not determine whether it is acute, sub-acute or chronic. An example of an acute condition is acute urinary tract infection, which usually recovers fairly quickly with antibiotic therapy. Repeated such infections can result in renal damage and chronic **renal failure**.

In most acute disorders, the person affected will return to their normal health and activity, although some will progress to a chronic state of disease or may die. Table 1.2 gives examples of some acute conditions.

Table 1.2 Examples of acute conditions

Acute myocardial infarction (heart attack)
Acute **bronchitis**
Acute **renal failure**
Acute **hepatitis**
Trauma

When severe, acute conditions often have considerable emotional implications for the individual concerned and for their family as they often require adaptation or lead to a major change in their lives. Independence may be reduced, they may fear further health complications and have a reduced ability to participate in enjoyable activities. While most people adjust over time, care and support are usually necessary to achieve such an adaptation.

APPLY

Long-term implications of acute conditions in families

The effect of an acute condition occurring in a close relative can be considerable, as Jack Garcia demonstrates. Jack, Thomas Bodie's partner, undertakes monthly testicular self-examination. His father has a history of testicular cancer and Jack wants to make sure that he identifies it early and gets immediate treatment if it develops. In this respect his health behaviour is healthy but underpinned by caution. Jack is aware of the potential for the condition to occur, causing him and his partner some anxiety. His behaviour also acts as an example for the Bodie family of the importance of regular checking for such acute conditions and the importance of support with them.

JACK GARCIA
CASE NOTES

Chronic

A chronic condition is one that persists over an extended period of time, described in terms of months and years rather than days and weeks, and usually longer than 3 months. A considerable number of organs or systems of the body can be affected (Table 1.3).

Table 1.3 Examples of chronic conditions

Physiological conditions	Hypertension (cardiovascular system)
	Chronic bronchitis (respiratory system)
	Chronic renal failure (kidneys)
	Chronic hepatitis (liver)
	Multiple sclerosis (nervous system)
	Diabetes mellitus (endocrine system – glucose regulation)
	Rheumatoid arthritis (joints)
	Epilepsy (brain)
	Osteoporosis (bones)
	Ulcerative colitis (large intestine)
Psychological conditions	Alzheimer's disease
	Bipolar disorder

Sometimes the condition is progressive, resulting in an increasing loss of independence and ability over time, for example, in chronic bronchitis. In some conditions, the disorder may plateau, e.g. hypertension can be well controlled with medication. However, in many progressive disorders the deterioration will progress and eventually result in permanent disability or death, e.g. in multiple sclerosis. However, the symptoms can often be kept under control with medication and a healthy lifestyle, thus extending the person's health-related quality of life through managing the condition, such as osteoporosis. This sometimes results in slowing its **progression**, and may result in a cure.

Some chronic conditions are largely related to health behaviours (see below) such as smoking or little exercise. According to WHO/Europe (2016) non-communicable chronic diseases are the greatest cause of **morbidity** and mortality in the European Region, an example of a highly developed part of the world with highly developed health services. In this region, the major chronic conditions of **cardiovascular disease**, diabetes, respiratory disease, **cancer** and mental health disorders result in an estimated 86% of the deaths and 77% of the disease incidence.

There are also some chronic conditions associated with infections. For example, **human immunodeficiency virus (HIV)** and **acquired immune deficiency syndrome (AIDS)** are an example of an infective chronic condition caused by a **virus**. Less developed parts of the world have much higher incidences of infective chronic disorders than advanced countries. For example, South Africa has the biggest **epidemic** of HIV/AIDS, with 19.2% of the population infected and with 48% of the adult population receiving antiretroviral medications (AVERT, 2016).

Another microbial grouping with an influence on chronic disease is the herpes virus. This is a complex group of viruses which, over time, have been identified as consisting of 97 species, divided into numerous groupings of families, subfamilies and genera. Of these, the most important in human disease is HHV-6, otherwise known as human herpes virus 6 with two main species, HHV-6A and HHV-6B (discussed jointly as HHV-6). Humans acquire this virus early in life, some as early as one month, and the virus can initiate an active infection, often with a high temperature, **inflammation** of the tympanic membrane, and **malaise** and irritability. It then becomes latent in salivary glands, blood-forming stem cells and others, and remains established within the host for the individual's lifetime. It can become reactivated at intervals to promote spread of the infection. It is found worldwide in almost 100% of the population (Braun et al., 1997). A range of other infections are associated with this virus including: hepatitis, febrile **convulsions** and **encephalitis**. It has also been found in people with multiple sclerosis, and is associated with various other disorders, e.g. chronic fatigue **syndrome**, **fibromyalgia**, AIDS, optic neuritis, temporal lobe **epilepsy** and cancer (Challoner et al., 1995; Komaroff, 2006).

An individual or individuals with chronic illness in the family may have a significant effect on the way of life of the family. As those around us in our daily lives are often our first line of support, it is paramount that the impact of illness on all involved is considered so that their health and provision of social support are not adversely affected. Maintaining as healthy a lifestyle as possible, promoting activity and enhancing quality of life are crucial. Health services need to be exactly that – services that promote health and minimise the occurrence of ill-health. Unfortunately, the majority of health services are focused on managing illness after it has occurred rather than on proactively preventing it or slowing its onset and progression.

APPLY

Chronic conditions in the Bodie family

In the Bodie family, the grandparents both have chronic health issues but they live active, happy lives. George is on medication to limit his raised **cholesterol** level. Maud has had an acute myocardial infarction (heart attack) which has resolved but she now has heart failure, managed effectively with medication, and also takes thyroid hormones for low thyroid function.

Among the next generation, Richard has type 2 diabetes, while Derek has asthma; both men are managing their conditions well. In the following generation, Margaret has hay fever, again managed effectively when the pollen count is high. However, the similarities in immune response with hay fever, asthma and **eczema** (the atopic triad) mean that she may also develop asthma as she gets older (Huovinen et al., 1999).

Acute on chronic

The term **acute on chronic** describes the situation where someone with a chronic condition has an acute exacerbation of their condition, requiring more intensive treatment.

APPLY

Managing risk of acute on chronic attacks

There are a number of chronic conditions in which the individual affected may have an acute episode on top and may need admission to hospital or emergency care to enable them to return to their normal stable condition. For example, it is not uncommon for someone to have to be taken to hospital with an acute attack of asthma - a condition that Derek in the Bodie family suffers from. Although most people with asthma become knowledgeable about their condition, Derek's medical experience gives him an advantage in managing his condition so that, as yet, he has not had an acute on chronic attack. A number of conditions demonstrate this picture of acute on chronic presentation, including chronic bronchitis, liver disease, **chronic kidney disease**, and **rheumatoid arthritis**.

DEREK BODIE
CASE NOTES

Sub-acute

This term refers to conditions that fall between acute and chronic in nature. The illness cannot be regarded as acute but more than meets the criteria for chronic. A classic example here is when an older person develops a **subdural haematoma** (a type of blood clot on the brain). Often there is a delay in presentation as the impact in the initial stage is not overly symptomatic. However, as the clot begins to break down (from solid into a more liquid state) it increases in mass and signs and symptoms become more obvious. This can be over a week from the onset and at this stage is referred to as sub-acute subdural haematoma. Table 1.4 identifies a number of sub-acute conditions.

Table 1.4   Examples of sub-acute conditions

Sub-acute thyroiditis
Sub-acute endocarditis
Sub-acute combined degeneration of the cord (vitamin B_{12} deficiency)

CAUSES OF DISEASE (AETIOLOGY)

Diseases can be either **congenital** or **acquired**.

- Congenital disorders (defect or anomaly) are conditions which are present at birth. They may be genetically determined (e.g. **cystic fibrosis**) or may be due to some other factor in the uterine environment up to the time of birth. An example of this is the abnormalities resulting from thalidomide, given to women in early pregnancy in the late 1950s and early 1960s to treat morning sickness (McBride, 1961).
- Acquired diseases are those that develop after birth although they may still be due to pre-natal influences. One example of this is **Huntington's chorea** (or Huntington's disease) which is genetically determined, so is pre-determined at conception, but does not become manifest until much later in life.

Diseases can also be **communicable** or **non-communicable**.

- Communicable disorders (also described as infectious or contagious) are caused by microbes transmitted to people from other people, from animals (zoonoses), or from other reservoirs of infection in the environment. They can be spread through the air, through contact with bodily fluids, or through ingesting infected food or fluids.
- Non-communicable disorders are not contracted by communication with others or by infection, but occur as a result of a range of risk factors. Many of these can be limited through interventions that encourage modification of lifestyle and treatment of physiological factors which can result in disease (Chapter 2). A non-communicable disorder can be traumatic in nature or can develop from unhealthy lifestyle factors such as smoking, poor diet, repeated physical stress on the body, and chronic stress/anxiety.

A wide range of factors can result in or predispose to disordered function which may lead to disease and we will look at these in outline (Table 1.5). Later chapters which focus on disorders of specific body systems will consider these as relevant.

FACTORS INFLUENCING DISEASE PRESENTATION

In the section above, causes of disease were examined. A number of issues that influence the presentation of disease are considered next.

Table 1.5 Causes of disordered physiological function

Cause		Examples
Trauma	Acute	Head injury leading to brain trauma
	Chronic	Repetitive **strain** injury (e.g. wrist)
Infection		Pneumonia (lungs), **pyelonephritis** (kidneys), AIDS/HIV
Immune response		Hay fever, anaphylactic shock, autoimmune disorders
Heat or cold		Burns, frostbite
Ionising radiation		Radiation sickness
Poisons		Alcohol – **cirrhosis** of the liver
		Drugs – hepatitis
		Tobacco smoke – carcinoma of the lung
		Chemicals – asbestosis (lungs), bladder cancer
Inadequate nutrient intake		Kwashiorkor (due to protein deficiency)
		Pernicious anaemia (due to inadequate vitamin B_{12} **absorption**)
		Anorexia nervosa (nutrient intake restricted due to mental illness)
Excessive nutrient intake		Cardiovascular disease
		Diabetes mellitus type 2
		Obesity (risk of diabetes and other diseases)
Lack of oxygen supply to part of body		**Gangrene** (e.g. of foot or leg)
		Stroke
Altered cell division		Carcinoma of epithelial tissues (e.g. lungs)
		Sarcoma of connective tissues (e.g. bone)

Physiological mechanisms in disease

A number of physiological mechanisms can play a role in disease and are discussed here.

Disordered negative feedback

From your knowledge of physiology (Boore et al., 2016, Chapter 1), you should already understand the way in which negative feedback acts to maintain a steady state (i.e. **homeostasis**) in the various physiological parameters. From a biological perspective, disease can be considered as disordered homeostasis. Under normal circumstances any disturbance from the normal results in changes to minimise that disturbance. Thus, the body compensates for and adapts to any disturbances which threaten the steady state and homeostasis is maintained.

In certain diseases, negative feedback fails and deviations from normal persist or extend. Two examples are:

* in oversecretion of the thyroid gland hormones, the normal feedback mechanisms which inhibit further secretion of the thyroid hormones fail and high levels of hormone secretion continue
* in carcinoma, the contact inhibition which controls cell division through negative feedback fails and cell division continues unchecked.

Stress

Stress is both a response and a causative factor in disease. It is how one's body responds to any demand or threat and the causes or effects may be physiological or psychological in nature. It is caused by a wide range of circumstances – physical illness, social factors, etc. – known as stressors. Under these circumstances the body automatically activates its defences in the fight-or-flight reaction (initiated through the sympathetic nervous system) or the stress response. There are a number of models of stress but the one we are focusing on is that described by Selye (1976) and used by other authors, including Cox (1978). Much of the literature is relatively old but is still relevant and used by many authors.

From a physiological perspective, the stress response is mediated through the **hypothalamus** and links from this to the limbic system, and thus to the cerebral cortex, ensuring that emotional states influence the stress response. It has a short-acting and a longer-acting aspect and occurs through the action of specific hormones. The secretion of many hormones is influenced in stress but the major ones are:

short-acting (acute) response: involves mainly **catecholamines** (adrenaline and noradrenaline from the adrenal medulla)

longer-acting response: involves **glucocorticoids** (e.g. **cortisol**, cortisone etc., from the adrenal cortex) as well as other hormones.

The activities in both aspects of the stress response are to prepare the body to cope with any extra demands placed upon it. In moderation, it is an essential adaptive response (an inability to respond effectively may lead to death), but in excess or prolonged it can result in changes which contribute to the presentation of disease. Selye (1976) described the stress response in three stages (Figure 1.1): the Alarm Reaction, the Stage of Resistance, and the Stage of Exhaustion.

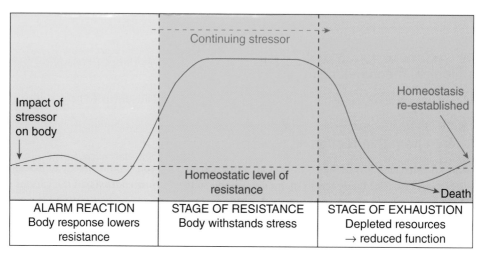

Figure 1.1   The stress response

The acute response to stress overlaps with the Alarm Reaction described by Selye and is also known as the fright, flight or fight response. The physiological changes that occur enable the body to respond rapidly to threat (perceived or actual) (see Table 1.6) and may also occur when people are stressed in illness. Frequent episodes can result in hypertension (high blood pressure) and the changes that occur can result in acute exacerbations in people with chronic conditions.

The changes associated with the longer-lasting stress response are mainly due to increased glucocorticoid secretion and can also have deleterious effects on the person's health (Table 1.6). Some of the changes identified are very important in enabling the body to cope with extra demands. However, if they are prolonged they can lead to changes which are harmful to the body.

Table 1.6 The alarm reaction /acute stress response

System	Physiological changes	Physical changes	Signs and symptoms
Cardiovascular	Increased cardiac rate and output	Tachycardia, full pulse, raised BP	Palpitations, chest pains, headache
Respiratory	Can lead to low PO_2 causing **vasodilation**, fall in BP, low Ca^{2+}	Increased rate and depth of **ventilation** Tetany (muscle spasm)	Dizziness, fainting, panic (in extreme circumstances) Tingling of extremities Tetany (in extreme circumstances)
Gastrointestinal	Reduced blood supply and reduced secretion in gastrointestinal tract (GIT) Decreased or increased motility	Vomiting, diarrhoea, constipation, anorexia or overeating	Dry mouth, indigestion/dyspepsia (see previous column)
Skin	Contraction of pilomotor muscles Cholinergic sweating Reduced blood supply	Erection of skin hair Sweating Pallor	Clammy palms
Eye	Contraction of radial muscles	Dilated pupils	Blurred vision
Muscle	CNS arousal	Muscle tension, tremor Muscle spasm in severe cases Lack of coordination	Headache, back pain Muscle tension, tremor, twitching Lack of coordination
General	CNS arousal Increased metabolic rate	Insomnia, restlessness Low grade pyrexia	Insomnia, restlessness Fatigue/weakness Feeling hot or cold

Diabetes mellitus has been identified in Table 1.7 as a condition influenced by the stress response. The evidence for stress causing diabetes (type 1 or 2) is mixed: some studies have demonstrated a link between stressful events and the development of type 1 and type 2 diabetes, but other studies have found no such relationship (Lloyd et al., 2005). However, a number of studies demonstrate a relationship between stress and metabolic control in those with diabetes and the development of complications.

Table 1.7 Main effects of glucocorticoids in long-lasting stress response

Body function	Effect of corticosteroids	Physiological changes	Pathological changes
Carbohydrate metabolism	↑ gluconeogenesis ↑ blood glucose level Antagonises **insulin's** peripheral effects	Increased plasma glucose Glycosuria (if renal threshold exceeded)	Diabetes mellitus
Protein metabolism	Protein: ↑ breakdown, ↓ synthesis ↑ amino acid deamination	↑ amino acids in blood ↑ nitrogen content of urine Negative nitrogen balance	Muscle wasting, thinning of skin Loss of hair Depressed immune response

(Continued)

Table 1.7 (Continued)

Body function	Effect of corticosteroids	Physiological changes	Pathological changes
Lipid metabolism	↑ fat breakdown	↑ fatty acid and cholesterol levels ↑ ketone production and **ketonuria**	Adipose tissue redistributed from periphery to head and trunk
Calcium metabolism	Vitamin D metabolites antagonised	↓ calcium absorption from gut ↑ renal **excretion** of calcium	Reduced calcium levels → potential for osteoporosis
Inflammatory response	Lysosomes in cells stabilised **Phagocytosis** suppressed ↓ **collagen** formation ↓ histamine and bradykinin released	Inhibits inflammation ↓ formation of granulation tissue ↓ allergic response	Potential for gastric **ulceration** Reduced rate of wound healing
Immune response	↓ immunoglobulin formation ↓ levels of white blood cells **Atrophy** of lymphoid tissue	Decreased white cell count Immunosuppression	Decreased resistance to infection
Fluid and **electrolyte** balance	↑ Na⁺ and H₂O resorption in kidneys ↑ K⁺ and H⁺ excretion	Increased extracellular fluid (ECF)	Potential for **oedema** (fluid in tissues)
Blood	↑ coagulability, ↓ white cells	Reduced blood clotting time	Haemoconcentration, blood clotting
Central nervous system	Emotional changes	Increased rate of learning	Emotional changes with illness

Source: Adapted from Boore, 2000

'Stressful experiences have an impact on diabetes self-care behaviour' (Lloyd et al., 2005: 124). More recently, Williams et al. (2013) provided evidence that perceived stress predicted abnormal glucose **metabolism** in women but not in men.

APPLY

Stress and diabetes

RICHARD JONES CASE NOTES

Within the Bodie family, Richard demonstrates a possible link between stress and diabetes. He was successfully treated by cognitive behavioural therapy (CBT) for stress some time ago and has had type 2 diabetes for the last 5 years. CBT may have focused on stress management as identified by Lloyd et al. (2005), who described three stages:

- Removing or minimising the source of stress
- Changing the response to stress
- Modifying the longer-term effects of stress

If this was the focus of treatment, it is likely to have enhanced Richard's management of stress and his diabetes, resulting in better blood glucose control. He is managing his diabetes well, with blood glucose levels remaining within acceptable levels. The diet taken by him and Hannah facilitates diabetes management and her support helps him.

Many of the physiological mechanisms involved in stress are identified in Tables 1.6 and 1.7 but also important are behavioural mechanisms, which may be extremely varied, and the cause or result of stress. As part of reactions to stressors, emotional distress can lead to unhealthy behaviours; these can include smoking, drinking alcohol excessively, excessive eating (often of sweet things) to provide comfort, with potentially harmful effects on the body. Other chronic disorders may also be influenced by stress and stress management is an important aspect of person-centred nursing.

Circadian rhythm is the normal 24-hour rhythm that occurs in many physiological parameters such as body temperature, hormone secretion etc. Disturbed circadian rhythm can also result in a stress response.

ACTIVITY 1.1: UNDERSTAND

Circadian rhythm

Watch this video to better understand circadian rhythm. If you are using the eBook just click on the play button. Alternatively go to **https://study.sagepub.com/essentialpatho/videos**

As you watch, think about the Bodie family: enforced change in circadian rhythm, such as working night shifts, can result in stress as already considered. As an airline pilot, this is an important issue for Thomas Bodie, who finds himself working a range of different hours and across time zones. Circadian rhythm is also a factor which may influence the presentation or severity of disease or the efficacy of drug therapy.

CIRCADIAN RHYTHM (11:19 MINS)

Ageing

Variation between individuals increases with ageing as the rate of decline of physiological functions differs. The causes of ageing are still being researched but Wang et al. (2013) have discussed the effects of **oxidative stress** response due to mitochondrial dysfunction on ageing.

UNDERSTAND

Reactive oxygen species and ageing

Reactive oxygen species (ROS) are oxygen-containing molecules formed as a by-product of normal oxygen metabolism and which play important roles in cell signalling and homeostasis.

A mild oxidative stress response from the **mitochondria** is important in regulating adaptation and having an anti-ageing function. However, excessive ROS can result in damage to cellular components and initiate **apoptosis** (programmed cell death) through action of the mitochondria. (Wang et al., 2013).

An older person's physiology may be affected in various ways. For example, deficiencies in endocrine function can occur in older people, particularly in the hormones associated with the reproductive systems and growth hormone. The endocrine functions essential for life (controlled by the adrenal and thyroid glands) show minimal overall changes with ageing although there are changes in the **hypothalamic-pituitary-adrenal**/thyroid axis (Chahal and Drake, 2007).

An older person may have very little reserve capacity for maintaining homeostasis and even a minor event such as a cold can initiate a series of physiological disturbances and result in disease. The person may, or may not, achieve a new equilibrium. The physiological changes that occur in ageing will influence the presentation of disease. Table 1.8 indicates some of the changes that occur with normal ageing and the major clinical implications.

Table 1.8   Ageing and its clinical implications

System	Physiological changes	Clinical implications
Nervous system	**Neuron** numbers lessened Reaction time slower Spinal cord neurons lost Eyes: lens rigid and opaque Ears: degeneration of cochlea	Reduced memory, dementia Reduced balance and increased risk of falls Cataract → reduced vision Loss of high-tone hearing
Endocrine system	Deterioration of beta-pancreatic cells → reduced insulin secretion Reduced vitamin D function Reduced sex hormones	Impaired glucose tolerance ? diabetes mellitus Reduced Ca^{2+} in bone Changes in metabolism and physiological function
Gastrointestinal system	Reduced motility of gut Weakened cardiac **sphincter**	Constipation Oesophageal reflux
Respiratory system	Reduced elasticity and increased rigidity of lungs and chest Reduced **cough** and cilia function Mismatch of ventilation/**perfusion**	Reduced lung function with activity and exercise Increased risk of infection Reduced oxygen saturation
Renal system	Nephron numbers down Glomerular filtration rate down Tubular function diminished	Fluid balance impaired **Dehydration** or fluid overload risk Drug excretion impaired
Cardiovascular system	Reduced maximum heart rate Aortic dilation Reduced elasticity of arteries Reduced function sinoatrial node	Reduced exercise tolerance X-ray shows widened aortic arch Postural **hypotension** more likely Increased risk of atrial fibrillation
Musculoskeletal system	Reduced calcium in bones Ageing changes in bone, cartilage, ligaments Vertebrae shrink	Osteoporosis (↑ risk of **fractures**) Contribute to **osteoarthritis** development Loss of height
Skin	Photoageing Atrophy, wrinkling, dryness Decreased inflammatory response	Skin disorders Cancers Slow healing
Immune system	Reduced B and T cell **lymphocytes** Reduced immune response	Increased vulnerability to **antigens** - new or previously encountered

Source: Adapted from Blume-Peytavi et al., 2016; Chahal and Drake, 2007; Colledge et al., 2010; De Tata, 2014; Loeser, 2010; Montecino-Rodriguez et al., 2013; Montero-Odasso and Duque, 2005

DIAGNOSIS OF DISEASE

A diagnosis is important because it enables provision of the correct treatment for the particular condition. The diagnosis is determined through:

- *History taking*: involves gaining information from the person and perhaps family members to help diagnosis by finding out as much as possible about the person and their condition, including factors which worsen or improve it, and the time-line of its development. In traumatic conditions, the history of the trauma is central to the direction of clinical thinking and is often provided by witnesses to the incident and emergency personnel.
- Physical examination including:
  - *Signs*: are indicators of disordered function that can be readily observed: for example, rash or blue coloration of the skin, wheezing with respiration.
  - *Symptoms*: are indicators of disordered function that the person reports: for example, pain, pain on urination, confusion or loss of memory.
- *Non-invasive tests*: there are a number of tests which can be carried out easily to aid diagnosis (Table 1.9).

Table 1.9   Examples of non-invasive tests for diagnosis

Measurement of physiological parameters	Vital signs (temperature, pulse, respiration rate) Blood pressure Respiratory function: SpO_2 (peripheral oxygen saturation) Respiratory volumes
Urine testing (clinical setting)	Glucose, **ketones** Protein pH
Microbiological testing	From secretions, wounds etc. Urine, sputum, faecal samples

In addition, a wide range of additional tests, many invasive in some degree, are carried out to assist or confirm diagnosis (Table 1.10). The key element in the process is to achieve the appropriate differential diagnosis, i.e. the correct diagnosis is identified through differentiating it from other conditions with similar signs and symptoms. A clear diagnosis carries with it information about the cause of the disease and recommended treatments.

Table 1.10   Types of additional tests for diagnosis

Haematological	Blood cells and proteins, antigens, blood types, etc.
Biochemical	Chemical/biochemical substances in body fluids and tissues
Cytological (biopsies)	Small samples of tissues for examination of cells
Microbiological	Infected tissues or exudate examined for identification of specific microbes
Radiological (X-rays) and other scans, e.g. MRI, ultrasound	Used to examine the structure of internal organs (e.g. bones, fetal development), soft tissues
Electrocardiograph (ECG) Electroencephalograph (EEG)	ECG: electrical activity indicating function of the heart EEG: electrical activity indicating function of the brain
Physiological	Tests of function of specific organs/systems, e.g. renal function
Endoscopies	Examining body cavities by insertion of flexible tube, often with a camera attached

Syndromes

A syndrome is a set of signs and symptoms that occur together and sometimes indicate a specific condition. In the past, a considerable number of these groups of signs and symptoms were named after the clinician who described them or the first person identified with the condition. The cause was often not known but the description has led to a hypothesis and guided research, which, with scientific developments, often result in identification of the cause and appropriate treatment. A wide range of syndromes occur that, between them, can affect every system of the body with a number of different causes: Table 1.11 identifies some examples.

Table 1.11 Examples of syndromes

Carpal tunnel syndrome	Tingling and numbness, followed by sudden, sharp, piercing pain through the wrist and up the arm
Chronic fatigue syndrome	Extreme, prolonged tiredness with muscle pain, memory problems, headaches, pain in multiple joints, sleep problems, sore throat and tender lymph nodes
Cushing's syndrome	Upper body obesity, thin arms and legs, fatigue and muscle weakness, hypertension, hyperglycaemia. Due to prolonged raised cortisol level
Down (or Down's) syndrome	Mental and physical disability, slow growth, characteristic facial features, may have other health problems, e.g. heart disease. Genetic disorder
Fetal alcohol syndrome	Physical abnormalities: wide-set and narrow eyes, growth problems, nervous system abnormalities. Behavioural difficulties: daily living, learning, emotions, etc.
Marfan (or Marfan's) syndrome	Affects connective tissue, variable presentation. Often tall, thin and loose jointed, may have problems with heart and blood vessels, bones, eyes, skin, nervous system and lungs. Genetic disorder
Sudden infant death syndrome (SIDS)	'Cot death' – unexplained death during first year. Cause unknown but firm mattress and positioning on back for sleep reduces incidence
Sudden arrhythmic death syndrome (SADS)	Genetic heart conditions that can cause sudden death in apparently healthy people, often young and active

CONCLUSION

This chapter provides an introduction to disease and the factors that influence the development and presentation of disorders. Individuals vary considerably both biologically and behaviourally and the variation that occurs influences how disease presents. You have learnt about the different types of disease and will be able to think about the implications for those with the different types of disorder and their families.

A number of the pathological mechanisms involved in the development of disease have also been considered. Amongst these, stress and ageing are major factors that influence disorders and how individuals and families respond. Understanding these is central to working with those requiring person-centred care.

- Individuals can vary in anatomy, physiology, biochemistry and development, resulting in differences in susceptibility to disease and how it presents. In addition, emotional responses and lifestyle behaviours also influence disease and the person-centred care required.

- Diseases can be acute, chronic or sub-acute with differing disease pathways. In addition, someone with a chronic disorder can present with an acute exacerbation of their chronic illness. Diseases can also be congenital (i.e. existing from birth) or acquired (occurring after birth).

- Disease can be communicable (which can be passed onto someone else, e.g. infective) or non-communicable. In addition, there is a wide range of other causes of illness.

- There are a number of physiological mechanisms which influence disease presentation, including stress and ageing. Stress can present in an acute (Alarm Reaction) stage in which changes are due to the action of catecholamine hormones, or a chronic state resulting primarily from the action of glucocorticoid hormones. The changes that occur in ageing can also influence the body function and how disease presents.

- Achieving an accurate diagnosis is essential for appropriate treatment. History, physical examination and a range of haematological, biochemical, radiological and other tests enable this to be achieved. A syndrome is a specific set of signs and symptoms.

Studying this chapter will help you to understand the causes of disease and, thus, identify the sorts of problems with which people in your care may need help. Revise the different sections in turn then try to answer the questions below.

Answers are available online. If you are using the eBook just click on the answers icon below. Alternatively go to **https://study.sagepub.com/essentialpatho/answers**

1 Explain what you understand by 'normal' in relation to physical and behavioural function and how you can apply this understanding in providing high-quality care.

2 Describe five aspects of biological variation and how they vary in different individuals. Discuss the implications of these variations for planning and person-centred care.

3 Analyse and evaluate the implications for family-centred care of four aspects of behaviour that influence the development of chronic diseases.

4 State the main characteristics of each of the following categories of disease:

    i. Acute
    ii. Chronic
    iii. Sub-acute
    iv. 'Acute on chronic'

5 Differentiate between congenital and acquired disorders, and between communicable and non-communicable disease:

    i. Congenital
    ii. Acquired
    iii. Communicable
    iv. Non-communicable

6   Briefly explain, with examples, how disordered negative feedback can result in disease.

7   Describe the endocrine changes that occur in the acute stress response and evaluate their implications for the physiological changes in disease.

8   Identify the stages of the long-lasting stress response, the key physiological changes that occur and consider how you can plan family-centred care to facilitate quality of life.

9   What are the common effects of ageing on an individual's structure and function? How will these influence the development of physiological disorders as they age?

10   Discuss the importance of diagnosis and evaluate the contribution of the person's history, signs and symptoms, and additional tests in assisting diagnosis.

REVISE

ACE YOUR ASSESSMENT

- Further revision and learning opportunities are available online
- Test yourself away from the book with **extra multiple choice questions**
- Learn and revise terminology with **interactive flashcards**

If you are using the eBook access each resource by clicking on the respective icon. Alternatively go to **https://study.sagepub.com/essentialpatho/chapter1**

CHAPTER 1
ANSWERS

EXTRA
QUESTIONS

FLASHCARDS

REFERENCES

American Heritage (2016) *Dictionary of the English Language*, 5th edn. Geneva: Houghton Mifflin Harcourt Publishing Company.

AVERT (2016) *Global Information and Education on HIV and AIDS*. Brighton, UK: AVERT. (Last full review: 1 December 2016.) Available at: www.avert.org/professionals/hiv-around-world/sub-saharan-africa/south-africa (accessed 29 May 2017).

Blume-Peytavi, U., Kottner, J., Sterry, W., Hodin, M.W., Griffiths, T.W., Watson, R.E.B. et al. (2016) Age-associated skin conditions and diseases: current perspectives and future options. *The Gerontologist, 56* (Suppl 2): S230–S242.

Boore, J. (2000) Stress. In S.M. Hinchcliff, S.E. Montague and R. Watson (eds), *Physiology for Nursing Practice*, 2nd edn. Edinburgh: Harcourt Publishers.

Boore, J., Cook, N. and Shepherd, A. (2016) *Essentials of Anatomy and Physiology for Nursing Practice*. London: Sage.

Braun, D.K., Dominguez, G. and Pellett, P.E. (1997) Human herpesvirus 6. *Clinical Microbiology Reviews, 10* (3): 521–67.

Chahal, H.S. and Drake, W.M. (2007) The endocrine system and ageing. *Journal of Pathology, 211*: 173–80.

Challoner, P.B., Smith, K.T., Parker, J.D., MacLeod, D.L., Coulter, S.N., Rose, T.M. et al. (1995) Plaque-associated expression of human herpesvirus 6 in multiple sclerosis. *Proceedings of the National Academy of Sciences of the United States of America*, 92 (16): 7440–4.

Colledge, N.R., Walker, B.R. and Ralston, S.H. (2010) *Davidson's Principles and Practice of Medicine*, 21st edn. Edinburgh: Churchill Livingstone/Elsevier.

Collins English Dictionary (2012) Complete and Unabridged Digital Edition. London: HarperCollins Publishers.

Cox, T. (1978) *Stress*. Macmillan: Basingstoke.

Daanen, H.A.M. and Lichtenbelt, W.D.V.M. (2016) Human whole body cold adaptation. *Temperature*, 3 (1): 104–18 Available at: https://doi.org/10.1080/23328940.2015.1135688 (accessed 12 June 2018).

Deng, Y., Misselwitz, B., Dai, N. and Fox, M. (2015) Review: Lactose intolerance in adults – biological mechanism and dietary management. *Nutrients*, 7: 8020–35 Available at: www.mdpi. com/journal/ nutrients (accessed 28 May 2017).

De Tata, A. (2014) Age-related impairment of pancreatic beta-cell function: pathophysiological and cellular mechanisms. *Frontiers in Endocrinology* (online journal), 5 (Sept): article 138 Available at: www.ncbi.nlm.nih.gov/pmc/articles/PMC4153315/pdf/fendo- 05-00138.pdf (accessed 24 March 2016).

Foster, F. and Collard, M. (2013) A reassessment of Bergmann's Rule in modern humans. *PLoS ONE, 8* (8): e72269 Available at: https://doi.org/10.1371/journal. pone.0072269 (accessed 12 June 2018).

Huovinen, E., Kaprio, J., Laitinen, L.A. and Koskenvuo, M. (1999) Incidence and prevalence of asthma among adult Finnish men and women of the Finnish twin cohort from 1975 to 1990, and their relation to hay fever and chronic bronchitis. *Chest*, 115 (4): 928–36.

Komaroff, A.L. (2006) Is human herpesvirus-6 a trigger for chronic fatigue syndrome? *Journal of Clinical Virology*, 37: S39–S46.

Lloyd, C., Smith, J. and Weinger, K. (2005) Stress and diabetes: a review of the links. *Diabetes Spectrum*, 18 (2): 121–7.

Loeser, R.F. (2010) Age-related changes in the musculoskeletal system and the development of osteoarthritis. *Clinics in Geriatric Medicine, 26* (3): 371–86.

McBride, W.G. (1961) Thalidomide and congenital abnormalities (Letter to the Editor). *The Lancet, 278* (7216): 1358.

McCormack, B. and McCance, T. (2019) The Person-Centred Nursing Framework 2010 Revised. Belfast: Ulster University. Available at: https://www.ulster.ac.uk/nursingframework (accessed 15 April 2019).

Montecino-Rodriguez, E., Berent-Maoz, B. and Dorshkind, K. (2013) Causes, consequences, and reversal of immune system ageing. *Journal of Clinical Investigation, 123* (3): 958–65.

Montero-Odasso, M. and Duque, G. (2005) Vitamin D in the aging musculoskeletal system: an authentic strength preserving hormone. *Molecular Aspects of Medicine, 26*: 203–19.

Overfield, T. (2017) *Biologic Variation in Health and Illness: Race, Age and Sex Differences*, 2nd edn. Menlo Park, CA: Addison–Wesley.

Sanders, L.F. and Duncan, G.E. (2006) Population-based reference standards for cardiovascular fitness among U.S. adults: NHANES 1999–2000 and 2001–2002. *Medicine and Science in Sports and Exercise, 38* (4): 701–7.

Selye, H. (1976, reissued 1978) *The Stress of Life*. New York: McGraw–Hill.

Wang, C.H., Wu, S-B., Wu, Y-T. and Wei, Y-H. (2013) Oxidative stress response elicited by mitochondrial dysfunction: implication in the pathophysiology of aging. *Experimental Biology and Medicine, 238* (5): 450–60.

Williams, E.D., Magliano, D.J., Tapp, R.J., Oldenburg, B.F. and Shaw, E.D. (2013) Psychosocial stress predicts abnormal glucose metabolism: The Australian Diabetes, Obesity and Lifestyle (AusDiab) Study. *Annals of Behavioural Medicine, 46* (1): 62–7.

World Health Organisation (WHO) (1948) Preamble to the Constitution of WHO as adopted by the International Health Conference, New York, 19 June – 22 July 1946; signed on 22 July 1946 by the representatives of 61 States. Official Records of WHO, no. 2, p. 100. Entered into force on 7 April 1948. (Note: The definition has not been amended since 1948.)

World Health Organisation (WHO) (2018) *Health Topics: Disabilities*. Geneva: WHO.

World Health Organisation (WHO) Europe (2016) *Health Topics: Noncommunicable Diseases*. Copenhagen, Denmark: World Health Organisation Regional Office for Europe. Available at www. euro.who.int/en/health-topics/noncommunicable-diseases/noncommunicable-diseases.

HEALTH AND DISEASE IN SOCIETY

Watch the following video to ease you into this chapter. If you are using the eBook just click on the play button. Alternatively go to **https://study.sagepub.com/essentialpatho/videos**

PUBLIC HEALTH (5:33)   EPIDEMIOLOGY (7:20)

LEARNING OUTCOMES

When you have finished studying this chapter you will be able to:

1. Understand the principles of public health and the relevance to person-centred nursing.
2. Recognise the importance of epidemiology in recognising causes of diseases and how this understanding can be used to promote person-centred care.
3. Discuss how epidemiology contributes to diagnosis and treatment of disease and to prevention through public health.
4. Describe the main approaches used in epidemiological studies to confirm the causes of disease and to control its development.
5. Understand the value of cohort and case-control studies in following up progression of people with particular conditions.
6. Illustrate how epidemiology integrates with ethical and political considerations.

INTRODUCTION

Most of this book is about disorders affecting individuals and their management. However, this chapter has a much broader perspective: public health building on the science of **epidemiology**. This is currently defined by WHO as:

> the science and art of preventing disease, prolonging life and promoting health through the organized efforts of society. (Acheson, 1988 cited by WHO Europe, 2012)

This is also described as:

> the branch of medicine which deals with the incidence, distribution, and possible control of diseases and other factors relating to health. (Oxford Dictionaries, 2018)

More concisely:

> Epidemiology is the study of health and disease in populations. (Saracci, 2010: 2)

Together these definitions identify the key concepts with which this chapter is concerned: epidemiology is the basic science underpinning public health.

Epidemiology enables us to begin to understand the range of factors that influence the distribution of **disease** through the population and how it spreads between populations. Understanding the principles of epidemiology enables us to recognise the relationship between different factors – genetic, social class, environment, behaviour, **nutrition**, education and others – and the presentation of disease. It has a key role in identifying necessary public health measures and assists in identifying the appropriate person-centred care. Central to this is facilitating individuals in making appropriate choices about lifestyle and thus influencing disease incidence in the population.

PERSON-CENTRED CONTEXT: THE BODIE FAMILY

BODIE FAMILY
CASE NOTES

Some members of the Bodie family provide examples of epidemiology in practice. George and Maud are examples of generally healthy elderly people with medical conditions that epidemiological research has identified as relatively common in their age group and public health interventions are prescribed.

George was diagnosed with raised **cholesterol** (**hypercholesterolaemia**) when he was 73 (9 years ago), since then he has been taking **statins**. He has also received guidance on lifestyle issues to reduce the risk of heart disease.

GO DEEPER

Atherosclerosis

Atherosclerosis is very common among the population at large. The consensus statement of the European Atherosclerosis Society (Nordestgaard et al., 2013) identifies that 1 in 500 of the general population are heterozygous for the relevant gene for familial hypercholesterolaemia, which increases the risk of

ischaemic heart disease due to atherosclerosis (Humphries et al., 2006). We do not know whether George's form runs in the family or not.

However, there is evidence that there is considerable underdiagnosis and undertreatment of this condition in a number of developed and less developed countries (Ahn et al., 2015; Nordestgaard et al., 2013). For example, Pearson (2004) identified a considerable gap between those with a diagnosis of this condition and those receiving treatment in the USA. To improve this situation, OTC (Over-The-Counter) statins were being encouraged.

In the UK, only low-intensity OTC statins can be purchased. However, on-line pharmacies enable individuals to access statins via medical practitioners employed by these pharmacies. These doctors question people at a distance and tend to prescribe moderate intensity statins delivered by post. Most GPs will carry out a more comprehensive assessment, including blood tests, before prescribing appropriate treatment, which is likely to be higher density statins than OTC drugs. The majority of those taking statins in the UK are diagnosed and treated in the National Health Service by their General Practitioners and local pharmacies.

Maud also has some conditions which are more common in older people, including heart failure, which is being managed effectively, and **hypothyroidism**. She is an example of the incidence of hypothyroidism in areas which have adequate iodine, where it is higher among the elderly and 10 times more common in women than men (Vanderpump, 2011). These results are mainly from Caucasian populations (McGrogan et al., 2008).

Jack Garcia lives in New York and has a generally healthy lifestyle. However, his father had testicular **cancer** which was treated effectively. This condition is the commonest malignancy worldwide among young men (15–34 years), particularly Caucasians, and is usually curable, particularly when diagnosed early. In addition, epidemiological research with families has found that men with fathers with a history of testicular cancer are four times more likely to develop this than men in the general population (Manecksha and Fitzpatrick, 2009). Jack, at 28, is wisely performing self-examination monthly to ensure rapid treatment if anything abnormal is detected.

The siblings Derek and Margaret Jones both have conditions associated with **atopy**: Derek has asthma and Margaret hay fever. Atopy is the genetic tendency to develop the classic allergic diseases: atopic **dermatitis**, allergic **rhinitis** (hay fever) and asthma. Familial grouping of phenotypes is found, although different conditions may present – in this case one has asthma, the other hay fever. There are several chromosomal regions associated with atopic responsiveness (Koppelman et al., 2002), which may explain that two siblings are affected but neither parent is.

Danielle has been receiving the **immunisations** recommended at this stage in her life. George, Maud and Derek receive their **influenza** immunisations annually because they are all at increased risk of developing complications from flu. Other family members receive immunisations when going abroad. Epidemiological research has provided the knowledge identifying the value of these interventions and helped promote public health.

EPIDEMIOLOGY

The overall role of epidemiology has been outlined above. In addition, however, understanding the statistical analysis is important in being able to use the findings to plan future services. Statistics helps us to understand and interpret the world, including individuals with disorders with whom we work, and thus enhance the quality of care. However, the detail of statistics is not studied in this book.

Three main types of study within epidemiology can be identified: descriptive, analytical and intervention studies each contribute to our understanding of disease within populations (Carr et al., 2007). The findings contribute to understanding public health and planning health and other services to promote the health status of the community.

In addition, the field of epidemiology has been described in five areas, as shown in Table 2.1.

Table 2.1 Five major areas in epidemiology

Descriptive epidemiology	Health and disease and their trends over time in specific populations
Aetiological epidemiology	Searches for factors (hazardous or beneficial) influencing health status (e.g. toxins, poor diet, pathogenic microorganisms, health-promoting behaviours)
Evaluative epidemiology	Evaluates preventative interventions, estimates risks of specific diseases for people exposed to hazards
Health services epidemiology	Describes and analyses work of health services
Clinical epidemiology	Describes natural course of a disease in patient population and evaluates effects of diagnostic procedures and treatment

Source: Saracci, 2010: 11

Descriptive epidemiology

This branch of epidemiology examines the incidence of disease in relation to person, place and time. It aims to understand the patterns of health and disease within a population and to generate possible explanations for the findings. The sorts of questions asked in relation to a particular disorder are as follows:

- *Person*: what are the demographic details of those affected, i.e. age, gender, occupation, ethnic background, socioeconomic status, lifestyle factors such as smoking, diet, exercise? This sort of study can provide information about diversity within the population and enable the specific areas to be identified which need consideration with different groups (Lowth, 2015). For example, behaviours associated with certain religious and cultural practices may have potential health implications (Laird et al., 2007). Some examples include:
  - ritual fasting and potential implications for those with chronic diseases such as **diabetes mellitus**
  - potential exposure to infectious diseases when participating in the Haj (the major pilgrimage to Mecca that all Muslims are expected to undertake during their lifetime)
  - a high incidence of consanguineous marriage (i.e. marriage between relatives) increasing the risk of some genetic disorders
  - female genital mutilation (also known as cutting), in which a surgical procedure damages the female genital organs with no medical benefits, and possibly bleeding, infections and other complications including in childbirth (WHO, 2018a), and childhood marriage occur in some groups. While illegal in many countries (including the UK) both of these are often undertaken when girls whose families are living in Western countries are taken back to their ancestral homes and families during long holidays for the surgery and/or to marry (often) a relative whom they have never met. Efforts to minimise this practice include preparing teachers and training airport staff to identify potential girls at risk and putting 'stickers' up in toilet cubicles with advice on

how to get help (Iqbal, 2015). Nursing and midwifery professionals need to be able to recognise potential health issues associated with diversity and to intervene appropriately.

- *Place*: is there a difference in the incidence of the condition in some areas, e.g. related to geography, the condition of various parts of a city, the availability of local facilities?
- *Time*: does the incidence of the disease being considered vary over a number of years, at different times of the year, in different weather/climatic conditions, etc.?

Routinely available data

A significant amount of data related to diseases is available through routinely collected information; for example, death certificates must be completed by the attending doctor and the data becomes available to the Office for National Statistics (in the United Kingdom) and can be used to review changes in the incidence of specific diseases over time. A range of administrative data sets are also used and the Office for National Statistics coordinates the national decennial (10-yearly) census, next due in 2021.

GO DEEPER

Cholera and epidemiology

An example of an early epidemiological study was carried out by John Snow in 1854 when an area of London supplied by two water companies (the Lambeth Water Company and the Southwark and Vauxhall Company) had a cholera epidemic. Snow identified that the relative proportion of cholera deaths in parts supplied by the Southwark and Vauxhall Company was significantly higher than elsewhere, in particular in those areas where people got their water from the Broad Street Pump. Snow approached the Board of Guardians and reported that he believed that the cholera was spreading in the water from the Broad Street Pump. While this was an incredible suggestion in those times, they agreed to remove the pump handle. The cholera epidemic died down. His hypothesis that cholera was transmitted by contaminated water is now generally accepted by epidemiologists and his action recognised by the installation of the John Snow Memorial marking the epicentre of the outbreak (Rossignol, 2007).

Data on cardiovascular incidence and mortality is collected in numerous countries and parts of the world and demonstrates improving results. The epidemiological statistics enable the changes occurring and the effects of interventions on **morbidity** to be identified.

APPLY

Changes in cardiovascular morbidity

These are diseases of the heart and blood vessels, causing a range of disorders through central and peripheral parts of the circulatory system and are the primary cause of death worldwide. Over three-quarters of these deaths occur in low- and middle-income countries where they cause 37% of premature deaths (under 70 years) from non-communicable diseases (WHO, 2018b).

(Continued)

(Continued)

However, it is also important to recognise the developments occurring and approaches to reducing morbidity (illness rate) and mortality (death rate) since they peaked in the 1960s (Luepker, 2016). In Europe these disorders have been diminishing in incidence since the 1980s but they are still the main cause of mortality and major cause of morbidity, but with considerable variability across the region. Central and Eastern Europe have higher death rates from these conditions than in Northern, Southern and Western Europe. These results tend to be linked with minimal levels of primary health care related to smoking and other lifestyle factors and inadequate approaches to early detection and treatment. While smoking has diminished across Europe, the highest rates are found in the countries of the old Soviet Union which also have high levels of cardiovascular diseases (CVDs) (Wilkins et al., 2017).

There is still progress to be made through **health promotion** activities to promote an appropriate diet to reduce **obesity**, limit smoking, encourage exercise and moderate drinking. In addition, conditions which increase risk, and therefore should be identified and treated effectively, include diabetes mellitus, **hypertension** and hypercholesterolaemia (WHO, 2018c).

Cross-sectional surveys

In this type of study, information is collected about the health status and other factors of interest in the population being studied. The aim is to identify the proportion of the population which has the disease being studied (i.e. the prevalence of the disorder is determined). This enables adequate planning of appropriate health services to be carried out.

Analytical studies

Analytical studies aim to identify associations between the diseases of interest and possible causes. There are four types of study in this group.

Ecological studies

These studies are different from most others considered here as data is collected on the whole population. Routinely collected disease data are compared with other factors in the population which could be causes of these diseases.

Cross-sectional studies

These have been mentioned above. In this context they are trying to identify the prevalence of disorders and association with various factors. For example, this type of study has demonstrated a relationship between obesity and diabetes mellitus, and behaviour.

Case-control studies

In these studies, one group of cases (who have the condition of interest) is compared with a group of controls (who do not have the condition). The individuals involved are screened by interview, survey or previous records to determine their exposure. The exposure to potential cause of those in the two groups is compared to see if the exposure of the group of cases differs from that of the control group. If so, these variables may influence the **progression** and eventual disease outcomes (Rossignol, 2007).

ACTIVITY 2.1: UNDERSTAND

Social interventions for health

Read the following article to enhance your understanding of the relationship between physical activity, obesity and diabetes: Creatore et al. (2016) 'Association of neighborhood walkability with change in overweight, obesity, and diabetes.' This particular paper (set in Ontario, Canada) examines the suitability of the neighbourhood for walking and the incidence of obesity and diabetes. Although more research is needed, it suggests that these factors are related.

If you are using the eBook you can access the article directly by clicking the icon.

ARTICLE: PHYSICAL
ACTIVITY, OVERWEIGHT
AND DIABETES

Cohort studies

Two groups similar in characteristics relevant to the study (except for the condition of interest) are selected and the outcome of interest is compared. Cohort studies can assess a range of outcomes, allowing an exposure to be rigorously assessed for its impact in developing disease, although these studies are lengthy and expensive, especially if the follow-up period is extensive. They are useful for studying exposure to rare conditions such as radiation from the Chernobyl nuclear power plant in 1986. The study can be retrospective or prospective; in either case the groups are similar apart from the condition being studied.

Retrospective

In this case both groups have been exposed to similar conditions except in relation to the key issue being studied and outcomes have occurred. One group has been exposed to the condition being studied while the other has not. The data has already been collected and the results will be studied.

Prospective

In these studies, all the participants come from the same study population and are divided into two groups, one of which will have been exposed to the characteristic under study, and the other will not. As far as possible, the two groups are comparable on other relevant characteristics. Those in both groups are then followed for a specified period to identify the individuals who develop the expected outcome/disease.

Intervention (or experimental) studies

The difference between these and the previous types of study is that in this situation the researcher intervenes to change the exposure of the participants to the factor being studied.

Clinical trials

In these studies, one group of people with a particular condition receive a specified treatment and their progress is compared with a second control group who are not receiving the active intervention. One of the key issues is to prevent bias so that the participants are randomly assigned to a group in what is known as a *randomised double-blind controlled trial*. The 'double-blind' part of this term indicates that neither the participant nor the person managing the trial knows which group the participant is in.

When a drug is being tested, the control group of participants normally receives a tablet that appears similar to the active treatment but is not active; it is what is known as a placebo. In some circumstances the study is aiming to compare a new treatment with the one currently in use.

Community trials

In these studies the study is examining the effect of an intervention on a community as the unit of study, not individuals. Because social, cultural and environmental conditions may be key factors in the incidence of disease, a **community trial** tries to alter these conditions community-wide and then evaluate the effect. However, it is not usually feasible to undertake double-blind controlled trials.

Contribution of epidemiology

Epidemiology plays an extremely important role in identifying conditions that contribute to health or disease, and in providing you with an enhanced understanding of how to contribute to person-centred care. In addition, it provides the knowledge and understanding that politicians and officials need to undertake the planning and implementation of conditions for optimum health for individuals and the community through public health. An example is the identification of particular conditions which are more common in those from particular ethnic groups or geographical areas than other members of the population.

PUBLIC HEALTH

Public health is underpinned by the science of epidemiology and the WHO definition has already been presented. An earlier US description, still widely quoted and as relevant as ever, is below.

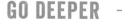 GO DEEPER

Public health

In 1920, Winslow, an American public health specialist of his time, defined public health as follows:

> Public Health is the science and the art of preventing disease, prolonging life, and promoting physical health and efficiency through organized community efforts for the sanitation of the

environment, the control of community infections, the education of the individual in principles of personal hygiene, the organization of medical and nursing services for the early diagnosis and preventive treatment of disease, and the development of the social machinery which will ensure to every individual in the community a standard of living adequate for the maintenance of health.

(C.E.A. Winslow, 1920, cited in Evans, 2011)

The key issue in relation to public health is that it is 'public' and focused on enhancing the health of the whole population. The World Federation of Public Health Associations (WFPHA) developed a Global Charter for the Public's Health (GCPH) (Lomazzi, 2016), which identifies core services (protection, prevention, promotion) and functions to enable these services (governance, advocacy, capacity and information) (Figure 2.1). These largely overlap with the areas considered below.

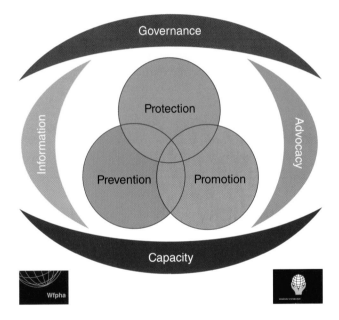

Figure 2.1 Illustration of the Global Charter for the Public's Health (Lomazzi, 2016)

Within each country the health system is determined by government involving public, private and voluntary sector organisations contributing to health maintenance, and activities influencing health behaviour and status. The structure and interaction within such organisations vary across different countries of the world. In the UK, the four countries of England, Scotland, Wales and Northern Ireland manage most of the public health issues independently, although with some coordination from national government.

Areas of public health practice

Organisations with public health remits have identified three areas of public health practice, shown in Figure 2.2. These are largely the same for different organisations but with some differences (FPH, 2010; Gray et al., 2006).

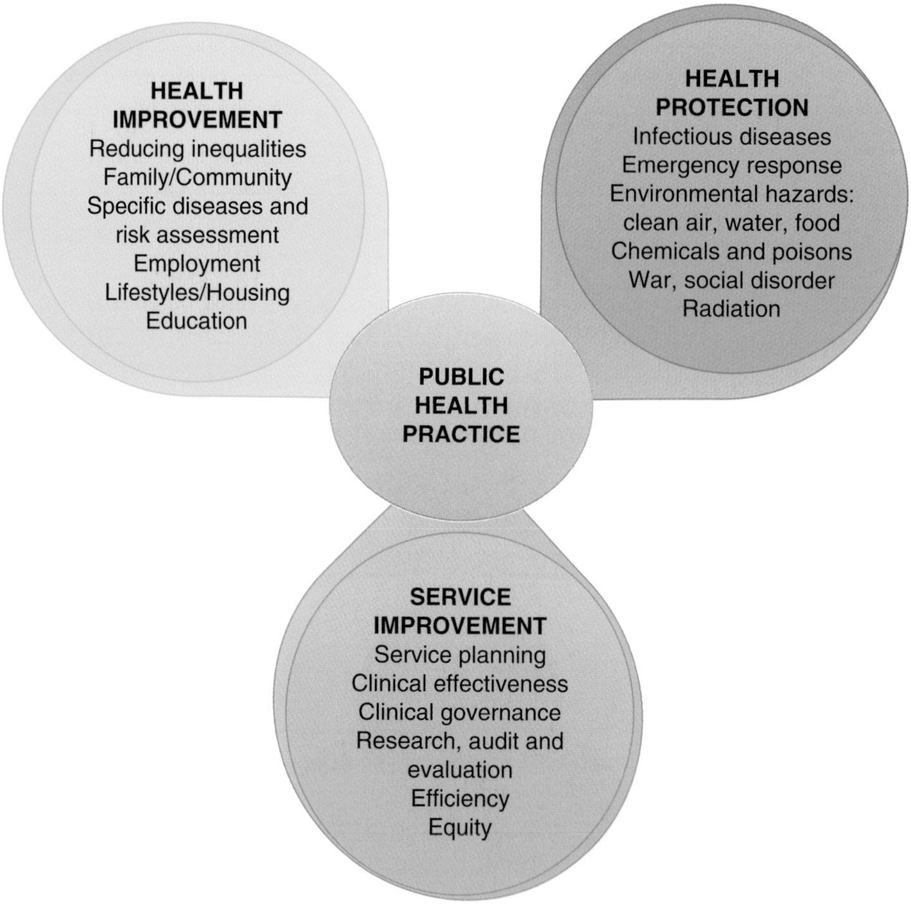

HEALTH IMPROVEMENT
Reducing inequalities
Family/Community
Specific diseases and
risk assessment
Employment
Lifestyles/Housing
Education

HEALTH PROTECTION
Infectious diseases
Emergency response
Environmental hazards:
clean air, water, food
Chemicals and poisons
War, social disorder
Radiation

PUBLIC HEALTH PRACTICE

SERVICE IMPROVEMENT
Service planning
Clinical effectiveness
Clinical governance
Research, audit and
evaluation
Efficiency
Equity

Figure 2.2   Public health practice

Health protection

This area of public health practice is concerned with actions to reduce exposure to factors that can impact on the development of ill-health. In general, these requirements require tackling at different levels. While normally there are adequate emergency services which undertake rescue and safety activities as necessary, circumstances can arise in which additional support is required and members of the public may contribute as they are able. The box below discusses unusual conditions in the UK which increased the health risks to the population and in which members of the public contributed to **health protection**.

APPLY

Health protection provided by the public

In the winter of 2017/18 some parts of the UK had very severe snow with potential public health risks. This sort of extreme weather is uncommon in the UK and resources for dealing with these conditions are limited. Severe snow drifts, yellow and amber, and some red weather warnings, and disrupted transport by road, rail and air, caused considerable disturbances and potentially placed some citizens at risk. A number of individuals and various organisations endeavoured to contribute to health protection for members of the population at large.

Food and drink supplies were affected and the RAF (Royal Air Force) and other emergency services delivered supplies to villages cut off from the usual supply routes. Water supplies to many houses were cut off and families had to thaw snow for drinking (after boiling for 10 minutes) and washing. People living near roads where cars were stuck for many hours supplied food and water to those in the cars. Some companies were asked by power providers to shut down factories to make gas available for heating homes, particularly to ensure that older people could keep warm.

The conditions were such that a number of individuals died of hypothermia or other diseases aggravated by the very cold weather, for example the increased risk of having a heart attack (myocardial infarction). Hospitals were overloaded. Many health care staff had difficulty getting to work. Some of the armed forces and owners of 4x4 vehicles helped to move staff to work. Farmers used tractors to help community staff reach their patients. Without the contribution of many individuals, the effects of the severe weather could have been much worse.

National government officials and ministers deal with major social issues such as war and severe social disorder, and ensure that suitable emergency response equipment and facilities are available. Regulations are introduced to ensure that hazards such as chemicals, poisons and radiation are dealt with in industry or elsewhere, in a way that limits the exposure of members of the public, and that those working with these risks are trained and equipped appropriately to maintain their safety. Local authorities have responsibility for ensuring the provision of clean air, water and food. Medical authorities carry the responsibility for ensuring that appropriate measures are taken to limit exposure to or to be immunised against infectious diseases.

Health improvement

This aspect of public health aims to

> improve the health and wellbeing of individuals or communities through enabling and encouraging healthy lifestyle choices as well as addressing underlying issues such as poverty, lack of educational opportunities and other such areas. (NHS Scotland, 2018)

Much of the work in this area is guided by regional government through organisations with different areas of expertise and responsibilities. The key issue is to reduce inequalities at individual, family and community level through a range of different initiatives which enhance the quality of life, life opportunities and well-being:

- *Housing*: is it possible for individuals and families to find accommodation that provides enough water, heating, space for children to play, and access to shops selling affordable items central to optimal health? Is there a library nearby? These are key issues for a satisfactory quality of life. Policies are often determined at government level and implemented locally.
- *Education*: is essential for development in life. The local education authority carries overall responsibility for the education services at primary and secondary level. Third-level education

(i.e. post-18) is mainly independent and carries a major responsibility for preparation for the professions and skilled trades. Clearly this is central to the opportunities available for life through employment. In addition, friends made at this stage in life can influence lifestyle choices later. Education for health is also valuable although introduced in very different ways in schools of various types.

- *Employment*: an adequate income is essential for a satisfactory lifestyle. Are there opportunities in the area? What is local government doing to encourage additional employment in the area?
- *Lifestyles*: the factors considered above all influence the scope for lifestyle choices in relation to social, recreational, cultural and literary activities.
- *Specific diseases and risk assessment*: this aspect of public health is managed under the direction of central and local health authorities. It aims to carry out a range of activities to identify conditions associated with differing work conditions, such as asbestos in buildings being demolished being a risk factor for mesothelioma. The local building authorities are responsible for ensuring safe asbestos disposal. The local health services arrange influenza and other immunisations, breast cancer screening, maternal and child health clinics.

The range of issues above can influence quality of life, minimise risks to health and provide necessary information about health risks and how to promote health. Education, housing and traffic conditions, and lifestyles can all contribute to undertaking adequate exercise and limiting obesity. Some key factors need consideration which are central to the quality of health. Some particular examples are:

- Obesity has already been mentioned but is one of the key factors in health. Obesity has a major influence on the risk of disorders including **cardiovascular disease** and diabetes mellitus, which both have the potential to cause serious physical damage.
- Mental ill-health can have a major impact on the quality of life and the provision of mental health services for those at all ages with such problems is essential.
- Air quality is also crucial. Air pollution is identified as the world's largest environmental health risk (WHO, 2018d). Of those living in urban areas, more than 80% are exposed to air quality levels that exceed the WHO limits, with those in low-income cities in contact with higher levels. Developments in vehicle manufacture with reduced impact on air quality are receiving considerable attention with the aim of reducing this factor.

Service improvement

This component of public health is concerned with the provision of a range of services which contribute to health in different ways.

- Research, audit and evaluation is concerned with identifying risks to health and the incidence, morbidity and mortality concerned with different disease processes. Advances in treatment are developed and resulting changes in epidemiological data are identified and used in decision-making about implementation in new treatments. The research carried out must be available for service managers.
- Service planning involves the research outputs evaluated by first-rate researchers and efficient managers who plan implementation to ensure clinical effectiveness and equity in access to care. The Cochrane Collaboration exists to improve health care decisions by gathering and summarising the best evidence involving a worldwide network of researchers, professionals and others involved in health care (Cochrane, 2018).
- Clinical governance has been described as 'the system through which NHS organisations are accountable for continuously improving the quality of their services and safeguarding high standards of care by creating an environment in which clinical excellence will flourish' (Public Health England, 2018).

Value of public health and health promotion

The discipline of public health has tended to be seen as having two major directions:

- 'a broad focus on the underlying social and economic causes of health and disease and their variation in populations'
- 'a narrower medical focus with treatment of ill health at its centre' (Carr et al., 2007: 6).

The list of achievements in public health (Table 2.2) includes important examples from both these directions and also relates to the three areas of public health practice discussed above.

Health promotion is a key element in the three aspects of public health discussed above. It has been defined as enabling

> people to increase control over their own health. It covers a wide range of social and environmental interventions that are designed to benefit and protect individual people's health and quality of life by addressing and preventing the root causes of ill health, not just focusing on treatment and cure. (WHO, 2016a: 1)

Table 2.2 Ten important public health achievements

Vaccination	Eradication of smallpox; polio almost eliminated; immunisation against a wide range of diseases
Control of infectious diseases	Control of typhoid, cholera through clean water and sanitation Tuberculosis and sexually transmitted disease controlled by antibiotics
Decline in mortality from **coronary heart disease** and **stroke**	Risk factor modification (cessation of smoking, control of B/P) Improved access to early detection and treatment
Healthier mothers and babies	Better hygiene and nutrition, access to health care and technological advances in neonatal and maternal health care
Family planning	Altered socioeconomic role of women, reduced family size, improved maternal and child health, barrier contraceptives, reduced unwanted pregnancies and STD transmission
Safer and healthier foods	Decreased microbial contamination, increased nutritional content, nutritional deficiency diseases (e.g. rickets, goitre, pellagra) almost eliminated
Fluoridation of drinking water	Leading to reduction in tooth decay and loss of teeth
Recognition of tobacco use as health risk	Changes in social norms leading to reduced smoking and mortality from smoking-related disease
Safer workplaces	Reduction in fatal occupational injuries; control of pneumoconiosis and silicosis
Motor vehicle safety	Fall in motor vehicle-related deaths due to engineering improvements, vehicles and roads Changed behaviours – use of seat-belts, reduction in drink-driving, lowered use of mobile phones

Source: Gray et al., 2006, after Center for Communicable Disease Control, Atlanta, GA

Three key elements for health promotion have been identified (WHO, 2016a), which are discussed below:

* *Good governance for health*: involves health becoming central to government policy; being considered in relation to all decisions and policies aiming to prevent illness and injuries. Regulations introduced need to relate private activities with public goals, e.g. tax policies to dissuade unhealthy behaviours such as eating high salt food products, or seat-belt and other safety regulations. Local authorities have requirements laid upon them to promote healthy living conditions.
* *Health literacy*: people need knowledge, abilities and understanding to be able to make choices that promote health, for example about healthy food and accessing health care appropriately. They also need to be in a setting in which members of the community can influence policy.
* *Healthy cities*: play an important role in facilitating population health, contributing to healthy countries and, thus, a healthy world. High-quality functioning of local government makes an important contribution to urban planning and developing measures to promote community health and primary and emergency health care.

Public health activities are considered necessary in all parts of the world, although application will vary according to environmental, government and economic factors. The WHO Regional Office for Europe has identified essential operations for the implementation of public health (Table 2.3).

Table 2.3   Ten essential public health operations (EPHOs)

1	Surveillance of population health and well-being
2	Monitoring and response to health hazards and emergencies
3	Health protection including environmental, occupational, food safety and others
4	Health promotion including action to address social determinants and health inequity
5	Disease prevention, including early detection of illness
6	Assuring governance for health and well-being
7	Assuring a sufficient and competent public health workforce
8	Assuring sustainable organisational structures and financing
9	Advocacy, communication and social mobilisation for health
10	Advancing public health research to inform policy and practice

Source: World Health Organisation Europe, 2012

Worldwide public health

We have been looking at some of the principles of public health and now we are examining some issues around public health worldwide or global health. This is defined as:

> an area for study, research, and practice that places a priority on improving health and achieving health equity for all people worldwide. (Koplan et al., 2009: 1995)

An important role in promoting worldwide health has been identified by WHO (2016b) in the Global Strategic Directions for Strengthening Nursing and Midwifery, as outlined in Figure 2.3.

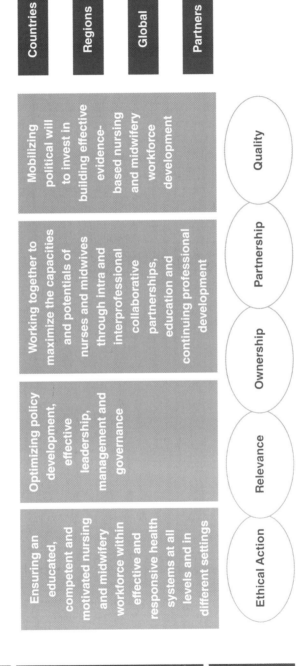

Figure 2.3 Global strategic directions for strengthening nursing and midwifery, 2016–2020

Source: WHO (2016b)

Vision, thematic areas and principles are identified which aim to achieve high-quality nursing care for all to meet population needs through supporting UHC (Universal Health Coverage) and SDGs (Sustainable Development Goals). Clearly nurses and midwives have the potential to make substantial contributions to these goals.

Key areas of inequalities, challenges and health disorders are discussed below.

Inequalities

One of the key issues in considering global health is about inequalities beginning early in life. The effects of relative poverty during pregnancy are marked and long-lasting, with deleterious influences on childhood illness and behavioural problems. In particular, the limited resources diminish inputs that influence child development, including reduced reading and stimulation limiting language and cognitive development and, often, less value placed on education. Overall, these children frequently achieve lower educational outcomes and socioeconomic status (Larson, 2007). It is abundantly clear that poverty is a major determinant of the quality of health within and between developed and less developed countries (Stuart and Soulsby, 2011a).

The differences in health between those living with greater or lesser social and economic resources are marked, with a wide range of such inequalities influencing health and well-being. The social, psychosocial, material and biological factors all influence behaviours and position in society which, in turn, are modified by education, occupation, income and political beliefs. The term 'structural violence' is sometimes used in describing the social factors that cause harm to individuals and populations. This term was originally devised by Galtung (1969, cited by Farmer et al., 2006): they are described

> as structural because they are embedded in the political and economic organization of our social world; they are violent because they cause injury to people. (Farmer et al., 2006: 1686)

In general, health care professionals are not prepared to deal with these factors which are primarily the responsibility of government and regional officials plus those working within the relevant local organisations. However, health professionals do need to be able to understand the relevance of these issues and collaborate with those responsible for these areas.

Challenges

Much of the effort in reducing health inequalities worldwide is about broadly identifying the issues involved and planning across a range of organisations. For example, housing, agriculture, social services, education, infrastructure and engineering, all involving finance, are outside the responsibility of health ministries. Although countries may organise them differently, they are usually within government departments without a health remit. However, planning to enhance the health status of a country has to take account of all these issues (Clift, 2013), which fall into a number of categories:

* *Infrastructure*: in considering developing countries, this group of concerns includes health-related developments but also more general concerns such as roads, dams and power stations, schools and universities.
* *Population growth*: uncontrolled population growth, with the related increased need for food, antenatal and postnatal care, increases the high risks associated with childbirth (see Chapter 18, Female reproductive system), especially in circumstances where midwives and obstetricians may be in short supply. Family planning is crucial.

- *Agriculture and livestock*: if agriculture and livestock are not managed effectively, then poverty will limit access to adequate nutrition, clean water and sanitation, and education. Livestock may be exposed to diseases, which limits healthy animals for nutrition and for providing a living for families (Stuart and Soulsby, 2011b).

Health disorders

Another major area in enhancing global health is collaboration and funding in dealing with various specific health disorders, falling into two main groups – infectious diseases and **non-communicable disorders** (Stuart and Soulsby, 2011c).

- *Infectious diseases*: these are caused by organisms (**bacteria**, **viruses**, **fungi** or **parasites**), many of which compose the **microbiome** living in or on our bodies and are mainly harmless. However, in certain conditions they can cause disease and be transmitted between individuals. Some conditions are known as zoonoses in which the infecting agent is transmitted from animals to humans: 61% of human pathogens are said to be zoonotic and up to 75% of recently identified pathogens are in this group (WHO, 2018e). Terms used to describe distribution include:
  - ○ **Endemic**: a condition that is generally present in a group or area, such as a cold
  - ○ **Epidemic**: a widespread distribution of a condition in an area at a specific time, such as influenza
  - ○ **Pandemic**: a condition that spreads worldwide. When a new influenza virus emerges, it often spreads widely among populations, most of whom do not have immunity.

It is clear that the issue of promoting and maintaining public health within a country or worldwide requires the combined efforts of different organisations, both health services and those with wider responsibilities. Education and leadership within the different areas of activity are also essential and the qualities of fortitude and resilience are crucial.

APPLY

Pandemic spread

The speed of spread of pandemics is strongly related to the transport methods used. Thus, the spread of plague was largely through ship travel and then horse-drawn travel on land and was thus fairly slow. Nowadays, air travel can facilitate rapid transport of infection around the world. It is crucial to understand the diseases which may become pandemic, e.g. Ebola, and how to screen travellers and implement quarantine methods as necessary.

GO DEEPER

Non-communicable disorders

WHO estimates that this group of diseases make up 59% of the 56.5 million deaths on this planet per year (Marshall, 2004). It is creating a growing problem for middle and lower income countries to deal with while

(Continued)

(Continued)

still trying to meet the problems associated with infectious diseases. These non-communicable disorders include conditions related to obesity such as cardiovascular diseases, diabetes and cancers. Most of the cardiovascular diseases are related to major risk factors such as high cholesterol, high blood pressure, low fruit and vegetable intake, inactive lifestyle and tobacco use, and obesity is becoming a major problem in many developing countries. WHO's strategy for tackling this worldwide problem recognises the importance of all sectors contributing, including governments, NGOs (non-governmental organisations), the private sector and stakeholders (including the food industry) (WHO, 2018b).

Communicable Disorder (Pandemic)

Probably the most well-known pandemic in human history is the plague, known as the Black Death, of the mid-14th century (1346–1353). It was caused by a bacterium (carried by rats), *Yersinia pestis*, named after Alexandre Yersin, who isolated the bacterium. It is transmitted by the carrier biting someone and regurgitating the gut's contents into the bloodstream of the human. There have been a number of outbreaks of plague over the years and this bacterium is still found in the American Southwest and parts of Asia.

There are three variants of this disease:

- Bubonic: large swollen areas (buboes) appear around lymph nodes. 18% survival rate for individuals. Pus released is unpleasant to see and smell.
- Pneumonic: affected respiratory system. Easily transmitted between people. Patient drowns in own blood. Survival rate 1%, dies within 2 days.
- Septicaemic: least common form. Disseminated intravascular coagulation (DIC) occurs: blood clots and causes necrosis, then loses ability to clot properly.

This pandemic is said to have reduced the world population by about 50%. The social organisation of the population changed radically, with the size of the labouring population shrinking. Thus, the workers were able to be much more selective in the work they would undertake. The merchant class grew and became wealthier. The nobles became less wealthy and the noble and merchant classes began to intermarry (Armstrong, 2016).

It is thought that the disease originated in China and was transmitted around the world by sailing ships to sea ports. The bacteria were carried in fleas on rats and by jumping from rats to humans, transmitted to humans and carried inland. However, recently, it appears that the plague bacteria were carried by lice and human fleas (although further research is needed to confirm this) (Benedictow, 2004; Dean et al., 2018).

CHAPTER SUMMARY

In this chapter we have looked at two major concepts that influence person-centred care: epidemiology and public health. Epidemiology uses research methodology to provide the data to facilitate understanding of the context of health and disease, and to identify factors that influence the presentation of disease in populations. These data are used to enable public health services and approaches to promote health of populations through health protection, **health improvement** and **service improvement**. All these contribute to health promotion by preventing the key causes of ill-health, rather than just focusing on treatment and cure.

- Epidemiology plays an important role in identifying factors that influence health and disease and provides the understanding necessary to plan and implement conditions for optimum health for individuals and communities.

- There are three major areas of study in epidemiology: descriptive, analytical and intervention, with a number of sub-groups within them.

- Public health is underpinned by the science of epidemiology and it is defined by WHO as the science and art of preventing disease, prolonging life and promoting health through the organised efforts of society.

- Areas of public health practice are health protection, health improvement and service improvement, and health promotion is a key element in all three of these.

- The three key elements of health promotion have been identified by WHO as: good governance for health, literacy and healthy cities which together enable people to increase control over their own health.

- Worldwide public health requires the application of public health principles worldwide and is known as Global Health which aims to improve health and achieve health equity worldwide.

- Global health is achieved by acting within three main areas: inequalities in relation to socioeconomic status and poverty; challenges related to infrastructure, population growth and agriculture and livestock; and health disorders falling into two main groups – infectious diseases and non-communicable disorders.

The content of this chapter will help you understand the principles of epidemiology underpinning public health, and approaches to enhancing the health of the public and individual communities. Revise the different sections in turn then try to answer the questions.

Answers are available online. If you are using the eBook just click on the answers icon below. Alternatively go to **https://study.sagepub.com/essentialpatho/answers**

1   What is epidemiology and how does it contribute to public health?

2   Identify the main types of epidemiological studies and their contribution to an understanding of the distribution of disease.

3   Discuss what is meant by a double-blind controlled trial and their contribution to planning health care interventions.

4   Define and explain public health and the importance of the three areas of public health practice.

5   Explain why public health is valuable and evaluate five examples of public health achievements.

6   Analyse the importance of health promotion in influencing the health of the population.

7   Identify and evaluate the main elements of public health.

8   Discuss the importance of global health and the major groups of issues in promoting worldwide health.

REVISE

ACE YOUR ASSESSMENT

- Further revision and learning opportunities are available online
- Test yourself away from the book with **Extra multiple choice questions**
- Learn and revise terminology with **Interactive flashcards**

If you are using the eBook access each resource by clicking on the respective icon. Alternatively go to **https://study.sagepub.com/essentialpatho/chapter2**

CHAPTER 2
ANSWERS

EXTRA
QUESTIONS

FLASHCARDS

REFERENCES

Acheson, D., Chairman (1988) *Public Health in England*. The Report of the Committee of Inquiry into the Future Development of the Public Health Function. London: HMSO.

Ahn, S.H., Lee, J., Kim, Y.J., Kwon, S.U., Lee, D., Jung, S.C., Kang, D.W. and Kim, J.S. (2015) Isolated MCA disease in patients without significant atherosclerotic risk factors: a high-resolution magnetic resonance imaging study. *Stroke*, *46* (3): 697–703.

Armstrong, D. (2016) *The Black Death: The World's Most Devastating Plague*. The Great Courses, Virginia: The Teaching Company.

Benedictow, O.J. (2004) *The Black Death, 1346–1353: The Complete History*. Woodbridge, Sussex: The Boydell Press.

Carr, S., Unwin, N. and Pless-Mulloli, T. (2007) *An Introduction to Public Health and Epidemiology*, 2nd edn. Maidenhead: Open University Press, McGraw-Hill.

Clift, C. (2013) *The Role of the World Health Organization in the International System*. Centre on Global Health Security Working Group Papers. London: Chatham House. Available at: www.chathamhouse.org/sites/default/files/publications/research/2013-02-01-role-world-health-organization-international-system-clift.pdf (accessed 4 June 2018).

Cochrane (2018) About us [Homepage]. Available at: http://www.cochrane.org/about-us (accessed 11 March 2018).

Creatore, M.I., Glazier, R.H., Moineddin, R. et al. (2016) Association of neighborhood walkability with change in overweight, obesity, and diabetes. *JAMA*, *315* (20): 2211–20.

Dean, K.R., Krauer, F., Walløe, L., Lingjærde, O.C., Bramanti, B., Stenseth, N.C. et al. (2018) Human ectoparasites and the spread of plague in Europe during the Second Pandemic. *PNAS (Proceedings of the National Academy of Sciences of the United States of America)*, *115* (6): 1304–9.

Evans, M.W. (2011) Basic concepts in public health. In M.T. Haneline and W.C. Meeker, *Introduction to Public Health for Chiropractors*. Sudbury, MA: Jones and Bartlett Publishers. Available at: http://samples.jbpub.com/9780763758226/58226_CH02_FINAL.pdf (accessed 9 March 2018).

Farmer, P.E., Nizeye, B., Stulac, S. and Keshavjee, S. (2006) Structural violence and clinical medicine. *PLoS Medicine*, *3* (10): 1686–91.

FPH (2010) *What Is Public Health?* London: The UK's Faculty of Public Health Available at: www.fph.org.uk/what_is_public_health (accessed on 9 March 2018).

Galtung, J. (1969) Violence, peace, and peace research. *Journal of Peace Research, 6* (3): 167–91.

Gray, S., Pilkington, P., Pencheon, D. and Jewell, T. (2006) Public health in the UK: Success or failure. *Journal of the Royal Society of Medicine, 99*: 107–11.

Humphries, S.E., Whittall, R.A., Hubbart, C.S., Maplebeck, S., Cooper, J.A., Soutar, A.K. et al. (2006) Genetic causes of familial hypercholesterolaemia in patients in the UK: relation to plasma lipid levels and coronary heart disease risk. *Journal of Medical Genetics, 43* (12): 943–49.

Iqbal, N. (2015) How border guards are trained to spot potential FGM victims. BBC Newsbeat, 22 July 2015. www.bbc.co.uk/newsbeat/article/33626605/how-border-guards-are-trained-to-spot-potential-fgm-victims.

Koplan, J.P., Bond, T.C., Merson, M.H., Reddy, K.S., Rodriguez, M.H, Sewankambo, N.K. and Wasserheit, J.N. (Consortium of Universities for Global Health Executive Board) (2009) Towards a common definition of global health. *Lancet, 373* (9679): 1993–5.

Koppelman, G.H., Stine, O.C., Xu, J., Howard, T.D., Zheng, S.L., Kauffman, H.F. et al. (2002) Genome-wide search for atopy susceptibility genes in Dutch families with asthma. *Journal of Allergy and Clinical Immunology, 109* (3): 498–506.

Laird, D.L., Amer, M.M., Barnett, E.D. and Barnes, L.L. (2007) Muslim patients and health disparities in the UK and the US. *Archives of Disease in Childhood, 92* (10): 922–6.

Larson, C.P. (2007) Poverty during pregnancy: its effects on child health outcomes. *Paediatrics and Child Health, 12* (8): 673–7.

Lomazzi, M. (2016) A Global Charter for the Public's Health – the public health system: role, functions, competencies and education requirements. *European Journal of Public Health, 26* (2): 210–12.

Lowth, M. (2015) Diseases and different ethnic groups. Patient: Health information you can trust. Available at: https://patient.info/doctor/diseases-and-different-ethnic-groups (accessed 6 October 2018).

Luepker, R.V. (2016) Falling coronary heart disease rates: a better explanation. *Circulation, 133* (1): 8–11.

Manecksha, R.P. and Fitzpatrick, J.M. (2009) Epidemiology of testicular cancer. *British Journal of Urology International (BJUI), 104*: 1329–33.

Marshall, S.J. (2004) Developing countries face double burden of disease. *Bulletin of the World Health Organization, 82* (7): 556.

McGrogan, A., Seaman, H.E., Wright, J.W. and de Vries, C.S. (2008) The incidence of autoimmune thyroid disease: a systematic review of the literature. *Clinical Endocrinology, 69*: 687–96.

NHS Scotland (2018) *Public Health: Health Improvement*. Edinburgh: NHS Education for Scotland. Available at: www.nes.scot.nhs.uk/education-and-training/by-theme-initiative/public-health/health-improvement.aspx (accessed 11 March 2018).

Nordestgaard, B.G., Chapman, M.J., Humphries, S.E., Ginsberg, H.N., Masana, L., Descamps, O.S. et al. (2013) Familial hypercholesterolaemia is underdiagnosed and undertreated in the general population: guidance for clinicians to prevent coronary heart disease: consensus statement of the European Atherosclerosis Society. *European Heart Journal, 34* (45): 3478–90.

Oxford Dictionaries (2018) Epidemiology. *English Oxford Living Dictionaries* [online]. Available at: https:// en.oxforddictionaries.com/definition/epidemiology (accessed 2 March 2018).

Pearson, T.A. (2004) The epidemiological basis for population-wide cholesterol reduction in the primary prevention of coronary artery disease. *American Journal of Cardiology, 94* (Suppl): 4F–8F.

Public Health England (2018) Guidance: 4. Clinical Governance [online]. Available at: www.gov.uk/government/publications/newborn-hearing-screening-programme-nhsp-operational-guidance/4-clinical-governance (accessed 3 November 2018).

Rossignol, A. (2007) *Principles and Practice of Epidemiology: An Engaged Approach*. New York: McGraw-Hill.

Saracci, R. (2010) *Epidemiology: A Very Short Introduction*. Oxford: Oxford University Press.

Stuart, K. and Soulsby, E. (2011a) Reducing global health inequalities: Part 1. *Journal of the Royal Society of Medicine, 104* (8): 321–6.

Stuart, K. and Soulsby, E. (2011b) Reducing global health inequalities. Part 2: Myriad challenges. *Journal of the Royal Society of Medicine, 104* (10): 401–4.

Stuart, K. and Soulsby, E. (2011c) Reducing global health inequalities. Part 3: Collaboration and funding. *Journal of the Royal Society of Medicine, 104* (11): 442–8.

Vanderpump, M.P.J. (2011) The epidemiology of thyroid disease. *British Medical Bulletin, 99*: 39–51.

Wilkins, E., Wilson, L., Wickramasinghe, K., Bhatnagar, P., Leal, J., Luengo-Fernandez, R. et al. (2017) *European Cardiovascular Disease Statistics 2017*. Brussels: European Heart Network.

Winslow, C.E.A. (1920) The untilled fields of public health. *Science, 51* (1306): 23–33.

World Health Organisation (WHO) (2016a) What is health promotion? [Online Q&A]. Available at: www.who.int/features/qa/health-promotion/en/ (accessed 12 March 2018).

World Health Organisation (WHO) (2016b) *Global Strategic Directions for Strengthening Nursing and Midwifery 2016–2020*. Geneva: Health Workforce Department, World Health Organisation Available at: www.who.int/hrh/nursing_midwifery/global-strategic-midwifery2016-2020.pdf (accessed 6 October 2018).

World Health Organisation (WHO) (2018a) Fact Sheet: Female genital mutilation [online]. Available at: www.who.int/news-room/fact-sheets/detail/female-genital-mutilation (accessed 6 October 2018).

World Health Organisation (WHO) (2018b) Fact Sheet: Noncommunicable diseases [online]. Available at: www.who.int/news-room/fact-sheets/detail/noncommunicable-diseases (accessed 14 June 2018).

World Health Organisation (WHO) (2018c) Health Topics: Cardiovascular disease [online]. Available at: www.who.int/cardiovascular_diseases/en/ (accessed 30 September 2018).

World Health Organisation (WHO) (2018d) WHO Global Urban Ambient Air Pollution Database (update 2016) [online]. Available at: www.who.int/phe/health_topics/outdoorair/databases/cities/en/ (accessed 30 September 2018).

World Health Organisation (WHO) (2018e) Neglected zoonotic diseases [online]. Available at: www.who.int/neglected_diseases/zoonoses/infections_more/en/ (accessed 17 March 2018).

World Health Organisation (WHO) Europe (2012) European Action Plan for Strengthening Public Health Capacities and Services. Copenhagen: World Health Organisation Regional Office for Europe Available at: www.euro.who.int/__data/assets/pdf_file/0005/171770/ RC62wd12rev1-Eng.pdf (accessed 9 March 2018).

INTEGRATED HEALTH CARE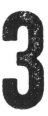

LEARNING OUTCOMES

When you have finished studying this chapter you will be able to:

1. Clarify the implications of statutory and voluntary regulation of different practitioners within person-centred nursing.
2. Describe the principles of surgical interventions, radiotherapy, chemotherapy and other approaches in the medical treatment of disease.
3. Understand the effects on the person undergoing such treatments.
4. Discuss the contribution to health recovery and maintenance of the range of non-medical health and social care professionals.
5. Differentiate between Complementary and Alternative Medicine (CAMs) (often referred to as therapies) and consider how the therapies and the practitioners contribute to health.
6. Recognise the importance of collaboration between health and social care professionals to provide person-centred care.

INTRODUCTION

This chapter will consider the major types of interventions used in the treatment of the disorders of mental and physical health which are the foci of this book and the roles of the different professionals involved in health care in achieving the anticipated outcomes. The understanding acquired will help you appreciate how to collaborate with others in providing person-centred care.

Person-centred nursing aims to provide holistic care through helping with the different facets of physical and mental health with professional interventions. The model (see Preface) endeavours to meet biological, psychological, social and spiritual needs while incorporating the person's values and beliefs, engaging authentically, sharing decision-making and demonstrating sympathetic presence.

Such care involves the input of a range of health and social care practitioners, all with a specific area of expertise; most supported by evidence (Figure 3.1). Nurses play an important role in integrating these inputs and facilitating the recipient of care in utilising the clinical knowledge and skills of these practitioners.

———— PERSON-CENTRED CONTEXT: THE BODIE FAMILY ————

BODIE FAMILY
CASE NOTES

Various members of the Bodie family and their friends and colleagues have received care from different members of the multidisciplinary team in the recent past. A few examples are:

- Following her heart attack (**myocardial infarction** [MI]) 3 years ago, Maud attended a rehabilitation course at her local hospital involving several different specialists including the following:
  - ○ Dietitians helped her to select appropriate changes to her diet.
  - ○ A physiotherapist taught her specific exercises and the importance of taking regular aerobic exercise (e.g. walking) to promote heart strength.
  - ○ The cardiac nurse specialist kept in touch with her over the next year to ensure that she was managing the lifestyle changes to minimise her risk of a repeat MI.
- A friend and ex-colleague of George's had a cerebral **thrombosis** (a type of **stroke**) about 4 months ago. He is fortunate in that he appears cognitively unaffected. He is receiving physiotherapy to help him regain mobility, and the occupational therapist visited his home with other members of the care team to assess what changes could help him manage more easily.
- Richard has found the help of the dietitian particularly valuable in managing his diet to reduce the risk of complications associated with diabetes. He contacts the diabetic nurse specialist with any queries about managing his condition.

REGULATORY POSITION OF PRACTITIONERS

This section is based on the current position within the United Kingdom. These practitioners fall into two major groups: health and social care professionals; and complementary and alternative therapists.

The Professional Standards Authority for Health and Social Care (PSA) was set up by the UK Parliament in 2002 with modifications at later dates. It is independent of government and has three main aspects of work:

- reviewing the work of the regulators of health and social care professionals
- accrediting organisations that register health and care practitioners in unregulated occupations
- giving policy advice to Ministers and others and encouraging research to improve regulation (PSA, 2017).

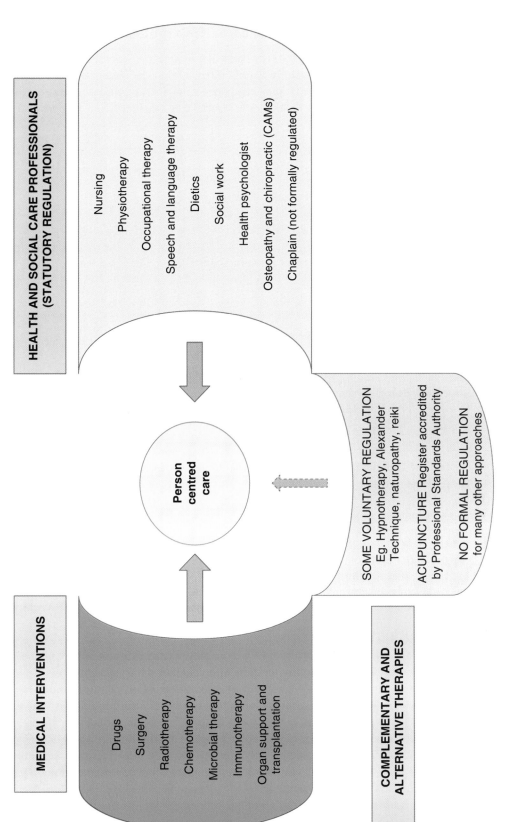

Figure 3.1 Provision of person-centred care

Statutory regulation of health and social care (HSC) professionals

Practitioners included within this group are regulated by statute (i.e. by law) by one of the nine Regulatory Bodies of the UK (Table 3.1) under the oversight of the PSA. Many of these professionals work in various settings but primarily within the NHS. Two of the disciplines considered as **Complementary and Alternative Medicine** (CAMs) (see below) are statutorily regulated, i.e. osteopathy and chiropractic.

Table 3.1   UK health and social care regulators

General Medical Council (GMC)	Doctors, i.e. medical practitioners
Nursing and Midwifery Council (NMC)	Nurses and midwives
General Dental Council (GDC)	Dentists, dental care professionals, e.g. nurse, hygienist, technician, orthodontic therapist, clinical dental technician
Health and Care Professions Council (HCPC)	Arts therapists, biomedical scientists, chiropodists/podiatrists, clinical scientists, dietitians, hearing aid dispensers, nutritionists, occupational therapists, operating department practitioners, orthoptists, paramedics, physiotherapists, practitioner psychologists, prosthetists/orthotists, radiographers, social workers, speech and language therapists
General Chiropractic Council (GCC)	Chiropractors
General Osteopathic Council (GOsC)	Osteopaths
General Optical Council (GOC)	Opticians (optometrists and dispensing opticians)
General Pharmaceutical Council (GPhC)	Pharmacists, pharmacy technicians and pharmacy premises
Pharmaceutical Society of Northern Ireland (PSNI)	Pharmacists and pharmacy premises in Northern Ireland

The PSA oversees the Professional Regulators (PSA, 2016a) to help protect patients, service users and the public. The different regulators carry out the following activities for their own discipline(s):

* Set standards of competence and conduct that health and care professionals must meet in order to be registered and practise.
* Check the quality of education and training courses to make sure they give students the skills and knowledge to practise safely and competently.
* Maintain a register that everyone can search.
* Investigate complaints about people on their register and decide if they should be allowed to continue to practise or should be struck off the register – either because of problems with their conduct or their competence (PSA, 2016b).

Statutory regulation means that the professionals concerned can only practise if they are entered on their professional register; there is no such requirement for those with voluntary self-regulation.

Growing numbers of nurses are accessing higher education to achieve advanced nursing qualifications, including preparation for nurse prescribing, specialised community nursing roles, advanced nurse practitioner (ANP), as well as specialist qualifications in specific areas of practice such as emergency care nursing, intensive care nursing, care of older people, etc. The Nursing and Midwifery Council (NMC) and the Royal College of Nursing (RCN) in the UK work in partnership, including with the health departments of the four countries of the UK, to promote approaches to improve safety. The RCN accredits Advanced Nurse Practitioner (ANP) programmes offered in Higher Education Institutions in the UK against approved standards and has defined the level of practice expected of ANPs (Table 3.2).

Table 3.2 Level of practice of Advanced Nurse Practitioner (ANP)

- Making professionally autonomous decisions, for which they are accountable
- Receiving people with undifferentiated and undiagnosed problems and making an assessment of their health care needs, based on highly developed nursing knowledge and skills, including skills not usually exercised by nurses, such as physical examination
- Screening people for **disease** risk factors and early signs of illness
- Making differential diagnoses using decision-making and problem-solving skills
- Developing with the person an ongoing nursing care plan for health, with an emphasis on health education and preventative measures
- Ordering necessary investigations, and providing treatment and care both individually, as part of a team, and through referral to other agencies
- Having a supportive role in helping people to manage and live with illness
- Having the authority to admit or discharge people from their caseload, and refer people to other health care providers as appropriate
- Working collaboratively with other health care professionals and disciplines
- Providing a leadership and consultancy function as required

Source: Royal College of Nursing, 2012: 4

Practice at this level is grounded in direct care but also incorporates education, research and management. Those holding such qualifications play important and growing roles in working in partnership with medical and other staff. In particular, they contribute to individualising the care provided and help the family to recognise ways to promote quality of life for all (RCN, 2012).

Voluntary regulation of Complementary and Alternative Medicine (CAMs) practitioners

The term Complementary and Alternative Medicine (CAMs) is applied to the range of different therapies within these areas of practice. This is a complex area but, in essence, these are therapies outside mainstream medicine (i.e. medical approaches to care which originated in Western civilisation). The practitioners of two CAMs that work under statutory regulation have already been mentioned above (osteopathy and chiropractic). The other CAMs disciplines do not have statutory regulation but may have voluntary regulation. However, some of the HSC professionals discussed above may also use CAMs; for example, acupuncture is used by some physiotherapists and anaesthetists in pain management. Some individuals receiving care from HSC professionals may also be being treated by CAMs practitioners for symptom management and quality of life issues. Most HSC professionals are unlikely to be working often or closely with CAMs as they are not usually fully integrated in health and social care within mainstream health care provisions.

While **complementary** and **alternative therapies** are separately defined, there is overlap with some approaches used within both categories. Differentiating between them is not straightforward but the following is the most usual approach:

- *Complementary therapies*: when a non-mainstream practice is used together with conventional medicine; for example, chiropractic, osteopathy and acupuncture may be used alongside mainstream orthopaedics, physiotherapy and pain management. Another example is aromatherapy, which has a developing evidence base alongside its millennia of use. Aromatherapy uses essential oils that have reputed physiological and psychological benefits and are often used to complement other therapies, such as when used in massage and pain control.

- *Alternative therapies*: when a non-mainstream practice is used instead of conventional medicine (NHS Choices, 2016a). Some individuals choose to receive alternative therapies, although, on occasion, there is little evidence to support their use. An example is homeopathy where practitioners and receivers follow the philosophy that 'like cures like' based on highly dilute substances. Homeopathy is not legally regulated but products used are regulated by the Medicines and Healthcare Products Regulatory Agency (NHS, 2018a).

Many HSC practitioners have reservations about using alternative therapies with people suffering from serious diseases (e.g. **cancer**) when mainstream approaches are available. However, a number of complementary therapies are evidence-informed; their rejection is often because they are culturally different approaches and because regulation does not yet fully ensure the standardisation of approaches. Additionally, some argue that the power and influence of the pharmaceutical industry is a factor; if CAMs approaches are very successful, this could see a decline in uptake in conventional drug therapies.

Regulation is complex in relation to CAMs. Many CAMs have individual professional associations which share information within their own area and collaborate in determining preparation for practice. Some of these health and care occupations have chosen voluntary regulation and are accredited by the PSA to endeavour to protect the public by meeting the standards for education, ethics and professional conduct, and disciplinary processes. At present (PSA, 2016c) there are 24 voluntary registers covering 30 occupations, some of which are particularly relevant to nurses, including:

- *The British Acupuncture Council* (BAcC, 2016): in 2013 it was entered on the Accredited Voluntary Register of PSA. Originally created from an amalgamation of several acupuncture associations.
- *Complementary and Natural Healthcare Council* (CNHC, 2017): covers a wide range of CAMs, including Alexander Technique teaching; aromatherapy; Bowen therapy; craniosacral therapy; healing; hypnotherapy; massage therapy; microsystems acupuncture; naturopathy; nutritional therapy; reflexology; reiki; shiatsu; sports therapy; yoga therapy.
- *UK Public Health Register* (UKPHR, 2015): professional regulation for public health specialists and practitioners from various backgrounds with similar knowledge and skills involved in promoting public health, particularly those with no other regulatory body.
- *Genetic Counsellor Registration Board* (see Chapter 5).

In contrast to the situation with statutory regulation, there is no formal legal protection for the public against incompetent or unqualified practitioners of CAMs. However, following government guidance, professional associations in a number of CAMs have been working to agree appropriate standards and requirements for each therapy.

In addition to those professions with statutory or voluntary regulation with PSA, there are a number of other voluntary registers for CAMs professionals. The General regulatory Council for Complementary Therapies (GRCCT, 2016) is one covering a number of different disciplines. It aims to ensure the quality of practitioners and practice within each area. Those entered on the register maintained must: abide by a Code of Professional Conduct and Ethics; answer to the GRCCT Complaints Disciplinary procedures; maintain knowledge and competent practice through continuing professional development; and hold professional indemnity and public liability insurance.

No formal regulation

In addition to the disciplines already considered, there are some CAMs which are not considered potentially harmful and, while they have professional associations, they have no formal regulatory structure. Formally homeopathy belonged in this group but it is still, to a limited extent, available within the NHS in the UK, although its availability is diminishing.

In addition, hospital chaplains have no statutory regulation but they play an important role within the health care team. There are some voluntary associations for chaplains in differing settings or religious groups. The College of Health Care Chaplains is one of these; it is:

> a professional organisation for chaplains and pastoral carers of all faith and belief groups. It is open to all recognised healthcare Chaplaincy and spiritual care staff, paid and voluntary, as well as those with an interest in Chaplaincy. It works to promote the professional standards of chaplaincy and to support its members, both nationally and within health and social care organisations. (CHCC, 2018)

MEDICAL INTERVENTIONS

Numerous interventions prescribed and undertaken by doctors are available and, as scientific knowledge advances, new ones are being developed and implemented by specialist medical staff and researchers. The principles underpinning each intervention and the specific approaches to treatment of the condition presented are introduced. Often more than one approach is used in combination. Chapter 4 will consider **pharmacology** – the use of drugs which are molecules that alter the physiology or biochemistry of cells, tissues, organs or organisms. Administration of medication is the most common form of treatment and is often used in combination with other approaches.

Surgery

Surgery involves an operative approach using special techniques manually or with instruments to undertake: treatment of disease, injury or deformity; investigation; and improvement of bodily function or appearance.

Surgery has been undertaken for millennia but only in recent centuries have scientific developments permitted more complex surgery. **Homeostasis** was first described by Claude Bernard in the 19th century (Virtanen, 2016), enabling understanding of the basic principles of physiology. Principles underpinning surgery developed from these.

In essence, an operation (depending on type) consists of various stages to achieve a satisfactory result:

* preparing the person and equipment for the procedure
* achieving access to the appropriate body part
* undertaking the procedure
* repairing tissues layer by layer
* promoting healing.

GO DEEPER

History of surgery

* The practice of surgery to treat injuries and trauma appeared in pre-historic times. Evidence exists for suturing or draining and cauterising open wounds, amputation of badly injured limbs, and setting **fractures**. There is archaeological evidence that in Neolithic times trepanation (scraping a hole in the skull to treat various health problems, e.g. epileptic **seizures**, **migraines**, mental health disorders) was used and often the hole healed, indicating the person survived.

(Continued)

(Continued)

- More sophisticated techniques were developed in various ancient civilisations. In Egypt, Imhotep (around 2600 BC) was a renowned doctor later deified and merged with the Greek God of Healing (Asklepios) and eventually introduced into Rome (Encyclopaedia Britannica, 2016). Galen (2nd century AD) was a Greek physician and surgeon who worked on the basis of four humours identified by Hippocrates (460–370 BC): blood, phlegm, yellow bile and black bile. Based on these, Galen identified four types of personality: sanguine, phlegmatic, choleric and melancholic (Nutton, 2014).
- Galen's influence on medicine lasted until the mid-17th century. Only after this time did modern surgery develop when **haemostasis**, **anaesthesia** and **asepsis** enabled more complex surgery.

The types of surgery can be classified based on different characteristics, such as urgency, method of access, procedure performed (Table 3.3), including laparoscopic and endoscopic approaches. The use of laparoscopy and endoscopy have considerably increased and these both reduce the time needed in hospital for recovery and minimise the risk of complications associated with bed rest. The use of an endoscope enables examination inside the person's body by inserting a thin, flexible tube with a powerful light and a camera on the end. Originally only the oesophagus, stomach and colon were accessed this way, but now many other areas including ENT, heart, urinary system and bronchi are viewed through this method. A rigid tube can be used to view joints. Laparoscopy permits surgery inside the abdomen or pelvis by inserting a slender instrument with a light and camera to permit delicate surgery while the surgeon can see what is happening.

Three main areas of development have enabled surgery to progress to the high standard now achieved: management of bleeding; controlling pain of surgery; and prevention of infection. These achievements and, more recently, developments in techniques, instrumentation and understanding of bodily functions, have enabled advances in surgery.

Table 3.3 Classification of surgery

URGENCY	
Emergency	Prompt action necessary to save life, limb, or functional capacity
Semi-elective	Avoidance of permanent disability or death. Procedure can be temporarily postponed
Elective	For non-life-threatening condition at patient's request, and availability of surgeon and resources
PURPOSE	
Diagnosis	Exploratory – for a differential diagnosis, e.g. biopsy
Therapeutic	Alteration of physiological function or anatomical structure
Cosmetic	Improvement of appearance
DEGREE OF INVASIVENESS	
Via body opening	Endoscope (normally) inserted via normal anatomical opening, e.g. gastroscopy, sigmoidoscopy
Minimally invasive (keyhole surgery)	Small incision to insert, e.g. laparoscope through which surgery performed
Open surgery	Large incision to access area requiring surgery

PROCEDURE	
Excision	Removal of organ or tissue, e.g.: • Amputation of body part, usually limb or digit • Resection - removal of all or part of internal organ/part of body
Reconstruction	• Repair of injured, mutilated, or deformed part of the body • Reattaching a severed body part
Transplant	Replacement of organ/body part by one from different person
By body part	Specifies organ or system involved
EQUIPMENT	
Conventional	Usual surgical instruments
Endoscopic	Camera and miniature instruments inserted through endoscope
Laser surgery	Laser for cutting tissue instead of scalpel or similar instruments
Microsurgery	Operating microscope for seeing small structures
Robotic surgery	Surgical robot controls instrumentation under direction of surgeon

Source: Adapted from Meeker and Rothrock, 1999

Haemostasis

Haemostasis has always been essential in surgery in minimising the risk of intra- and postoperative haemorrhage. During surgery, bleeding is treated by: diathermy (heat produced by electricity) to cut tissue and seal blood vessels; ligatures to tie off the larger blood vessels; and pressure to encourage clotting in small blood vessels.

In preparation for surgery, the nurse aims to minimise complications associated with intrinsic blood clotting (usually in the deep veins of the leg) by ensuring adequate hydration and teaching leg exercises to prevent circulatory stasis. Providing psychological care to minimise **stress** can help prevent infection; stress reduces the effectiveness of the immune system (Boore, 1978). Developments in blood transfusion enable safe blood replacement and safer surgery.

Anaesthesia and analgesia

Pain is a common occurrence following surgery and the physiological mechanisms of nociception are considered in Boore et al. (2016). Minimising the pain experienced makes surgical interventions much more acceptable. **Anaesthetics** are medications that numb sensation locally (local anaesthetic) or render the person unconscious (general anaesthetic), permitting tests and operations without (or with minimal) pain or discomfort.

Conditions for pain-free surgery have been sought since history began. However, it is only in recent (e.g. 19th) centuries that anaesthetics began to replace strong drink and physical strength to restrain people for operations (e.g. amputations). In addition to effective anaesthetics, there have been major developments in airway management and maintaining adequate oxygen supply to the lungs.

A range of analgesic drugs provide pain relief in different situations. The opioid drugs (synthetic or derived from poppies) are strong and used in moderate to severe pain, e.g. postoperatively, after a heart attack or severe trauma. The non-opioid drugs include aspirin (acetylsalicylic acid), paracetamol and other non-steroidal anti-inflammatory drugs (NSAIDs) used in milder pain, such as musculoskeletal conditions. Paracetamol can be very effective when combined with other analgesics (i.e. used as an adjunct).

Asepsis

The risk of infection is always present when the body's protective mechanisms are disrupted, as when the skin is breached for surgery. Cleanliness and asepsis are essential in preventing microorganisms infecting the wound and appropriate preoperative preparation can reduce infection rates (Boore, 1978). Semmelweis was the pioneer who recognised the importance of handwashing in reducing cross-infection: however, his work was not recognised until the germ theory of infection and antiseptic techniques were identified (e.g. by Pasteur, Koch and Lister) (Best and Neuhauser, 2004). Aseptic Non-Touch Technique (ANTT) is now a key skill in many aspects of nursing and medical care to prevent infection.

───────────────── **GO DEEPER** ─────────────────

Developments in asepsis

Ignaz Semmelweis (1818-1865) (Hungarian): identified that the death rate of women following delivery by medical students or doctors (coming straight from performing post-mortems) was much higher than in those delivered by midwives. He introduced compulsory hand-washing and dramatically reduced the death rate in those delivered by medical students or doctors. His work was not recognised by his peers and he eventually died in an insane asylum (Best and Neuhauser, 2004).

Louis Pasteur (1822-1895) (French): disproved the theory of spontaneous generation of microorganisms. His experiments convinced his peers of the truth of germ theory and he is regarded as one of the fathers of germ theory (Ullmann, 2016).

Robert Koch (1843-1910) (German): described as the founder of modern bacteriology, with Koch's postulates outlining the link between cause and effect in infection (Colledge et al., 2010: 132, Box 6.1):

1. The same organism must be present in every case of the disease.
2. The organism must be isolated from the diseased host and grown in pure culture.
3. The isolate must cause the disease when inoculated into a healthy, susceptible animal.
4. The organism must be re-isolated from the inoculated diseased animal.

However, other infectious agents have since been identified where these postulates do not apply (e.g. prions, viruses) (Colledge et al., 2010). Koch was awarded the Nobel Prize for Medicine or Physiology in 1905.

Joseph Lister (1827-1912) (British): was a surgeon and scientist when the death rate from **sepsis** following amputation was between 45 and 50% (1861 to 1865). He introduced antisepsis into surgery using carbolic acid as a barrier between the wound and the air (thought to be the mode of transmission), which also protected the wound from the hands and instruments being used. He was the founder of antiseptic surgery. That **bacteria** should never enter a wound is the basis of surgery today (Cartwright, 2016).

Radiotherapy

Radiotherapy uses high-energy radiation to destroy **tumours**, mainly of **malignant** cells (about 50% of those with cancer receive such treatment) but sometimes treating non-malignant tumours. It is used in three different situations (NHS Choices, 2015a):

*   alone or in combination with **chemotherapy** in aiming to cure cancers
*   for **adjuvant therapy** to shrink a tumour before or to destroy small amounts of tumour left after surgery
*   to minimise symptoms and enhance quality of life in someone with an incurable malignancy.

The high-energy radiation damages the DNA of cancer cells, which then die. Some surrounding healthy cells are also damaged but usually repair their DNA and survive.

The dose of radiation administered is determined by size, type and position of the tumour and the anticipated outcome. The dose, and its administration, is carefully planned to control the radiation spread beyond the diseased tissue, and thus minimise side-effects. Avoiding gaps in treatment whenever possible prevents cell multiplication, which reduces the cure probability (Barrett et al., 2009). Therapeutic radiographers play an important role in planning and delivering the course of treatment and provide ongoing support and monitor progress (Society of Radiographers, 2016).

Radiotherapy can be administered in different ways. External beam radiotherapy is administered by a number of doses of high-energy radiation beams directed at the affected body part and spread over a number of days or weeks. The positioning and stillness of the person receiving treatment is essential to ensure that the major dose is focused on the tumour. Internal radiotherapy is performed by inserting very precisely a small amount of a radioactive substance near to the malignant growth, or by administering orally or by injection some radioactive liquid which is absorbed by the malignant cells and acts on them. Other people need protection from the radiation emitted.

Proton beam therapy is now being used in some situations instead of the more usual radiotherapy. This uses protons, the positively charged particles from the nucleus of atoms, which are directed very precisely and disintegrate with a burst of energy when they contact the target spot – the tumour being treated. This minimises damage to the surrounding tissues. This form of treatment is used when it is particularly important to minimise exposure to radiation; examples are with children and some tumours of the brain and spinal cord (Cancer Research UK, 2017).

The side-effects of radiotherapy caused by DNA damage to the healthy tissues are usually temporary, although permanent infertility can result from radiotherapy to the pelvic area or genitals. However, the more common side-effects (e.g. sore skin, hair loss, tiredness, gastrointestinal reactions) are changes that can cause distress and emotional upset in the person concerned and need attention in person-centred care to improve the physical and emotional state and quality of life (Porritt and Gilleece, 2013).

Chemotherapy

Chemotherapy is the other major therapy used in non-surgical treatment of malignant disease or following surgery: drugs are used to kill the cancer cells. Different types of drugs are used depending on the type and stage of development of the condition. These are administered orally or by injection, used individually or sometimes in combination.

The division and spread of cancer cells are prevented by the drugs used. If the malignancy has already spread or it is suspected that it might spread, chemotherapy is often the treatment of choice with one of the following objectives (NHS Choices, 2015b):

* to cure the cancer (i.e. curative chemotherapy)
* to complement other treatments, for example before or after radiotherapy, to increase the efficacy of the main treatment
* to minimise the likelihood of the cancer returning after radiotherapy or surgery
* to contribute to palliative treatment and reduce the rate of spread and severity of symptoms.

Certain non-malignant chronic conditions, for example, **rheumatoid arthritis**, may be treated by similar drugs.

Chemotherapy acts on fast-growing cells, crucial in killing cancer cells which are dividing rapidly, but also damaging other fast-growing cells such as those of the skin, gastrointestinal lining, blood cells and hair follicles. Thus, side-effects may occur during a course of treatment (Table 3.4), with most of those receiving such treatment feeling weak and tired, nauseated, and suffering hair loss. They need person-centred care to minimise the ill effects and help them cope with their symptoms and how they may feel about themselves in terms of body image and potential loss of social role and independence. People need reassurance to know that, after completion of treatment, the side-effects usually disappear.

Table 3.4 Side-effects of chemotherapy

System	Effect on body	Side-effects
Gastrointestinal tract	Pain and **inflammation** of cells lining tract	Mouth **ulcers**, **diarrhoea**, **nausea** and vomiting, bloating, loss of appetite
	Reduced function	Constipation
Blood formation	Reduced red cells	**Anaemia**, fatigue
	Reduced platelets	Bruising, nose bleeds, bleeding gums
	Reduced white cells	Increased risk of infection
Skin and nails	Reduced hair follicle activity	Hair loss, distress
	Skin cell replacement slowed	Dry, sore skin, sensitivity to sunlight
	Nail growth slowed	Brittle, flaky nails, white lines may develop
Central nervous system	Activity altered	Problems with short-term memory, concentration and attention span, insomnia, **depression**
	Sleep problems	
	Unpleasant treatment	
Sexuality and fertility	Reduced libido	Lack of desire for sexual activity
	Reduced fertility	Sometimes infertility

Source: Adapted from NHS Choices, 2015b

Microbial therapy and immunotherapy

Microbial therapy and **immunotherapy** are treatments based on the interaction between people and microorganisms. The human microbiota is the conglomerate of microorganisms that live in and on the human body, primarily in the gut, skin, mouth, respiratory tract and vagina. It is important in maintaining bodily health. Research and development in treatment are continuing in this area.

──────────── **REVISE: A&P RECAP** ────────────

The human microbiota

The human microbiota plays an important role in health and disturbances can result in ill-health. For a full discussion see Chapter 4, The Human Microbiome and Health, in *Essentials of Anatomy and Physiology for Nursing Practice* (Boore et al., 2016).

The immune system plays the major role in protecting the body against microbes, toxins and malignant (i.e. cancer) cells. Its development is partly controlled by the gut microbiota. Immunotherapy can be considered as modulation of the immune response, altering its ability to fight infection, cancer or other disease described as:

- activation immunotherapy when the immune response is enhanced
- immune suppression and tolerance when it is reduced. (Murphy, 2012)

Microbial therapy

Microbial therapy modifies physiological function, at present mainly through influencing the human gut microbiota. Some microbial therapies are already in use.

Faecal microbial therapy

This is used with about a 90% success rate for individuals with persistent *Clostridium difficile* colonic infection. About 50g of faecal material from a healthy donor is liquefied in an acceptable liquid. Bowel lavage largely clears microbes from the person's gut, and the faecal transplant is administered by retention enema, colonoscopy or nasoduodenal infusion (Merenstein et al., 2014). Antibiotic therapy can disrupt the normal microbial content of the gut with ill effects and Relman (2013) emphasises the importance of restoring the normal microbial makeup within the human ecosystem to promote health.

Microbial therapy for allergies

Normally, the body develops tolerance to food **antigens** (i.e. a substance that produces an immune response). However, some individuals, particularly if they have had courses of antibiotics which altered the balance of microbes within the gut, become allergic to certain food antigens (e.g. peanuts). These cause an **allergic reaction** when encountered. Restoring the normal microbiota by inserting commensal *Clostridia* (i.e. not the pathogenic *C. difficile*) into the GI tract is effective and relates to the suggestion that:

> a new paradigm in which both antigen-specific tolerance and a bacteria-induced barrier protective response are required to prevent sensitisation to food antigens. (Stefka et al., 2014: 13149)

Activation immunotherapy with cancer

Malignant tumours develop because of genetic and epigenetic changes in the cells' DNA, altering the antigens on the cell membrane. If these altered antigens are recognised by the immune system as 'non-self', the immunological cells will respond by attacking the abnormal cells. Nevertheless, many cancer cells replicate and, while having some abnormalities, may be similar enough to normal that the immune system is ineffective in eliminating them. Immunotherapy is still being developed for treatment of these tumours.

REVISE: A&P RECAP

Genetics and epigenetics

For a full discussion of genetic and epigenetic changes and their role in disease see Chapter 4, The Human Microbiome and Health, in *Essentials of Anatomy and Physiology for Nursing Practice* (Boore et al., 2016).

GO DEEPER

DNA damage

DNA damage causing **mutation** is often a result of environmental factors such as UV radiation, or occurs in DNA replication. The cell has numerous mechanisms for repairing DNA and returning it to normal. However, sometimes repair enzymes and other mechanisms are not fully effective and the cell may become malignant and continue to multiply.

In addition, **obesity** can cause DNA damage. A raised BMI (body mass index) is related to **oxidative stress** which increases the risk of DNA damage. Oxidative stress occurs when cell function is disturbed and causes the production of reactive molecules such as oxygen-containing molecules, including peroxides. These molecules cause damage to all cell components, including the bases that form DNA. Obesity is related to type 2 **diabetes mellitus**, **atherosclerosis** and some other disorders (Al-Aubaidy and Jelinek, 2011).

Autologous immune enhancement therapy (AIET)

In this mode of treatment, immune cells (**natural killer (NK) cells**, cytotoxic **T-lymphocytes** and others) from the individual's own body are extracted and treated to increase their efficacy against cancer. They are cultured and infused back into the affected person's bloodstream where the immune cells will attack the malignant tissues. This is also used against some non-malignant conditions including **hepatitis** C and chronic fatigue **syndrome**. This approach to treating cancers has produced some beneficial results, particularly when using NK cells (with numbers expanded) for the immune system contribution. Cancers of a number of different organs were treated with **AIET** in combination with chemotherapy and hyperthermia with generally positive results on prognosis (Terunuma et al., 2013). An anthracycline drug has been used as chemotherapeutic treatment for breast cancer and one of these, epirubicin (EPI), has been used in combination with NK cells. The treatment of breast cancer with EPI and NK cells was more effective than either treatment alone, and produced better results than the sum of the two therapeutic modalities (Feng et al., 2016).

UNDERSTAND

Drug in cancer chemotherapy

Anthracyclines are a type of drug derived from the *Streptomyces* bacterium. It is used in cancer chemotherapy.

Monoclonal antibodies to treat cancer

Antibodies are specialised proteins produced by immune cells to target specific antigens. They move through the bloodstream until they meet the relevant antigen, attach to it and attract other components of the immune system to destroy the cells with that particular antigen. **Monoclonal antibodies** are made in the laboratory to target a specific antigen and numerous copies are produced. The antibody must match the specific antigen and they are available to treat some cancers.

Cancer vaccines

The immune response to malignant cells can be enhanced by **vaccination** against the antigens on the cell membranes (Murphy, 2012), particularly when the cancer is caused by a **virus**. While most vaccines aim to *prevent* infection, some of those in relation to cancer may also act *against* the disease. Work on vaccines to prevent or treat cancer is progressing and various types of vaccine have been made from cancer cells, parts of cells, or pure antigens (Cancer Research UK, 2014).

The human papilloma virus (HPV) is the major cause of cervical cancer and a vaccine against it has been developed. **Clinical trials** have demonstrated that administration of this vaccine to teenage girls results in a significant reduction in the incidence of carcinoma of the cervix and this is now policy in the UK (NHS Choices, 2014a). It appears likely that Australia will become the first country to eradicate cervical cancer due to its effectiveness in increasing the immunisation rate (The Guardian, UK, 2018). It is hoped that vaccines for other viral conditions will be developed.

Vaccines developed to treat cancer are different from those that work against viruses. These aim to get the immune system to attack cancer cells in the body by attacking specific antigens, instead of preventing the disease. It is hoped that the **memory cells** in the immune system will maintain the function of these vaccines.

Immune checkpoint inhibitors to treat cancer

The normally functioning immune system has numerous hardwired inhibitory pathways which maintain **self-tolerance**, preventing the body destroying its own cells. Some of these immune-checkpoint pathways are co-opted by the tumour resulting in immune resistance, particularly to the T-cells specific to the tumour antigens, enabling division and spread of the malignant cells. There has been some development, and research is continuing, of drugs that interrupt these checkpoints and promote the body's immune response against the tumour, which regresses (Topalian et al., 2015).

Non-specific activation immunotherapy

Adjuvant therapy

A number of chemicals produced by the immune system can be used to stimulate the immune system. These may be used alone against cancer or to act as an adjuvant (to enhance the body's immune response to an antigen) along with other types of immunotherapy. These include such substances as:

* **cytokines**: essential in controlling the growth and activity of cells of the immune system and include **interleukins** which carry signals between white blood cells
* **interferons**: help the body attack viruses and cancers.

Vaccination

Vaccination for promoting activity of the immune system against infections minimises the incidence of a considerable number of infectious diseases.

Immunosuppression and immune tolerance

These treatments diminish abnormal immune responses in, for example, autoimmune disease or allergies. They are also used to prevent the rejection of transplanted organs or tissues.

Drugs that inhibit function of the immune system are used for those receiving organ transplants, and for those with autoimmune disorders. **Glucocorticoids** inhibit lymphocyte activity and are used quite commonly in these situations. However, the side-effects of these drugs means that care must be taken with the regime prescribed.

Immune tolerance therapies modify the immune system to prevent it attacking its own body cells in autoimmune disease or the foreign cells after organ transplant.

Allergen immunotherapy is an approach used to manage allergies. While symptomatic treatment may be wholly or partly effective, those with extreme allergies, e.g. severe hay fever (allergic **rhinitis**) or asthma, or who cannot avoid the allergens to which they are sensitive, need additional treatment. Treatment to minimise or stop their symptoms starts with minute amounts of the allergen/antigen with increasing doses as the individual becomes de-sensitised.

Organ support and transplantation

A number of people at some time have an organ or organs malfunctioning and require long- or short-term support to maintain homeostasis during recovery or while waiting for curative treatment. This is prescribed medically but requires significant nursing input to monitor the person receiving support and the function of the equipment used.

The range of organ support is shown in Table 3.5. Technological developments enable support of homeostasis through complex methods and equipment for achieving balance in the extracellular fluid by administering the substances needed by the body or eliminating excess and waste from the body. **Extracorporeal life support (ECLS)** is equipment external to the body which carries out the functions of the non-functioning organ. Critically ill and injured individuals may develop multi-organ dysfunction and 'ECLS (for cardiac, respiratory, renal or liver failure) supports the other organs and may support the haematological, coagulation and central nervous system' (McCunn and Reed, 2009: 557). These authors also discuss the 'concept of a single "organ support" machine' (p. 558) initiated before multi-organ failure develops.

The other group of approaches is transplantation of organs to replace those no longer functioning well enough to support homeostasis. Often such support will be supplemented by drug therapy to prevent immune rejection of the organ.

Much of this level of care will be provided in hospital but increasingly people requiring some of this support may be living at home supported by family members following the necessary training, and/or by community and/or specialist nursing staff.

Table 3.5 Organ support

Organ	Conditions	Support (* = organ replacement)
Respiratory	Protect the airway, remove secretions	Regular suction
	Profound hypoxaemia, e.g. acute respiratory distress syndrome	O_2 therapy by face mask
	Postoperative care – major surgery	Continuous positive airways pressure/ biphasic positive airway pressure (BiPAP)
	Severe **asthma**: rest	Full ventilatory support with endotracheal intubation
	Hypercapnia: e.g. chronic obstructive airways disease	Heart and lung transplant[1]*
		(e.g. cystic fibrosis)

Organ	Conditions	Support (* = organ replacement)
Cardiovascular	Severe heart failure Cardiac arrhythmias Reduced cardiac output	Invasive monitoring of pressures Intra-aortic balloon pumping etc. Cardiac pacemaker Heart transplant*
Renal	Acute or chronic renal failure	Renal dialysis Renal transplant*
Neurological	Severe CNS depression Therapeutic hypothermia	Invasive neurological monitoring IV medication
Gastrointestinal	Oral intake inadequate	**Parenteral** or **enteral** nutrition
Dermatological	Major rashes, burns, exfoliation: more than 30% body surface	Complex dressings (e.g. vacuum, open wounds, multiple dressings) Skin grafts*
Liver	Hepatocellular failure: coagulopathy and/ or **portal hypertension**	Liver purification and detoxification Liver transplant*

¹Transplanting a lung is very complex; it is easier to transplant a heart. Thus, when new lungs are needed the heart and lungs are replaced in this person and his/her heart is transplanted into someone needing a new heart.

Source: Adapted from Health and Social Care Information Centre, 2016

NON-MEDICAL PRACTITIONERS IN HEALTH CARE

Figure 3.1 in the chapter introduction identifies the range of health workers (other than medical practitioners) in person-centred care, the HSC professionals and the complementary and alternative therapists (CAMs).

This section considers the HSC professionals who specialise in depth in particular aspects of care. In the UK, these professionals now qualify at degree level, acquiring a high degree of knowledge and skills and developing their own area of practice through research. The care of an individual is enhanced by the contribution of the different professionals. Collaboration between the different members of the health care team can increase the chances of meeting the different components of the Person-Centred Nursing Framework (PCNF). While each of the different professional groups has their own specific expertise, the role of nurses in focusing on the overall quality of care and comfort of both the individual affected and their family is vital.

Physiotherapy

Physiotherapists primarily use physical methods of treatment within a holistic framework to help restore function in people with reduced movement or pain due to disease, injury or deformity. They involve those with such disorders in their own treatment and care to minimise risk of recurrence in the future. They work in a range of settings including hospitals, community health centres, clinics or GPs' surgeries, various workplaces, clubs etc. as well as making some home visits.

Types of disorders treated and approaches used are shown in Figure 3.2 and Table 3.6.

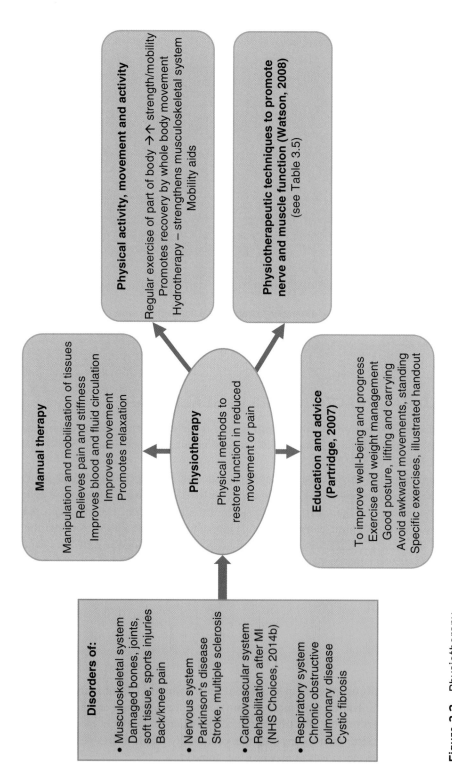

Figure 3.2 Physiotherapy

Source: Mangusan, 2011; NHS Choices, 2016b

Table 3.6 Physiotherapeutic techniques

Techniques	Therapeutic applications and effects
MANUAL THERAPIES	
Education and advice	General advice on enhancing well-being by, e.g., regular exercise, maintaining appropriate weight, good posture, good techniques for lifting, carrying, standing
Movement and exercise	To improve mobility and function:
	Focusing on specific part of body or whole body (e.g. walking)
	Hydrotherapy or aquatic therapy to relax and support muscles and increase strength
	Increasing/maintaining physical activity
	Providing mobility aids
Manual therapy	Manipulation, mobilisation and massage of body tissues:
	Relieves pain and stiffness, improves blood circulation, promotes fluid drainage from parts of the body, improves movement of different parts of the body, promotes relaxation
ELECTROTHERAPEUTIC TECHNIQUES	
Neuromuscular and muscular electrical stimulation	Non-neurological conditions: strengthening atrophied or weakened muscle
	Neurological: improving motor function, reduced spasticity, increased muscle strength and range of movement
TENS (transcutaneous electrical nerve stimulation)	Non-invasive technique for **analgesia** in acute and chronic pain. Electric current stimulates nerves below skin and triggers natural pain-relieving mechanisms
Interferential currents	Two medium-frequency electrical circuits of slightly different cycles per second create interference at intersection. Blocks pain transmission at spinal cord
OTHER TECHNIQUES	
Acupuncture	Used in combination with other treatments to alleviate pain and promote recovery
Ultrasound (high-frequency sound waves)	Speeds progress through inflammatory and other phases of tissue repair – pain relief, carpal tunnel syndrome
Cryotherapy (cold therapy)	Ice pack, ice massage or other application. Minimises pain and swelling, especially if soon after injury
Heat therapy: contact or radiant	Hot packs, paraffin wax bath, hydrotherapy, infrared radiation etc. improve blood flow and speed healing, relieve pain
Pulsed and continuous shortwave therapy (electrical/ magnetic field)	(Can produce heat) improves flow of essential nutrients and ions in and out of cells, increases blood flow. Therapeutic effects: pain relief, peripheral nerve repair, recovery of soft tissue injuries, wound healing

Source: Adapted from Watson, 2008; NHS, 2018b

Occupational therapy

Occupational therapists (OTs) work with people of all ages who need support to carry out the activities of daily living (note that the Activities of Daily Living model that OTs use is different to the Roper (2000) Activities of Living model that nurses use) in all settings (home, school, work, etc.). They help individuals identify their strengths and weaknesses, and activities that they cannot manage alone, and together work out methods to enable the person to achieve those activities. They may identify different techniques, suggest changes to the environment and supply equipment to help (NHS Choices, 2015c).

OTs work with a range of people, in various situations, and with different conditions due to accident, age or disease, or which may be **congenital**: they may have a physical disorder, learning disability or mental health condition (Table 3.7).

Table 3.7 Examples of conditions benefiting from occupational therapy

System/type of condition	Adults	Children
Musculoskeletal conditions	Arthritis (rheumatoid or osteo-) Fractured hip	Achondroplasia Duchenne muscular dystrophy
Neurological conditions	Multiple sclerosis Parkinson's disease Stroke Dementia	Cerebral palsy Spina bifida
Mental health conditions	Depression Schizophrenia	Bipolar disorder Depression Autism Other disorders affecting mental health
General	Chronic fatigue syndrome Dyspraxia Ageing	Down syndrome Learning disability

Having identified the difficulties experienced, the OT uses various approaches to achieve the hoped-for outcomes:

* identifying manageable stages in the activity and practising them (e.g. to get out of bed)
* identifying a different way to undertake the activity (e.g. different ways of getting clothes on)
* suggesting changes to methods or equipment to make it easier (e.g. fitting a seat to facilitate taking a shower)
* providing aids and appliances to make activities easier (e.g. large-handled cooking or eating utensils).

OTs also contribute to rehabilitation following surgery or illness (physical such as arthritis or mental such as depression). An OT aims to enable the individual to carry out the activities necessary for all parts of life including work (paid or voluntary), education, leisure and social activities. Figure 3.3 identifies the major factors in occupational therapy for work.

Rehabilitation for leisure and social activities is equally important in helping the individual to achieve a work–life balance and enhance their quality of life. A similar process is carried out as in Figure 3.3, but with the focus on activities for enjoyment by the individual concerned and how these can be accessed.

Speech and language therapy

Speech and language therapists (SLTs) make an important contribution within the health and social care team, as well as within the education services. SLTs work with people with problems of communication or ingestion, including:

* Infants: difficulties in drinking, swallowing, early play and communication
* Children: speech, language and communication difficulties, e.g. stammering and other communication problems due to learning disabilities and hearing loss

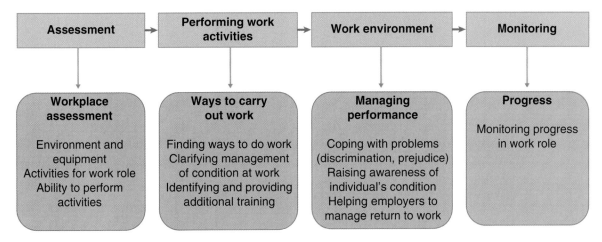

Figure 3.3 Occupational therapy for work

- Adults with learning disabilities: developmental problems including autism and Down syndrome
- Adults: communication and/or swallowing problems due to acquired brain injuries (e.g. following stroke, head injury, neurodegenerative disease and cognitive impairment) (RCSLT, 2016).

The SLT aims to provide holistic care: the PCNF, originally designed for nursing, is synergistic with speech and language therapy, as exemplified in the core values of Connect (the communication disability network in London and the south-west of England) (Table 3.8).

Table 3.8 Connect's core values

Respect	We value difference, diversity and dialogue
Communication	We believe in communication that is clear, open and accessible to all
Creativity	We enjoy being open to and developing new ideas and practices
Excellence	We offer long-term services that are high-quality, effective and efficient
Participation	We believe people have the right to participate fully in choices and decisions about therapy and life.

Source: Anderson and Van Der Gaag, 2005: 18

SLTs work through stages of assessment, therapy and enabling to provide the care required (Bray and Todd, 2006). As in other disciplines, assessment of the individual requiring care is crucial to enable appropriate therapy to be planned and implemented.

APPLY

Speech therapy with dementia

Dementia presents many complexities and can be used to illustrate the range of expertise required by speech therapists. Several conditions can lead to dementia and an accurate diagnosis enables the identification of potential difficulties. These fall into two main groups: communication difficulties, i.e. speech and language; and ingestion, i.e. eating, drinking and swallowing (RCSLT, 2014).

Communication difficulties

For the SLT to provide appropriate intervention for the particular person requiring care, it is important to identify the specific diagnosis of the speech disorder. This enables the therapist to determine the appropriate treatment and predict the likely progress. The severity and nature of speech and language difficulties influence the individual's ability to understand and communicate. An inability to communicate effectively can result in challenging behaviour, and has an important psychological and social impact on daily living for the individual, family members and carers. Some major problems that occur in people with neurodegenerative disorders are shown in Table 3.9.

The SLT identifies and works with the communication network of people and places to enhance opportunities for communication. The individual's capacity for decision-making and the SLT's skills in identifying strategies to enable this are important (RCSLT, 2014).

Eating, drinking and swallowing

The SLT also identifies the type and seriousness of difficulties in eating, drinking and swallowing, and implications for **nutrition** and hydration, as well as enjoyment. The risks of choking and inhalation are identified and meals and drinks managed to reduce this risk and ensure that adequate food and drink are taken. This guidance continues when **enteral** nutrition becomes necessary for a variety of reasons in progressive disease. Involving the family and carers in decision-making about care is important. However, we must always remember that the nurse must advocate for the wishes of the person in their care; at times this may differ from the views of their family members and carers.

Table 3.9 Communication disorders in neurodegenerative disorders

Aphasia and/or	Aphasia - severe difficulty with producing or understanding language and/or speech. Usually due to left-sided brain damage. May be unable to speak
Dysphasia	Dysphasia - less severe. Those affected partially lose speech or understanding
	Both are of two types:
	Expressive - partial or total loss of producing language in different modes (spoken, manual, or written), comprehension usually intact
	Receptive - people have difficulty understanding written and spoken language
	Most people with aphasia have some trouble with speaking, and a mixture of problems with writing, reading and perhaps listening
Dysarthria	Difficulty in speaking, may be due to difficulty in tongue and lip movements resulting in disturbed speech sounds (loud or quiet, strained or hoarse, slurred, hesitations, etc.). May be associated with **dysphagia**
Dysphagia	Swallowing difficulties. Some have problems swallowing certain foods or liquids, others cannot swallow at all. May **cough** or choke when eating or drinking.

Nutrition and dietetics

Nutrition is the branch of science that deals with nutrients and nutrition, particularly in humans (OED, 2016) and is the scientific foundation for dietetics (Lutz et al., 2015). Registered dietitians are the only qualified health professionals that assess, diagnose and treat dietary and nutritional problems at an individual and wider public health level (BDA, 2016a). They adjust the nutrition of individuals depending on their medical disorder and individual requirements.

Adequate nutrition is essential for human health and many disorders have specific requirements for recovery or maintenance of health. Dietitians work with healthy and sick people to help them make sensible and clinically appropriate choices about the food they eat. They work in a wide range of settings, within the NHS and privately, in community or hospital settings and in public health, with people with acute or chronic physical illness, mental health problems or learning disabilities. They are important in the multidisciplinary team looking after adults and children with conditions that alter gastrointestinal function or have special nutritional needs (see Table 3.10).

Dietitians use up-to-date research knowledge of nutrition converted into guidance to facilitate sensible dietary choices. They assist those with nutritional issues to undertake and evaluate appropriate interventions, including exclusion diets, nutritional supplements, or other dietary intervention. They carry out other activities, including:

* calculating nutritional requirements for those requiring enteral and **parenteral** nutritional support
* advising on food choices for those in hospitals, nursing homes or other care settings
* helping public health professionals minimise the risk of nutrition-related disorders and promote health
* educating health and social care professionals and support staff to enhance their contribution to good nutrition.

Dietitians' expertise also enables them to advise on interactions between drugs and diet (BDA, 2016b).

Table 3.10   Conditions with dietitians' involvement

Matter of concern	Examples
Disease with specific dietary requirements	Diabetes mellitus (dietary advice to regulate blood glucose)
	Renal failure
	Liver disease
	Hypertension
	Metabolic disorders
	Acquired brain injury
Disorders of gastrointestinal tract	Digestive problems
	Coeliac disease
	Irritable bowel syndrome
Weight and health issues	Overweight/obesity – need to lose weight
	Loss of weight due to illness needs replacement
	Improve general fitness or athletic performance
	Chronic fatigue syndrome
Eating disorders	Anorexia nervosa
	Bulimia nervosa
	Binge eating disorder (BED)
Pregnancy related	Preparation for pregnancy (e.g. folic acid before pregnancy)
	Breastfeeding and weaning
Food intolerance	Food allergy
	Lactose intolerance

RICHARD JONES
CASE NOTES

APPLY

Nutrition support in diabetes

Richard Jones was diagnosed with type 2 diabetes mellitus 5 years ago. With diabetes it is very important to manage the diet so that the glucose level remains within the normal level. If the glucose varies high or low the person concerned can become unwell. A number of complications can develop if blood glucose level is high. It is important that anyone with diabetes learns about their diet and how to manage it.

Richard was referred to the dietitian when he was first diagnosed and she spent some time with Richard and his wife, Hannah. She helped them to understand the types of nutrients in different foods and how to balance them to ensure a diet that meets their nutritional needs and keeps Richard's blood glucose at a balanced level. She sees them at intervals to help them adjust their meals at different times of the year and if they are unwell at any time.

Social work

Health and social care are separated in many organisational structures for supporting members of the population requiring help, although in some places (for example, Northern Ireland) they are integrated.

Social workers have been described by the British Association of Social Workers as professionals working with individuals and families, from babies to older people, to help improve conditions in their lives (BASW, 2016). Their work is based on the international definition agreed in 2014 by the International Federation of Social Workers (IFSW) and the International Association of Schools of Social Work (IASSW):

> Social work is a practice-based profession and an academic discipline that promotes social change and development, social cohesion, and the empowerment and liberation of people. Principles of social justice, human rights, collective responsibility and respect for diversities are central to social work. Underpinned by theories of social work, social sciences, humanities and indigenous knowledge, social work engages people and structures to address life challenges and enhance wellbeing. (IFSW, 2016)

Here we are focusing on health care social workers, who help those involved with health care services. Assessment of the individual's needs through contact with the person concerned, the family and appropriate health care professionals is the first stage of the social worker's involvement. They then begin to identify the support needed by those requiring assistance to manage their life within the constraints of their health status and help them access that help. Social workers assist those with physical or mental health problems through a range of activities: providing advice using a range of communication approaches, problem-solving and critical thinking skills; referring an individual to appropriate facilities or resources; acting as an advocate in negotiating the health care system; helping to complete documentation; and providing guidance to access financial support as necessary. They will often find it necessary to inform people of their rights.

Pharmacist

Pharmacists are experts in medicines and how to use them and have usually completed a 4-year combined under- and postgraduate Master's degree. They contribute to patient care by advising prescribers on the most appropriate medicines and potential drug interactions, and by collaborating with other health care professionals. They also help to ensure people take their drugs safely by providing information in relation to both prescribed and over-the-counter (OTC) drugs. They can also advise on the management of long-term disorders.

Pharmacists may work in hospitals, in pharmacy chains or in their own business. A number of them are now undertaking courses to become prescribers and can thus limit the burden on General Practitioners and other prescribers (National Careers Service, 2018).

Health psychologist

Health psychology is an area of clinical psychology that:

> applies the tools of the discipline to the prevention of illness, the enhancement and maintenance of health, the identification of the correlates of illness and health, the treatment of individuals in the health care system, and the formulation of health care policy. (Trull and Prinstein, 2013: 511)

It is highly relevant to the influence of lifestyle on health and well-being. It focuses on the psychosocial perspective on health and disease complementing the biomedical perspective, a more common focus for medical personnel. The combination of these perspectives as the biopsychosocial model is important within the PCNF.

As infectious diseases have become less important in relation to **morbidity** (diseased state, disability, or poor health) and mortality (the number of deaths in a given population), the emphasis has moved to lifestyle factors. Stress and health have already been discussed (Chapter 1) and are relevant to the work of the health psychologist. They are also involved with behaviours that influence the incidence of **chronic illnesses** (Table 3.11).

In addition, they design approaches to help those with mental ill-health or learning disability, assisting those awaiting treatments such as surgery or complying with regimes to manage their condition. Primarily, counselling psychologists focus on improving health-related quality of life through enabling people to address psychological factors that impact on their health and well-being (e.g. social anxiety, self-consciousness) and to become able to manage their emotions while addressing any maladaptive behaviours in their lives (NICE, 2013).

Table 3.11   Lifestyle and disease conditions

Behaviour	Related conditions
Cigarette smoking	Cardiovascular disease, pulmonary disease, cancer
Alcohol abuse and dependence	Liver and neurological disease, some cancers, cardiovascular problems, fetal alcohol syndrome, physical aggression, suicide, motor accidents
Obesity	Diabetes, cardiovascular disease, hypertension, certain cancers

Source: Barr and Low, 2011. Reproduced with permission of the Centre for the Advancement of Interprofessional Education (CAIPE)

APPLY

Mental ill-health

Two of the members of the Bodie family have experienced mental ill-health.

Richard had an episode of stress some time ago which was treated by a psychologist who took him through a six-week course of Cognitive Behavioural Therapy. This is a 'talking treatment' which helps someone with problems to understand how thoughts, beliefs and attitudes influence the way they feel and behave. They learn how to cope with their problems through combining thinking with doing (Blenkiron, 2018). As Richard has not had periods of stress since then, it appears that he has learnt how to manage stressful situations.

(Continued)

(Continued)

Matthew suffers from depression which he has had for almost 15 years. Initially he received some psychological therapy in the form of short CBT and antidepressants (**SSRIs**, i.e., **selective serotonin reuptake inhibitors**), which had some effect, but did not completely eliminate his symptoms (Timonen and Liukkonen, 2008). Since then he has continued with antidepressant drugs and has joined a DIY (Do It Yourself) local group which provides regular meetings with like-minded people. He also collaborates with his father on restoring vintage cars. He achieves a satisfactory quality of life.

Hospital chaplain

While chaplains are not registered HSC professionals, they play an important role in supporting those requiring health care, their families and carers, as well as NHS staff as needed. The chaplaincy team usually involves individuals from a range of faiths or none to reflect the religious makeup of the population (e.g. a range of Christian denominations, Muslim (different sects), Hindu, Sikh, Buddhist, Jewish, Pagan, Humanist). It is relatively common to have one or a few full-time chaplains reflecting the predominant faiths in the population, with others to be called on as appropriate; some receive remuneration, others act in a voluntary capacity (Ryan, 2015).

Individual chaplains focus mainly on providing religious and spiritual support for those of their own faith and denomination, but also work as a team interacting with anyone who needs help. Some are qualified religious professionals, while others are lay people. They see people in hospital or in their own homes to help them deal with life and death, illness or injury. In addition, they are available to provide pastoral and welfare support.

They can mediate and calm individuals in difficult situations or where there is misunderstanding between recipients of care and health care professionals; for example, when the religious background of the person concerned has beliefs that are contrary to the medical treatment recommended. In mental health care, they can be particularly valuable in facilitating interaction. As 'outsiders' they can also provide independent feedback to health care organisations.

COMPLEMENTARY AND ALTERNATIVE MEDICINE (CAMS)

There are a considerable number of different disciplines included within CAMs, some of which have been shown earlier in this chapter.

CAM disciplines

The two disciplines with statutory regulation (osteopathy and chiropractic) and acupuncture, used by some HSC professionals, are considered below. In addition, some of the other complementary therapies are introduced.

Osteopathy and chiropractic

NICE guidelines

NICE (2016) guidelines for practice within the NHS in the treatment of back pain include the statement:

Consider manual therapy (spinal manipulation, mobilisation or soft tissue techniques such as massage) for managing low back pain with or without sciatica, but only as part of a treatment package including exercise, with or without psychological therapy. (NICE, 2016)

These approaches are performed by different professionals including osteopaths and chiropractors, as well as physiotherapists and doctors with specialist training (NICE, 2016). It is used to a significant extent, with some evidence, in the management of musculoskeletal disorders. However, evidence for its efficacy in other conditions is minimal (NHS Choices, 2015d).

These manual therapies by chiropractors, osteopaths or physiotherapists are also recommended by NHS Choices (2017).

Osteopathy

> Osteopathy is a system of diagnosis and treatment for a wide range of medical conditions. It works with the structure and function of the body, and is based on the principle that the well-being of an individual depends on the skeleton, muscles, ligaments and **connective tissue**s functioning smoothly together. (GOsC, 2016)

Osteopaths aim to improve one's physical health by increasing joint mobility, muscle tension and blood and nerve supply to tissues through physical techniques such as touch, manipulation, stretching and massage. Guidance on exercises and posture also aim to promote recovery. There is evidence for the efficacy of spinal manipulation in relieving back pain in adults, migraine, headache and dizziness due to damage to the cervical spine, and joint pain in the upper and lower limbs. Massage is also effective for chronic lower back pain and neck pain. There is limited evidence for the value of osteopathy in numerous other conditions (Bronfort et al., 2010).

Chiropractic

Chiropractic is described as:

> a health profession concerned with the diagnosis, treatment and prevention of mechanical disorders of the musculoskeletal system, and the effects of these disorders on the function of the nervous system and general health. (GCC, 2010)

Chiropractors also treat conditions of the musculoskeletal system (bones, muscles and joints) using a range of techniques (some including acupuncture), particularly working on the spine, and advice on exercises, diet and lifestyle for the individual concerned. However, the evidence for its effectiveness is limited (NHS Choices, 2014c), but see NICE Guidelines below.

Acupuncture

Acupuncture is derived from ancient Chinese medicine and is believed to enhance the flow of energy (or life force) through meridians of the body and stimulate the nerves causing release of endorphins, which relieve pain. Very fine needles are inserted into the body at specific points. These may be rotated and left in position for some minutes. It is used for a range of conditions including chronic pain, such as neck pain, joint pain, dental pain and postoperative pain (NHS Choices, 2016c). NICE have removed their recommendation that acupuncture be used in treatment for back pain (NICE, 2016). However, there is still some dispute about this (Kligler et al., 2016; Yeganeh et al., 2017).

Other complementary therapies

There are a wide number of other therapies which may be used by people receiving health care (see Voluntary Regulation of CAMs Practitioners), with or without the advice of the health professional involved. Table 3.12 identifies a number of these (three of which have already been discussed), some of whom work within the NHS (NHS Health Education England, n.d.).

Table 3.12 Complementary and Alternative Medicine (CAMs) in the NHS

Osteopathy	Moving, stretching and massaging the muscles and joints
Chiropractic	Manipulating joints
Acupuncture	Inserting fine needles into the body
Aromatherapy	Using natural oils
Homeopathy	Using very small amounts of substances to cure symptoms
Clinical hypnotherapy	Directing the imagination using verbal communication
Massage	Manipulation of soft tissues (muscles, ligaments, etc.)

Source: NHS Health Education England, n.d.

Aromatherapy is one of those therapies where use within the NHS is growing. Essential oils are extracted from all parts of the plant, including the flowers, bark, stem, leaves, roots and fruits, and are used in aromatherapy by inhalation or application to the skin locally or in a bath (Cancer Research UK, 2018). These oils are used in various combinations to relieve symptoms occurring with numerous conditions including 'depression, indigestion, headache, insomnia, muscular pain, respiratory problems, skin ailments, swollen joints, urine associated complications etc.' (Ali et al., 2015: 601). Aromatherapy is more effective when aspects of lifestyle and diet are also enhanced. In combination with appropriate drugs, these oils can contribute to the treatment of nervous system disorders. Further research is needed but some of the ways in which these oils affect the nervous system have been identified (Cook and Lynch, 2008).

INTERPROFESSIONAL COLLABORATION IN ACHIEVING PERSON-CENTREDNESS

The overall aim of understanding pathophysiology is to be able to contribute to the provision of high-quality care. The practitioners considered in this chapter each contribute to the care provided but collaboration between the members of the team is essential for person-centredness to be provided. Here we are going to look briefly at some factors which enhance the likelihood of effective holistic care through appropriate preparation. Collaboration between different professionals to improve care requires preparation and a clear understanding of how to work effectively as a team.

The Centre for the Advancement of Interprofessional Education (CAIPE) has the overall aim to:

> Promote health and wellbeing and to improve the health and social care of the public by advancing interprofessional education. (CAIPE, 2018)

It endeavours to enhance collaboration between professions and organisations but also with service users, families and carers. It believes that it is only through interprofessional education that effective collaboration for high-quality care can be provided. It describes:

> interprofessional education as occasions when members or students of two or more professions learn with, from and about each other to improve collaboration and the quality of care and services. (CAIPE, 2018)

This organisation provides guidance on the academic and practice-based education for preparing professionals, both during and after qualification, to function in this way. Figure 3.4 illustrates the major achievements of values, process and outcomes of such education. Table 3.13 specifies approaches to education to achieve these characteristics.

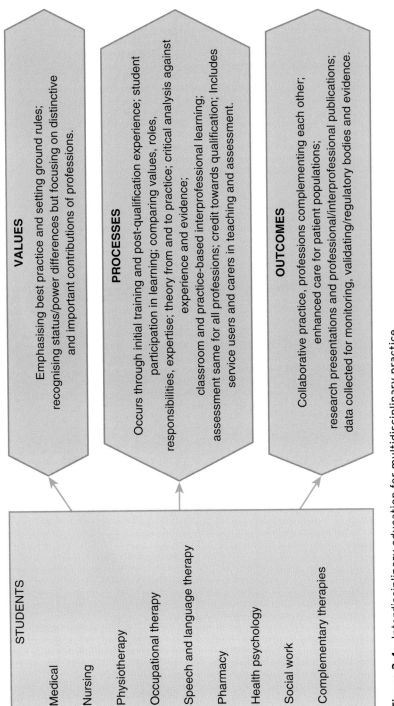

Figure 3.4 Interdisciplinary education for multidisciplinary practice

Table 3.13   Interprofessional education approaches

VALUES
Focuses on the needs of individuals, families and communities to improve their quality of care, health outcomes and wellbeing
Applies equal opportunities within and between the professions and all with whom they learn and work
Respects individuality, difference and diversity within and between the professions and all with whom they learn and work
Sustains the identity and expertise of each profession
Promotes parity between professions in the learning environment
Instils interprofessional values and perspectives throughout uniprofessional and multiprofessional learning
PROCESS
Comprises a continuum of learning for education, health, managerial, medical, social care and other professions
Encourages student participation in planning, progressing and evaluating their learning
Reviewing policy and practice critically from different perspectives
Enables the professions to learn with, from and about each other to optimise the exchange of experience and expertise
Deals in difference as it searches for common ground
Integrates learning in college and the workplace
Synthesises theory and practice
Grounds teaching and learning in evidence
Includes discrete and dedicated interprofessional sequences and placements
Applies consistent assessment criteria and processes for all the participant professions
Carries credit towards professional qualifications
Involves service users and carers in teaching and learning
OUTCOMES
Engenders interprofessional capability
Enhances practice within each profession
Informs joint action to improve services and instigate change
Improves outcomes for individuals, families and communities
Disseminates its experience
Subjects developments to systematic evaluation and research

Source: Adapted from Barr and Low, 2011. Centre for the Advancement of Interprofessional Education

The outcomes of such a programme should be demonstrated in the characteristics of a good interdisciplinary team identified by Nancarrow et al. (2013) (Table 3.14). Such a team will be likely to provide high-quality person-centred care.

Table 3.14 Characteristics of a good interdisciplinary team

	Themes	Description
1	Leadership and management	Having a clear leader of the team, with clear direction and management; democratic; shared power; support/supervision; personal development aligned with line management; leader who acts and listens
2	Communication	Individuals with communication skills; ensuring appropriate systems to promote communication within the team
3	Personal rewards, training and development	Learning; training and development; training and career development opportunities; incorporates individual rewards and opportunity, morale and motivation
4	Appropriate resources and procedures	Structures (for example, team meetings, organisational factors, team members working from the same location) Ensuring that appropriate procedures are in place to uphold the vision of the service (for example, communication systems, appropriate referral criteria and so on)
5	Appropriate skill mix	Sufficient/appropriate skills, competencies, practitioner mix, balance of personalities; ability to make the most of other team members' backgrounds; having a full complement of staff, timely replacement/cover for empty or absent posts
6	Climate	Team culture of trust, valuing contributions, nurturing consensus; need to create an interprofessional atmosphere
7	Individual characteristics	Knowledge, experience, initiative, knowing strengths and weaknesses, listening skills, reflexive practice; desire to work on the same goals
8	Clarity of vision	Having a clear set of values that drive the direction of the service and the care provided; portraying a uniform and consistent external image
9	Quality and outcomes of care	Patient-centred focus, outcomes and satisfaction, encouraging feedback, capturing and recording evidence of effectiveness of care and using that as part of a feedback cycle to improve care
10	Respecting and understanding roles	Sharing power, joint working, autonomy

Source: Nancarrow et al. (2013): BioMed Central Ltd 2013. Reproduced with permission under the terms of the Creative Commons Attribution License (http://creativecommons.org/licenses/by/2.0).

CONCLUSION

This book on pathophysiology aims to give you the understanding of diseases that you need to be able to provide appropriate care. However, equally useful is some understanding of the different modes of treatment so that you can provide the support and care needed to optimise the individual's recovery.

Nurses do not work in isolation; they collaborate with a number of other professionals who bring their own specific skills to the overall programme of person-centredness. To work effectively with these different experts, you need some knowledge of their expertise and the standards to which they conform.

In addition, some individuals receiving care from health and social care professionals may be, or have been, receiving therapy from CAMs, some complementary to mainstream treatment, some replacing it.

- The types of medical management used in the treatment of conditions considered in this book include: surgery, radiotherapy, chemotherapy, microbial and immunotherapy, and organ support. Pharmacology (drug treatment) is considered in the next chapter. All such treatments have physiological effects on the person, and some may cause adverse effects of which you need to be aware.

- There are numerous professionally qualified and statutorily regulated health and social care professionals who contribute to recovery from illness and maintenance of health. These interventions include physiotherapy, occupational therapy, speech and language therapy, nutrition and dietetics, social work and health psychology. Osteopathy and chiropractic are also included in this group although they are also CAMs.

- The Complementary and Alternative Therapies (CAMs) are a considerable number of therapies which aim to enhance health and well-being. Apart from osteopathy and chiropractic, a number of disciplines come under the aegis of voluntary regulation or accreditation, while some only have professional associations but with no regulatory system.

- The contribution of the chaplaincy team within health care is also briefly considered.

- In order to provide person-centred care, collaboration between the members of the team is essential and the importance of appropriate education is necessary to enable effective team-working.

REVISE

TEST YOUR KNOWLEDGE

Studying this chapter will help you understand the implications of the different types of treatment mentioned in later chapters. Revise the sections in turn. How well do you remember the different types of treatment and the effects on the individuals concerned? How do the different professionals contribute to person-centred care? Then try to answer the questions below.

Answers are available online. If you are using the eBook just click on the answers icon below. Alternatively go to **https://study.sagepub.com/essentialpatho/answers**

1   What do you understand by statutory regulation and identify six of the statutory regulators and indicate the professions for which they are responsible.

2   What is the difference between statutory and voluntary regulation?

3   In relation to surgery, differentiate between the following terms:

   o   emergency and elective surgery
   o   diagnostic and therapeutic surgery
   o   minimally invasive and open surgery
   o   endoscopic, conventional and microscopic surgery

4   Outline the three major areas of development in surgery.

5   What are the three main uses of radiotherapy?

6   List the main side-effects of chemotherapy affecting the gastrointestinal tract, blood, skin and nails, and nervous system.

7 What do you understand by the following terms and can you give one example of the application of each?

o   Microbial therapy
o   Activation immunotherapy
o   Suppression immunotherapy

8 Identify five statutorily regulated non-medical health and social care professionals. For each of these, outline their contribution to person-centred care.

9 What do you understand by CAMs and how are the two groups of practitioners defined? Identify four such practitioners and their contribution to person-centred care.

- Further revision and learning opportunities are available online

- Test yourself away from the book with **Extra multiple choice questions**

- Learn and revise terminology with **Interactive flashcards**

If you are using the eBook access each resource by clicking on the respective icon. Alternatively go to **https://study.sagepub.com/essentialpatho/chapter3**

REVISE
ACE YOUR ASSESSMENT

CHAPTER 3 ANSWERS

EXTRA QUESTIONS

FLASHCARDS

REFERENCES

Al-Aubaidy, H.A. and Jelinek, H.F. (2011) Oxidative DNA damage and obesity in type 2 diabetes mellitus. *European Journal of Endocrinology*, 164 (6): 899–904.

Ali, B., Al-Wabel, N.A., Shams, S., Ahamad, A., Khan, S.A. and Anwar, F. (2015) Essential oils used in aromatherapy: a systemic review. *Asian Pacific Journal of Tropical Biomedicine*, 5 (8): 601–11.

Anderson, C. and Van Der Gaag, A. (2005) *Speech and Language Therapy: Issues in Professional Practice*. London: Whurr Publishers.

BAcC (2016) *The British Medical Acupuncture Society*. Northwich, Cheshire. www.medical-acupuncture. org.uk.

Barr, H. and Low, H. (2011) *Principles of Interprofessional Education*. Fareham, UK: Centre for the Advancement of Interprofessional Education (CAIPE) Available at: www.caipe.org/resources/publications/barr-low-2011-principles-interprofessional-education (accessed 22 July 2017).

Barrett, A., Dobbs, J., Morris, S. and Roques, T. (2009) *Practical Radiotherapy Planning*, 4th edn. Boca Raton, FL: CRC Press/Taylor and Francis.

BASW (2016) Social work careers. British Association of Social Workers [online]. Available at: www.basw.co.uk/social-work-careers/#whatissocialwork (accessed 10 April 2016).

BDA (2016a) Careers in dietetics. British Dietetic Association: The Association of UK Dietitians [online]. Available at: www.bda.uk.com/careers/career (accessed 9 April 2016).

BDA (2016b) What do dietitians do? British Dietetic Association: The Association of UK Dietitians [online]. Available at: www.bda.uk.com/improvinghealth/yourhealth/dietitians (accessed 9 September 2016).

Best, M. and Neuhauser, D. (2004) Ignaz Semmelweis and the birth of infection control. *BMJ Quality and Safety*, 13: 233–4.

Blenkiron, P. (2018) *Improving the Lives of People with Mental Illness: Cognitive Behavioural Therapy*. London: Royal College of Psychiatrists.

Boore, J.R.P. (1978) *Prescription for Recovery*. London: Royal College of Nursing.

Boore, J., Cook, N. and Shepherd, A. (2016) *Essentials of Anatomy and Physiology for Nursing Practice*. London: Sage.

Bray, M. and Todd, C. (2006) *Speech and Language: Clinical Process and Practice*, 2nd edn. Chichester: Whurr Publishers.

Bronfort, G., Haas, M., Evans, R., Leininger, B. and Triano, J. (2010) Effectiveness of manual therapies: the UK evidence report. *Chiropractic & Osteopathy*, 18: 3. (Open access journal: http://doi.org/10.1186/1746-1340-18-3.)

CAIPE (2018) Centre for the Advancement of Interprofessional Education: About us [online]. Available at: www.caipe.org/about-us (accessed 8 July 2018).

Cancer Research UK (2014) Cancer vaccines [online]. Available at: www.cancerresearchuk.org/about-cancer/cancer-in-general/treatment/biological-therapy/types/cancer-vaccines (accessed 23 July 2017).

Cancer Research UK (2017) Proton beam therapy is arriving in the UK: what does that mean for patients? [online]. Available at: http://scienceblog.cancerresearchuk.org/2017/07/17/proton-beam-therapy-is-arriving-in-the-uk-what-does-that-mean-for-patients/ (accessed 6 July 2018).

Cancer Research UK (2018) *General Cancer Information: Aromatherapy*. London: Cancer Research UK. Available at: https://www.cancerresearchuk.org/about-cancer/cancer-in-general/treatment/complementary-alternative-therapies/individual-therapies/aromatherapy (accessed 3 October 2018).

Cartwright, F.F. (2016) Joseph Lister, Baron Lister of Lyme Regis. Encyclopaedia Britannica [online]. Available at: www.britannica.com/biography/Joseph-Lister-Baron-Lister-of-Lyme-Regis (accessed 30 November 2018).

CHCC (2018) College of Health Care Chaplains. Available at: [homepage] www.healthcarechaplains.org (accessed 7 October 2018).

CNHC (2017) Complementary and Natural Healthcare Council's Strategic Objectives January – December 2017 [online]. Available at: www.cnhc.org.uk/sites/default/files/Downloads/Strategic-objectives-2017.pdf (accessed 9 July 2017).

Colledge, N.I., Walker, B.R. and Ralston, S.H. (2010) *Davidson's Principles and Practice of Medicine*. Edinburgh: Churchill Livingstone, Elsevier.

Cook, N. and Lynch, J. (2008) Aromatherapy: reviewing evidence for its mechanisms of action and CNS effects. *British Journal of Neuroscience Nursing*, 4 (12): 595–601.

Encyclopaedia Britannica (Editors) (2016) Imhotep: Egyptian architect, physician, and statesman [online]. Available at: www.britannica.com/biography/Imhotep (accessed 30 November 2018).

Feng, H., Ying Dong, Y., Wu, J., Qiao, Y., Ge Zhu, G., Jin, H. et al. (2016) Epirubicin pretreatment enhances NK cell-mediated cytotoxicity against breast cancer cells in vitro. *American Journal of Translational Research*, 8 (2): 473–84.

GCC (2010) Code of Practice and Standards of Proficiency. General Chiropractic Council [online]. Available at: www.gcc-k.org/UserFiles/Docs/COPSOP_2010.pdf (accessed 29 March 2016).

GOsC (2016) General Osteopathic Council website [online]. Available at: www.osteopathy.org.uk/home/ (accessed 28 April 2016).

GRCCT (2016) Welcome to the GRCCT. General Regulatory Council for Complementary Therapies [online]. Available at: www.grcct.org/about-us/ (accessed 16 May 2016).

Health and Social Care Information Centre (2016) Organ System Supported: Critical Care Period [online]. Available at: www.datadictionary.nhs.uk/data_dictionary/attributes/o/org/organ_system_supported_de.asp?shownav=0 (accessed 20 March 2016).

IFSW (2016) Global definition of social work. International Federation of Social Workers [online]. Available at: http://ifsw.org/get-involved/global-definition-of-social-work/ (accessed 7 October 2016).

Kligler, B., Teets, R. and Quick, M. (2016) Complementary/integrative therapies that work: a review of the evidence. *American Family Physician*, *94* (5): 369–74.

Lutz, C.A., Mazur, E.E. and Litch, N.A. (2015) *Nutrition and Diet Therapy*, 6th edn. Philadelphia: F.A. Davis.

Mangusan, D. (posted 2011) Types of physiotherapy treatments – physiotherapy interventions [online]. Available at: www.physiotherapynotes.com/2011/03/physiotherapy-treatments-types-of.html (accessed 10 January 2019).

McCunn, M. and Reed, A.J. (2009) Critical care organ support: a focus on extracorporeal systems. *Current Opinion in Critical Care*, *15* (6): 554–9.

Meeker, M.H. and Rothrock, J.C. (1999) *Alexander's Care of the Patient in Surgery*, 11th edn. St Louis, MO: Mosby.

Merenstein, D., El-Nachef, N. and Lynch, S.V. (2014) Fecal microbial therapy: promises and pitfalls. *Journal of Pediatric Gastroenterology and Nutrition*, *59* (2): 157–61.

Murphy, K. (2012) *Janeway's Immunology*, 8th edn. New York: Garland Science/Taylor & Francis.

Nancarrow, S.A., Booth, A., Ariss, S., Smith, T., Enderby, P. and Roots, A. (2013) Ten principles of good interdisciplinary team work. *Human Resources for Health*, *11*: 19 Available at: http://human-resources-health.biomedcentral.com/articles/10.1186/1478-4491-11-19 (accessed 21 March 2016).

National Careers Service (2018) Pharmacist: dispensing chemist, community pharmacist, hospital pharmacist [online]. Available at: https://nationalcareersservice.direct.gov.uk/job-profiles/pharmacist (accessed 8 October 2018).

NHS (2018a) Homeopathy [online]. Available at: www.nhs.uk/conditions/homeopathy (accessed 3 October 2018).

NHS (2018b) Techniques – Physiotherapy [online]. Available at: www.nhs.uk/conditions/physiotherapy/how-it-works/ (accessed 4 January 2019).

NHS Choices (2014a) Vaccinations [NHS online]. Available at: www.nhs.uk/conditions/vaccinations/pages/who-should-have-hpv-cervical-cancer-cervarix-gardasil-vaccine.aspx (accessed 22 April 2016).

NHS Choices (2014b) Heart attack – Recovery [NHS online]. Available at: www.nhs.uk/Conditions/Heart-attack/Pages/Recovery.aspx (accessed 22 April 2016).

NHS Choices (2014c) Chiropractic [NHS online]. Available at: www.nhs.uk/Conditions/chiropractic/Pages/Introduction.aspx (accessed 28 April 2016).

NHS Choices (2015a) Radiotherapy [NHS online]. Available at: www.nhs.uk/conditions/Radiotherapy/Pages/Introduction.aspx) (accessed 6 April 2016).

NHS Choices (2015b) Chemotherapy – Side effects [NHS online]. Available at: www.nhs.uk/Conditions/Chemotherapy/Pages/Definition.aspx (accessed 20 March 2016).

NHS Choices (2015c) Occupational therapy [NHS online]. Available at: www.nhs.uk/conditions/occupational-therapy/Pages/introduction.aspx (accessed 18 April 2016).

NHS Choices (2015d) Osteopathy [NHS online]. Available at: www.nhs.uk/conditions/osteopathy/pages/introduction.aspx (accessed 22 April 2016).

NHS Choices (2016a) Complementary and alternative medicine [NHS online]. Available at: www.nhs.uk/Livewell/complementary-alternative-medicine/Pages/complementary-alternative-medicines.aspx (accessed 22 April 2016).

NHS Choices (2016b) Physiotherapy – Techniques [NHS online]. Available at: www.nhs.uk/Conditions/Physiotherapy/Pages/How-does-it-work.aspx (accessed 5 April 2016).

NHS Choices (2016c) Acupuncture [NHS online]. Available at: www.nhs.uk/conditions/acupuncture/ (accessed 7 July 2018).

NHS Choices (2017) Back pain [NHS online]. Available at: www.nhs.uk/conditions/back-pain/treatment/ (accessed 7 July 2018).

NHS Health Education England (n.d.) Health careers – Complementary and Alternative Medicine (CAM) [NHS Careers website]. Available at: www.healthcareers.nhs.uk/explore-roles/wider-healthcare-team/roles-wider-healthcare-team/clinical-support-staff/complementary-and-alternative-medicine-cam (accessed 8 July 2018).

NICE (2013) Depression in adults: recognition and management. Clinical Guideline [CG90] [new version expected December 2019]. The National Institute for Health and Care Excellence. Available at: www.nice.org.uk/guidance/cg90 (accessed 8 October 2018).

NICE (2016) Low back pain and sciatica in over 16s: assessment and management. NICE guideline [NG59]. The National Institute for Health and Care Excellence. Available at: www.nice.org.uk/guidance/ng59/chapter/Recommendations (accessed 8 July 2018).

Nutton, V. (2014) Galen of Pergamum: Greek physician. Encyclopaedia Britannica [online] Available at: www.britannica.com/biography/Galen-of-Pergamum (accessed 30 November 2018).

OED (2016) Nutrition. Oxford English Dictionary: the definitive record of the English Language [online]. Available at: www.oed.com/view/Entry/129332?redirectedFrom=Nutrition#eid (accessed 9 April 2016).

Partridge, C. (ed.) (2007) *Recent Advances in Physiotherapy*. Chichester: Wiley.

Porritt, B.M. and Gilleece, T. (2013) Radiotherapy-related treatment reactions. In A. Ramlaul and M. Vosper (eds), *Patient Centred Care in Medical Imaging and Radiotherapy*. Edinburgh: Churchill Livingstone, Elsevier.

PSA (2016a) Professional Standards Authority – About us [online]. Available at: www.professionalstandards.org.uk/about-us (accessed 14 July 2017).

PSA (2016b) About regulators [online]. Available at: www.professionalstandards.org.uk/what-we-do/our-work-with-regulators/about-regulators (accessed 6 July 2018).

PSA (2016c) Our work with accredited registers – Find an accredited register [online]. Available at: www.professionalstandards.org.uk/what-we-do/accredited-registers/find-a-register (accessed 6 July 2018).

PSA (2017) Review of professional regulation and registration with annual report and accounts 2016/17. London: PSA. Available at: www.professionalstandards.org.uk/publications/detail/review-of-professional-registration-and-regulation-2016-17-with-annual-report-accounts (accessed on 20 July 2017).

Relman, D.A. (2013) Restoration of the gut microbial habitat as a disease therapy. *Nature Biotechnology, 31* (1): 35–7.

RCN (2012) RCN competences: advanced nurse practitioners. *An RCN guide to advanced nursing practice, advanced nurse practitioners and programme accreditation.* London: Royal College of Nursing. Available at: ww.rcn.org.uk/professional-development/publications/pub-003207.

RCSLT (2014) *Speech and Language Therapy for People with Dementia.* RCSLT Position Paper 2014. London: Royal College of Speech and Language Therapists.

RCSLT (2016) *What Is Speech and Language Therapy?* London: Royal College of Speech and Language Therapists.

Roper, N. (2000) *The Roper–Logan–Tierney Model of Nursing: Based on Activities of Living.* Edinburgh: Churchill Livingstone.

Ryan, B. (2015) *A Very Modern Ministry: Chaplaincy in the UK.* London: Theos (Cardiff Centre for Chaplaincy Studies). Available at: www.theosthinktank.co.uk/files/files/Modern%20Ministry%20combined.pdf (accessed 20 July 2017).

Society of Radiographers (2016) *A Career in Radiography.* London: Society of Radiographers. Available at: www.sor.org/about-radiography/career-radiography (accessed 16 May 2018).

Stefka, A.T., Feehley, T., Tripathi, P., Qiu, J., McCoy, K., Mazmanian, S.K. et al. (2014) Commensal bacteria protect against food allergen sensitization. *Proceedings of the National Academy of Sciences of the United States of America (PNAS), 111* (36): 13145–50.

Terunuma, H., Deng, X., Nishino, N. and Watanabe, K. (2013) NK cell-based autologous immune enhancement therapy (AIET) for cancer. *Journal of Stem Cells and Regenerative Medicine*, *9* (1): 9–13.

The Guardian, UK (2018) Australia on track to wipe out cervical cancer within 20 years. *The Guardian*, 3 October 2018.

Timonen, M. and Liukkonen, T. (2008) Management of depression in adults. *BMJ*, *336* (7641): 435–9.

Topalian, S.L., Drake, C.G. and Pardoll, D.M. (2015) Immune checkpoint blockade: a common denominator approach to cancer therapy. *Cancer Cell*, *27* (4): 450–61.

Trull, T.J. and Prinstein, M.J. (2013) *The Science and Practice of Clinical Psychology*, 8th edn. Boston, MA: Wadsworth, CENGAGE Learning.

UKPHR (2015) UK Public Health Register. Available at: ww.ukphr.org/about-us/ (accessed 20 July 2017).

Ullmann, A. (2016) Louis Pasteur: French chemist and microbiologist. Encyclopaedia Britannica [online]. Available at: www.britannica.com/biography/Louis-Pasteur (accessed 30 November 2018).

Virtanen, R. (2016) Claud Bernard: French scientist. Encyclopaedia Britannica [online]. Available at: https://www.britannica.com/biography/Claude-Bernard (accessed 30 November 2018).

Watson, T. (ed.) (2008) *Electrotherapy Evidence-Based Practice*, 12th edn. Edinburgh: Churchill Livingstone, Elsevier.

Yeganeh, M., Baradaran, H.R., Qorbani, M., Moradi, Y. and Dastgiri, S. (2017) The effectiveness of acupuncture, acupressure and chiropractic interventions on treatment of chronic nonspecific low back pain in Iran: a systematic review and meta-analysis. *Complementary Therapies in Clinical Practice*, *27*: 11–18.

PRINCIPLES OF PHARMACOLOGY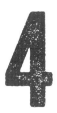

UNDERSTAND: CHAPTER VIDEOS

Watch the following videos to ease you into this chapter. If you are using the eBook just click on the play buttons. Alternatively go to: **https://study.sagepub.com/essentialpatho/videos**

PHARMACOKINETICS (5:49)   PHARMACODYNAMICS (4:03)   PROCESSING MEDICINE (4:12)

LEARNING OUTCOMES

When you have finished studying this chapter you will be able to:

1. Explain the concept of pharmacodynamics, i.e. what drugs do to the body through their interaction with receptors and the alteration of cell function.
2. Explain the four processes of pharmacokinetics, i.e. what the body does to drugs, how drugs are absorbed into and distributed throughout the body, metabolised and excreted.
3. Identify factors which influence the action of drugs.
4. Recognise adverse drug reactions and understand approaches to prevention.
5. Recognise the legal and professional parameters for drug prescription.
6. Identify the key issues for safety in relation to drug prescribing and administration, and in drug use with older people or children.

INTRODUCTION

This chapter progresses from Chapter 3 on major approaches to treatment of ill-health to consider the principles of drug therapy. As a registered nurse you will have considerable involvement in administering, and perhaps prescribing, drugs in a way that will ensure their effective action. Therefore you need an understanding of **pharmacology** and medicines management. In this chapter, you will learn about drug types, how they act and side-effects which may occur, and the understanding acquired will help you to collaborate with others in providing safe person-centred care. This chapter is written for those preparing for initial registration as a nurse but will also assist those revising the key concepts of pharmacology.

The administration of medications (also known as drugs) is the commonest form of treatment of disorders. The use of particular drugs in the treatment of different conditions will be considered in the relevant chapters throughout the book.

Drugs have been defined as:

> A chemical substance of known structure, other than a nutrient or an essential dietary ingredient, which, when administered to a living organism, produces a biological effect. (Rang et al., 2016: 1)

However, some dietary constituents such as vitamins or iron, are also given as medications.

There are two major aspects of pharmacology to be considered:

* **Pharmacodynamics**: what drugs do to the body
* **Pharmacokinetics**: what the body does to drugs

Legal issues related to pharmacology are briefly considered in this introduction.

Legal issues

Drug classification

All jurisdictions have legal standards for the management of drugs. In the UK, The Human Medicines Regulations (2012) replaced and simplified the various Acts and Statutory Instruments dealing with the preparation, storage, prescribing etc. of medicines (Appelbe and Wingfield, 2013). This section is based on the situation in the UK but almost all countries have regulations related to the management of medications – if applicable to you, undertake the activity below.

ACTIVITY 4.1: APPLY

Pharmaceutical regulations

Those of you reading this in countries other than the United Kingdom, look up the regulations related to drug prescription and administration which apply in your own country. You should be able to find this on the Web under: pharmaceutical regulations [name of your country]

There are three groups of medications (Appelbe and Wingfield, 2013):

- General Sales List (GSL) drugs can be sold without supervision, e.g. in a supermarket or shop.
- Pharmacy (P) medicines are those which are not included in the GSL or the POM (below) groups and can only be sold over the counter (OTC) in registered premises under the supervision of a pharmacist. They do not need a prescription.
- Prescription Only Medicines (POM) can only be provided by a pharmacist in registered premises in response to a prescription written by an authorised prescriber. The premises are usually a chemist's shop or hospital pharmacy, although some doctors, usually in rural communities, act as dispensing doctors and are permitted to provide drugs to some people in their care.

In providing person-centred care it is important to be aware of all the drugs being taken by the person, including the OTC (i.e. both P and GSL) medications as they may interact with those prescribed.

Drugs which can be prescribed within the UK National Health Service (NHS) are determined by NICE (the National Institute for Health and Care Excellence). Information about these drugs and others which must be self-funded (with a prescription and consultant's agreement) and considerable additional information is contained within the British National Formulary (BNF, 2018). This is an essential reference for prescribers and those who administer medications. It is published in print twice a year (March and September), with monthly updates online. The drugs that may be prescribed by registered nurses, with an additional prescribing qualification, are identified within an agreed formulary.

Prescribers

There are two main groups of prescribers in the UK.

Independent prescribers

Independent prescribers are able to prescribe medicines on their own initiative from the BNF and include doctors, dentists and some non-medical health professionals (including nurses, pharmacists and, more recently, registered chiropodists/podiatrists, physiotherapists, optometrists and registered therapeutic radiographers). The non-medical health professionals must have completed appropriate education and supervision in preparation for this role, in addition to their standard professional education. They then have their names entered on the appropriate prescribers register and are permitted to prescribe within their area of expertise.

Supplementary prescribers

These include the non-medical health professionals (not usually independent prescribers) identified above and dietitians who have completed the appropriate training. They are permitted to prescribe within the limits of a clinical management plan agreed for a specific group of people by the supplementary prescriber, doctor (independent prescriber) and recipient. The recently published NMC (Nursing and Midwifery Council) (2018) standards of proficiency for registered nurses now require nurses to be equipped to progress to the completion of a prescribing qualification after registration.

Whoever the prescriber, nurses administer medication to those in hospital and other residential settings and play a role in ensuring that those in the community take their medications correctly. It is thus essential that you understand the principles underpinning drug action.

Nurse prescribers

The role of nurses in prescribing is increasing. At present there are three main groups (Dowden, 2016):

- Independent prescribers can prescribe anything from the BNF on their own initiative (within their area of competence).
- Community practitioner nurse prescribers can prescribe independently but only from the Nurse Prescribers Formulary for Community Practitioners.
- **Supplementary prescribers** can only prescribe drugs (from the BNF) agreed as part of the patient's clinical management plan.

In addition, all nurses have to learn to undertake the necessary accurate calculations to administer drugs safely (see later).

PERSON-CENTRED CONTEXT: THE BODIE FAMILY

BODIE FAMILY
CASE NOTES

Among a family group of the size and range of ages of the Bodies, you would expect to find a number of them taking drugs for chronic or acute disorders, and indeed this is the case with this family. Indeed, they may also take medications irregularly for symptom management not necessarily related to a disorder (e.g. paracetamol for an occasional headache).

As is fairly common with their age group, the oldest members of the family, George (84) and Maud (77), are both taking drugs to manage chronic conditions. For her **heart failure** Maud is taking digoxin to regulate the cardiac cycle and warfarin to limit the associated risk of blood clotting, and thyroxine for her below normal level of activity of the thyroid gland. George is prescribed **statins** to lower his raised blood cholesterol levels.

ACTIVITY 4.2: APPLY

Lowering blood cholesterol

Spend some time searching the Internet for different approaches to lowering blood cholesterol levels. Some of these will involve natural substances and changes in lifestyle. The title above will help you to begin your search.

In the next generation, two members of the family, Hannah and Sarah, are going through the menopause and HRT (Hormone Replacement Therapy) has been used to help minimise the symptoms often associated with this stage of life. Sarah stopped taking these recently after 2½ years while Hannah is gaining relief from symptoms by using HRT patches.

Edward has chronic low back pain and, when it is particularly problematic, uses OTC pain-relieving drugs and visits an osteopath as necessary. In addition, Matthew is receiving anti-depressant medication on a long-term basis.

Amongst the grandchildren, Derek has mild asthma and Margaret has hay fever. Both manage their conditions themselves under the overall guidance of their General Practitioner. They request prescriptions for the necessary inhalers or oral medication to control symptoms as necessary.

PHARMACODYNAMICS

A drug molecule acts by interacting with specific molecules in the body known as receptors (see below) which regulate the activity of the target cells. Drugs can be of different types, including (Katzung and Trevor, 2015):

- **Agonists**: (activators), which through binding with the receptor alter the cell activity in some way such as enhancing the action of an enzyme which alters a specific mechanism within the cell
- **Antagonists**: (inhibitors) also interact with a receptor and, by so doing, prevent other molecules binding with that receptor and activating the particular mechanism. For example, atropine is an antagonist which blocks the acetylcholine agonist site and reduces acetylcholine function.

They can also be described in the following terms:

- Chemicals normally synthesised within the body, e.g. hormones
- Substances not created within the body, called xenobiotics
- Poisons: substances that are almost always harmful; however, almost any substance can be harmful in large enough dosages
- Toxins: poisons created by biological organisms; some toxins can be used for beneficial results (e.g. botulinum toxin for hyperspasticity).

Drug receptors

Most receptors are in the cell membrane and usually interact with molecules formed within the body to regulate cell function, but drugs also interact with them. The drug molecule has to be the specific size and shape to interact (like a lock and key) with the precise receptor it is to affect, and can vary considerably in size, complexity and duration of action. Each drug works by modifying a particular aspect of cell function (Figure 4.1).

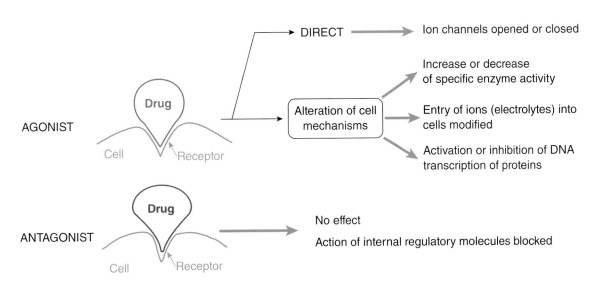

Figure 4.1 Drug-receptor interaction and activity

In addition, less than 10% of receptors are within the cell cytoplasm and interact with a range of molecules, mostly hydrophobic, with a major role in the regulation of endocrine function, but also involvement in sensing lipids. A considerable number of drugs, with a structure enabling entry to the cell, combine with such receptors (nuclear receptors) and the drug–receptor combination enters the nucleus of the cell and influences the transcription of DNA (Rang et al., 2016).

ACTIVITY 4.3: UNDERSTAND

Drug receptors

Watch this video to help better understand drug receptors. If you are using the eBook just click on the play button. Alternatively go to **https://study.sagepub.com/essentialpatho/videos**

(▷)

DRUG RECEPTORS (6:54)

PHARMACOKINETICS

The degree of drug action is dependent on the level of drug in the general bloodstream and thus available to interact with the appropriate cell receptors (see Distribution below).

The level at which the drug is effective is the therapeutic level, while the toxic (i.e. poisonous) level is the concentration at which toxicity occurs. The difference between these levels is the therapeutic index. A small therapeutic index means that there is little difference between the therapeutic and the toxic levels and side-effects can occur fairly easily. Digoxin is an example of a drug with a small therapeutic index, used to strengthen the heart beat in people with heart failure.

The concentration of the drug in the tissue fluids and, thus, their level of activity is determined by the balance between the four pharmacokinetic processes of **absorption**, **distribution**, **metabolism** and **excretion** (Figure 4.2).

Figure 4.3 illustrates how these processes act on a single drug dose to achieve and then decline from the therapeutic range and the shaded area shows the therapeutic concentration and duration of action of the drug.

To maintain the concentration within the therapeutic range, repeated doses are administered to ensure that the concentration rises and remains within this zone as the trajectories of successive doses overlap (Figure 4.4). The timing of doses is determined by the half-life of the drug, i.e. the time taken for the plasma concentration of the drug to fall by half as it is distributed through the body and then metabolised and excreted from the body.

Absorption

Absorption is the first of the pharmacokinetic processes in which drugs move from the site of administration into the bloodstream. The speed and effectiveness of absorption, and thus **bioavailability** (i.e. the proportion of a dose that reaches the systemic circulation and is thus available to act on the target organs [McGavock, 2016]), varies with the structure of the drug itself and the route of administration, considered in three groups: **enteral**, **parenteral** and **topical** (Lilley et al., 2017).

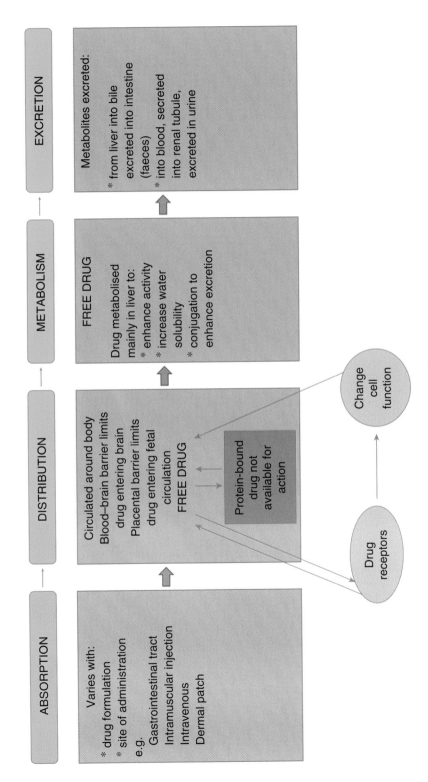

Figure 4.2 Pharmacokinetic mechanisms determining drug concentration

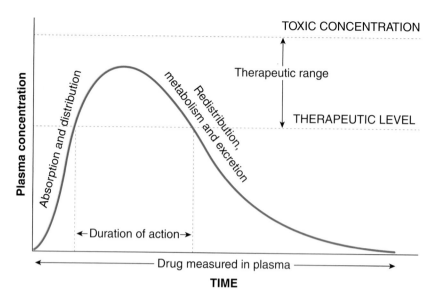

Figure 4.3 Plasma concentration of drug following a single dose

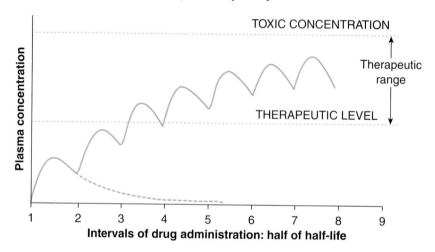

Figure 4.4 Achieving steady state drug concentration

Enteral route (gastrointestinal tract)

This route enables absorption through the mouth, stomach or intestine. The gastrointestinal tract (GIT) is a major route for administration of medications although various drugs are administered for absorption at different points of the GIT. The majority of orally administered drugs are absorbed in the stomach or intestine into the bloodstream. The acidity of the stomach, which can vary with age, time of day, presence of food and liquid, and presence of medications, can alter the dissolving and absorption of the drug. Some drugs must be taken with water on an empty stomach, others with food. Some drugs are produced with an enteric coating to prevent dissolving of the coating in the stomach, thus protecting the stomach lining from the active drug which will only be released in the intestine.

First-pass metabolism

Following absorption in the stomach, small intestine or part of the large intestine, the drugs enter the portal circulation which carries the drug molecules to the liver. Here some of the drug is converted into inactive molecules through **first-pass metabolism**, resulting in a smaller proportion of the active drug passing into the general circulation. The proportion of some drugs that would be metabolised in this way means that they need to be absorbed where they will bypass the liver and directly enter the general circulation to reach their site of action.

Sublingual (i.e. under the tongue) and buccal (between the cheek and the gum) sites for absorption have rich blood supplies and drugs (e.g. glyceryl trinitrate) enter the general blood circulation directly, thus bypassing the liver and rapidly reaching the site of action.

Rectal administration of drugs is also sometimes used although this may cause some embarrassment. This approach (along with parenteral routes – see below) bypasses some of the first-pass metabolism (Lilley et al., 2017).

Parenteral routes

These include a variety of routes outside the GIT where drugs are administered usually by injection, as in Table 4.1. The routes indicated within the NMC core competencies are: intramuscular, subcutaneous, intradermal and intravenous.

Table 4.1   Injection routes

Intravenous	Directly into the venous circulation with rapid onset of action
Intramuscular	Into muscle tissue from which it is absorbed more slowly and randomly
Subcutaneous	Into subcutaneous tissue (i.e. under the skin), e.g. **insulin** administration
Intradermal	Very small volumes into the dermis of the skin, mainly diagnostic testing
Intraarterial	Into arteries supplying specific organs
Intrathecal	Into the **cerebrospinal fluid** (CSF) at 3rd–4th lumbar vertebral space, or intraventricularly, bypassing blood–brain barrier
Epidural	Same level as intrathecal injection but not into CSF, e.g. local **anaesthesia**
Intrapleural	Into the pleural space
Intraarticular	Into a joint cavity, e.g. treating **inflammation** of joint

Topical routes

Topical administration involves the application of a medication to a body surface. The drugs may be in different forms, e.g. liquid, cream, powder, but these routes usually deliver a specific amount of drug over a longer period than enteral and parenteral routes, and most also bypass first-pass metabolism. They also minimise systemic side-effects. Topical routes include the following (Table 4.2):

Table 4.2   Topical routes of administration

Skin (transdermal)	Adhesive patches enable a drug to pass through the skin into the systemic circulation at a steady rate
Intravaginal	Drugs administered may have a local effect or a systemic action
Eyes, ears, nose	Drops are usually administered for a local effect; nasal sprays may have a systemic action
Lungs	Inhalation of very small drug particles delivers drugs to alveoli of the lungs where they are rapidly absorbed in the treatment of pulmonary disorders

Absorption processes

The dosage and way the drug is formulated determines the rate of dissolution and absorption of the drug. Drugs in liquid form in solution or suspension are absorbed more rapidly than solid drugs in tablets, capsules etc. The particle size also influences the rate of dissolution and absorption, with small particles being absorbed more rapidly than larger ones. Table 4.3 indicates how the speed of absorption varies with the formulation of medications.

Table 4.3 Speed of absorption of different enteral drug formulations

Speed	Dissolution	Site of absorption	Type of formulation
Fastest			
	Mouth	Mouth: avoids first-pass metabolism	Oral disintegration: Sublingual tablets Buccal tablets Oral soluble wafers
	Stomach	Some drugs, particularly liquids, are absorbed. Solid formulations begin absorption in stomach	Liquids, elixirs, syrups Suspensions Powders, capsules, tablets
	Intestine	Absorption continues in the intestine. Coated and enteric coated tablets absorbed here	Coated tablets Enteric coated tablets
Slowest			

Distribution

This second stage in pharmacokinetics is the transport of drugs through the circulation to distribute them to their active site. Drugs are distributed first to organs with the biggest blood supply but then to almost all parts of the body. A proportion of the drug molecules in the bloodstream combines with plasma proteins – mainly albumin – and some of the drug remains 'free' or unbound. **Malnutrition** can result in low albumin levels, and thus reduces the amount of bound drug and increases the free drug molecules. The two forms, combined and free, are in equilibrium. It is only the free drug which is small enough to pass through the capillary walls to enter the extracellular fluid and pass from there to the cells of the body where they react with the drug receptors (see Pharmacodynamics below) (Figure 4.1).

Drug molecules cannot readily enter parts of the body with restricted blood supply or having specific barriers. For example, bones have a limited blood supply while the blood–brain barrier restricts the passage of drugs into the brain (Lilley et al., 2017).

The blood–brain barrier is a semipermeable membrane barrier that separates blood in the general circulation from circulation of blood and extracellular fluid in the brain. The 'tight junctions' between the cells of the brain **epithelium** prevent most substances in the blood from reaching the brain cells. The effectiveness of this barrier is reduced in a number of conditions including **stroke** (cerebrovascular accident) and neuroinflammatory disorders such as HIV-induced dementia, **multiple sclerosis** and **Alzheimer's disease** (Ballabh et al., 2004).

Metabolism

This stage of pharmacokinetics involves biochemically altering the drug molecule into a different form which may be an inactive, a more or less active metabolite, or a more soluble substance which can be excreted readily. The liver is the organ with the greatest contribution to drug metabolism, but other tissues also contribute, including kidneys, skeletal muscle, lungs, plasma and intestinal **mucosa**.

Lipid-soluble drugs are difficult to excrete from the body and this stage of metabolism is crucial in converting the molecule into a water-soluble substance that is readily excreted. There are two main types of conversion:

- Chemical changes (oxidation, reduction or hydrolysis): carried out by hepatic enzymes known as p450 or microsomal enzymes, which make molecules more water-soluble and less active.
- Conjugation or combination with an additional molecule (e.g. sulphate, glucuronic acid, glycine, etc): form less toxic, less active substances which are more readily excreted.

Both types of conversion are dependent on healthy liver function.

Excretion

The main organs of **excretion** are the kidneys, although the liver and gut also have a role.

Many drugs are metabolised in the liver before release into the general circulation and carriage to the kidney but others will have bypassed hepatic metabolism and retain their original structure. In the kidney they pass through the processes of filtration, some tubular reabsorption, and active secretion into the renal tubules before excretion in the urine.

Some other drugs are excreted into the biliary system of the liver and pass into the small intestine in the bile. They may pass through enterohepatic recirculation by reabsorption and repeated biliary excretion until passed out in faeces.

Factors influencing pharmacokinetics

Disturbances in function of the GIT will disrupt drug absorption. For example, **vomiting** will prevent gastric dissolution and absorption as the drugs are eliminated from the stomach. Surgery which has shortened the small intestine or reduced the size of the stomach will increase the speed with which gut contents, including the administered drug, pass through to the rectum and are eliminated, and will reduce the time for the drug to be absorbed into the circulation. **Diarrhoea** has a similar effect.

Disorders of the circulation may disrupt distribution of drugs around the body and to the individual organs or tissues on which they should be working. Disorders of the liver will reduce drug metabolism, thus causing a higher level of drug in the body and increased action on the body. Kidney disorders may also reduce excretion.

In addition to changes in body function influencing drug action, interaction between drugs can also influence their activity (see below).

ISSUES IN ADMINISTRATION

Patient safety

As indicated earlier, drugs used in the treatment of **disease** can be harmful if administered incorrectly or inappropriately; every nurse must know about, and must accurately perform, administration to ensure that drugs will function as anticipated. The nurse must also know when it is appropriate to omit a drug from administration. The essentials of drug administration are the necessary aspects of practice to ensure patient safety in relation to drugs, and are stated below. The basic principle is that the prescription is correct for the person/recipient and is administered as prescribed (except when it is not appropriate and should be omitted). Safe administration of medicines requires professional judgement and concentration on the part of the nurse. (See Apply: The essentials of drug administration, below.)

Most health care institutions have specific standards for drug administration. For example, student nurses can usually only administer drugs under the supervision of a registered nurse, and controlled drugs must normally be checked and administered by two registered nurses (a student nurse can sometimes be a third person in this situation).

APPLY

The essentials of drug administration

Correct person: The name and person's details on the prescription chart must correspond with the name on the patient's identification details (e.g. on their armband), including full name, identification number and age, and with the patient's verbal statement (when possible). Some patients with, for example, dementia may be confused and a photograph included with their prescription. Any allergies recorded must also be noted and considered.

Appropriate prescription: The drug details on the prescription must be correct. That is, the dosage prescribed must be appropriate for the person, taking account of the normal dose of the drug, the different strengths in which it is dispensed, and the person's condition and age. You should normally never find that you have to administer very large numbers of a tablet to give the prescribed dose. The dose, route and time should all be specified. The date of expiry of the prescription (e.g. for antibiotics) must be checked. Any queries must be checked with the prescriber. It is essential to use the BNF and the agreed formulary to check the information about the drug and its use before prescribing or administering a drug.

Administration: The administration of the drug must be correct. The prescription must be checked carefully against the drug container. Some drugs have similar (but not exactly the same) names, but completely different actions: great care is required.

- Check for any side-effects before administration.
- The dosage must match the prescription.
- The route of administration must be as specified.
- The correct time of administration must be adhered to. Some drugs are most effective if administered in the morning, others in the evening, some on an empty stomach, others with food.
- The drug must be administered in person to the appropriate recipient, and consumption witnessed (i.e. not left on the locker).

Recording: Accurate records of drugs administered must be completed and signed by the responsible person. Any adverse reactions must be reported and recorded.

(Lawson and Hennefer, 2010; Lilley et al., 2017)

Important notes:

- You should never administer drugs for another nurse unless you have been fully involved in all processes outlined in these principles; otherwise you cannot be certain what you are giving and whether it is appropriate.
- There will be occasions when it is not appropriate to give a prescribed drug. For example, you would not administer anti-hypertensive drugs to a person with very low blood pressure as you would lower it further, potentially causing them serious harm.

Adverse drug reaction profile

Watch this video and think about the importance of adverse drug reactions and how to recognise them. If you are using the eBook just click on the play button. Alternatively go to

https://study.sagepub.com/essentialpatho/videos

ADVERSE DRUG REACTION PROFILE (4:10)

Drug therapy through the life span

The person's stage in life is important in considering the dosage of drug being prescribed and administered. In development of drugs, most clinical testing does not include pregnant women, babies and children, the elderly, those taking other drugs, heavy drinkers and smokers, and those abusing drugs (McGavock, 2016). Thus, drug therapy in these groups must be managed with considerable care.

The four processes in pharmacokinetics function differently in children and older adults (Table 4.4). These changes mean that drug dosages at the two extremes of life need to be different from those administered to adults in general. The dosage guidelines for many drugs do not include details for the young and old, and specialist guidance is required. One of the considerations in drug therapy with older people is polypharmacy as many of these people may have a number of chronic diseases needing treatment.

Chronic conditions in the Bodie family

Maud is an example of an older person with a number of chronic conditions. As already mentioned, she is taking digoxin to increase the force of myocardial contraction and warfarin to reduce the risk of blood clotting. As aspirin could cause bleeding from the stomach and she is already taking warfarin, she is warned against taking aspirin (or any medication containing aspirin) for pain relief.

MAUD BODIE
CASE NOTES

Table 4.4 Pharmacokinetics in young and old

Stage	Babies and children vs. Adults	Older adults
Absorption	Peristalsis reduced Slower gastric emptying First-pass metabolism reduced Intramuscular absorption faster	Reduced absorption due to: Gastric pH reduced, emptying slowed Movement through GI tract slowed and blood flow reduced Villi flattening reduces absorption
Distribution	Total body water greater Fat content lower Protein-binding reduced More drugs enter brain	Total body water reduced Combining with plasma proteins lessened Decreased body mass → increased fat

(Continued)

Table 4.4 (Continued)

Stage	Babies and children vs. Adults	Older adults
Metabolism	Immature liver→low ability to metabolise drugs	Ageing liver produces lower levels of microsomal enzymes
	Older children with increased liver enzymes need higher doses	Blood flow through liver reduces over time → reduced liver metabolism
	Genetic factors, liver enzyme production, prenatal influences on mother alter metabolism	
Excretion	Kidney function reduced due to immaturity	Decreased blood flow → lower glomerular filtration
	Kidney perfusion may be decreased → reduced urine concentration and drug excretion	Reduction in numbers of nephrons

Source: Adapted from Lilley et al., 2017

ADVERSE DRUG EVENTS

This section is dealt with in three parts:

* Altered drug activity
* Preventing adverse effects
* Types of adverse drug events

Altered drug activity

Drugs are potentially hazardous in a number of different ways. Interactions can occur between drugs, between drugs and herbs (many drugs come from plant sources), between drugs and foods, and can alter activity at the stages in pharmacokinetics (i.e. absorption, distribution, metabolism, excretion) and in relation to binding with plasma proteins or receptors (pharmacodynamics) (FitzGerald, n.d.). When people are prescribed additional drugs, the risk of interactions must be considered and checked and the individual warned about the particular risks associated with their own drug regime. Specifically, polypharmacy places many ageing people at risk, as older people tend to be prescribed more drugs, which they have the potential to interact and also place high demand on the liver and organs involved in elimination (e.g. the kidneys).

In addition, some drugs which have a narrow margin of safety can have adverse effects alone or another drug can increase the drug level of the first one and result in an adverse reaction (Lynch, 2016). St John's Wort is a herb often taken by individuals independently of medical advice but which can interact in relation to the pharmacokinetics or pharmacodynamics of a number of drugs: individuals should be asked about their use of this herb when drugs are prescribed (Henderson et al., 2002). The risk of interactions is of particular concern in older people who may be receiving drugs for the treatment of several chronic conditions. The BNF has a useful section on drug interactions and a recent copy should be consulted. Adverse drug events will be considered first under the stages of pharmacokinetics and pharmacodynamics.

Absorption

Some interactions can affect drug absorption. For example, taking antacids may reduce the absorption of a number of drugs, including: some used in control of blood pressure; a number of commonly used antibiotics; digoxin; certain anti-epileptic drugs; and others.

A further example is an effect on metabolism that occurs in the gut and normally destroys some toxins (including certain drugs) before absorption. Grapefruit, grapefruit juice and Seville oranges inactivate some of the enzymes involved so that higher levels of the drugs concerned enter the body and may have a toxic effect (FitzGerald, n.d.). Examples of drugs affected include some antimalarial drugs, calcium-channel blockers, some statins regulating blood **cholesterol** level, and others (McGavock, 2016).

Distribution

The distribution of drugs varies according to blood perfusion through the tissues and is often uneven due to a variation in blood perfusion in different tissues. Poorly perfused tissues such as muscle and fat result in the slow distribution of drugs (Le, 2017a).

Metabolism

A number of drugs inhibit or induce (speed up) the activity of the drug-metabolising enzymes in the liver (McGavock, 2016). Inhibition of these enzymes will cause an increase in the drug levels in the blood and pharmacological activity. Induction of drug metabolising enzymes will result in faster metabolism and (normally) levels will fall more rapidly than usual. Some foods can alter drug metabolism, for example, a high protein diet can stimulate cytochrome P450 involved in drug metabolism in the liver (Youdim, 2016). In addition, some herbs can also influence drug metabolism (Marko, 2016). St John's Wort has been identified as causing the induction of enzymes.

Excretion

Most drugs are excreted through filtration by the kidneys following metabolism in the liver in which the drug molecules combine with other chemicals which prevent their reabsorption following filtration in the kidneys. In addition to filtration, the elimination of many drugs involves active tubular secretion in the proximal tubule which is dependent on energy and can be blocked by substances that block this process. The pH of urine varies considerably, altering the degree of excretion of drugs. Excretion through the kidneys decreases with age and by the age of 80 it is about 50% of its previous performance at 30 (Le, 2017b). Renal disorders will reduce drug excretion.

Binding

Drugs may compete for the same binding site on plasma proteins; this may cause the level of free (active) drug in the bloodstream to be raised. This may be of no significance but if a drug, e.g. digoxin, is displaced it can result in toxicity.

When two drugs compete for binding with the same cell membrane receptor, then an adverse reaction may occur. A molecule that binds to such a molecule is called a ligand and may be an agonist which activates the receptor or an antagonist which prevents receptor activity. If one drug acts as an antagonist it opposes the other's activity (Farinde, 2016).

Preventing adverse effects

Drug development

In the development of drugs, considerable efforts are taken to minimise the risk of adverse effects through a number of stages (see Go Deeper). Stage 4 in development is particularly important as most side-effects are identified after the drug has been released for prescription to the general public: it is essential that such effects are reported to the Medicines and Healthcare Products Regulatory Agency (in the UK, the Yellow Card Scheme can be used for reporting suspected adverse drug reactions [ADRs]).

Preventable adverse events

One of the major causes of adverse drug events is an error in administration. Care in complying with all the issues mentioned under 'The essentials of drug administration' (above) is essential. If an inadvertent error does occur, it is crucial that it is reported immediately so that any necessary remedial action can be implemented.

――――――――――― GO DEEPER ―――――――――――

Drug development

Table 4.5 Stages in drug development

Stage	Procedures and protocols
Research	Identification of potential chemicals for therapeutic use
Preclinical testing	Laboratory development involving in vitro ('in glass') and animal studies to clarify how the chemical works on the cells and organs, including identification of toxic effects on body organs
	Tests for mutagenesis (i.e. altered DNA) which can lead to **carcinogenesis** or teratogenesis (gross structural abnormalities arising during fetal development) or other fetal abnormalities
Clinical trials	Phase 1: Volunteer studies: up to 100 healthy volunteers (usually paid in recognition of risk involved) to investigate pharmacokinetic and metabolic properties, and safety
	Phase 2: A homogeneous group of up to 500 people with condition for which drug is designated, omitting old, children, pregnant women, heavy drinkers, smokers, drug abusers, those on other drugs
	Usually double-blind controlled trials (50% get active drug, 50% placebo or usual treatment) to test efficacy, safety and dosage
	Phase 3: Further testing of safety and efficacy in a heterogeneous group of up to 3000 people for a longer period (3 months to one year)
	Application submitted to licensing authority for approval. Further testing required or rejection
	Phase 4: Drug available for prescribing, but post-marketing surveillance necessary to examine:
	Further safety and adverse effects
	Efficacy of drug in the general population
	Cost-effectiveness
	Unexpected therapeutic actions

Source: Adapted from McGavock, 2016; Rang et al., 2016

Types of adverse drug events

Known effect of drug

These adverse effects are similar to but stronger than the normal effects of the drug and are related to the dose administered and the individual's susceptibility to the drug (Rang et al., 2016). Accurate administration and careful observation of the effects of the drug are the first essential aspects of management. Many such adverse effects are reversible if the dosage is reduced. **Iatrogenic** reactions are caused by medical examination or treatment.

Unrelated to known action of drug

In some cases, adverse effects may be unrelated to the therapeutic action of the drug and can range from mild to very severe. Some ADRs are predictable if the drug is taken in excess, for example, an excessive dose of paracetamol results in liver damage (hepatotoxicity).

However, there are several major groups of ADRs unrelated to therapeutic actions which may occur with a normal dose.

Idiosyncratic reactions

Idiosyncratic reactions tend to be serious, unpredictable and uncommon. Unexpected chemical reactions can occur in susceptible people due to individual variation in DNA (nuclear or **mitochondrial**). They may cause damage to organs, e.g. liver, kidneys.

Immunological reactions

A number of drugs can cause an **allergic reaction** in some individuals. It is important that those affected are aware of the drugs to which they are allergic, compounds within which they may be contained, and understand that they must not take them. These individuals are often recommended to carry an adrenaline pen (an Epipen) for emergency treatment in, for example, **anaphylactic shock**. They may also be advised to wear a Medic Alert bracelet. In addition, the In Case of Emergency (ICE) function on most smart phones often hosts the information (Rang et al., 2016).

Allergic reactions can be of various types, ranging from life-threatening to relatively minor, and include:

- Anaphylactic shock: this occurs due to the release of histamine and other mediators causing a rash, tissue swelling, **bronchospasm** and hypotension, and may be lethal (anaphylactoid reactions are similar changes but occur due to nonimmune-mediated release of mediators from **mast cells** and/ or **basophils** or by direct complement activation)
- Haematological reactions
- Allergic liver damage
- Other reactions including skin eruptions which can range from mild rashes to life-threatening skin loss.

Carcinogenesis and fetal abnormalities

As indicated in the Go Deeper box, some drugs can cause **mutations** in DNA, resulting in the initiation of cancers.

Some drugs, if given during pregnancy, can result in a range of fetal abnormalities, as can German measles (rubella). The best-known example of a drug causing major abnormalities is the use of thalidomide in the late 1950s and 1960s in the treatment of early morning sickness. Eventually the increased incidence of major abnormalities in newly born infants was linked to this drug. There have been considerable changes in the testing required in the development of new drugs to reduce the risk of occurrence of similar tragedies. The terms used for such abnormalities are:

* **Carcinogenic**: has the potential to cause **cancer**
* **Teratogenic**: the drug can disturb embryonic or fetal development and result in a birth defect.

In more recent years, a commonly used anti-epileptic drug, sodium valproate, has also been associated with fetal abnormalities and has led to a new **syndrome** called fetal valproate syndrome (Dodou and Whiteley, 2014). This has led to a considerable review of how epilepsy is managed in pregnant women and those planning a pregnancy.

CHAPTER SUMMARY

This chapter has considered some of the broad issues involved in the pharmacological treatment of disorders. It aims to enable you to be safe practitioners in relation to drug administration and prescription through using your knowledge and understanding, professional judgement, concentration and sense of responsibility.

KEY POINTS

* Drugs are available in three groups in the UK: General Sales List, Pharmacy and Prescription Only Medicines. The last group can only be provided if prescribed by an independent prescriber or a supplementary prescriber within a clinical management plan.

* Drugs link with receptors within the cells of the target organs. The drugs may be agonists (activators) or antagonists (inhibitors).

* The level of drug action depends on the concentration of the drug in the bloodstream. This is determined by the pharmacokinetic stages of:

   a. Absorption – by enteral (first-pass metabolism must be taken into account), parenteral or topical routes. The speed of absorption varies with route of administration and formulation of the drug.

   b. Distribution – a proportion of the drug will be carried in combination with plasma proteins. The free drug is available for combining with receptors and modifying cell function.

   c. Metabolism – drug molecules are mainly metabolised in the liver to an inactive or more active substance, or to a more water-soluble form which can be readily excreted.

   d. Excretion – the kidneys are the main organ for drug excretion but some drugs are excreted into the bile, thence into the small intestine and pass out in the faeces.

- The basic principle of drug administration is that the correct person gets the correct drugs. Dosages vary in the young and older adults due to variation in the pharmacokinetics.

- A range of adverse drug events can occur and are particularly common in older adults due to polypharmacy and a reduction in organ function. They can be due to the known effects of the drug, idiosyncratic in nature, or due to immunological reactions, or mutagenic changes in the DNA.

REVISE

TEST YOUR KNOWLEDGE

The content of this chapter will help you understand the principles of drug therapy. Revise the different sections in turn then try to answer the questions below.

Answers are available online. If you are using the eBook just click on the answers icon below. Alternatively, go to **https://study.sagepub.com/essentialpatho/answers**

1   Outline the different classes of drugs and the two groups of prescribers.

2   Identify and briefly describe the main terms used to describe types of drugs.

3   Outline how drugs act on the body.

4   Identify and briefly describe the four stages of pharmacokinetics.

5   Specify the main routes for administration of drugs.

6   What do you understand by first-pass metabolism? How can it be avoided?

7   Outline the essentials of drug administration.

8   Briefly discuss the potential difficulties in drug administration with older people.

9   Outline the types of adverse drug effects that can occur and consider how these can be limited.

REVISE

ACE YOUR ASSESSMENT

- Further revision and learning opportunities are available online
- Test yourself away from the book with **Extra multiple choice questions**
- Learn and revise terminology with **Interactive flashcards**

If you are using the eBook access each resource by clicking on the respective icon. Alternatively go to **https://study.sagepub.com/essentialpatho/chapter4**

CHAPTER 4 ANSWERS

EXTRA QUESTIONS

FLASHCARDS

REFERENCES

Appelbe, G.E. and Wingfield, J. (eds) (2013) *Dale and Appelbe's Pharmacy and Medicines Law*, 10th edn. London: Pharmaceutical Press.

Ballabh, P., Braun, A. and Nedergaard, M. (2004) The blood–brain barrier: an overview – structure, regulation, and clinical implications. *Neurobiology of Disease, 16* (1): 1–13.

BNF (2018) *British National Formulary*, 76th edn. London: BMJ Group and Royal Pharmaceutical Society.

Dodou, K. and Whiteley, P. (2014) Concerns with using sodium valproate to treat epilepsy in pregnant women. *The Pharmaceutical Journal, 292* (7808): 482.

Dowden, A. (2016) The expanding role of nurse prescribers. *Prescriber*, 20 June. Available at: www.prescriber.co.uk/article/expanding-role-nurse-prescribers/ (accessed 20 August 2018).

Farinde, A. (2016) *Clinical Pharmacology, Drug–Receptor Interactions*. Kenilworth, NJ, USA: MSD Manual, Professional Version Available at: www.msdmanuals.com/professional/clinical-pharmacology/pharmacodynamics/drug%E2%80%93receptor-interactions (accessed 9 October 2018).

FitzGerald, R. (n.d.) *Important Drug Interactions*. University of Liverpool, Wolfson Centre for Personalised Medicine/MRC Centre for Drug Safety Science. Available at: https://tinyurl.com/yd5dh68t (accessed 3 December 2018).

Henderson, L., Yue, Q.Y., Bergquist, C., Gerden, B. and Arlett, P. (2002) St John's wort (*Hypericum perforatum*): drug interactions and clinical outcomes. *British Journal of Clinical Pharmacology, 54* (4): 349–56.

Katzung, B.G. and Trevor, A.J. (2015) *Basic and Clinical Pharmacology*, 13th edn. New York: McGraw-Hill Education.

Lawson, E. and Hennefer, D.L. (2010) *Medicines Management in Adult Nursing*. Exeter: Learning Matters.

Le, J. (2017a) *Clinical Pharmacology: Drug Distribution to Tissues*. Kenilworth, NJ: MSD Manual, Professional Version. Available at: www.msdmanuals.com/en-gb/professional/clinical-pharmacology/pharmacokinetics/drug-distribution-to-tissues (accessed 9 October 2018).

Le, J. (2017b) *Clinical Pharmacology: Drug Excretion*. Kenilworth, NJ: MSD Manual, Professional Version. Available at: www.msdmanuals.com/en-gb/professional/clinical-pharmacology/ pharmacokinetics/ drug-excretion (accessed 9 October 2018).

Lilley, L.L., Collins, S.R. and Snyder, J.S. (2017) *Pharmacology and the Nursing Process*, 8th edn. St Louis, MO: Mosby.

Lynch, S.S. (2016) *Clinical Pharmacology: Drug Interactions*. Kenilworth, NJ: MSD Manual, Professional Version. Available at: www.msdmanuals.com/en-gb/professional/clinical-pharmacology/factors-affecting-response-to-drugs/drug-interactions (accessed 9 October 2018).

Marko, M.G. (2016) *Special Subjects: Overview of Dietary Supplements*. Kenilworth, NJ: MSD Manual, Professional Version Available at: www.msdmanuals.com/en-gb/professional/ special-subjects/dietary-supplements/overview-of-dietary-supplements#v1126015 (accessed 9 October 2018).

McGavock, H. (2016) *How Drugs Work: Basic Pharmacology for Health Professionals*, 4th edn. Boca Raton, FL: CRC Press.

Nursing and Midwifery Council (2018) *Future Nurse: Standards of Proficiency for Registered Nurses*. London: NMC.

Rang, H.P., Ritter, J.M., Flower, R.J. and Henderson, G. (2016) *Rang and Dale's Pharmacology*, 8th edn. London: Churchill Livingstone, Elsevier.

Youdim, A. (2016) *Nutrient–Drug Interactions*. Kenilworth, NJ: MSD Manual, Professional Version Available at: www.msdmanuals.com/en-gb/professional/nutritional-disorders/ nutrition-general-considerations/nutrient (accessed 9 October 2018).

GENETIC DISORDERS

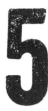

UNDERSTAND: CHAPTER VIDEOS

Watch the following video to ease you into this chapter. If you are using the eBook just click on the play button. Alternatively go to **https://study.sagepub.com/essentialpatho/videos**

HUMAN GENETICS (5:55)

LEARNING OUTCOMES

When you have finished studying this chapter you will be able to:

1. Understand the approaches used in the diagnosis of genetic disorders including completion of a family history.
2. Identify the approaches used in genetic screening.
3. Describe the key factors which influence the expression of an altered gene in single gene disorders.
4. Clarify the main types of chromosomal aneuploidy (presence of an altered number of chromosomes in a cell).
5. Differentiate between polygenic and multifactorial diseases.
6. Outline the cause of mitochondrial disease and how it can be treated.
7. Discuss the importance of genetic counselling and genetic services and consider ethical implications.

INTRODUCTION

In this chapter you will consider the genetic basis of **disease**, the patterns of inheritance, and how genetic disorders are diagnosed and treated. Some genetic disorders are evident at birth while others manifest much later in life. Genetic disorders are caused by **mutations** or alterations in genes, leading to a disorder or to a predisposition to certain diseases, such as **cancer**, **diabetes**, **cardiovascular disease** and mental disorders (WHO, 2018). Advances in genetic research and technology have changed the way such disorders are managed and, for many people, have increased their life expectancy.

In this chapter we are going to outline some of the principles involved in caring for people with genetically determined conditions and their families. Each person has a unique genetic makeup encompassed within the **chromosomes** and **mitochondria** of the body cells and changes in the genetic makeup can result in a range of different disorders. This chapter introduces a number of different disorders caused by changes in the genetic makeup of the individual and the implications this may have for them and their families.

REVISE: A&P RECAP

Genetic and epigenetic control

To help you through this chapter, you might find it useful to revise your background knowledge of genetic and epigenetic control.

For a full discussion see Chapter 3, Genetic and Epigenetic Control of Biological Systems, in *Essentials of Anatomy and Physiology for Nursing Practice* (Boore et al., 2016).

PERSON-CENTRED CONTEXT: THE BODIE FAMILY

BODIE FAMILY
CASE NOTES

Within members of the Bodie family, a number of different disorders occur which are or may be influenced by genetic factors. These include some conditions that are definitely known to have a genetic component. Some examples are discussed here.

Maud has **hypothyroidism**. Panicker (2011) suggests that up to 67% of circulating thyroid-stimulating hormone (TSH) and thyroid hormone concentrations are genetically determined. While there is still much to discover about the genes involved, susceptibility to autoimmune hypothyroidism is largely genetically determined with alterations in immune regulation-associated genes (Chapter 13). Genetic alterations can affect thyroid development causing **congenital** hypothyroidism distinct from hypothyroidism caused by iodine deficiency in the diet (Maitra, 2015).

Two of the family have allergic conditions: Derek has asthma and Margaret has hay fever. These, along with **dermatitis**, are known as atopic conditions and individuals may be diagnosed with one, e.g. hay fever (**allergic** rhinitis), and later in life may develop another such condition such as asthma. **Atopy** is defined as:

> the genetic tendency to develop allergic diseases such as allergic rhinitis, asthma and atopic dermatitis (eczema). Atopy is typically associated with heightened immune responses to common allergens, especially inhaled allergens and food allergens. (AAAA, 2018)

Diabetes type 2, which Richard has, is also known to have a genetic component.

Jack Garcia's father had testicular cancer and it is now known that 49% of the risk of developing this is due to genetic factors (Institute of Cancer Research (ICR), 2015). Jack is well aware of this and undertakes regular (monthly) self-examination of his testes to ensure that any changes are identified and treated early.

GO DEEPER

Genetics and diabetes

If you are interested in learning more about the work on genetics and diabetes watch this video. If you are using the eBook just click on the play button. Alternatively go to

https://study.sagepub.com/essentialpatho/videos

GENETICS AND DIABETES (4:22)

Principles of inheritance and genetic disorders

UNDERSTAND

Laws and modes of inheritance

Tables 5.1 and 5.2 present a brief recap of some of the key aspects of genetics (Boore et al., 2016).

Table 5.1 The three laws of inheritance

Law of Dominance	An organism (person) with at least one dominant allele in their cells will display the effect of the dominant allele
Law of Segregation	During gamete formation, the pair of alleles for each gene segregate from each other so that each gamete carries only one allele for each gene
Law of Independent Assortment	Genes for different traits can segregate independently during the formation of gametes

Table 5.2 Modes of genetic inheritance in disease

Single gene inheritance	**Dominant**: Gene carried by one parent. At each pregnancy there is a 50% chance of the condition being inherited and demonstrated in offspring
	Recessive: Both parents carry the gene. If inherited from both parents, the offspring will have the condition. In each pregnancy, the offspring will have a one in four chance of having the condition.
	Sex-linked: One parent carries the abnormal gene on one of the sex chromosomes, usually the X (female) chromosome as this is larger than the Y (male) chromosome. Condition most commonly shown in males and carried in females
Polygenic inheritance	These conditions require the presence of several or many genes, each having a small effect on presentation of the condition
Multifactorial inheritance	This type of condition usually involves more than one gene in combination with environmental factors
Chromosomal abnormality	Some relatively rare conditions occur due to disturbances in the normal number of chromosomes. A chromosome may be lost or gained or its structure altered
Mitochondrial DNA	**Mitochondria**, organelles in the cytoplasm of the cell, contain about 1% of the total DNA and are concerned with energy **metabolism**. They are inherited solely from the mother

SINGLE GENE DISORDERS

These disorders are caused by a single altered nucleotide (building blocks of DNA) in the three main types of single gene inheritance: dominant, recessive and sex-linked (most usually X-linked). Less common variants occasionally occur but are not being discussed here. An example of each of the three main types is discussed in some detail:

UNDERSTAND

Patterns of inheritance

The modes of inheritance (dominant, recessive and X-linked) are discussed fully in Chapter 3 of *Essentials of Anatomy and Physiology for Nursing Practice* (Boore et al., 2016).

Family trees for the different types of condition are included.

Autosomal dominant: Huntington's disease

Huntington's disease (HD) affects 5–10 per 100,000 of the European population, affecting men and women equally. It is a disease of the central nervous system which is progressive, with symptoms usually appearing in adulthood in the fourth or fifth decade of life or earlier. As an autosomal dominant disorder, a mutated gene from one parent is sufficient for its development. In 1993 the mutated gene was first identified on chromosome 4 and is now known as the *Huntingtin* gene or *HTT*. This gene codes for the protein Huntingtin (in genetics italic is used to differentiate the gene name from the protein). Normally this gene has repeated sequences of the bases cytosine, adenine and guanine (CAG). Up to 35 copies are made and normally about 17 in a person without HD. In the mutated gene the number of repeats increases beyond 35 and Huntington's disease will develop. The more repeats of the protein, the earlier the age of onset of the condition. The average repeat for a person with Huntington's disease is 44 (Stuitje et al., 2017). This results in an abnormal protein with increased glutamine amino acids which damage the person's normal cells, particularly neurons.

In this disease degeneration of neurons in the striatum leads to progressive deterioration of movement, cognition and behaviour and, eventually, causes dementia. Early symptoms are often behavioural, including mood changes, irritability, anger, lack of concentration and depression. Movement is also affected, resulting in uncontrollable jerky movements of the face and limbs which become more frequent as the condition progresses. The person's posture, balance and gait are affected. Cognitive symptoms include impairment in concentration and memory.

While it is possible to identify people who carry the altered gene, it is not possible to indicate the age of onset of symptoms. Currently there is no cure for Huntington's disease and treatment is based on the management of symptoms. Ongoing research is focusing on creating drugs that reduce the level of the abnormal protein in the nervous system of patients with HD and this has shown encouraging results to date (Tabrizi, 2017).

Autosomal recessive disorder: Cystic fibrosis

Cystic fibrosis is an autosomal recessive condition that occurs because of mutations in the *Cystic Fibrosis Transmembrane Conductance Regulator* (*CFTR*) gene. This gene codes for the production of a protein that regulates ion transport across epithelial membranes. A mutation in the gene leads to reduced production or abnormal function of the protein, thus affecting ion transport. Each parent transmits one gene to the child with this condition who thus carries two altered genes. It is the most common genetic disorder among Caucasians and, in the UK in 2015, 10,800 people had CF (Cystic Fibrosis Registry, 2015).

Transport of salt and water across sodium and chloride channels in the cell membranes is disrupted, resulting in highly viscous (sticky) secretions being produced, which obstruct tubules and ducts and disrupt the activity of a number of organs. In the sweat glands there is decreased reabsorption of sodium, resulting in the production of salty sweat. In the gastrointestinal and respiratory epithelium there is reduced chloride secretion into the lumen and increased **absorption** of sodium and water. This results in thick viscid secretions on the surface **mucosa** (Kumar et al., 2018). Organs affected include the pancreas in 85–90% of people affected, disrupting digestion and sometimes blocking the pancreatic ducts. The liver and the salivary glands are also affected. In the lungs, thick secretions can obstruct the airways and increase the risk of giving rise to severe chronic bronchitis and bronchiectasis, in which destruction of smooth muscle and elastic tissue results in permanent dilation of bronchi and bronchioles.

X-linked disorder: Haemophilia A

This hereditary disorder can result in life-threatening bleeding, due to abnormal factor VIII, one of the essential factors for coagulation (Moreira and Das, 2018). It is inherited as an X-linked recessive trait, mainly affecting males carrying one altered gene, but also occurs in homozygous females carrying two altered genes on the X chromosomes. In about 30% of persons affected, there is no family history of the condition; it occurs due to a new genetic mutation.

People with **haemophilia** bruise easily and trauma or **surgery** can lead to severe haemorrhage. Injury to joints can lead to bleeding into the joints and progressive deformities. The severity of the condition depends on the level of deficiency of factor VIII, with activity levels of <1% of normal causing severe haemophilia A (Kumar et al., 2018).

Gene expression

There are three factors which influence the expression of an altered gene:

* *Germline mosaicism*: the person affected has more than one genetically different cell-line. This arises when there is a mutation in the germ cells (ovum or spermatozoa) of one parent, but not in the **somatic** (body) cells.
* *Penetrance*: relates to the extent that the trait carried in the abnormal gene presents the disorder.
* *Reduced penetrance*: this is when the trait does not present even though the abnormal gene is carried.
* *Age-dependent penetrance*: this is when a genetic disorder is only expressed later in life. Children carrying the mutated gene may be born before the disease has presented in the parents. An example is Huntingdon's disease.
* *Variable expression*: this refers to the degree of severity of the presentation of the condition. Environmental factors or other genes may alter the degree of expression.

Table 5.3 clarifies some of the differences between these modes of inheritance and identifies some examples.

Table 5.3 Characteristics of single gene disorders

Dominant	Recessive	X-Linked
One parent carries altered gene	Both parents carry altered gene	One parent (usually mother) carries altered X-chromosome
Condition occurs equally in either gender	Condition occurs equally in either gender	Usually shown in males, carried in females
50% chance of occurrence in each pregnancy	1 in 4 chance of occurrence in each pregnancy	Carrier mother, father not affected → son has 50% chance of disease, daughter 50% chance of carrier
Either parent (with altered gene) can transmit condition to child		Affected father, mother not a carrier → 0 males, 100% females affected
		Affected father, carrier mother → 50% males affected, 50% females affected, 50% female carrier
No skipping of generations. Vertical transmission of disease phenotypes	Clustering of disease around siblings. Vertical transmission not usually clear. Consanguinity increased risk	Transmitted through carrier female. Gaps seen in family tree where disease has skipped generations
Some examples of conditions		
Achondroplasia: short, long bones **Marfan syndrome**: tall, long limbs Familial **hypercholesterolaemia**: high blood **cholesterol** → early cardiovascular disease Hereditary spherocytosis: red blood cells prone to rupture	Sickle cell **anaemia**: abnormal-shaped red blood cells, carrier protected against malaria Phenylketonuria: → risk of intellectual disability if not diagnosed early or managed with special diet **Neimann–Pick disease**: metabolic disorder, varied age of penetrance Spinal muscular atrophy: nerve/muscle deterioration	Duchenne muscular dystrophy: early death Haemophilia B: Christmas disease - blood clotting deficiency Red-green colour blindness, 7–10% of men and 0.49% to 1% of women are affected Male pattern baldness X-linked agammaglobulinaemia (low levels of immunoglobulins)

TP53 mutations

One single gene mutation of particular interest affects a **tumour** suppressor gene, *TP53*. The majority of mutations of this gene are known as missense mutations. These have been defined as:

> A genetic alteration in which a single base pair substitution alters the genetic code in a way that produces an amino acid that is different from the usual amino acid at that position. (NCI, 2017, on-line Dictionary of Genetics Terms)

TP53 prevents excessive **proliferation** of cells. It has been described as '*the guardian of the genome*' (Surget et al., 2014: 57) because of its importance in preventing **malignant** change and spread. It is an important gene which is activated by cellular **stress** and changed cellular homeostasis occurs due to damage to the DNA, inadequate **nutrition**, excessive heat, change in pH, **hypoxia**, **virus** infection or activation of an **oncogene**.

An oncogene has been defined as:

> A gene that is a mutated (changed) form of a gene involved in normal cell growth. Oncogenes may cause the growth of cancer cells. Mutations in genes that become oncogenes can be inherited or caused by being exposed to substances in the environment that cause cancer. (NCI, 2017, on-line Dictionary of Genetics Terms)

A mutation in *TP53* is common in most human cancers (>50%) (Surget et al., 2014). Mutations in the germline cells result in early onset cancers. Mutations in somatic *TP53* can result in numerous cancers including: breast cancer, bone and soft tissue sarcomas, brain tumours, adrenocortical carcinomas, and less commonly leukaemia, stomach and colorectal cancer. The presence of this mutation can be a factor in the prognosis of cancer and the response to treatment (Petitjean et al., 2007).

DISORDERS DUE TO CHROMOSOMAL ALTERATIONS

These conditions involve disturbances in the number or structure of chromosomes. Normal chromosomal makeup is shown in the individual **karyotype**. A normal karyotype has 23 pairs of chromosomes, 46 in total, 22 pairs of autosomes and two sex chromosomes, XX for female and XY for male. The gametes, ovum and sperm, carry 23 chromosomes, 22 plus a sex chromosome (X or Y). The fertilised zygote has 46 chromosomes including 2 sex chromosomes.

REVISE: A&P RECAP

Karyotype

If you are unsure as to what a karyotype is, it may be helpful to look this up quickly. A normal karyotype is illustrated in Chapter 2, The Human Cell, in *Essentials of Anatomy and Physiology for Nursing Practice* (Boore et al., 2016).

There are a number of different types of chromosomal abnormalities which are considered here (see Table 5.4). Most are examples of aneuploidy, which is an altered number of chromosomes in a cell, for example 45 or 47 instead of the usual 46 chromosomes. However, a difference of one or more complete sets of chromosomes is called euploidy.

Table 5.4 Types of chromosomal abnormalities

Aneuploidy	An abnormal number of chromosomes in a cell (not an exact multiple of the haploid number)
Euploidy	Any number of complete chromosome sets in a cell (an exact multiple of the haploid number)
Monoploidy	One member of the chromosome pair is missing
Polyploidy	When a cell contains more than two paired (homologous) sets of chromosomes

Polyploidy

Cells containing multiples of the normal chromosome count are called polyploid. A human triploid cell contains 69 chromosomes (including three sex chromosomes), while a tetraploid cell has 92 chromosomes in each cell nucleus and is much rarer. Most of these fetuses are miscarried and those that survive birth typically die shortly after delivery (Jorde et al., 2016).

Autosomal aneuploidy

This term is used when individual autosomal chromosomes are missing or an extra one is present. These arise during the formation of gametes or fertilisation of the egg and such embryos make up at least 10%

of human pregnancies (Nagaoka et al., 2012) and are mainly due to disturbances in the maternal gametes. The incidence increases with maternal age, with one explanation linking this to the deterioration of a substance (cohesin) which holds together the two chromatids (which form each chromosome) (Jessberger, 2012).

The commonest types are:

- **Monosomy**: only one copy of a specific chromosome instead of the normal two. Usually autosomal monosomies are not compatible with a live birth.
- **Trisomy**: three copies of a specific chromosome. These are more likely to be compatible with life.

The commonest autosomal aneuploidies are trisomies of chromosomes 21, 18 and 13 (Table 5.5), a large proportion of which are lost spontaneously during the pregnancy. The risk of these conditions occurring increases with maternal age. **Mosaicism** is the presence of more than one line of genetically identical cells within the body and occurs in a small proportion of infants born with these trisomies.

Table 5.5 Autosomal chromosomal aneuploidies

Genetic abnormalities	Name	Characteristics
Trisomy 21	Down syndrome	75% of fetuses with Trisomy 21 abort spontaneously. 1 in 700–1000 live births have Trisomy 21
		People with this condition have characteristic facial features – small ears, flattened face, slanting eyes, slightly enlarged tongue. 50% have single palmar crease
		Moderate to mild intellectual disability
		Various anatomical abnormalities may occur, including 40% with heart defects which may lead to reduced length of life
		People with Trisomy 21 now have a greatly increased life expectancy with modern health care (50% live longer than 50 years). See Activity 5.2 for more context on Down Syndrome
Trisomy 18	Edwards syndrome	This occurs every 1 in 6000 live births; many are stillborn
		There is prenatal growth deficiency, and the person has characteristic facial features (small ears, small mouth), and hand features (index finger overrides third finger)
		Major effects can include congenital heart defects, missing radius, omphalocele (bowel protrudes into umbilical cord) and marked developmental delays. See Activity 5.3 for more context on Edwards Syndrome
Trisomy 13	Patau syndrome	1 in 10,000 births: ~95% spontaneously abort and 95% of babies born alive die in first year
		Characteristics include developmental disability, distinctive facial features (small eyes, wide nose)
		Abnormalities of central nervous system, heart and kidneys
		Post-axial polydactyly in which an additional digit occurs on ulnar margin of the hand, or lateral to the 5th toe

Source: Jorde et al., 2016

ACTIVITY 5.1: APPLY

Having a child with Down syndrome

This website introduces Meriel's story, 'Having a child with Down syndrome':
www.tellingstories.nhs.uk/index.php/joys-story?id=230

ACTIVITY 5.2: APPLY

Having a child with Edwards syndrome

This website introduces Marianne, who tells the story of her son, who has Edwards syndrome, 'He happens to have an extra chromosome - it makes him extra special':
www.tellingstories.nhs.uk/index.php/joys-story?id=289

Sex chromosome aneuploidy

These conditions are much more common among live-born infants than the autosomal aneuploidies. Monosomies and trisomies and additional variations occur, most due to errors in meiosis in the mother related to increasing maternal age (Nagaoka et al., 2012). The effects of these aneuploidies are all (except the complete absence of the X chromosome) compatible with life. Mosaicism also occurs in this group of aneuploidies.

As many as 1 in 400 people carry one of these aneuploidies and Table 5.6 summarises the main sex chromosome aneuploidies and the effects on the person affected. In addition, these aneuploidies cause disturbances to the brain and language development. Males with 47XXY and females with 47XXX have been shown to have reduced brain volume, while those with further additional X chromosomes have more markedly diminished brain size (Lenroot et al., 2009). In addition, an increased incidence of sex chromosome aneuploidies was found in people with language and reading impairment and normal IQ (Simpson et al., 2014). Early identification of people with these aneuploidies could assist in providing appropriate management and support.

Table 5.6 Sex chromosomal aneuploidies

Genetic abnormalities	Name	Characteristics
Monosomy X (45,X)	Turner syndrome	Female. High incidence of **spontaneous abortions**
Mosaicism in 30-40% e.g. 45X/46XX, rarely 45X/46XY		Short in height and no adolescent growth spurt occurs (often treated with growth hormone). Characteristic shaped face, broad 'webbed' neck. **Lymphoedema** of hands and feet at birth
		Lack of sexual development and most people are infertile. Major and minor malformations occur including congenital heart defects. About 50% have defects in renal structure
Trisomy X (47XXX)		In 1 in 1000 females, with minor effects
4, 5 or more X chromosomes can occur		Sometimes women affected are sterile with menstrual irregularity
		Some have mild intellectual disability
		Additional X chromosomes (e.g. 4 or 5) - increased intellectual and physical disability

(Continued)

Table 5.6 (Continued)

Genetic abnormalities	Name	Characteristics
47XXY 48XXXY 49XXXXY	Klinefelter syndrome	1 in 500 to 1 in 1000 male births
		Taller than usual, with long arms and legs
		Post-puberty, testes are small, most people are infertile with low testosterone
		About 1 in 3 develop gynaecomastia (breast development) with increased risk of breast cancer
		May show learning disability and reduced verbal IQ
		Additional X chromosomes lead to increased intellectual and physical disability. See Activity 5.4 for more context on Klinefelter Syndrome
47,XYY		1 in 1000 males
		Taller than most men and lower than usual IQ (10-15 points lower)
		Increased incidence of relatively minor behavioural problems, e.g. intellectual disabilities, hyperactivity, attention deficit disorder

Source: Jorde et al., 2016

ACTIVITY 5.3: APPLY

Living with Klinefelter syndrome

Go to this website to read Andrew's story of living with Klinefelter syndrome 47XXY, 'The buck stops with me':

www.tellingstories.nhs.uk/index.php/all-stories/133-andrews-story?highlight=WyJrbGluZWZlbHRlciJd

POLYGENIC AND MULTIFACTORIAL DISEASES

The genetic disorders already considered have been relatively straightforward in biological terms, based on the individual chromosomes and single genes. We are now going to examine some more complex situations, starting with the pathogenesis of polygenic and multifactorial diseases which are more complex and varied.

REVISE: A&P RECAP

Polygenic and multifactorial disorders

These aspects of polygenic and multifactorial disorders are introduced fully in Chapter 3 on genetics and epigenetics in *Essentials of Anatomy and Physiology for Nursing Practice* (Boore et al., 2016).

Polygenic inheritance is when the characteristic concerned occurs as a result of the effects of a number of genes interacting: traits inherited in this way demonstrate a variable range of the characteristic occurring including height, intelligence, eye colour and skin colour. The traits concerned frequently show a continuous distribution pattern.

--- **REVISE: A&P RECAP** ---

Polygenic inheritance

Polygenic inheritance of skin colour is illustrated clearly in Figure 3.7 in Chapter 3 on genetics and epigenetics in *Essentials of Anatomy and Physiology for Nursing Practice* (Boore et al., 2016).

Multifactorial conditions result from a combination of genetic changes, as in polygenic disorders, and environmental factors such as diet, including high salt and high sugar content, exercise, stress and smoking (Table 5.7). Loktionov (2003) has reviewed links between nutrition and multifactorial **chronic illnesses. Obesity** is a particular risk factor for a number of disorders. What is clear is that individuals can eliminate or reduce a number of these risk factors and thus minimise the development of a number of these conditions.

Table 5.7 Examples of multifactorial disorders

Disorder	Characteristics	Risk and management
Neural tube defects (NTDs)	**Spina bifida** (spinal tissue protrudes through vertebral column) (Chapter 16) **Anencephaly** (complete or partial absence of cranium and cerebral hemisphere) (Chapter 16)	Folic acid supplementation before conception and during early pregnancy reduces risk of NTDs
Some cancers	Many cancers cluster in families – shared genes and environmental factors Breast, ovarian, prostate, colorectal cancers	Smoking a major environmental risk factor. Infectious agents cause some cancers, e.g. human papilloma virus causes cervical cancer. Screening can identify and permit treatment at early stage
Heart disease	Narrowing of arteries by **atherosclerosis** → **myocardial infarction**. Family history common	Obesity, **hypertension**, cigarette smoking, raised cholesterol. Reduce risk by exercise, low salt and sugar diet
Stroke	Loss of blood to brain (clot or haemorrhage). Causes include single gene disorders + other conditions	Family history increases risk with factors as above. Management to reduce risk
Hypertension	Raised blood pressure – increases risk of cardiac (heart) disease or stroke	Manage risk as for heart disease
Type 2 diabetes	Some **insulin** resistance → raised blood glucose. Often obese. Family history, mainly older (40 years +)	Exercise, reduced calorie diet to reduce obesity
Alzheimer's disease	60-70% of progressive cognitive decline in older people with amyloid plaques and tangles in the brain. Family history common	Variation in modes of inheritance
Narcolepsy	Sudden sleeping episodes. Associated with specific **human leucocyte antigen** (HLA) or MHC (**major histocompatibility complex**) genes	See in Chapter 7, Disorders of Immunity and Defence
Psychiatric disorders	Schizophrenia, **bipolar disorder, autism spectrum disorder**: tend to cluster in families and have genetic factors involved	Treatment aims to modify **neurotransmitter** receptors, ion channels and relevant enzymes

Source: Adapted from Boore et al., 2016; Jorde et al., 2016; Mosaad, 2015; Pitkin, 2007; Strachan et al., 2015

GO DEEPER

Genetics and psychiatric disorders

If you are interested in more on the genetics of psychiatric disorders watch the following short video. If you are using the eBook just click on the play button. Alternatively go to

https://study.sagepub.com/essentialpatho/videos

GENETICS OF PSYCHIATRIC
DISORDERS (4:28)

MITOCHONDRIAL DISEASES

Mitochondria play a vital role in energy management for body function with several hundred mitochondria in each cell of the body. Each mitochondrion contains mitochondrial DNA, with the total mitochondrial DNA comprising a very small amount of the total DNA of the body. These organelles play their role in energy management through producing ATP (adenosine tri-phosphate), the source of energy for all cellular metabolism. Highly active organs have high ATP requirements, thus needing large numbers of mitochondria with their DNA: as such these organs are most seriously affected by mitochondrial diseases.

Each mitochondrion contains several copies of the mitochondrial genome. All the mitochondria and their DNA come from the ovum from the mother. Only the head of the sperm enters the ovum, the middle piece and the tail are left outside the ovum and the middle piece contains all the mitochondria in the sperm. Each body cell contains a population of mitochondria and mutations (i.e. changes in the DNA sequence) can occur in any of them, although leaving some unaffected. The mutation rate of mitochondrial DNA is some 10 times greater than nuclear DNA.

There can be considerable variation in the distribution of mutations through each cell and the different tissues, known as **heteroplasmy**, which can result in considerable variation through the body (Jorde et al., 2016). A range of types of mutation can occur, comparable to those that happen in nuclear DNA. A wide range of mitochondrial disorders can occur, some resulting in severe disabilities. However, heteroplasmy can influence the severity of the mitochondrial disorder. Hundreds of different mitochondrial disorders have been identified (Jorde et al., 2016) (Table 5.8).

Mitochondrial mutations have also been associated with some common human diseases. These include late-onset deafness and **Alzheimer's disease**. It has also been suggested that mitochondrial mutations occurring through life may make a possible contribution to ageing.

Table 5.8 Examples of mitochondrial diseases

Missense mutation (causes a different amino acid to be produced)	
Leber hereditary optic **neuropathy** (1 in 10,000)	Optic nerve death, rapid loss of vision in central visual field. Age of onset 7–75. Visual changes are irreversible
Single base mutation	
Myoclonic **epilepsy** with ragged red fibre syndrome	Epilepsy, dementia, ataxia (uncoordinated muscle movement), myopathy (muscle disease). Presents variably
Mitochondrial encephalomyopathy	Stroke-like episodes. Highly variable presentation
Duplications and deletions	

Missense mutation (causes a different amino acid to be produced)

Kearns–Sayre disease	Muscle weakness, damage to cerebellum, **heart failure**
Pearson syndrome	Infantile pancreatic insufficiency, pancytopenia, lactic **acidosis**

Source: Adapted from Jorde et al., 2016

GO DEEPER

Mitochondrial disorder

Chronic progressive external **ophthalmoplegia** is another mitochondrial disorder.

Symptoms include: weakness of eye muscles, typically appearing in adults 18–40 years, slowly worsening. The first sign is typically drooping eyelids.

APPLY

Mitochondrial replacement therapy

In 2015, the UK became the first country to pass laws to permit the use of mitochondrial replacement therapy to prevent the birth of babies with fatal mitochondrial diseases (BBC, 2015). This process involves three-person IVF developing what is known as three-parent babies and is approved by the Human Fertilisation and Embryology Authority (HFEA). The term three-parent baby is somewhat misleading as, within each cell, between 1 and 0.1% of the DNA is from the mitochondria of the donor with the remainder, within the nucleus, from the parents. Figures 5.1 and 5.2 clarify the two possible processes for producing a healthy embryo, embryo repair or egg repair.

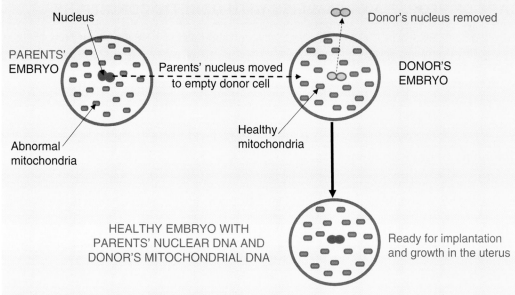

●● = Nuclear DNA from both parents

Figure 5.1 Repair of embryo

(Continued)

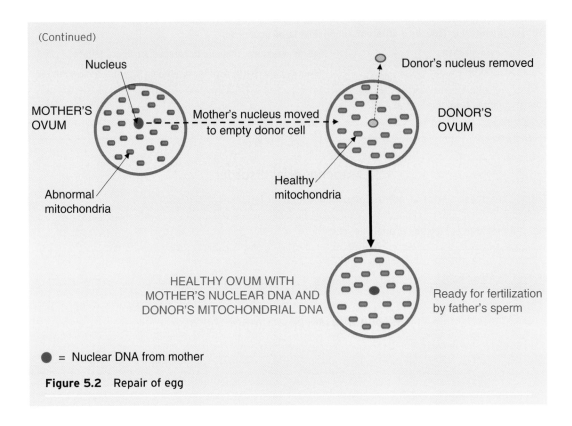

Figure 5.2 Repair of egg

CARE OF PEOPLE AND FAMILIES WITH GENETIC CONDITIONS

Individuals and families with genetic disorders need different types of assistance to facilitate living as normal a life as possible. These fall into three main areas:

* Diagnosing and managing the care of people with genetic conditions
* Genetic counselling
* Management of genetic conditions.

Diagnosis of genetic disorders

The first stage in working with individuals with genetic disorders and their families is identification of the particular disorder and how it is transmitted through generations. A major technique used is development of a family tree (genogram).

Family histories

A family tree is the foundation for assessment of genetic disorders and it is important that this is documented clearly and accurately. Information about the symbols used and some examples of family trees are included in Chapter 3 of *Essentials of Anatomy and Physiology for Nursing Practice* (Boore et al., 2016). A family tree needs to be well organised and a number of recommendations will help to achieve this (Table 5.9).

Table 5.9 Preparing family trees

1	Obtain details about the person affected followed by family members (parents, children, siblings)
2	Collect information about one side of the family and then the other side, as far as grandparents or further back if possible
3	Specifically find out about deceased relatives, including perinatal deaths
4	Include non-biologically related relatives (i.e. step-siblings, in-laws, adoptees), making the relationship clear on the pedigree
5	Ask about consanguinity (relationship by blood) (common in some cultures but not in others)
6	Private and sensitive information may be needed, e.g. pregnancies including terminations, paternity
7	Separating family trees for different branches of the family will enable identification of shared information
8	Check whether there is any further information that may be useful. At each meeting check whether there have been any changes

Source: Adapted from Skirton et al., 2005: 37–9

Careful completion of the family tree is the first step in identification of genetic disorders. The pattern of presentation of the condition in different family members through generations enables the type of inheritance to be identified. Along with the specific signs and symptoms, and often a number of blood and other clinical tests, the individual disease can usually be identified. However, when achieving a diagnosis it is necessary to take account of the fact that the same condition may present with varying severity and at different stages in life.

ACTIVITY 5.4: UNDERSTAND

Creating a family tree (genogram)

Try to draw your family tree. This will help you to understand the process for times when you may need to help patients produce their own genogram. Use the resources below to guide you:

www.scotgen.org.uk/learning-objects/drawing-a-family-history/

www.genome.gov/pages/education/modules/yourfamilyhealthhistory.pdf

Risk assessment

Completion of a family history and achievement of a diagnosis will usually enable risk assessment for the particular condition, i.e. the chance of occurrence of the condition in an individual, their offspring, or in other relatives will be estimated. This can be calculated when three conditions are met:

1. The diagnosis is certain.
2. The mode of inheritance is understood.
3. The biological relationship between those concerned is known. (Skirton et al., 2005)

In relation to occurrence of a genetic condition, it is important that parents are quite clear that the risk identified is for each pregnancy. For example, if the risk of a particular condition occurring in a baby born of particular parents is 1 in 4 (as with a recessive condition when both parents carry one gene for the condition), then every future offspring from those parents also has a risk of recurrence of 1 in 4. As important as the numerical risk of recurrence is the importance placed by those concerned on personal factors such as previous experience of the condition (e.g. in other family members) and their understanding of the rate of occurrence in the population at large of this condition.

As knowledge of genetics and epigenetics and disease has developed, and continues to increase (see Boore et al., 2016), the potential for helping people with such conditions is also enhanced. Thus, risk assessment is carried out on a greater scale than previously, focusing on several different groups (Skirton et al., 2005). In addition to the family history, two key aspects of structure and function are examined:

1. Disturbances of metabolism or structure which may be diagnostic of the specific condition.
2. The genetic makeup of the cell, i.e. the chromosomes (made of DNA) of the cell (normally 22 pairs of autosomes and one pair of sex chromosomes: XX (female) or XY (male) – 46 in total) and the chromosomes within the mitochondria of the cell. Genetic analysis allows abnormalities of the DNA to be identified.

Pre-symptomatic screening

There are a number of genetic alterations which can give rise to disorders later in life and which are usually suspected as a result of the family history. Examination of the DNA of individuals in these families can now enable such conditions to be diagnosed before symptoms develop and clinical surveillance used to identify pathological changes early. Table 5.10 shows examples of tests used in such surveillance.

Table 5.10 Some tests used for clinical surveillance in certain genetic disorders

Tests	Conditions	Inheritance	Notes
Colonoscopy (Using a thin, flexible tube, a colonoscope, to look at the colon)	Familial adenomatous polyposis	Autosomal dominant	Colorectal cancer syndrome, hundreds of adenomatous colorectal polyps, almost inevitably progresses to colorectal cancer at about 35-40 years. Screening performed from 10 to 12 years for early diagnosis and treatment. Recessive version less serious
	Hereditary non-polyposis colorectal cancer (Lynch syndrome)	Autosomal dominant	With high risk of colon cancer and range of other cancers, e.g. ovary, stomach, small intestine, hepatobiliary tract, upper urinary tract, brain and skin. It is a type of cancer syndrome
	Peutz–Jeghers syndrome	Autosomal dominant	Malformations resembling polyps, usually **benign**, in gastrointestinal tract and hyperpigmented macules (discoloured areas) on the lips and oral mucosa. May develop into cancer
Mammogram (X-ray picture of breast - breast cancer check)	Familial breast and ovarian cancer	Autosomal dominant	Genes *BRCA1* and *BRCA2* are associated with hereditary breast (female and male) and ovarian cancer syndrome, ovarian cancer (includes fallopian tube and primary peritoneal cancers), and some other cancers e.g. **prostate cancer**, pancreatic cancer and melanoma. Some patients have surgery (e.g. double **mastectomy**) before malignancy develops

Tests	Conditions	Inheritance	Notes
Echocardiogram (high-pitched ultrasound waves echo of parts of heart)	Marfan syndrome	Autosomal dominant	Variable disorder of **connective tissue**. Those affected are tall and thin, with long arms, legs, fingers and toes, flexible joints and **scoliosis**. The heart, blood vessels, bones, joints and eyes; lungs, skin and nervous system may be affected. Aortic enlargement can be life-threatening
	Hypertropic cardiomyopathy	Autosomal dominant	Enlarged heart muscle. An important cause of disability and death in patients of all ages, sudden and unexpected death in young people is the most devastating presentation
Renal ultrasound (sound waves make images of the kidneys, ureters and bladder)	Adult polycystic kidney disease	Autosomal dominant	Causes small, fluid-filled sacs (cysts) to develop in the kidneys, usually diagnosed in adults over 30 years of age: abdominal pain, hypertension, **haematuria**, calculi → **renal failure**
	Tuberous sclerosis	Autosomal dominant	Multisystem disease causing benign tumours in brain and other vital organs, e.g. kidneys, heart, liver, eyes, lungs and skin. Symptoms may include **seizures**, intellectual disability, developmental delay, behavioural problems, skin abnormalities, and lung and kidney disease
	von Hippel–Lindau syndrome	Autosomal dominant	Mutation in tumour-suppressing gene. Development of vascular tumours, e.g. retinal and cerebellar haemangiomas, **phaeochromocytomas**, renal and liver cysts, renal cell carcinoma
Serum iron studies (concentration of iron in blood and body)	Hereditary haemochromatosis (adult, juvenile and neonatal forms)	Autosomal recessive (types 1, 2, 3) Autosomal dominant (type 4)	Both copies of the gene in each cell have mutations. The parents of an individual with this condition each carry one copy of the mutated gene but do not show signs and symptoms of the condition
			One copy of the altered gene in each cell is sufficient to cause the disorder. In most cases, an affected person has one parent with the condition
			Inappropriate absorption of iron by small intestine leads to iron deposited in viscera, endocrine organs, and other sites, causing structural injury and impaired function; e.g. lens of eye, **basal ganglia** of brain, or range of tissues including liver, heart and endocrine system. Prompt diagnosis and depletion of tissue iron by chelating agents and venesection may be life-saving

Source: Adapted from Galiatsatos and Foulkes, 2006; Griffiths and Cox, 2015; Maron, 2002; Petrucelli et al., 2016; Skirton et al., 2005

Postnatal screening

The commonest and easiest screening is carried out shortly after birth in many countries. A range of metabolic disorders (mostly rare) are tested for by obtaining a blood sample from a heel prick.

Many conditions can be treated effectively if caught early. Table 5.11 lists a number of conditions routinely tested for in the UK (Great Ormond Street Hospital, 2012).

Table 5.11 Examples of conditions tested for on a postnatal heel prick in the UK

Phenylketonuria (PKU)

Congenital hypothyroidism (CHT)

Sickle cell disease (SCD)

Cystic fibrosis (CF)

Medium-chain acyl-CoA dehydrogenase deficiency (MCADD)

Homocystinuria (HCU)

Maple syrup urine disease (MSUD)

Glutaric acidaemia type 1 (GA1)

Isovaleric acidaemia (IVA)

APPLY

DANIELLE ZUMA
CASE NOTES

Heel prick test

Danielle is the youngest member of the Bodie family and was born in hospital in Brussels.

A heel prick test shortly after birth checked Danielle for a range of metabolic conditions which can be treated effectively if diagnosed early. If any abnormal results are found, the baby and parents concerned are referred for specialist treatment. However, Danielle's results were all normal, causing relief to her parents, Michelle and Kwame Zuma.

Prenatal diagnosis

Prenatal testing is carried out with the overall aim of identifying the risk of a child with a genetic condition and variation being born, thus enabling the parents to make informed choices about the continuation of the pregnancy. At this stage, it is important to consider the ethical implications of prenatal testing, and nurses and health care professionals must be educated and adequately prepared to offer support and information to women and couples in making an informed autonomous decision. It must also be noted that difference and disability must be valued and disabled people treated equally and fairly.

ACTIVITY 5.5: APPLY

Ethics and prenatal screening

It is important that you are well-versed on the ethical issues that accompany genetic screening. Read this article to develop your insight and reflect on the dilemmas that are faced by people in this position:

Reid, B., Sinclair, M., Barr, O., Dobbs, F. and Crealey, G. (2009) A meta-synthesis of pregnant women's decision-making processes with regard to antenatal screening for Down syndrome. *Social Science & Medicine, 69* (11): 1561-73.

If you are using the eBook you can access the article directly by clicking the icon.

ARTICLE: ETHICS OF
PRENATAL SCREENING

A number of techniques are used to identify a range of genetic disorders in the fetus (i.e. before birth) (Table 5.12).

Table 5.12 Techniques for prenatal diagnosis

Type	Specific methods	Notes
Visualisation of anatomical disturbances	Ultrasound (sonogram)	High-frequency sound waves bounce off different parts of the body and create 'echoes' which probe turns into a moving image of internal organs. Diagnosis of genetic syndromes identifies fetal, placenta and amniotic abnormalities, followed by invasive testing. Most accurate during 2nd trimester but also useful earlier and later. Cranial changes allow spina bifida diagnosis. Increased thickness of fluid in nuchal fold at back of the neck often indicates Down syndrome
	Magnetic resonance imaging	Fetal MRI complements an ultrasound examination either confirming the findings or acquiring additional information about fetal abnormality. Not used as a primary screening tool in prenatal care; better reserved for later in 2nd or 3rd trimester when pathologies can be seen more readily. MRI may help parents decide on the future of their pregnancy
	Radiography (rarely)	10 weeks' gestation onwards, fetal skeleton visibility enables diagnosis of inherited skeletal dysplasia, particularly disorders of bone and cartilage development, in 2nd and 3rd trimesters. Rarely used – dangers of radiation to fetus
Invasive genetic analysis of fetal cells	Amniocentesis	15-17 weeks' gestation: with ultrasound guidance, 20-30 ml of amniotic fluid is aspirated via a needle through the abdominal wall. Fetal cells in the fluid are grown and genetic analysis performed
	Chorionic villus sampling	10-11 weeks' gestation: sample of chorionic villi cells are aspirated via cervical or abdominal approach for genetic analysis. Early examination enables termination of pregnancy during first trimester
	Non-invasive prenatal testing (NIPT)	9-10 weeks' gestation: blood sample from pregnant woman. No risk of miscarriage. Accurate prenatal screening test for Down, Edwards and Patau syndromes
	Percutaneous umbilical cord blood sampling (PUBS)	With ultrasound guidance, 20 or 22 gauge spinal needle is inserted through the abdominal wall into a relatively stable segment of the umbilical cord and a blood sample taken. Contraindicated in a fetus under the age of 18 weeks due to risk of complications. Typically reserved for pregnancies at high risk for genetic defect

(Continued)

Table 5.12 (Continued)

Type	Specific methods	Notes
Genetic analysis before pregnancy initiated	Pre-conception	Carried out when a genetic condition is known to occur in the family or ethnic group, or for some reason, a family history has been performed and indicates that there may be some inherited disease or deformity. The parents are tested before conception to identify their carrier status to guide appropriate decision-making
	Pre-implantation	Used with in vitro fertilisation (IVF) when an ovum is fertilised by a sperm in a laboratory. About 3 days after fertilisation
		The embryo contains 6–8 cells (blastomeres), one or two of which can be removed and examined with two techniques:
		1. FISH (fluorescence in situ hybridisation) which can determine whether part of a chromosome is missing
		2. PCR (polymerase chain reaction) – replication of short, specific DNA sequence allows examination of very small amounts of DNA to assess genetic variation and diagnose disease
		Diagnosis of genetic conditions enables implantation of unaffected embryos. See section on heterozygote screening

Source: Adapted from Chaoui and Nicolaides, 2010; Conner et al., 2014; Jorde et al., 2016; Kaback, 2000; Krakow et al., 2009; Mastenbroek et al., 2007; Mastenbroek et al., 2011; Prayer et al., 2017; Schneider et al., 2009; Skirton et al., 2005; Strachan et al., 2015

GO DEEPER

Pregnancy screening

During pregnancy it is common practice to undertake scans to examine the stage of pregnancy and anatomical disturbances. If you are interested in more detail watch the following video. If you are using the eBook just click on the play button. Alternatively go to

https://study.sagepub.com/essentialpatho/videos

PREGNANCY SCREENING (2:34)

Heterozygote screening

Pre-conception genetic analysis is useful when there is a known possibility of carrier status in the planned parents. There are various conditions which are transmitted in an autosomal recessive manner. **Heterozygote screening** enables the genetic status to be identified pre-conception with relevant education and counselling facilitating people in their decision-making (Kaback, 2000).

When both parents are carriers of the gene, prenatal diagnosis using amniocentesis (obtaining a sample of amniotic fluid around the fetus) or chorionic villus sampling (obtaining a small sample of cells from the placenta) can identify a fetus with the condition. Alternatively, using preimplantation genetic diagnosis linked with in vitro fertilisation, the embryo is tested prior to implantation. Healthy embryos are transferred into the mother's uterus. One condition where this is possible is **Tay–Sachs disease**.

--- **GO DEEPER** ---

Tay-Sachs disease

Tay-Sachs disease is a neurological autosomal recessive disorder. It was relatively common among Ashkenazi Jews (i.e. descendants from France, Germany and Eastern Europe comprising the majority of the Jewish population of North America and the UK) who have a carrier frequency of about 1 in 30 in their population.

Carriers of one Tay-Sachs gene do not have signs and symptoms of the disease. However, they do appear to have some protection against **tuberculosis** (TB) and populations with this genetic trait have a lower death rate from TB than non-Jewish groups in similar areas. It appears that they have a selective advantage (Withrock et al., 2015). Similar relationships occur with some other conditions where carrier status can provide a protective status for particular infectious diseases.

To minimise the incidence of Tay-Sachs disease, heterozygote screening among the Jewish community has become standard using various approaches. An organisation called Dor Yeshorim, also called the Committee for Prevention of Jewish Genetic Diseases, has offices worldwide and offers mate selection screening to members of the Jewish community globally (Ekstein and Katzenstein, 2001). It aims to reduce, and eventually eliminate, the incidence of serious genetic disorders common among the Jewish population. It works to achieve this by avoiding marriage between carriers through screening, information and counselling early in a potential relationship. This population screening approach has developed since the 1970s and the worldwide incidence of Tay-Sachs disease has reduced by 90% (Schneider et al., 2009).

The following video provides additional information about Tay-Sachs disease. If you are using the eBook just click on the play button. Alternatively go to

https://study.sagepub.com/essentialpatho/videos

TAY-SACHS DISEASE (4:33)

Genetic counselling

This area of work is based on precise diagnosis and understanding of human genetics and is derived from this rather than from the behavioural sciences as is the more usual counselling. However, high-quality communication skills are essential for working with those affected with genetic conditions. Genetic counselling was defined by the American Society for Human Genetics (ASSH, 1975) and this definition is still accepted in North America, the UK and many other countries.

Genetic counselling is defined as:

> a communication process which deals with human problems associated with the occurrence, or the risk of occurrence, of a genetic disorder in a family. (ASHG, 1975: 240)

The aims of genetic counselling are to help the individual or family:

- Understand the information about the genetic condition
- Appreciate the inheritance pattern and risk of recurrence
- Understand the options available
- Make decisions appropriate to their personal and family situation
- Make the best possible adjustment to the disorder or risk of recurrence.

The overall aim is to help people to gain sufficient understanding of their situation so that they can make informed decisions about what they wish to do (Skirton et al., 2005). In addition to the genetic counselling as considered above, those working with people with genetic disorders and their families will need to be able to provide more individual counselling to help them adapt to living with the condition that they have. In addition, there are always going to be individuals receiving care who will have restricted life spans and both the individuals and their families need access to resources and support to adjust to the expected change in their lives.

Genetic services in the UK are normally provided within regional specialist centres where teams of medical and non-medical specialists apply their specific expertise. A considerable proportion of the genetic counsellors are nurses by background and recognised as such by the Association of Genetic Nurses and Counsellors (AGNC, 2015). This organisation represents genetic counsellors, genetic nurses and other non-medical staff working with patients in the UK and Ireland within Clinical Genetics, NHS Genomic Medicine Centres and other relevant health care settings. This organisation expects that its members are registered with the Genetic Counsellor Registration Board (GCRB, 2017) whose vision is *'ensuring expertise to serve families with genetic conditions'*. It aims to:

> establish, maintain and improve standards of practice in genetic counselling to assure public safety in the United Kingdom and Republic of Ireland through accepting responsibility for:
>
> * Setting and monitoring standards for entry to the profession
> * Establishing and maintaining open and transparent systems of professional accreditation
> * Maintaining and improving standards of professional practice, to protect and promote the professional reputation for the benefit of the profession and public alike. (GCRB, 2017: 1)

Having reviewed the principles of genetic counselling, it is also important to consider briefly the range of other activities involved in working with those with genetic disorders and their families.

Management of genetic conditions

Professional practice

Working within genetic services will mainly involve dealing with a number of people, with a range of relatively common conditions. However, every so often someone will be diagnosed with a rare complex condition who may need intervention from a number of different specialist teams. The genetic team will usually take on the coordinating role with the different specialists (Skirton et al., 2005). Those working in genetic services also take responsibility for arranging genetic screening and for maintaining clinical registers. Such registers can be used to contact individuals when a new treatment is introduced or to ensure that appropriate support services are being made available. This may include offering screening to individuals within affected families at relevant stages in life.

Confidentiality is one of the key ethical principles when maintaining such registers and when working with those with these conditions. If a family history identifies someone else within the family who is at risk of having the condition, then permission must be obtained from the initial person identified to let others in the family know the situation. Application of the range of activities of professional practice can greatly influence the incidence of genetic disorders and the quality of life of people affected.

Boundaries of practice

In most countries, those working as professionals within any field of health care are required to hold professional statutory registration. They must have received appropriate education for the role they are undertaking and are responsible for working within the limits of their ability. Often a senior colleague may act as a supervisor to enable relatively inexperienced staff to continue to develop their own expertise, and protect the patient from mistakes.

Within this specialist area of work, the practitioners will take responsibility for ensuring that their practice is based on the latest evidence. In addition, they are likely to be involved in collaborating with others to undertake research to contribute to the development of that evidence.

Treatment approaches

Gene therapy

We have already looked at approaches to dealing with mitochondrial disorders. The Go Deeper box below introduces some issues related to developments in management of genetically related conditions.

GO DEEPER

Developments in the management of genetic conditions

A number of developments have occurred which relate to the content of this chapter and are introduced here.

Watch the three videos below. The first is on Iceland's 'Genetic Goldmine' and how Iceland is proving an invaluable resource for genetic research. The second explores an approach to editing DNA called CRISPR. If you are using the eBook just click on the play buttons. The third introduces new approaches to individualised care under the banner of Precision Health. Alternatively go to:

https://study.sagepub.com/essentialpatho/videos

GENETIC RESEARCH
IN ICELAND (2:25)

EDITING DNA (4:12)

PRECISION HEALTH (2:26)

CHAPTER SUMMARY

We hope that you now understand how important genetic inheritance can be in the presentation of disease. Many disorders result from a balance between nature (genetics and some environmental factors) and nurture (lifestyle and behavioural factors). Understanding this will help you recognise the importance of person-centredness in enabling individuals and their families to adjust their lifestyle to recognise and make personal decisions about the risk of the particular disease developing and to manage the situation for the optimum quality of life.

- The three laws of Dominance, Segregation and Independent Assortment summarise how genes are transmitted between generations.

- There are a number of different modes of genetic inheritance shown in the section on the principles of inheritance and genetic disturbances at the beginning of this chapter.

- Completion of a family history is central to understanding the mode of inheritance and, with additional examination and tests, helps to achieve a diagnosis.

- There are a number of approaches used in assessment of the risk of developing a genetic disorder. Some can be used to prevent conception or birth of an affected child, others to diagnose a potential metabolic or other diagnosis and give treatment to control development, or to diagnose early changes and treat before manifestation of the full disease, e.g. colon or breast cancer.

- Chromosomal abnormalities can result in a number of disorders. The main groups are autosomal aneuploidy, when the number of autosomes is abnormal, and sex chromosome aneuploidy, when the sex chromosome number is altered. Autosomal aneuploidies tend to have more serious effects than sex chromosomal disorders.

- There are three factors which influence the expression of single gene disorders: germline mosaicism, penetrance and variable expression. The three main modes of inheritance are dominant, recessive and X-linked.

- Polygenic inheritance involves a number of genes. Multifactorial inheritance is based on a combination of genes and environmental factors and is often involved in chronic diseases. Management of environmental factors is key in these disorders.

- Mitochondrial diseases are passed only through the mother and can result in varying severity of disease, some very severe. The so-called 'three-parent child' is a recent approach to developing a healthy offspring through embryo or egg repair when the abnormal mitochondria are replaced by healthy mitochondria from a donor.

- Genetic counselling is important in helping parents to understand the condition and make informed decisions about their future. Those working in this field are also involved in the range of provision and activities within the genetic services.

REVISE

TEST YOUR KNOWLEDGE

Studying this chapter will help you to understand the genetic causes of disease and, thus, identify the sorts of problems with which your patients and families may need help. Revise the different sections in turn then try to answer the questions below.

Answers are available online. If you are using the eBook just click on the answers icon below. Alternatively go to **https://study.sagepub.com/essentialpatho/answers**

1. Discuss the major recommendations for completing a family history and indicate the importance in helping to identify genetic disorders.

2. Identify how screening is used in risk assessment in relation to genetic disorders, giving some examples of the approaches used for diagnosing different disorders.

3. Clarify the differences between autosomal and sex hormone aneuploidy, and give some examples from the two groups and their implications for quality of life.

4   What are the three factors which influence expression of an abnormal gene? Differentiate between the characteristics of dominant and recessive gene disorders and give some examples of each.

5   Differentiate between polygenic and multifactorial disorders. Discuss the importance of environmental factors in multifactorial chronic diseases.

6   Summarise your understanding of mitochondrial diseases and clarify how three-parent babies are created and their importance.

7   Discuss the contribution of health care workers in working within genetic services.

- Further revision and learning opportunities are available online

- Test yourself away from the book with **Extra multiple choice questions**

- Learn and revise terminology with **Interactive flashcards**

REVISE

ACE YOUR ASSESSMENT

If you are using the eBook access each resource by clicking on the respective icon. Alternatively go to **https://study.sagepub.com/essentialpatho/chapter5**

CHAPTER 5 ANSWERS

EXTRA QUESTIONS

FLASHCARDS

REFERENCES

AAAA (American Academy of Allergy, Asthma and Immunology) (2018) Atopy defined. Available at: www.aaaai.org/conditions-and-treatments/conditions-dictionary/atopy (accessed 4 December 2018).

AGNC (Association of Genetic Nurses and Counsellors) (2015) About us. Available at: www.agnc.org.uk/about-us/ (accessed 8 May 2017).

ASHG (American Society of Human Genetics Ad Hoc Committee on Genetic Counseling) (1975) Genetic counseling. *American Journal of Human Genetics*, 27: 240–42.

BBC (2015) UK approves three-person babies. By J. Gallagher (Health Editor), BBC News, 24 February 2015. Available at: www.bbc.co.uk/news/health-31594856 (accessed 17 May 2017).

Boore, J., Cook, N. and Shepherd, A. (2016) *Essentials of Anatomy and Physiology for Nursing Practice*. London: Sage.

Chaoui, R. and Nicolaides, K.H. (2010) From nuchal translucency to intracranial translucency: towards the early detection of spina bifida. *Ultrasound in Obstetrics and Gynecology*, 35 (2): 133–8.

Conner, S.N., Longman, R.E. and Cahill, A.G. (2014) The role of ultrasound in the diagnosis of fetal genetic syndromes: best practice and research. *Clinical Obstetrics and Gynaecology*, 28 (3): 417–28.

Cystic Fibrosis Registry (2015) Annual Data Report. www.cysticfibrosis.org.uk/registryreports (accessed 4 October 2018).

Ekstein, J. and Katzenstein, H. (2001) The Dor Yeshorim story: community-based carrier screening for Tay–Sachs disease. *Advances in Genetics*, 44: 297–310.

Galiatsatos, P. and Foulkes, W.D. (2006) Familial adenomatous polyposis. *American Journal of Gastroenterology*, 101: 385–98.

GCRB (Genetic Counsellor Registration Board) (2017) Home page. Available at: www.gcrb.org.uk (accessed 5 August 2017).

Great Ormond Street Hospital (2012) *Newborn Blood Spot Screening.* London: Great Ormond Street Hospital for Children NHS Foundation Trust.

Griffiths, W.J.H. and Cox, T.M. (2015) Hereditary haemochromatosis. In D.A. Warrell, T.M. Cox and D. John (eds), *Oxford Textbook of Medicine*, 5th edn. Oxford: Oxford University Press. Available at: Oxford Medicine Online, doi: 10.1093/med/9780199204854.003.120701_update_003 (accessed 26 May 2017).

ICR (Institute of Cancer Research) (2015) Nearly half of testicular cancer risk comes from inherited genetic faults. Available at: www.icr.ac.uk/news-archive/nearly-half-of-testicular-cancer-risk-comes-from-inherited-genetic-faults (accessed 18 November 2017).

Jessberger, R. (2012) Age-related aneuploidy through cohesion exhaustion. 'Exploring aneuploidy: the significance of chromosomal imbalance' review series. *European Molecular Biology Organization Reports*, pp. 539–46.

Jorde, L.B., Carey, J.C. and Bamshad M.J. (2016) *Medical Genetics.* Philadelphia, PA: Saunders, Elsevier.

Kaback, M.M. (2000) Population-based genetic screening for reproductive counselling: the Tay–Sachs disease model. *European Journal of Pediatrics, 159* (Suppl. 3): S192–5.

Krakow, D., Lachman, R.S. and Rimoin, D.L. (2009) Guidelines for the prenatal diagnosis of fetal skeletal dysplasias. *Genetics in Medicine, 11*: 127–33.

Kumar, V., Abbas, A.K. and Aster, J.C. (eds) (2018) *Robbins and Cotran Pathologic Basis of Disease,* 9th edn. Philadelphia, PA: Saunders, Elsevier.

Lenroot, R.K., Lee, N.R. and Giedd, J.N. (2009) Effects of sex chromosome aneuploidies on brain development: evidence from neuroimaging studies. *Developmental Disabilities Research Reviews, Special Issue: Cognitive Profiles in Sex Chromosome Disorders, 15* (4): 318–27.

Loktionov, A. (2003) Common gene polymorphisms and nutrition: emerging links with pathogenesis of multifactorial chronic diseases (Review). *Journal of Nutritional Biochemistry, 14*: 426–51.

Maitra, A. (2015) The endocrine system. In V. Kumar, A.K. Abbas and J.C. Aster (eds), *Robbins and Cotran Pathologic Basis of Disease*, 9th edn. Philadelphia, PA: Saunders, Elsevier.

Maron, B.J. (2002) Hypertrophic cardiomyopathy: a systematic review. *JAMA, 287* (10): 1308–20.

Mastenbroek, S., Twisk, M., Echten-Arends, J.V., Sikkema-Raddatz, B., Korevaar, J.C., Verhoeve, H.R. et al. (2007) In vitro fertilization with preimplantation genetic screening. *New England Journal of Medicine, 357*: 9–17.

Mastenbroek, S., Twisk, M., van der Veen, F. and Repping, S. (2011) Preimplantation genetic screening: a systematic review and meta-analysis of RCTs. *Human Reproductive Update, 17* (4): 454–66.

Moreira, A. and Das, H. (2018) Acute life-threatening hemorrhage in neonates with severe hemophilia A: a report of 3 cases. *Journal of Investigative Medicine High Impact Case Reports, 6*: 1–5.

Mosaad, Y.M. (2015) Clinical role of human leukocyte antigen in health and disease. *Scandinavian Journal of Immunology, 82* (4): 283–306.

Nagaoka, S.I., Hassold, T.J. and Hunt, P.A. (2012) Human aneuploidy: mechanisms and new insights into an age-old problem. *Nature Reviews/Genetics, 13*: 493–504.

NCI (2017) NCI Dictionary of Genetics Terms. USA, National Cancer Institute at the National Institutes of Health Available at: www.cancer.gov/publications/dictionaries/genetics-dictionary?cdrid=460164 (accessed 6 May 2017).

Panicker, V. (2011) Genetics of thyroid function and disease. *Clinical Biochemist Reviews, 32* (4): 165–75.

Petitjean, A., Achatz, M.I.W., Borresen-Dale, A.L., Hainaut, P. and Olivier, M. (2007) TP53 mutations in human cancers: functional selection and impact on cancer prognosis and outcomes. *Oncogene, 26*: 2157–65.

Petrucelli, N., Daly, M.B. and Pal, T. (2016) *BRCA1*- and *BRCA2*-associated hereditary breast and ovarian cancer. In R.A. Pagon, M.P. Adam, H.H. Ardinger et al. (eds), *GeneReviews* [Internet]. Seattle, WA:

University of Washington, Seattle (1998 Sep 4; updated 2016 Dec 15). Available at: www.ncbi.nlm.nih.gov/books/NBK1247/ (accessed 25 April 2017).

Pitkin, R.M. (2007) Folate and neural tube defects. *American Journal of Clinical Nutrition*, 85 (1): 285S–288S.

Prayer, D., Malinger, G., Brugger, P.C., Cassady, C., De Catte, L., De Keersmaecker, B. et al. (2017) ISUOG Practice Guidelines: performance of fetal magnetic resonance imaging. *Ultrasound in Obstetrics and Gynecology*, 49 (5): 671–80. doi: 10.1002/uog.17412.

Schneider, A., Nakagawa, S., Keep, R., Dorsainville, D., Charrow, J., Aleck, K. et al. (2009) Population-based Tay–Sachs screening among Ashkenazi Jewish young adults in the 21st century: hexosaminidase A enzyme assay is essential for accurate testing. *American Journal of Medical Genetics, Part A, 149A*: 2444–7.

Simpson, N.H., Addis, L., Brandler, W.M., Slonims, V., Clark, A., Watson, J. et al. (SLI Consortium) (2014) Increased prevalence of sex chromosome aneuploidies in specific language impairment and dyslexia. *Developmental Medicine and Child Neurology*, 56 (4): 346–53.

Skirton, H., Patch, C. and Williams, J. (2005) *Applied Genetics in Healthcare: A Handbook for Specialist Practitioners*. New York/Abingdon: Taylor and Francis/T & F Informa.

Strachan, T., Goodship, J. and Chinnery, P. (2015) *Genetics and Genomics in Medicine*. New York/Abingdon: Garland Science/Taylor and Francis.

Stuitje, G., van Belzen, M.J., Gardiner, S.L., van Roon-Mom, W.M.C., Boogaard, M.W., REGISTRY Investigators of the European Huntington Disease Network et al. (2017) Age of onset in Huntington's disease is influenced by CAG repeat variations in other polyglutamine disease-associated genes. *Brain, 140* (7).

Surget, S., Khoury, M.P. and Bourdon, J.-C. (2014) Uncovering the role of p53 splice variants in human malignancy: a clinical perspective. *OncoTargets and Therapy*, 7: 57–68.

Tabrizi, S. (2017) Excitement as trial shows Huntington's drug could slow progress of disease. Press Release, 11 December, University College London.

Withrock, I.C., Anderson, S.J., Jefferson, M.A., McCormack, G.R., Mlynarczyk, G.S.A., Nakama, A. et al. (2015) Genetic diseases conferring resistance to infectious diseases. *Genes and Diseases, 2* (3): 247–54.

World Health Organisation (WHO) (2018) Human genomics in global health. World Health Organisation. Available at: www.who.int/genomics/about/commondiseases/en/ (accessed 12 January 2018).

MENTAL ILL-HEALTH

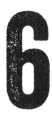

6

UNDERSTAND: CHAPTER VIDEOS

Watch this video to ease you into this chapter. If you are using the eBook just click on the play button. Alternatively go to **https://study.sagepub.com/essentialpatho/videos**

SCIENCE OF
DEPRESSION (3:45)

LEARNING OUTCOMES

When you have finished studying this chapter you will be able to:

1. Discuss the altered physiology of mood disorders, **schizophrenia** and **autism spectrum disorder** (ASD).
2. Apply the pathophysiology of mental ill-health to practice.
3. Appreciate the personal impact of mental ill-health and the centrality of person-centred care in successful management.

INTRODUCTION

In this chapter, you will examine the biological basis underpinning a small range of conditions that lead to mental ill-health. The disorders considered in this chapter are largely neurological in origin in that they originate at the time of the central nervous system developing (neurodevelopmental) or are as a result of dysfunction in the mood circuitry of the central nervous system. While disorders causing mental ill-health have not traditionally been viewed as neurological in origin, advances in science over recent years have enabled their origins to be tracked more definitely and this remains an area of emerging new knowledge. Considering the centrality of mental health in our health-related quality of life, understanding the origins of these disorders is central to providing holistic, person-centred care.

The connection between positive mental and physical health is well established; both are integral to maintaining **homeostasis** and health-related quality of life. The reverse is also true; altered physiological processes can impact on mental health. When we think of the key role that the nervous system plays in our identities and in the processing of our experiences, thoughts and feelings through life, it is logical that altered neurological functioning can lead to mental ill-health. Indeed, it may be exposure to **stress** and anxiety that is the precursor in some cases. There is therefore truth in the saying that there is no health without mental health. Indeed, mental ill-health places a person at greater risk of a general medical condition (Chesnaye and Kemp, 2016).

In 2010, depressive disorders accounted for around 40% of **disability-adjusted life years** (DALYs); 14.6% of these were anxiety disorders, 7.4% were related to schizophrenia and 7% related to **bipolar disorder** (Whiteford et al., 2013). Within this context, the likelihood of a nurse caring for a person experiencing or having experienced mental ill-health is high; this requires nurses to have sufficient understanding of common mental ill-health disorders in order to provide informed, person-centred care. Only through a collective understanding of mental ill-health can we begin to offset the human, personal, social and economic impact of mental illness (Vigo et al., 2016).

In this chapter, we are going to limit our focus to mood disorders (unipolar depression and bipolar disorder), schizophrenia and autism spectrum disorder (ASD). These disorders have been chosen as they have well-established pathophysiological origins in a field where research and understanding of the pathophysiological basis of mental ill-health are still emerging. We should make it clear that ASD is not traditionally viewed as a mental health disorder but more as a developmental disorder. However, you will learn that it is technically a neurodevelopmental disorder that has an initial common pathway with schizophrenia and it can have elements of mental ill-health. Thus, we are including it in this chapter. This chapter does not intend to cover the pathophysiology of all disorders leading to mental ill-health; those concerned with the mental health field of nursing will need to study further.

——— PERSON-CENTRED CONTEXT: THE BODIE FAMILY ———

BODIE FAMILY
CASE NOTES

If we consider the Bodie family, only one family member, Matthew, has a diagnosis of enduring mental ill-health; **depression** can be classified as a neurological disorder due to pathophysiological changes in the amygdala, **hippocampus** and **prefrontal cortex** (Savitz et al., 2013). Additionally, depression has been isolated as a risk factor for **Alzheimer's disease** (Xu et al., 2015) (Chapter 16). Matthew is fortunate in that his prescribed drug therapy is effective as he is concordant and vigilant in taking it as prescribed. As you will learn in this chapter, continuing treatment long term is essential for recovery. In addition, the exercise that Matthew undertakes will also help to promote his mental health.

While Matthew may be the only person with an enduring mental ill-health disorder, other members of the Bodie family are at risk. For example, you will learn in this chapter that stress and anxiety are two common triggers for developing depression (unipolar and bipolar). Richard Jones has experienced stress in the past that was successfully managed through cognitive behavioural therapy; if this had not been addressed, it may have led to the development of depression. Hannah Jones works as a social worker and may be exposed to social situations that are stressful and anxiety-provoking; being able to manage this is essential to prevent mental ill-health.

REVISE: A&P RECAP

The stress response

It will be helpful at this stage to revise your knowledge of the stress response; this will heighten your understanding of the impact of stress on physical health. For an effective summary look at Chapter 7, The Endocrine System, in *Essentials of Anatomy and Physiology for Nursing Practice* (Boore et al., 2016).

MOOD DISORDERS

Unipolar depression

When we refer to depression, we are largely referring to unipolar depression as opposed to the bipolar form, which we will look at separately. Depression affects approximately 17% of people at some stage in life (Duman, 2014). The impact of this on health-related quality of life is significant and can be experienced as immense suffering. Understanding the pathophysiological cause of depression is important in not only understanding its causes to maximise prevention, but also in understanding the basis for treatment. In this sense, this chapter will only consider the biological issues and will not deal with personal therapies and the evidence underpinning them. You will need to explore those issues separately while having an understanding of the biological elements.

Marcus et al. (2012) identify that depression is characterised by low mood, a loss of pleasure or interest, reduced energy and feelings of guilt or low self-worth. This is usually accompanied by sleep and/or appetite dysfunction, reduced concentration and, often, debilitating anxiety. The impact is profound in that depression can be debilitating, leaving the person unable to self-care and function effectively in society. In extreme cases it can lead to suicide. Considering the devastation that depression can cause in someone's life and to the lives of those who love and care for them, understanding its origins is paramount. As a person-centred nurse, regardless of what your field of practice is, you are likely to encounter people living with depression. While they need your compassion and support, they also need your understanding.

It is well established that mood is regulated by a circuit of **neurons** between the prefrontal cortex, hippocampus, **cingulate** cortex, amygdala and basal ganglia. When this circuitry is disrupted, the potential for a mood disorder arises, particularly when connections from the prefrontal cortex to other areas are reduced (Duman, 2014); hippocampal and prefrontal cortex volume reduction are classically seen in people with depression. Belzung et al. (2015) identify that the impairment in performance **cognition** seen in depression is also related to this mood circuitry in that it cannot de-activate, impairing cognition.

In the last 20 years, research has increasingly been able to identify the pathophysiological basis of depression. In 2002, Duman highlighted that stress and anxiety were key factors that could result in depression. Ongoing exposure to both stress and anxiety are known to result in **atrophy** of pyramidal neurons in the hippocampus; this leads to a reduction in dendrite numbers and length in the hippocampus and an associated decrease in hippocampal volume. The net result is impairment of neuronal connections in this part of the brain. Considering the role of the hippocampus in the limbic system, this is thought to be one key cause of depression. The hippocampus is one of the few areas of the brain where new neurons can be generated, and so this leads us to believe that hippocampal causes of depression are potentially reversible (Duman, 2002). In addition, there is a reduction in the volume of neurons and **neuroglia** of the subgenual prefrontal cortex of the brain in people with depression.

It is clear that the hippocampus and prefrontal cortex are areas of concern, but what leads to such degenerative changes? A number of factors have been identified and they include (Carvalho et al., 2014; Duman, 2002, 2014):

- **Hyperactivation** of the **hypothalamic–pituitary–adrenal** (HPA) axis; this has a major role in the response to stress and hyperactivation results in reduced support to neurons by neuroglia
- Overactivation of receptors for the excitatory **neurotransmitter glutamate**, leading to damage of intracellular organelles that can result in neuronal death
- Pathogenic destruction
- Genetic predisposition.

Essentially, altered **synaptogenesis** occurs in the neural circuits between the prefrontal cortex (PFC), hippocampus, cingulate cortex, amygdala and basal ganglia as a result of excess **glucocorticoids**, reduced glial support to neurons (trophic support) and inflammatory cytokine damage (Carvalho et al., 2014). Raised serum levels of proinflammatory **cytokines** can result in fatigue and suppressed appetite, symptoms often seen in those with depression (Duman, 2014). Stress also decreases the numbers of **astrocytes** and **oligodendrocytes** in the prefrontal cortex of those with depression, leaving neurons more vulnerable to **oxidative stress** and synaptic dysfunction.

In addition to these traditional views on the causes of depression, it is now identified that a biological stress response can lead to neuronal hypertrophy in the amygdala (Duman, 2014). This is thought to increase emotional responses to situations and also increase anxiety in those with depression. A reduction in hippocampal and prefrontal cortex volume and hypertrophy of the amygdala leads to increased activity in other areas of the limbic system (Duman, 2014), resulting in dysfunction in mood regulation. There is also thought to be a reduction in spinal synapses in those with depression. Młyniec et al. (2015) have also identified that a number of elements are essential to homeostasis of the neurotransmitters/ hormones involved in regulating mood:

- Calcium
- Chromium
- Copper
- Iodine
- Iron
- Lithium
- Magnesium
- Manganese
- Selenium
- Vanadium
- Zinc

Depression and neurotransmitters

The link between depression and neurotransmitter dysfunction has long been the basis of treatment. Anomalies in **dopamine** levels are thought to impair motivation and concentration, and reduced noradrenaline (norepinephrine) and dopamine levels are associated with fatigue and **hypersomnia**.

In addition, noradrenaline and serotonin dysregulation is associated with other physical symptoms. While many antidepressant medications focus on improving these levels, however, it is the return to homeostatic functioning of the HPA axis and enlargement of the hippocampus from its diminished size that are associated with recovery. This suggests that it is the effect of these neurotransmitters on **neurogenesis** and trophic factors that is key.

APPLY

Antidepressant therapy

Antidepressant therapy has become the mainstay of medical management of depression alongside other therapeutic interventions (e.g. psychotherapy, cognitive behavioural therapy). The main mode of action of antidepressants is to counter the actions of stress. For example, tianeptine prevents stress-related atrophy in pyramidal neurons (Duman, 2002). Other antidepressants (**serotonin and norepinephrine reuptake inhibitors [(SNRIs]**) result in increased cell production and inhibit the stress factors that block neurogenesis. Over time, it is thought that such effects reverse hippocampal atrophy and other neural damage caused by stress, leading to recovery of mood regulation (Duman, 2002, 2014).

In more recent years, N-methyl-D-aspartate (**NMDA) receptor antagonists**, such as ketamine, have been found to have swift and prolonged antidepressant actions by inducing new spinal synapses and reversing synaptic atrophy (Duman, 2014). This results in the reestablishment of the neuronal circuity that regulates mood.

Interestingly, the long-term use of antidepressant medication is also seen to result in an increased number of oligodendrocytes in the prefrontal cortex, resulting in greater trophic support to neurons (Duman, 2014). This is important as it stresses the necessity for antidepressant therapy to be continued if it is to have lasting effects.

Healy (2015) cautions us about the myth around the use of SSRIs. Read his views in the article 'Serotonin and depression: The marketing of a myth', available at https://davidhealy.org/articles

If you are using the eBook you can get to the article directly by clicking on the icon.

ARTICLE: SEROTONIN
AND DEPRESSION

ACTIVITY 6.1: APPLY

Signs and symptoms of depression

Watch this video to get an insight into the signs and symptoms of depression from those who have experienced it. Reflect on how open we are to acknowledging and responding to those who may have signs and symptoms. If you are using the eBook just click on the play button. Alternatively go to **https://study.sagepub.com/essentialpatho/videos**

SYMPTOMS OF
DEPRESSION (3:50)

Bipolar disorder

Bipolar disorder is a severe, enduring mood disorder whereby the person experiences periods of mania, **hypomania** (when someone is persistently disinhibited and euphoric) alongside periods of depression. The condition affects greater than 1% of the global population and it is considered to be the most heritable psychiatric disorder (Grande et al., 2016). As in other mood disorders, the condition is thought to be as a result of dysfunction in the neural circuitry that regulates mood, particularly the prefrontal cortex (see under Unipolar depression), as well as an imbalance in neurotransmitters within the circuitry, namely serotonin, noradrenaline and particularly dopamine (Grande et al., 2016). The **disease** process is thought

APPLY

Classifications of bipolar disorder

Bipolar disorder is clinically classified as follows by the American Psychiatric Association (APA) (2013):

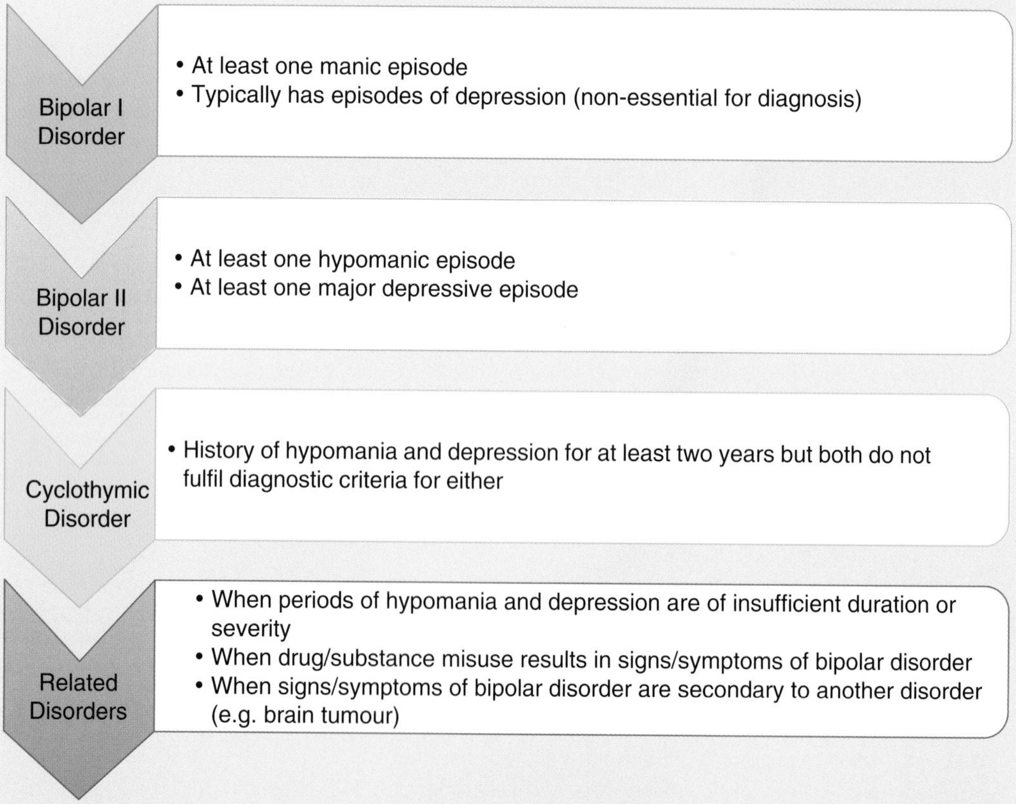

Bipolar I Disorder
- At least one manic episode
- Typically has episodes of depression (non-essential for diagnosis)

Bipolar II Disorder
- At least one hypomanic episode
- At least one major depressive episode

Cyclothymic Disorder
- History of hypomania and depression for at least two years but both do not fulfil diagnostic criteria for either

Related Disorders
- When periods of hypomania and depression are of insufficient duration or severity
- When drug/substance misuse results in signs/symptoms of bipolar disorder
- When signs/symptoms of bipolar disorder are secondary to another disorder (e.g. brain tumour)

Figure 6.1 Bipolar disorder DSM classification

It is important to highlight that recovery and exacerbation of symptoms are all part and parcel of mental ill-health and wellness. As a result, bipolar disorder can be cyclical in nature as the person moves between wellness and mental ill-health.

to be brought about by someone having a genetic susceptibility to the condition which, when combined with some form of environmental trigger (which is not yet fully understood), leads to a set of biochemical circumstances that cause and progressively exacerbate inflammatory and oxidative stress damage (Scaini et al., 2016). As with unipolar depression, **dendritic spine** loss is noted in those with bipolar disorder. Similarly, oxidative stress is implicated in neural damage, specifically as a result of reduced phosphates and pH along with lactate build-up (Callaly et al., 2015). These are linked to the hypothesised disruption to enzymes essential for cellular respiration in the **mitochondria**, particularly complex I (the largest enzyme involved), resulting in the neural disruption in bipolar disorder (Callaly et al., 2015; Scaini et al., 2016); remember, mitochondria are the powerhouses of cells and so have a central role in the neuron surviving or dying. This range of complex processes results in **apoptosis** and neurogenesis being deregulated in the neurons in the mood circuitry of the brain and in the supporting glial cells.

APPLY

Exercise and bipolar disorder

While it is well known that physical exercise is good for improving cardiovascular health, the evidence shows that it is one of the most effective non-pharmacological interventions for bipolar disorder. This is particularly the case when endurance training is engaged with as it promotes the production of new mitochondria and improved antioxidant supply to neurons, reducing stress damage from free radical production (Scaini et al., 2016).

ACTIVITY 6.2: APPLY

Signs and symptoms of bipolar disorder

Watch this video to get an insight into the signs and symptoms of bipolar disorder. Reflect on how exhausting and emotionally demanding it may feel to live feeling this way. If you are using the eBook just click on the play button. Alternatively go to

https://study.sagepub.com/essentialpatho/videos

SYMPTOMS OF BIPOLAR
DISORDER (1:00)

SCHIZOPHRENIA AND AUTISM SPECTRUM DISORDER (ASD)

The developing brain is vulnerable. Any form of attack from **pathogen**s or an autoimmune process has the potential to have enduring and pronounced effects on the person throughout their life span (Meyer et al., 2011). In recent decades, intrauterine infection and subsequent neonatal white matter inflammatory damage have been identified as key factors that give rise to both schizophrenia and autism spectrum disorder (ASD). While these terms are not synonymous, both conditions are known to have organisational and operational irregularities in multiple areas of the central nervous system (CNS): the cerebellum, insular cortex, fusiform gyrus, hippocampus, posterior cingulate, putamen, claustrum and left **thalamus** (Meyer et al., 2011).

Schizophrenia is a **syndrome** that occurs late in adolescence or early adulthood; it may occur earlier in life but the signs are not as apparent as younger people are in a state of development. Schizophrenia is characterised by signs of psychosis that include paranoid delusions and auditory hallucinations (Insel, 2010). Despite shared beginnings, ASD is very different to schizophrenia. ASD is a group of developmental disorders with symptoms that are seen on a continuum ranging from mild to severe. These symptoms include deficits in social reciprocity, communication challenges and repetitive behaviours that may be considered by some as unusual and restrictive (Hyman, 2013). It is considered to be a neurodevelopmental disorder, the reasons for which will become clear, with an onset early in life. *It is important to highlight that ASD is not considered a mental health disorder; its inclusion in this chapter is because of the shared origins with schizophrenia.*

A **glycoprotein** called **reelin** has been implicated in both conditions. Reelin is secreted into the extracellular matrix whereby it signals migrating neurons and their position in the developing brain. Its role is central in the development and lamination of the prenatal cortex (Bradshaw et al., 2017). Altered reelin expression is associated with impaired neuronal connectivity and synaptic plasticity; the cognitive impairment present in both schizophrenia and ASD is attributed, at least in part, to reelin-related developmental abnormalities (Folsom and Fatemi, 2013). The process of how this occurs is not yet fully understood.

In both schizophrenia and ASD, it is thought that there is an environmental factor that triggers a genetic susceptibility to the condition; the environmental factor is thought to be maternal infection during

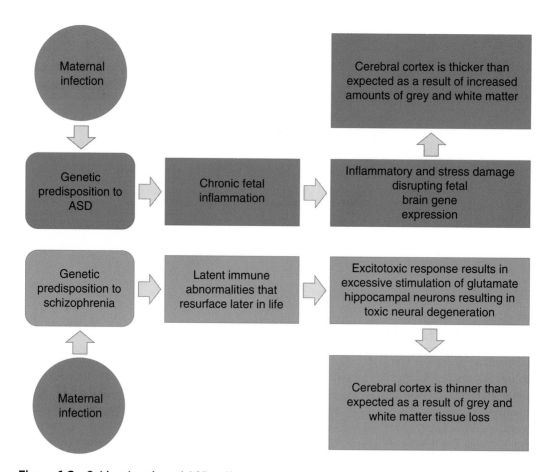

Figure 6.2 Schizophrenia and ASD pathways

pregnancy and, while a number of bacterial and viral illnesses are identified, it appears that the trigger is not pathogen-specific (Meyer et al., 2011). Rather, the issue appears to be that infection leads to increased levels of proinflammatory cytokines which negatively affect the developing fetal brain; cytokines can trigger cellular apoptosis and inhibit protein synthesis. They therefore have the potential to disrupt neurogenesis, neuronal plasticity and the survival of neurons (Meyer et al., 2011). While schizophrenia and ASD may have this initial common pathophysiological pathway, how they progress is different. Indeed, it is theorised that the response to the maternal infection and different genetic susceptibilities are key factors in whether ASD or schizophrenia occurs and this response is genetically determined (Figure 6.2).

Schizophrenia

Microcephaly is a common characteristic of schizophrenia. The cerebral cortex is found to be thinner than expected due to a loss of grey and white matter tissue. It is thought that once maternal infection occurs, anti-inflammatory and/or immunosuppressive activities may resolve the acute fetal inflammatory response but may also result in latent immune abnormalities that may resurface in later life when the person is exposed to stress or re-exposed to the original pathogen (Meyer et al., 2011). This is one explanation for why schizophrenia manifests later in life than ASD. Another variant on this theory is that the insult to the developing brain could be compensated for earlier in life, but this compensation failed as the child and the brain matured (Insel, 2010). As schizophrenia develops as the person grows and matures, it can present in stages (Figure 6.3).

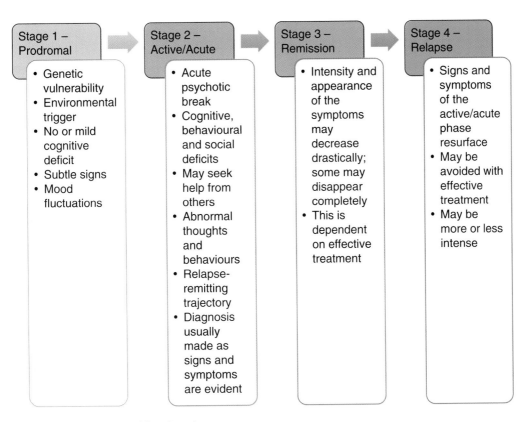

Figure 6.3 Stages of schizophrenia

As found in mood disorders, **excitotoxicity** is considered to cause excessive stimulation of glutamate hippocampal neurons, resulting in toxic degeneration; this is thought to explain the reduced volume in the **amygdala**, hippocampus and prefrontal cortex in schizophrenia. This neuronal loss results in reduced cognitive performance skills as the prefrontal cortex is not being activated. It also impairs sleep regulation. Other consequences of neural dysfunction are attributed to hormonal imbalances, particularly with regards to dopamine, serotonin and glutamate neurotransmitters. In particular, hyperactivity of **dopaminergic** neurons in the limbic system is thought to be the key imbalance. This is why medications blocking dopamine result in a reduction in psychotic symptoms and those that increase dopamine levels exacerbate symptoms.

ACTIVITY 6.3: APPLY

Signs and symptoms of schizophrenia

Watch this video to get an insight into how schizophrenia *may* be experienced by someone. Reflect on how insightful and aware we are of how someone may be affected. If you are using the eBook just click on the play button. Alternatively go to
https://study.sagepub.com/essentialpatho/videos

SYMPTOMS OF
SCHIZOPHRENIA (4:19)

ACTIVITY 6.4: UNDERSTAND

Pathophysiology of psychosis

Watch the following video to strengthen your understanding of psychosis and the pathophysiological causes. If you are using the eBook just click on the play button. Alternatively go to
https://study.sagepub.com/essentialpatho/videos

PATHOPHYSIOLOGY OF
PSYCHOSIS (9:42)

Autism spectrum disorder (ASD)

In ASD, **macrocephaly** is a prominent characteristic where there are increased amounts of grey and white matter, leading to thickening of the cerebral cortex (Meyer et al., 2011). In contrast to schizophrenia, maternal infection may result in persistent fetal **inflammation** that becomes chronic, resulting in inflammatory and stress damage to the developing brain. This maternal immune activation is thought to dysregulate fundamental elements of fetal brain **gene expression** that leads to ASD (Lombardo et al., 2017). The pathophysiology of ASD is not yet fully understood and remains an area of further research and investigation. ASD is genetically **heterogeneous** and the strength of its genetic influence results in a sibling recurrence risk of up to 50% in some populations (Sandin et al., 2014).

PERSON-CENTREDNESS AND MENTAL ILL-HEALTH

Laird et al. (2015) highlight that people are often exposed to vulnerability in the care experiences. When services, systems and care processes are not cohesive, people feel disempowered and experience an increase in vulnerability. Considering those with mental ill-health are often the most vulnerable and stigmatised in our society, it is essential that nurses ensure that the care they provide does not diminish self-worth. It is essential that nurses are affirmed in their person-centred values if their practice is to be compassionate and collaborative with those in their care (Schwind et al., 2014). Laird et al. (2015) highlight that this care should be experienced in a family-like atmosphere where there is a shared sense of belonging between nurses and those in their care.

While you have learned about the biological origins of selected disorders that cause mental ill-health, it is essential that you contextualise this knowledge alongside your professional values and the lived experience of having mental ill-health. This is necessary to ensure your care revolves around people, rather than the technicalities of the biological processes. Research shows that people living with mental ill-health feel they have an invisible disability (Kidd et al., 2015); if people cannot see it, they are less compassionate and considerate of how it affects those affected. People affected by mental ill-health are on a journey to find meaning in their lives and part of that journey is feeling accepted by those supporting them and learning to live with the stigma of mental illness. Pescosolido (2013) highlights that while neurobiology has made great gains in understanding mental ill-health, this knowledge has not reduced the stigma of having such disorders. It is therefore not neurobiological knowledge alone that will improve the care experience of people with mental ill-health; it is also the culture we create as nurses. Pescosolido (2013) highlights that stigma emanates from social relationships and therefore the solution to minimising stigma lies in an understanding that is wider than knowledge but extends to the nature of these social relationships, highlighted by Laird et al. (2015) and Schwind et al. (2014). The Apply sections below are intended to encourage you to engage with the lived experience of people so that the knowledge you gain in this chapter is considered in the context of understanding mental ill-health more fully.

ACTIVITY 6.5: UNDERSTAND

Living with depression

Unless you have experienced mental ill-health in your life, and you may well have, you may find that it is difficult to fully appreciate the experience of life with a condition such as depression. Watch this short video on living with depression that captures the lived experience. If you are using the eBook just click on the play button. Alternatively go to

https://study.sagepub.com/essentialpatho/videos

LIVING WITH
DEPRESSION (4:18)

ACTIVITY 6.6: APPLY

Supporting people with mental ill-health

The World Health Organisation (WHO) has produced a short video as a guide for partners, carers and sufferers of depression to provide advice for those living with and caring for people with depression on what to do, what not to do, and where to go for help. If you are using the eBook just click on the play button. Alternatively go to **https://study.sagepub.com/essentialpatho/videos**

DEPRESSION FOR
PARTNERS (5:56)

APPLY

Stress and cognition

Psychological stress has a well-documented relationship with impairing cognition (Oumohand and Breteler, 2017). When we are exposed to psychological distress, there is an increase in catecholamine levels as a result of the stress response. Within the prefrontal cortex, this raised level of catecholamines reduces neuronal activity (it is inhibitory), impairing cognitive processes (Arnsten, 2015). When stress becomes chronic, structural changes occur in the prefrontal cortex that lead to a progressive loss of function, including in relation to cognition. This is why people who have ongoing stress can find it hard to think or to source solutions, and can make poor judgements on occasion. Supporting people in finding ways to manage their levels of stress is central to preserving cognition function and therefore health-related quality of life.

CHAPTER SUMMARY

By now, you will be aware of the complexity of mental ill-health affecting people in society. Not only are the neurobiological elements of these disorders complex and still a focus of emerging science, the social complexity of how these disorders are perceived further challenges us as health care professionals in terms of supporting people and their families. These conditions negatively influence health-related quality of life and a compassionate and informed approach to care is needed, regardless of your field of nursing. Mental health is not something confined to mental health professionals; all nurses must acknowledge and address the mental health components of someone's health if we are to be holistic and person-centred in our care. As a nurse, you are highly likely to encounter a person who has experienced mental ill-health at some stage in their life. As a person-centred practitioner, it is important to remember that mental ill-health can change the life of a person and their family significantly and often for life. Understanding the conditions leads to better insights into appropriate care and such informed practice on your part will positively influence the care received.

- Depression (unipolar depression) and bipolar disorder are disorders that are primarily neurological in origin when there is inflammatory cytokine damage and destruction of neural tissue that result in a loss of volume in the hippocampus and prefrontal cortex. The mood circuitry of the brain is subsequently disrupted.

- Serotonin, dopamine and noradrenaline (norepinephrine) are the three key neurotransmitters central to the regulation of mood and the recovery of disrupted neural mood circuitry.

- Schizophrenia and ASD both share an initial common pathway in that maternal infection is thought to trigger an immune-related response that impacts negatively on neurodevelopment.

- In schizophrenia, the cerebral cortex is thinner than expected as a result of grey and white matter tissue loss secondary to latent immune abnormalities resurfacing later in life; the excitotoxic response that occurs results in excessive stimulation of glutamate hippocampal neurons, resulting in toxic degeneration.

- In ASD, the cerebral cortex is thicker than expected as a result of increased amounts of grey and white matter; persistent fetal inflammation as a result of maternal infection causes inflammatory and stress damage, disrupting fetal brain gene expression.

- Nurses need to appreciate the lived experience of people with mental ill-health in order to contextualise the neurobiology of disorders with the everyday challenges faced in managing life.

REVISE

In this chapter, you will have examined the biological basis underpinning a small range of conditions that lead to mental ill-health. Use the following questions to test your knowledge and understanding.

TEST YOUR KNOWLEDGE

Answers are available online. If you are using the eBook just click on the answers icon below. Alternatively go to **https://study.sagepub.com/essentialpatho/answers**

1 What is unipolar depression and what is thought to cause it?

2 What are the three main neurotransmitters associated with mood disorders?

3 What is bipolar disorder and what is thought to cause it?

4 What common pathophysiological pathway do ASD and schizophrenia share?

5 What is thought to cause schizophrenia after the initial common pathway?

6 What is thought to cause ASD after the initial common pathway?

7 What are the factors that people with mental ill-health feel positively influence their care?

REFERENCES

American Psychiatric Association (APA) (2013) *Diagnostic and Statistical Manual of Mental Disorders,* 5th edn (DSM-5). Washington, DC: American Psychiatric Publishing.

Arnsten, A.F. (2015) Stress weakens prefrontal networks: molecular insults to higher cognition. *Nature Neuroscience, 18* (10): 1376–85.

Belzung, C., Willner, P. and Philippot, P. (2015) Depression: from psychopathology to pathophysiology. *Current Opinion in Neurobiology, 30*: 24–30.

Boore, J., Cook, N. and Shepherd, A. (2016) *Essentials of Anatomy and Physiology for Nursing Practice.* London: Sage.

Bradshaw, N.J., Trossbach, S.V., Köber, S., Walter, S., Prikulis, I., Weggen, S. et al. (2017) Disrupted in Schizophrenia 1 regulates the processing of reelin in the perinatal cortex. *Schizophrenia Research.* Epub ahead of print. https://doi.org/10.1016/j.schres.2017.04.012.

Callaly, E., Walder, K., Morris, G., Maes, M., Debnath, M. and Berk, M. (2015) Mitochondrial dysfunction in the pathophysiology of bipolar disorder: effects of pharmacotherapy. *Mini Reviews in Medicinal Chemistry, 15* (5): 355–65.

Carvalho, A.F., Miskowiak, K.K., Hyphantis, T.N., Kohler, C.A., Alves, G.S., Bortolato, B. et al. (2014) Cognitive dysfunction in depression–pathophysiology and novel targets. *CNS & Neurological Disorders – Drug Targets* (formerly *Current Drug Targets – CNS & Neurological Disorders*), *13* (10): 1819–35.

Chesnaye, P. and Kemp, P. (2016) Integrating mental and physical healthcare. *Nursing Times, 112* (32): 20–3.

Duman, R.S. (2002) Pathophysiology of depression: the concept of synaptic plasticity. *European Psychiatry, 17*: 306–10.

Duman, R.S. (2014) Pathophysiology of depression and innovative treatments: remodeling glutamatergic synaptic connections. *Dialogues in Clinical Neuroscience, 16* (1): 11–27.

Folsom, T.D. and Fatemi, S.H. (2013) The involvement of Reelin in neurodevelopmental disorders. *Neuropharmacology, 68*: 122–35.

Grande, I., Berk, M., Birmaher, B. and Vieta, E. (2016) Bipolar disorder. *The Lancet, 387* (10027): 1561–72.

Healy, D. (2015) Serotonin and depression. *BMJ, 350*: h1771.

Hyman, S. (ed.) (2013) *The Science of Mental Health – Volume 2: Autism.* New York: Routledge.

Insel, T.R. (2010) Rethinking schizophrenia. *Nature, 468* (7321): 187–93.

Kidd, S., Kenny, A. and McKinstry, C. (2015) The meaning of recovery in a regional mental health service: an action research study. *Journal of Advanced Nursing, 71* (1): 181–92.

Laird, E.A., McCance, T., McCormack, B. and Gribben, B. (2015) Patients' experiences of in-hospital care when nursing staff were engaged in a practice development programme to promote person-centredness: a narrative analysis study. *International Journal of Nursing Studies, 52* (9): 1454–62.

Lombardo, M.V., Moon, H.M., Su, J., Palmer, T.D., Courchesne, E. and Pramparo, T. (2017) Maternal immune activation dysregulation of the fetal brain transcriptome and relevance to the pathophysiology of autism spectrum disorder. *Molecular Psychiatry*. Epub ahead of print. doi: 10.1038/mp.2017.15.

Marcus, M., Yasamy, M.T., van Ommeren, M., Chisholm, D. and Saxena, S. (2012) Depression: a global public health concern. *WHO Department of Mental Health and Substance Abuse, 1*: 6–8.

Meyer, U., Feldon, J. and Dammann, O. (2011) Schizophrenia and autism: both shared and disorder-specific pathogenesis via perinatal inflammation? *Pediatric Research, 69*: 26R–33R.

Młyniec, K., Gaweł, M., Doboszewska, U., Starowicz, G., Pytka, K., Davies, C.L. et al. (2015) Essential elements in depression and anxiety. Part II. *Pharmacological Reports, 67* (2): 187–94.

Oumohand, S.E. and Breteler, M.M. (2017) Characterizing the relation between stress, cognition, and brain health on population level in the Rhineland Study. *Psychoneuroendocrinology, 83*: 22–3.

Pescosolido, B.A. (2013) The public stigma of mental illness: what do we think; what do we know; what can we prove? *Journal of Health and Social Behavior, 54* (1): 1–21.

Sandin, S., Lichtenstein, P., Kuja-Halkola, R., Larsson, H., Hultman, C.M. and Reichenberg, A. (2014) The familial risk of autism. *JAMA, 311* (17): 1770–7.

Savitz, J., Frank, M.B., Victor, T., Bebak, M., Marino, J.H., Bellgowan, P.S. et al. (2013) Inflammation and neurological disease-related genes are differentially expressed in depressed patients with mood disorders and correlate with morphometric and functional imaging abnormalities. *Brain, Behavior, and Immunity, 31*: 161–71.

Scaini, G., Rezin, G.T., Carvalho, A.F., Streck, E.L., Berk, M. and Quevedo, J. (2016) Mitochondrial dysfunction in bipolar disorder: evidence, pathophysiology and translational implications. *Neuroscience & Biobehavioral Reviews, 68*: 694–713.

Schwind, J.K., Lindsay, G.M., Coffey, S., Morrison, D. and Mildon, B. (2014) Opening the black-box of person-centred care: an arts-informed narrative inquiry into mental health education and practice. *Nurse Education Today, 34* (8): 1167–71.

Vigo, D., Thornicroft, G. and Atun, R. (2016) Estimating the true global burden of mental illness. *The Lancet Psychiatry, 3* (2): 171–8.

Whiteford, H.A., Degenhardt, L., Rehm, J., Baxter, A.J., Ferrari, A.J., Erskine, H.E. et al. (2013) Global burden of disease attributable to mental and substance use disorders: findings from the Global Burden of Disease Study 2010. *The Lancet, 382* (9904): 1575–86.

Xu, W., Tan, L., Wang, H.F., Jiang, T., Tan, M.S., Tan, L. et al. (2015) Meta-analysis of modifiable risk factors for Alzheimer's disease. *Journal of Neurology, Neurosurgery and Psychiatry, 86* (12): 1299–306.

SECTION 2

KEY CAUSES OF DISEASE

This section builds on the previous one and examines some of the key physiological disturbances that can influence the presentation of disease in various systems of the body. Later sections look at the different systems of the body and their disorders, but this section focuses on the way these disturbances occur and affect body tissues, including:

Chapter 7. Disorders of Immunity and Defence. The ways in which microorganisms can cause infection and the way in which the body tissues and organs respond to infection and influence function are considered. The immune system is central to this function but can also be disrupted as introduced in Boore et al. (2016). Here we examine these conditions and relate their effects on person-centred care.

Chapter 8. Disorders of Blood and Blood Supply. Disturbances in the blood supply to organs and tissues will cause deterioration of their function and thus influence homeostasis. As this can affect any organ of the body, the causes and alterations that occur in the blood vessels in atherosclerosis are considered here along with the effect on some of the major organs. Additionally, this chapter considers disorders of blood which can also have a widespread impact on homeostasis in all systems of the body.

Chapter 9. Cellular Adaptation and Neoplastic Disorders. The different ways in which cells grow and differentiate, adapt, become atrophied, hypertrophic or hyperplastic, etc. and the causes of the different types of cellular adaptation are considered in the context of disease. In addition, this chapter examines conditions when cells proliferate out of control, differentiates between characteristics of benign and malignant neoplasia (new, abnormal growth) and considers the different causes of tumours.

Chapter 10. Disorders of Support and Protection. Disorders of systems involved with support of the body and protection from the external environment are examined, including causes and effects of major disorders of the musculoskeletal system and skin. The emotional/psychological and social implications of such disorders are a central element of person-centred nursing and are included.

DISORDERS OF IMMUNITY AND DEFENCE

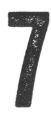

UNDERSTAND: CHAPTER VIDEOS

Watch the following videos to ease you into this chapter. If you are using the eBook just click on the play buttons. Alternatively go to **https://study.sagepub.com/essentialpatho/videos**

TYPES OF IMMUNE
RESPONSES (8:06)

B lymphocytes
(14:12)

LEARNING OUTCOMES

When you have finished studying this chapter you will be able to:

1. Explain the mechanisms of the immune response.
2. Describe the altered immune mechanisms that lead to hypersensitivity diseases.
3. Explain the mechanisms involved in autoimmune disease.
4. Discuss primary and secondary immunodeficiency disorders.
5. Outline the factors that make a microorganism pathogenic.
6. Identify measures that contribute to the control of sexually transmitted infections.
7. Discuss the signs of sepsis and how this can lead to septic shock.
8. Identify key challenges to infection prevention, control and treatment.

INTRODUCTION

Our defence system protects us from anything it perceives as foreign to the body and therefore a potential threat to **homeostasis**. The immune system is a finely tuned complex system that mounts a coordinated response to harmful substances such as infectious agents, and macromolecules such as proteins or chemicals. This is referred to as the immune response and it is essential to a healthy body. In certain circumstances some of the mechanisms of the immune response can break down, causing an ineffective response (immune deficiency), or an inappropriate response such as an exaggerated response to a substance or a response against the body's own cells. This can result in **disease**. In this chapter we start by reviewing the normal immune response mechanisms and then go on to look at what happens when the protective mechanisms of the immune response fail.

The immune system has evolved to protect and defend the body against infectious agents and foreign cells. Its finely tuned but complex mechanisms are effective in achieving this but sometimes it can react inappropriately, causing disease. In this chapter we will look at what happens when the immune system overreacts, resulting in a **hypersensitivity** disorder, reacts inadequately attacking the body's own tissue, resulting in autoimmune disorders, or fails to react, resulting in **immunodeficiency**. The subsequent effect on the body can range from mild to life-threatening illness.

REVISE: A&P RECAP

The immune system

Before reading this chapter, you may find it useful to revise the immune system. For a full summary see Chapter 13, The Immune System: Internal Protection, in *Essentials of Anatomy and Physiology for Nursing Practice* (Boore et al., 2016). Figure 13.1 (in Boore et al., 2016) clarifies the different aspects of the immune responses, and how the body responds through innate and adaptive immunity. The different lines of defence are demonstrated, including how the body removes infectious agents.

PERSON-CENTRED CONTEXT: THE BODIE FAMILY

BODIE FAMILY
CASE NOTES

Every day we come into contact with substances such as microorganisms or chemical toxins that require our immune systems to work to protect us against disease. Several factors such as our age, genetic makeup and the environment we live in can influence how we react to these substances and our risk of developing disease. Considering the Bodie family, George and Maud are now at an increased risk of acquiring infectious diseases because of their age and both get the flu vaccine every year to help reduce the risk of developing **influenza**. Derek Jones has asthma and takes anti-inflammatory medication as his immune system is over-reacting. Margaret Jones has hay fever which flares up and requires the use of anti-histamines to reduce her immune response to pollen. Kwame and Michelle Zuma travel to Africa frequently, requiring **vaccination** against microorganisms that they would not normally be exposed to. Their baby, Danielle, is currently having routine vaccinations to help her immune system protect her from childhood infections caused by **pathogens**.

IMMUNE DISORDERS

Disorders of the immune system result in homeostatic imbalances and fall into three broad categories: hypersensitivity, where the immune system overreacts; **autoimmunity**, where the immune system attacks the body's own tissues; and immunodeficiency, where components of the immune system fail (Figure 7.1).

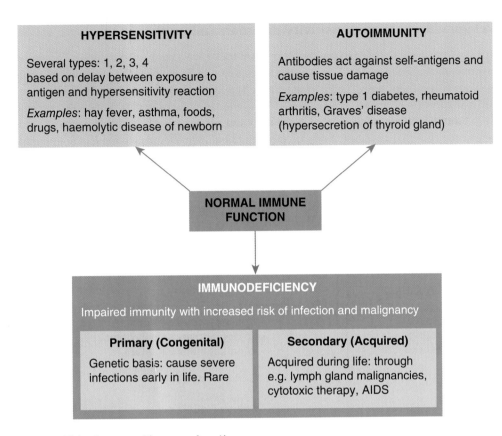

Figure 7.1 Disturbances of immune function

Source: Boore et al., 2016, Figure 13.10

HYPERSENSITIVITY

Hypersensitivity is when the immune response is altered, causing damage to cells, tissues and organs, and this is often in response to a substance that is normally harmless. Hypersensitivity diseases include allergy, autoimmunity (against **self-antigens**, failure of recognition) and **alloimmunity** (transplant tissue rejection). Hypersensitivity diseases are classified according to the type of immune response and the **antigen** responsible (Table 7.1).

Table 7.1 Classification of hypersensitivity diseases

Type of hypersensitivity	Immune mechanism	Mechanism of injury
Type I – immediate hypersensitivity	IgE antibody	Mast cells, eosinophils, mediators
Type II – antibody-mediated	IgM, IgG antibody against cell surface or extracellular matrix	Phagocytosis and opsonisation of cells
Type III – immune-complex-mediated	Immune complexes of circulating antigens and antibodies IgG or IgM	Complement-mediated activation of leucocytes
Type IV – T-cell-mediated	CD4⁺ T cells (helper T cells); CD8⁺ (cytotoxic/killer T cells)	Cytokine-mediated inflammation Direct target cell killing

Notes: IgE, Immunoglobulin E; IgM, immunoglobulin M; IgG immunoglobulin G.

Type I immediate hypersensitivity disorders (allergy)

A person has an allergy or type I hypersensitivity when they have a hypersensitive immune response to an environmental substance. This is one of the fastest growing conditions worldwide and is becoming a major public health problem (Tanno et al., 2016). This type of hypersensitivity is immediate and is known as an **allergic reaction**. The antigen, often referred to as the **allergen**, binds to immunoglobulin E (IgE) **antibodies** on the surface of **mast cells** and triggers a reaction specific to environmental antigens such as pollen, house dust, foods, shellfish, nuts and chemicals such as the antibiotic penicillin.

T-helper **lymphocytes**, or specifically T_h2 / CD4[+1] variant, are involved in allergic reactions and the production of IgE antibodies that trigger mast cells and **leucocytes**. These IgE antibodies bind to the mast cell on exposure to the antigen. This is called **sensitisation** and is the reason why this type of reaction occurs so rapidly on subsequent exposure to the antigen as the mast cell is now already coated with the IgE antibodies (Galli and Tsai, 2012). Mast cells are present in tissue, blood vessels and nerves, which is why many of the clinical features of an immediate reaction involve these sites due to vascular and smooth muscle stimulation. Once the mast cell is stimulated, it releases mediators and **cytokines** (Figure 7.2). The most potent mediator is **histamine** which causes bronchial smooth muscle contraction, **vasodilation**, increased vascular permeability and increased mucous production by nasal and bronchial glands.

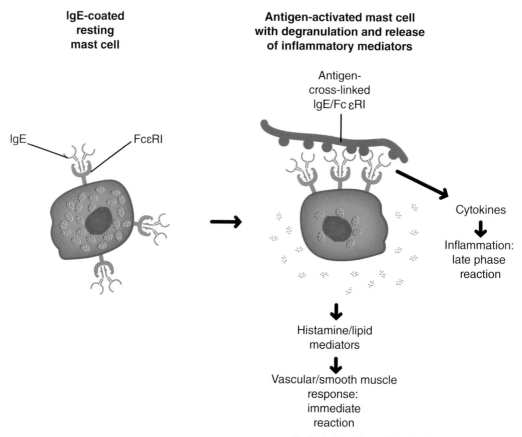

IgE-coated resting mast cell

Antigen-activated mast cell with degranulation and release of inflammatory mediators

Antigen-cross-linked IgE/Fc εRI

IgE

FcεRI

Cytokines

Inflammation: late phase reaction

Histamine/lipid mediators

Vascular/smooth muscle response: immediate reaction

Illustrated by Shaun Mercier © SAGE Publications

Figure 7.2 Activation of mast cells: IgE antibodies bind to receptors on the mast cell surface and stimulate degranulation and the release of histamine and cytokines

[1]FcεRI = high-affinity IgE receptor

[2]T_h1 cells and T_h2 cells differ in their function. T_h1 cells produce proinflammatory cytokines and mainly activate cell-mediate immunity whereas T_h2 cells produce anti-inflammatory cytokines and activate humoral immunity.

Histamine binds to **endothelial cells**, leading to increased vascular permeability and leakage of plasma into the tissues, resulting in **oedema**. Cytokines such as **tumour necrosis factor (TNF)** and **interleukins** are produced and are responsible for the **inflammation** associated with the delayed response. **Basophils** are also involved in type I hypersensitivity reactions in a similar way to mast cells.

There are two defined phases associated with many type I hypersensitivity reactions: a primary or immediate response and a late or delayed response. The immediate phase is associated with histamine release and usually occurs within minutes of exposure to the allergen. The tissues affected contain large numbers of mast cells and involve the skin, respiratory tract and gastrointestinal tract. Vasodilation of the vessels in the skin leads to oedema and **urticaria**, which is a skin reaction characterised by fluid-filled blisters known as wheals and surrounded by an area of redness known as flares (Figure 7.3). Bronchial smooth muscle spasm leads to bronchoconstriction and increased mucous secretion, causing difficulty in breathing. Inflammation of the mucous membranes of the nose (**rhinitis**) and membranes of the eyes (**conjunctivitis**) occurs and is a feature of allergic rhinitis (hay fever). The late phase response sustains the reaction and occurs hours later and can last for days, gradually subsiding. This phase involves **eosinophils** (white cells) which release **proteolytic enzymes** that damage tissue and is a feature of asthma.

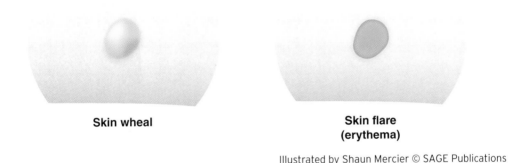

Skin wheal　　　　　　　　**Skin flare (erythema)**

Illustrated by Shaun Mercier © SAGE Publications

Figure 7.3 Skin reactions in allergy

Genetic susceptibility

Allergies often run in families and certain people are genetically predisposed to develop allergies, having higher than usual quantities of IgE. Patterns of inheritance are **multigenic**, leading to increased susceptibility for asthma and other atopic (allergy) diseases (Kaufmann and Demenais, 2012). Environmental factors have an impact on the development of allergy and exposure to microbes during early childhood is thought to reduce the risk of developing allergies later in life (Bufford and Gern, 2005).

APPLY

Antihistamines and asthma

Antihistamine use in allergic reactions can inhibit urticaria but in some allergic disorders, such as asthma, they are not effective at suppressing the reaction. In asthma, bronchoconstriction is more prolonged than the effects of histamine, suggesting that other mast-cell-derived mediators are involved.

Anaphylactic reactions

Anaphylactic reactions involve a systemic response to a hypersensitivity reaction, resulting in life-threatening clinical features such as difficulty in breathing due to severe bronchoconstriction, low blood pressure as a result of vasodilation and widespread oedema.

Anaphylactic reactions are type I hypersensitivities where the allergen is injected or absorbed across the epithelial membrane of the skin or gastrointestinal **mucosa**. This stimulates the mast cells in the area, resulting in the release of mediators which gain access to the vascular beds throughout the body (Reber et al., 2017). Systemic vasodilation and leakage cause oedema, decreased blood pressure and shock. There is constriction of the upper airways and laryngeal oedema, resulting in difficulty in breathing. This is accompanied by skin rash and itching. Gastrointestinal symptoms include **vomiting** and abdominal cramps. Anaphylactic reactions can be life-threatening and immediate management is to secure the airway and administer adrenaline/epinephrine to reverse the bronchoconstriction and vasodilation and improve **cardiac output**.

APPLY

Anaphylaxis and EpiPen

People with a known risk of **anaphylactic shock** need to carry an adrenaline/epinephrine 'pen' (EpiPen) with them at all times. This is to allow quick self-administration or administration by a bystander of adrenaline in the case of exposure to the allergen. Adrenaline binds to specific receptors on smooth muscle, reversing the effects of histamine, resulting in smooth muscle relaxation and reducing life-threatening bronchoconstriction.

Bronchial asthma

Bronchial asthma is an inflammatory disease of the airways caused by repeated immediate hypersensitivity and late phase allergic reactions (Abbas et al., 2015). The person with bronchial asthma will often have other allergic disorders, such as hay fever and **eczema**. The early phase response leads to reversible airway obstruction and difficulty in breathing due to bronchoconstriction and the production of thick **mucus**. There is also increased vascular permeability causing mucosal oedema. The late phase response leads to inflammation and increased airway responsiveness. Epithelial injury and changes in mucociliary function can result from chronic inflammation of the lung tissue. Mast cells, basophils and eosinophils produce mediators that cause constriction in airway smooth muscle. About 70% of asthma cases are associated with IgE-mediated reactions and 30% may be stimulated by non-immune stimuli such as cold air, exercise, **respiratory tract infections** or emotional upset (Abbas et al., 2015). See Chapter 14 for further information on bronchial asthma.

Allergic rhinitis (hay fever)

This is perhaps the most common allergic disease and is characterised by sneezing, itching and watery discharge from the nose and eyes. It is an immediate hypersensitive response to common allergens such as pollen, dust mites, fungal spores or animal hair and can occur all year round or seasonally when levels of the allergen are high, such as pollens in the summer months. There is mucosal oedema with leucocyte and eosinophil **infiltration**, and increased mucus secretion, resulting in coughing, sneezing and difficulty in breathing. This type of exposure is associated with intense symptoms. Management involves treating the symptoms and the use of antihistamines.

Food allergies

Food allergies are immediate hypersensitive responses to allergens in food. Common food allergens are contained in milk, eggs, nuts, particularly peanuts, fish and shellfish. Ingested food leads to the release of IgE-mediated factors from the gut mucosa, resulting in oedema, skin rash, itching, increased **peristalsis**, vomiting and **diarrhoea** (Sicherer and Sampson, 2018). A systemic response occurs more commonly with peanut and shellfish allergens and a person may be highly sensitive to these, so much so that they may not need to ingest them to develop a systemic response.

APPLY

Immunotherapy treatment for allergies

Immunotherapy treatment for allergies is aimed at altering the response of the immune system to the allergen where the person is gently exposed to a miniscule amount of the allergen through subcutaneous injections in repeated doses over a period of time. This is known as desensitisation and it appears to help reduce the response to the allergen, thus resulting in less severe symptoms (Larsen et al., 2016).

Watch this video clip to get a summary of type II hypersensitivity reactions. If you are using the eBook just click on the play button. Alternatively go to

https://study.sagepub.com/essentialpatho/videos

TYPE II HYPERSENSITIVITY
(9:04)

Type II antibody-mediated disorders

Antibodies IgG and IgM or immune complexes cause this type of immune response. The antibody binds to tissue-specific antigens on the cell surface, resulting in either cell dysfunction or destruction. This is often referred to as cytotoxic hypersensitivity. There are several processes by which type II reactions happen:

- Antibodies attach to antigens on the cell surface, causing the cell to be more vulnerable to **phagocytosis** by **macrophages**. **Complement proteins** are activated which facilitate phagocytosis, a process known as **opsonisation** (Boore et al., 2016). This leads to destruction of the cell. This mechanism is seen in autoimmune **haemolytic anaemia**, ABO blood group or Rhesus (Rh) incompatibility and mismatched blood transfusion reactions.
- Where antibodies bind to normal cell receptors they can cause the cell to malfunction, but they do not destroy the cell. The cell receptor (but not necessarily the cell) is inappropriately stimulated

or destroyed. For example, antibodies bind to and activate receptors for thyroid-stimulating hormone (TSH) on thyroid cells, leading to hyperthyroidism associated with **Graves' disease** (Justiz Vaillant and Zito, 2018).

- Complement- and antibody-mediated inflammation is another mechanism where antibodies stimulate **neutrophils** and macrophages to release toxins, including **lysosomal enzymes**, leading to inflammation and tissue injury. This mechanism is responsible for some forms of **glomerulonephritis**.

Type III immune complex-mediated disorders

Antigen–antibody complexes are formed when antibodies bind to either self-antigens or foreign antigens in the circulation and are then deposited in the vessel wall or tissues. Complement is activated, and neutrophils are attracted to the antigen–antibody complex and attempt to ingest it but often cannot as the complex is attached to a large area of tissue (Rote, 2017). This results in the release of large amounts of enzymes, leading to tissue damage. Features of the disorder depend on the tissue involved, rather than the cell as in other hypersensitivity reactions, and are often systemic, involving multiple tissues.

The tissues of the blood vessels, joints and glomerulus of the kidney are particularly vulnerable where antigen–antibody complexes are deposited and bind to the basement membrane of the vessels. Leucocytes and mast cells are activated to produce cytokines and vasoactive mediators which increase vascular permeability and blood flow, causing **vasculitis**. Characteristics of type III reactions include fever, enlarged lymph nodes, rash and pain at sites of inflammation. These features were originally described following injection for **immunisation** using animal serum and the term '**serum sickness**' was used to describe this type of reaction. Serum sickness is a systemic reaction and is usually short-lived unless there is repeated administration of the antigen. A localised reaction is known as an Arthus reaction, where there is repeated exposure to an antigen that reacts with a preformed antibody and forms an immune complex in the walls of the blood vessels (Abbas et al., 2015). This causes local vasculitis and **thrombosis** of the affected vessel and tissue necrosis. This can be observed following injection, ingestion or inhalation of allergens.

Type IV cell-mediated hypersensitivity disorders

This type of response is cell-mediated rather than antibody-mediated. T-cell lymphocytes induce inflammation and/or directly kill target cells in type IV hypersensitivity disorders (Abbas et al., 2015). There are two types of Type IV reactions: direct cell-mediated cytotoxicity and delayed-type hypersensitivity (Figure 7.4).

Direct cell-mediated response involves CD8+ cytotoxic T lymphocytes that directly kill target cells expressing foreign antigens. This can happen where persistent microbes, primarily viruses, have infected a cell and resist phagocytosis and antibody eradication. Cytotoxic T-lymphocytes kill the infected cell, causing tissue damage, regardless of whether the **virus** is harmful to the host. T cells can also react with self-antigens, leading to cytokine release, promoting inflammation and tissue injury. This is seen in many autoimmune disorders such as **multiple sclerosis**, type 1 diabetes and **rheumatoid arthritis**.

Delayed-type mediated hypersensitivity (DTH) involves the activation of CD4+ T-helper cells and the secretion of cytokines that promote an inflammatory reaction. This reaction occurs in people who have had previous exposure to the antigen and are therefore sensitised. The reaction is delayed as it develops 24–72 hours after exposure to the antigen and involves the activation of **T-helper cells** (T_h1 cells) that are ultimately responsible for the reaction. Cytokines, macrophages, **fibroblasts** and leucocytes are also involved in the process.

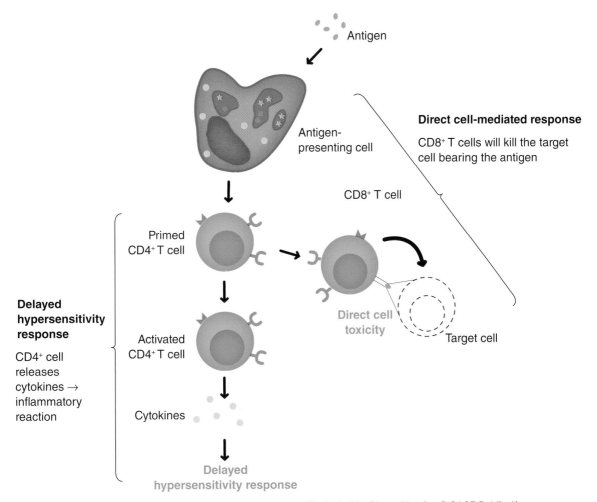

Illustrated by Shaun Mercier © SAGE Publications

Figure 7.4 Reactions in type IV cell-mediated hypersensitivity

The reaction can be illustrated in the tuberculin skin test (Mantoux), which uses this mechanism to identify if the person has been previously exposed to the tuberculin antigen. A small amount of the tuberculin antigen is injected under the skin and within 4 hours neutrophils accumulate around the injection site. Within 12 hours T cells infiltrate the area and blood vessels become permeable. **Fibrinogen** leaks from the plasma into the surrounding tissue and is converted into **fibrin**. The surrounding tissue becomes oedematous and appears firm (due to the fibrin) and inflamed. This indicates previous exposure to the **tuberculosis myco-bacterium**. This sequence of events leads to the formation of T_h1 cells, **memory cells** responsible for the reaction on subsequent exposure to the antigen. This is an example of the protective role of this mechanism, but it can also cause disease, for example contact hypersensitivity and **granulomatous hypersensitivity**.

Contact hypersensitivity is a type IV response to a wide range of substances such as metal, plants, chemicals or cosmetics and this response is confined to the skin. An incomplete lipid-soluble antigen, called a **hapten**, penetrates the epidermis where it combines with a protein carrier and is recognised as an antigen by sensitised CD4+ cells (Schrijvers et al., 2015). These cells release cytokines and stimulate the inflammatory response, resulting in oedema, pruritis and skin blisters. If no further exposure takes place, the reactions decrease after about 72 hours as the antigen is degraded (Young-Peterson, 2013). Contact dermatitis is a common example of delayed-type hypersensitivity (DTH) reaction.

ACTIVITY 7.1 APPLY

Mantoux test

Watch the following short video about the Mantoux skin test for TB delayed hypersensitivity. If you are using the eBook just click on the play button. Alternatively go to
https://study.sagepub.com/essentialpatho/videos

MANTOUX TEST
(8:35)

APPLY

Latex allergy

Natural rubber latex is used widely in health care environments and single-use disposable gloves are the most significant way health care workers are exposed to latex. Allergy to latex can be a type IV or type I reaction and therefore many health care employers have policies on or about the use of latex gloves (NHS-RCP, 2008).

If you are interested in finding out more on latex allergy, the British Association of Dermatologists (BAD) has produced a useful leaflet. You can find this by searching online using the terms BAD and latex allergy.

Granulomatous hypersensitivity

Granulomatous hypersensitivity reactions represent a chronic type IV reaction where macrophages are activated in response to microbial antigens. Microbes are localised in an area of tissue and are not destroyed by macrophages. T cells and macrophages produce cytokines and growth factors to increase the reaction, thus maintaining a prolonged inflammatory response which leads to the formation of **granuloma**s. These are a collection of inflammatory cells and **connective tissue** that eventually become fibrotic nodules and progressively change the local tissue environment. Granulomatous inflammation causes tissue damage and functional impairment. It is characteristic of persistent microbes such as *Mycobacterium tuberculosis*, which causes tuberculosis. T-cell-mediated (Type IV) hypersensitivity presents in autoimmune diseases of rheumatoid arthritis, multiple sclerosis and type 1 diabetes, which we will look at in the next section.

AUTOIMMUNE DISORDERS

Autoimmune disease is the result of the immune system reacting to the body's own antigens and its failure to recognise these as self-antigens. The immune system needs to be able to differentiate between self and foreign antigens so that it is unresponsive to the body's own tissue antigens. This is known as **self-tolerance**. In autoimmune diseases the mechanism of self-tolerance is lost.

Autoimmune disease can affect almost any cell or tissue in the body. The exact cause is unknown, but it is thought to be related to a combination of genetic susceptibility and environmental triggers such as infections or tissue injury (Farh et al., 2015). Genetic susceptibility can lead to autoimmune disease through the disruption of B-cell tolerance and T-cell tolerance pathways. Infections or tissue injury can expose self-antigens and activate **antigen-presenting cells** (APCs) and lymphocytes in tissues, leading to the creation of autoantibodies (Kumar et al., 2018).

Autoimmune diseases can be debilitating and progressive and have a huge impact on the person and their family. Some of the more common autoimmune diseases include **systemic lupus erythematosus (SLE)** and rheumatoid arthritis (RA) (Chapter 10).

Systemic lupus erythematosus (SLE)

SLE, also referred to as 'lupus', is an antibody-mediated autoimmune disease characterised by chronic inflammation of the tissues of the skin, kidney, blood vessels and other tissues. A large number of autoantibodies are found in the circulation, particularly **antinuclear antibodies (ANA)** which react against nucleic acid antigens, e.g. single-stranded and double-stranded DNA. In total, 180 autoantibodies have been isolated in people with SLE and it is thought their production could be antigen-driven (Gal et al., 2015). Approximately 95% of people with lupus are positive for ANA (Gordon et al., 2018). The autoantibody reacts with the circulating antigen and forms immune complexes which are deposited in the connective tissue anywhere in the body. This activates complement and the inflammatory process which can lead to tissue necrosis. Common sites of inflammation are the blood vessels, kidneys, lungs, heart, brain, skin and digestive tract. Some of the symptoms result from a type II hypersensitive reaction such as the destruction of erythrocytes, leading to anaemia, and some occur as a result of type III hypersensitivity reaction. Signs and symptoms can be mild to severe and can mimic other diseases (Frieri and Stampfl, 2016).

Epidemiology

Lupus can present at any age but most commonly affects women aged 17–55 years old. It affects almost 1 in 1000 of the population in the UK and is most frequently seen in women of Afro-Caribbean and Asian origin (Rees et al., 2016). In North America, the incidence is 23.2/100,000 person-years and the prevalence is 241/100,000 (Rees et al., 2017). The pathogenesis of SLE is multifactorial and includes genetic, environmental and hormonal factors. Genetic factors include the inheritance of particular **human leucocyte antigen (HLA) alleles** HLA-DR2 or HLA-DR3, increasing the risk of developing SLE. Family members of a person with SLE have an increased risk for development of the disease. Environmental factors such as exposure to UV radiation lead to **apoptosis** and an increased number of nucleic antigens which result in autoantibody formation.

Clinical signs and symptoms

The clinical presentation of SLE varies greatly because it is a multisystem disease. Often the person presents with a rash on the face referred to as a butterfly rash. Joint inflammation (arthritis) may cause joint pain (**arthralgia**) and there may be pleuritic chest pain and **photosensitivity**. Abnormal urinary findings, such as **haematuria** or **proteinuria**, may be present and anaemia and **thrombocytopenia** may be prominent. Coronary artery disease may develop. The person may go through periods of **remission** and exacerbation. Diagnosis is based on clinical features and diagnostic tests confirming the presence of antinuclear antibodies (ANAs) in the serum (Gordon et al., 2018). The common effects of SLE are shown in Table 7.2.

Table 7.2 Common clinical findings in SLE

Facial rash confined to cheeks
Discoid rash (raised patches, scaling)
Photosensitivity (development of a skin rash following exposure to sunlight)
Oral or nasopharyngeal **ulcers**
Non-erosive arthritis of at least two peripheral joints
Serositis (inflammation of the membranes of lung or heart)
Renal disorder
Neurological disorders
Haematological disorders
Immunological disorders
Presence of antinuclear antibody (ANA)

The treatment and management of SLE aim to control symptoms and prevent further damage to vital organs. Minimising exacerbations by avoiding triggers such as exposure to UV light and excessive fatigue can help. Non-steroidal anti-inflammatory drugs such as aspirin and ibuprofen reduce inflammation and relieve pain. **Corticosteroids** are used to reduce the immune response and inflammation. Cytotoxic immunosuppressive drugs should be considered in active lupus to reduce disease activity and treat severe symptoms where vital organs are involved (NICE, 2016). Advances in the understanding of SLE are improving and new approaches are focusing on antibody therapy (Abbas et al., 2015).

Rheumatoid arthritis (RA)

Rheumatoid arthritis, also discussed in Chapter 10, is an autoimmune disease characterised by inflammation of the joints and destruction of the joint cartilage and bone. Both cell-mediated and humoral immune responses may contribute to inflammation. T-helper cells (CD4⁺), activated B-lymphocytes, macrophages and proinflammatory cytokines are present in the inflamed joint (Abbas et al., 2015). Cytokines, particularly tumour necrosis factor, interleukin (IL)-1β, IL-6, IL-7 and IL-21, recruit leucocytes and cause the **synovial cells** to produce proteolytic enzymes such as **collagenase** that destroy the cartilage, ligaments and tendons of the joints. The synovial tissue becomes thickened and this is known as '**pannus**' (Figure 7.5). The pannus invades the bone and, along with increased osteoclast activity, leads to bone destruction with resultant pain, joint deformity and loss of function. The joints most commonly affected are the fingers, wrists, elbows, toes, ankles and knees.

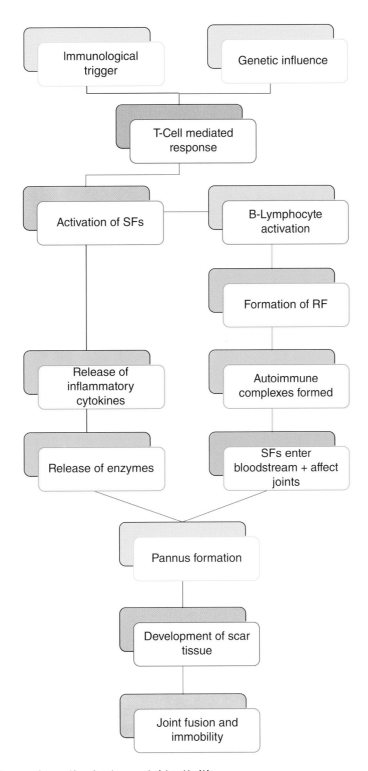

Figure 7.5 Pannus formation in rheumatoid arthritis

Note: SFs = synovial fibroblasts; RF = rheumatoid factors

Activated B cells, IgG or IgM antibodies react with their own molecules to become autoantibodies and are known as **rheumatoid factors (RF)**. The autoantibodies perpetuate inflammation and the continuous formation of immune complexes can be used in diagnostic testing. During inflammation the amino acid arginine is modified to citrulline, changing the structure of the protein (**citrullination**), and stimulates the autoimmune response through the production of specific antibodies by the immune system.

Like other autoimmune diseases, RA is a complex disorder in genetically susceptible people, triggered by an unknown environmental influence. There is breakdown of self-tolerance and activation of inflammatory processes. Genetic susceptibility is linked to human leucocyte antigen (HLA) areas of the **major histocompatibility complex (MHC)**. **Polymorphism**s in a gene called *PTPN22* which encodes for the protein tyrosine phosphate are associated with the development of RA. It is thought that this causes the protein to be defective, leading to excessive lymphocyte activation (McInnes and Schett, 2017).

Clinical features

RA can initially have general signs of fever and inflammation and generalised aching. Joints become tender and stiff, swollen and enlarged, leading to pain and loss of function. Limited mobility of the joints eventually leads to deformity. Rheumatoid nodules can form outside the joint in the subcutaneous tissue but may also invade the cardiac valves, pericardium, lung tissue and spleen. Systemic complications of RA include vasculitis and lung injury.

Treatment is aimed at slowing **progression** of the disease and reducing inflammation using corticosteroids and other immunosuppressants such as methotrexate. Antagonists against tumour necrosis factor (TNF) is a targeted treatment that reduces inflammation and slows joint destruction.

IMMUNODEFICIENCY DISORDERS

Immune deficiency disorders occur when there is failure of the immune system to function normally, resulting in an increased susceptibility to infections. This is either genetically determined (primary) or an **acquired** (secondary) disorder caused by another condition such as **cancer**, infection or ageing.

Primary (congenital) immunodeficiencies

Most **primary immunodeficiency** disorders are the result of a single gene **mutation** that results in immune dysregulation, autoimmunity and recurrent infection (Battersby and Cant, 2017). The onset of symptoms can occur early in life between 6 months and 2 years old and is manifested by recurrent infections and failure of the infant to gain weight or grow normally, also known as **failure to thrive** (Cant et al., 2013). Primary disorders vary depending on the component of the immune system that is affected but the major groups include **combined immunodeficiency**, antibody deficiencies and complement deficiencies.

Combined

Combined immunodeficiency is when T-lymphocyte and/or B-lymphocyte development is impaired. This can be X-linked, where there is a defect in the gene coding for interleukin cytokines, and results in impaired maturation of T cells and **natural killer (NK) cells**. An autosomal pattern of inheritance is characterised by a deficiency in an enzyme called **adenosine deaminase (ADA)** which causes the inhibition of DNA and immature lymphocytes (Shields and Patel, 2017). The most severe disorders are called severe combined immunodeficiencies (SCIDs) and serious life-threatening infections can develop frequently. **Pneumonia, meningitis**, chickenpox and gastrointestinal infections can be fatal. Immunisation using live vaccine, which is normally harmless in healthy children, may lead to infection in children with SCIDs. Di George **syndrome** is a form of SCID where there is **congenital** defect in the formation of the thymus gland and the parathyroid gland fails to develop. This results in decreased T-cell numbers and function and abnormal calcium regulation. Muscle twitching and abnormal development of facial features are characteristic of this syndrome.

Antibody deficiencies

Defects in B cells, either in their development or in their activation, and synthesis of antibodies results in disorders where antibody production is abnormal. This results in lower levels of circulating **immunoglobulins**, most commonly IgA (Shields and Patel, 2017). People may be asymptomatic but clinical signs include recurring sinus, pulmonary or GI infections.

Complement deficiencies

Several complement deficiencies are known and can result in reduced resistance to infection and increased frequency of bacterial or viral infections. The complement system consists of a large number of plasma proteins, mainly synthesised in the liver, which play an important role in promoting phagocytosis through opsonisation (it does this by combining with the pathogen and making it more readily identified by cells of the immune system).

Components of the complement pathway are referred to by the letter C and a number and C2 and C4 feature early in the complement pathway. Deficiency of these components results in reduced resistance to bacterial or viral infection and clearance of immune complexes which can result in autoimmune features (Notarangelo, 2010). Deficiency in C5–C9 causes increased susceptibility to the **bacteria** genus *Neisseria*, which causes localised infections, meningitis or **gonorrhoea** (Notarangelo, 2010). C3 has a central role in the complement pathway and loss of this component is severe and results in life-threatening infections with *Haemophilus influenzae* and *Streptococcus pneumoniae* bacteria. Deficiency in regulatory proteins results in excessive inflammatory responses and cell injury (Battersby and Cant, 2017).

Secondary (acquired) immunodeficiencies

Deficiencies of the immune system more commonly develop as a result of other conditions acquired during life where **immunosuppression** occurs secondary to another disease, as a side-effect of therapy for other diseases or due to infection of the immune system (Table 7.3).

Table 7.3 Causes of secondary (acquired) immunodeficiencies

Cause	Mechanism
HIV infection	Depletion of CD4⁺ helper cells
Protein-calorie **malnutrition**	Inhibition of lymphocyte maturation and function
Irradiation and chemotherapy for cancer	Decreased bone marrow leukocyte precursors
Involvement of bone marrow by leukaemia or **metastasis**	Reduced leucocyte development
Splenectomy	Decreased phagocytosis of microbes

Protein-calorie malnutrition adversely affects the maturation and functioning of cells of the immune system and is associated with increased susceptibility to infections and higher **morbidity** and mortality.

People with cancer affecting the bone marrow are susceptible to infections as the development and maturation of lymphocytes and leucocytes are affected. Treatment of cancer involves cytotoxic drugs which also arrest the development of lymphocytes and leucocytes, thus causing immunosuppression. Some drugs are given to cause immunosuppression, for example in the treatment of inflammatory diseases, or to prevent the rejection of transplanted tissue. Removal of the spleen results in the defective clearance of microbes and defective antibody responses to infections by encapsulated bacteria such as *Streptococcus pneumoniae*. These are examples of **iatrogenic** immunosuppression.

Infection of the immune system is also a secondary cause of immunodeficiency and one of the most prominent is **acquired immune deficiency syndrome (AIDS)** caused by infection of the immune system by **human immunodeficiency virus (HIV)**, which we will now discuss in more detail.

HIV and acquired immune deficiency syndrome (AIDS)

HIV is the human immunodeficiency virus which is transmitted by sexual activity, breast feeding, blood transfusion or injection. HIV infects and, if untreated, destroys the CD4$^+$ cells of the immune system and suppresses the immune response, leading to the development of acquired immune deficiency syndrome (AIDS). AIDS is a syndrome characterised by immunosuppression and opportunistic infections, **malignant** tumours, **cachexia** and central nervous system (CNS) degeneration.

Epidemiology

HIV/AIDS is a global **epidemic** with 36.9 million people living with HIV worldwide in 2017 (World Health Organisation [WHO], 2018). The African region is the most severely affected, with 4.1% of adults living with HIV infection, accounting for nearly two-thirds of people living with HIV worldwide. In 2017, 940,000 people died of HIV-related illness worldwide. In the same year, 1.8 million people were newly infected worldwide (WHO, 2018). These statistics reflect the global impact of HIV/AIDS and the morbidity and mortality associated with it. National HIV programmes have helped reduce the incidence of HIV and between 2000 and 2017 new HIV infections fell by 36% and HIV-related deaths fell by 38% (WHO, 2018). There is no cure for HIV/AIDS but education, prevention and access to antiretroviral treatment have resulted in HIV infection now being recognised as a **chronic illness** (Deeks et al., 2013) and will help save lives.

Pathogenesis

HIV is a **retrovirus**, which means that genetic information is carried on the RNA strand rather than DNA. An enzyme known as **reverse transcriptase** converts two identical strands of RNA into double-stranded DNA once inside the host cell.

The HIV retrovirus is spherical and contains a cone-shaped core surrounded by a lipid envelope (Figure 7.6). The core contains proteins, RNA and enzymes and the viral particle is covered in a lipid bilayer envelope with **glycoproteins (gp)** attached to its surface. The glycoproteins bind to receptors on the surface of the host cell and are essential for HIV infection. Glycoprotein gp120 (on the surface of the HIV envelope) binds to the CD4 molecule on the surface of T lymphocytes and promotes a secondary gp120 binding to a **chemokine receptor** on the cell surface. This induces gp41 to insert into the cell membrane, enabling the viral membrane to fuse with the target cell (Walker and McMichael, 2012).

Once inside the cell, the enzymes become active and viral reproduction commences. RNA undergoes reverse transcription to become viral DNA and enters the nucleus. The enzyme integrase from the HIV virus also enters the host cell nucleus and induces the integration of viral DNA into the genetic material of the host cell. This leads to the production of **virons** and ultimately cell death. Activation of T lymphocytes by antigens or cytokines enhances the process of viral transcription and replication and loss of CD4+ cells. Viral particles are released from the plasma membrane of the host cell and **lysis** occurs, causing destruction of the T cells. This is a cycle that ultimately results in the destruction of the immune system.

As viral production progresses, the rate of destruction of T cells is greater than they can be replaced, eventually leading to T cell immunodeficiency. Macrophages and **dendritic cells** can also be infected with HIV and can act as reservoirs of infection as these cells are not killed on viral replication like CD4+ cells.

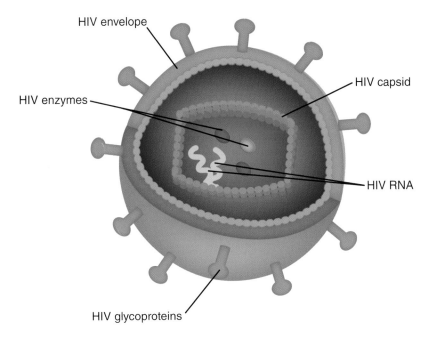

Illustrated by Shaun Mercier © SAGE Publications

Figure 7.6 HIV virus

Transmission of HIV infection

HIV is transmitted through body fluids that contain the virus via three major routes: sexual contact, inoculation with infected blood and mother to baby transmission.

Sexual contact is the most frequent mode of transmission where infected semen or vaginal fluid is exchanged and eventually gains entry to the bloodstream, for example through the mucosal lining of the vagina, anal mucosa, wounds or sores. Anti-retroviral treatment (ART) in a HIV-positive person can reduce the risk of transmitting the virus to an uninfected sexual partner (WHO, 2016).

Inoculation of infected blood or blood products is also a mode of transmission, particularly where needles are shared by intravenous drug users. The risk of transmission through blood transfusion is small as blood and blood products are screened for HIV in many countries. However, there is still a small risk due to a window where the infection is not detected; advanced testing of blood donors results in the risk as being 1 in 2 million. Mother to baby transmission occurs most frequently in utero, during childbirth or through breastfeeding.

Risk factors

Certain behaviour and conditions increase a person's risk of becoming infected, including having unprotected sex, having another sexually transmitted disease, sharing contaminated needles or any unsterile instrument that cuts or pierces the skin.

Diagnosis and testing

Blood serum tests can detect antibodies to HIV, however most people do not produce antibodies until around 28 days after infection. This period is known as the window where the infection can still be transmitted but antibodies are not detectable. The person may be asymptomatic or present with general flu-like symptoms. Testing for the virus itself is used in newborn babies of infected mothers.

Clinical features

The following clinical features are characteristic of HIV (Kumar et al., 2018):

* *Acute phase*: During this period the virus is infecting CD4+ T cells and progressing to the lymph tissue. The virus is disseminated through the blood and the host develops a response that manifests as a self-limiting acute illness with general flu-like symptoms such as headache, fatigue and fever. This can occur 3–6 weeks after infection. The number of circulating CD4+ cells falls. CD8+ T cells are detected in the blood.
* *Chronic phase*: This phase may last for years where the virus replicates and the destruction of CD4+ T cells in the lymphoid tissue continues. CD4+ T cell count declines. The person is generally asymptomatic during this phase but may develop symptoms of acute viral infection. This can stimulate HIV production through the activation of cytokines such as TNF in response to microbial infections.
* *Final phase*: HIV progresses to AIDS when CD4+ count drops below 200 cells/mm³; the person is susceptible to opportunistic infections and cancers such as lymphomas or **Kaposi sarcoma**. Cachexia (wasting syndrome), kidney failure and central nervous system degeneration are features of this stage of the disease. The immune system cannot mount a response to infections or oncogenic viruses. A diagnosis of AIDS is based on clinical manifestations and CD4 count.

Opportunistic infections and co-morbidities

Tuberculosis (TB) is the most common cause of death in HIV-positive adults and children and is responsible for about a third of deaths related to HIV (Gupta et al., 2015). Early diagnosis of TB through careful assessment of signs and symptoms and diagnostic tests can initiate anti-TB treatment as soon as possible and improve outcomes. Symptoms include fever, night sweats, cough and weight loss.

Cryptococcal meningitis is an opportunistic fungal infection that is not common in people with healthy immune systems. However, it is often seen in the later stage of HIV. It is diagnosed by lumbar puncture and treated with the antifungal drugs amphotericin B and fluconazole.

Kaposi sarcoma (KS) is a malignancy of the endothelial cells of blood and lymphatic vessels that initially manifests as a lesion on the skin and mucosal membrane of the mouth. It invades other organs including the GI tract, causing pain, bleeding and obstruction of the lungs with symptoms of **dyspnoea**, cough and **haemoptysis**. Kaposi sarcoma is caused by an oncogenic virus called Kaposi sarcoma herpes virus (KSHV) which is a latent herpesvirus infection. When HIV suppresses the immune system the KSHV becomes active and widespread, leading to KS.

Treatment and prevention

Major advances in the treatment of HIV have reduced the devasting effects of the progression of the disease. Treatment involves the administration of **antiretroviral drugs** that interfere with the viral life cycle and stop the progression of HIV. Once the virus is suppressed, the CD4$^+$ count gradually increases. Antiretroviral therapy (ART) is recommended for all people with HIV as soon as possible after diagnosis. Drugs used in combination are more effective and act in several ways (Table 7.4).

Table 7.4 Drugs used in HIV treatment

Class of drug	Mechanism of action
Nucleoside analogue	Inhibit the action of the enzyme reverse transcriptase
Viral **protease** inhibitors	Block the processing of viral proteins
Integrase inhibitor	Inhibit the viral entrance into the target cell
Entry inhibitor	Prevents viral attachment to the host cell by targeting CCR5 or CD4 molecules

Testing and counselling

Testing for HIV is advised for anyone exposed to the risk factors. This allows people to access treatment early and reduce the risk of transmission of the virus. When a person is diagnosed with HIV, it is recommended that they inform their sexual partner so that they too can be tested and commence treatment or preventative treatment. Antiretroviral therapy in noninfected high-risk individuals can block the acquisition of HIV and is used in pre-exposure prophylaxis (PrEP) in individuals who are at substantial risk of acquiring the virus (Ghosn et al., 2018).

HIV self-testing is a way to encourage people who do not know their HIV status to get tested. It has increased the uptake of testing among those at risk and should help identify more HIV-positive individuals (Johnson et al., 2017). Testing for TB early in a person with HIV infection is essential as TB is a leading cause of death. Prompt commencement of TB treatment and ART can reduce this.

Individuals can change their behaviour to limit exposure to risk factors, such as practising safe sex with consistent use of condoms and taking precautions against becoming infected through use of single sterile needles and syringes. Mother to child transmission can be prevented if both mother and baby are commenced on ARV drugs as early as possible in pregnancy and during breastfeeding (Payne et al., 2015).

ACTIVITY 7.2 APPLY

HIV testing

Listen to this podcast about early testing for HIV. If you are using the eBook just click on the play button. Alternatively go to

https://study.sagepub.com/essentialpatho/videos

HIV TESTING (8:24)

Alloimmunity: transplant rejection

Alloimmunity refers to the immune system reacting against the tissue of another individual and can be observed in blood transfusion reactions and transplanted tissue or in the fetus during pregnancy. The immune system recognises antigens on foreign tissue and mounts a response. The ABO and Rhesus (Rh) systems for blood groups are antigens expressed on the surface of red blood cells and can be targets of alloimmune reactions (Boore et al., 2016).

─────────────── **REVISE: A&P RECAP** ───────────────

Blood transfusion and potential reactions

Revise Chapter 12, The Cardiovascular and Lymphatic Systems in *Essentials of Anatomy and Physiology for Nursing Practice* (Boore et al., 2016) to refresh your knowledge about antibodies, and blood transfusion and the Rhesus system and pregnancy.

Transplanted tissue and organs are at risk of rejection due to the response of the immune system and rejection involves several of the immunological pathways that are seen in inflammatory diseases. Replacement of damaged non-functioning organs or tissues by healthy ones from a donor is a way of treating disease and prolonging life. Cells, tissues and organs can be transplanted from one person (the donor) to another person (the recipient). This process is known as transplantation and this type of transplanted tissue is known as an allograft. The immune system of the recipient can recognise the transplanted tissue as foreign and mounts a response to destroy the tissue. This is known as rejection and is a major barrier to transplantation.

Rejection is complex, involving a cellular response from T lymphocytes and antibodies and a humoral response, leading to inflammation and tissue necrosis. Major histocompatibility complex (MHC) molecules are expressed on the surface of all cells and are known as human leucocyte antigens (HLA). Their function is to enable the T lymphocytes CD4+ and CD8+ to recognise antigens. Donor tissue HLA can be recognised as foreign by host T lymphocytes and is the basis of rejection. The more similar two individuals are in their HLA types, the less risk of rejection. The recipient T lymphocytes recognise the donor antigens either directly or indirectly.

Direct pathway

Major histocompatibility complex (MHC) molecules on the surface of cells in the graft activate CD4+ and CD8+ cells and cause a type IV hypersensitivity reaction. Cytokines secreted by CD4+ cells cause increased vascular permeability and accumulation of macrophages, resulting in graft tissue damage.

Indirect pathway

T-cell lymphocytes recognise MHC antigens of the graft tissue when they are presented by the recipient's own antigen-presenting cells in the same way as in the recognition of other foreign antigens, such as microbes. This pathway also produces antibodies.

Bone marrow transplantation involves the transplantation of stem cells harvested from donor bone marrow or blood. This is used to replace cancerous blood cells and immunodeficiency disorders and involves the recipient requiring treatment to destroy malignant cells and create an environment where the grafted stem cells will develop. This type of transplant grafts immunological competent cells into an immunosuppressed individual. Rejection is mediated by T cells and natural killer cells (NK). Graft-versus-host disease (GVHD) is a condition where the donor T cells recognise the recipient tissue as foreign and react against it (Choi and Reddy, 2014). This involves the activation of CD4+ cells and CD8+ T cells in a type IV delayed-type hypersensitivity (DTH). Symptoms include skin rash and GI involvement with **nausea**, diarrhoea and abdominal pain.

Transplant rejection may be hyperacute, acute or chronic. Hyperacute rejection occurs immediately due to pre-existing antibodies to HLA antigens in the vascular **endothelium** of the grafted tissue. Acute rejection occurs within days to weeks following transplantation when the recipient develops a cell-mediated response to HLA antigens. Chronic rejection occurs over months and years and often involves damage to the vascular supply to the graft (Perkey and Maillard, 2018).

INFECTION

Infectious diseases are in the top 10 leading causes of death worldwide, with lower respiratory tract infections, HIV/AIDS and diarrhoeal diseases the top three leading causes of death in low-income countries. Overall, the global mortality rates due to infectious diseases have dropped (Global Health Estimates, 2018). Improvements in sanitation, the availability of clean drinking water, vaccination programmes and the use of antibiotics have played an important role in reducing the risk of infection occurring and improving the outcome if someone acquires an infection.

Infectious diseases are caused by pathogens such as bacteria, viruses, **fungi** and **protozoa** (Table 7.5). Humans have contact with these microorganisms every day but, due to our finely tuned defence systems, we do not often acquire an infectious disease. Microorganisms that cause disease in humans are referred to as pathogens.

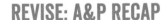

REVISE: A&P RECAP

Microbiome

Some microbes are beneficial to humans. You may find it useful to revise Chapter 4, The Human Microbiome and Health, in *Essentials of Anatomy and Physiology for Nursing Practice* (Boore et al., 2016).

General characteristics of microorganisms that cause disease

The microorganisms that cause infectious disease need to be capable of avoiding the immune system. They also need to be able to spread from one infected person to another. This is known as communicability. Certain microorganisms have high communicability and spread easily, making them difficult to control. They also need to be able to gain entry to the host and multiply (infectivity) and cause disease (pathogenicity) (Rote, 2017). These are known as virulence factors and when a microorganism possesses these it is said to be virulent.

Table 7.5   Main types of microbial organisms

Microbe type	Class of organism	Structure	Metabolism	Additional information
Bacteria	Prokaryotes	DNA or RNA within cell without membrane surrounding organelles. No nucleus	Varied oxygen requirements	
Archaea	Prokaryotes			Much research still required
Viruses	'At the edge of life'	RNA or DNA (genetic material), surrounded by a protein coat, sometimes with lipid coat	Dependent on host cell **metabolism** for replication	Non-active outside host Replicate only inside living cells of host using cell materials to produce proteins encoded in RNA or DNA and form viruses Each virus restricted to specific number/type of cell. Those infecting bacteria are known as 'phages'
Fungi	Eukaryotes	Separate from animals and plants with some characteristics of both Cell nuclei surrounded by membrane	Relies on carbon fixed by other organisms	Most grow from their tips as tubular filaments (hyphae) which branch producing a network of hyphae. Some grow by budding or binary fission as single cells: includes moulds, yeasts Some produce spores dispersed for reproduction. Further research to clarify role in microbiota needed
Protozoa/ protists	Eukaryotes	Eukaryote that is not animal plant or true fungus Independent cells or non-differentiated into tissues	Some use sunlight, others rely on organic compounds	Some are pathogens of animals, some of plants, some are non-pathogenic
Helminths	Eukaryotes	Worm-like **parasites** living in animal hosts	Feeding on living hosts	Can cause weakness and disease but can also reduce incidence of allergy and autoimmune conditions. Uncommon in developed countries

Source: Boore et al., 2016

Portal of entry

Microorganisms are able to gain entry through direct contact, inhalation, ingestion, penetration of the skin or by sexual transmission.

Direct contact

Some pathogens are transmitted directly from infected tissue or secretions to mucous membranes. Sexually transmitted infections are transmitted in this way.

Indirect contact

Microorganisms can gain access to the body via the gastrointestinal tract from the ingestion of infected food and water. The microorganism needs to overcome the acidic environment of the stomach, the resident microorganisms (flora), pancreatic enzymes and secreted IgA antibodies produced by plasma cells located in the mucosa-associated lymphoid tissue (MALT) (Brooks et al., 2013). Microorganisms can enter the host from the intestinal lumen.

Respiratory inhalation is another route of entry to the host and, like GI entry, the microorganism needs to overcome the defences of the respiratory system. The surface of the respiratory system is lined with ciliated mucous **epithelium** that sweeps any particles away from the lungs. The coughing mechanism removes particles form the lower respiratory tract and respiratory secretions contain antibodies and enzymes that can destroy invading microorganisms.

Penetration of the skin

A breech of the skin, the first line of defence, will allow microorganisms to enter and invade the tissue. Wounds, surgical incisions, burns, **pressure ulcers**, puncture of the skin with needles, sharp objects or insect or animal bites all breech the skin integrity.

Dissemination within the body

The portal of entry does not necessarily dictate the site of infection as once the microorganism has gained access it will either proliferate locally or cause infection at a distant site. The microbe may travel in the blood or lymph systems to spread to distant sites in the body. Viruses, bacteria, fungi and protozoa are transported in the plasma, however some viruses, such as herpes virus and HIV, are transported in leucocytes and some parasites, such as the *Plasmodium* species, use the red blood cells as a means of transport. Many viruses spread from cell to cell and some bacteria, fungi and helminths secrete enzymes that destroy tissue, allowing direct invasion (Kumar et al., 2018).

Transmission

Transmission of infections from one individual to another can occur via direct or indirect contact. For example, secretions from saliva, respiratory droplets from coughing and sneezing, faeces, blood, urine, genital mucosa and secretions, and vertical transmission from mother to fetus or newborn through the placenta, during childbirth or through breastfeeding.

Bacterial infection

Bacteria are single-celled prokaryotes (without membrane-bound organelles) that exist in a variety of shapes and sizes (see Boore et al., 2016, Chapter 4). They contain both DNA and RNA and many contain small extra chromosomal pieces called **plasmids** that are associated with the development of resistance to antibiotics. The cytoplasm of the bacterial cell is surrounded by the cytoplasmic membrane and this is surrounded by a rigid cell wall. The physical and chemical structure of the cell wall differentiates bacteria based on the Gram stain. Bacteria will either stain Gram positive (stain blue/green by the crystal violet dye) or Gram negative (stain red) when the dark Gram stain is not absorbed by the cell wall. The Gram stain is the most widely used technique for staining and identifying bacteria according to the structure of their cell wall. (See Table 7.6 for characteristics of gram-positive and gram-negative bacterial cells.) Most bacterial cell walls have a distinctive polymer known as peptidoglycan which is a carbohydrate protein structure that is unique to bacteria. This is why many antimicrobial drugs target the cell wall.

Table 7.6 Relative characteristics of gram-positive and gram-negative bacteria

Gram-positive bacteria	Gram-negative bacteria
Stain blue	Stain red
Thick layer of peptidoglycan in cell wall	Thin layer of peptidoglycan in cell wall
No outer membrane	Cell wall has an outer membrane of proteins and phospholipids known as **lipopolysaccharides** (LPS)
Secrete proteins out of the cell (exotoxins)	LPS released from cell wall outer membrane on cell death (**endotoxin**)

Bacteria's pathogenicity depends on the effectiveness of the immune system and the ability of the bacteria to overcome it. Once bacteria have gained access to the host, they must attach to host cells through surface molecules called **adhesins** or by structures called **pilli** found on the surface of the bacterial cell. The bacterial cell can produce toxins which destroy normal functioning of the host cell. Toxins are classified into two main types: endotoxins, which are components of the bacterial cell, and exotoxins, which are proteins secreted by the bacteria.

An endotoxin is a lipopolysaccharide (LPS) component of the outer membrane in gram-negative bacteria. LPS binds to the surface of the host leucocytes and activates the inflammatory response. This response induces cytokine production and T-lymphocyte activation. However, in larger doses, LPS has detrimental effects through excessive levels of cytokines, as seen in **septic shock** (discussed later).

Exotoxins are proteins secreted from the bacterial cell that cause cell injury and death. They can be classified according to their mechanism of action. Some act as enzymes on specific tissue cells, for example proteases (break down protein), **lipase**s (break down fats) and coagulases (cause blood clots). A–B toxins alter regulatory pathways; there is an active (A) component that is an enzyme and a binding (B) component that binds to the cell surface receptors and delivers the A protein into the cytoplasm. A–B toxins include the toxin of *Bacillus anthracis*, otherwise known as anthrax and *Vibrio cholerae*. **Neurotoxins** are exotoxins produced by *Clostridium botulinum* and *Clostridium tetani* that inhibit the release of **neurotransmitters**, leading to paralysis. **Enterotoxins** are specific exotoxins that affect the gastrointestinal tract, causing vomiting and diarrhoea, for example the exotoxin produced by *Clostridium difficile*.

Some bacteria produce **endospore**s when exposed to extreme conditions such as lack of nutrients or water. Endospores are highly resistant structures that can remain dormant for many years and are resistant to desiccation, toxic chemicals and UV irradiation. When conditions become favourable, the endospore exits the dormant stage to become a vegetative cell (germination). *Bacillus anthracis* (anthrax) and *Clostridium botulinum* (botulism) produce endospores when required.

Biofilms

Biofilms are complex multicellular masses consisting of interactive bacterial cells attached to a solid surface or to each other (Brooks et al., 2013). They are associated with urinary tract infections related to indwelling urinary catheters, foot **ulcer**s, burns, pneumonia and infections of the oral cavity due to dental plaque. They offer a survival advantage for the microorganism as they can evade the immune system and exposure to antibiotics and show increased tolerance to nutrient deprivation and the host immune response (Scherr et al., 2015).

Viral infection

Viruses cause infection and disease in humans and some can transform normal cells into cancerous cells (oncogenic virus). A virus is an obligate intracellular parasite that depends on the cell machinery for its replication. It consists of a piece of genetic material (DNA or RNA which can be double- or single-stranded) inside a protein coat. Viruses are acellular and have no structures for metabolism/reproduction and are therefore completely dependent on the host cells for existence. The host cell provides energy, synthetic machinery and materials for synthesis of viral proteins and nucleic acids. Viral replication takes place and new viral particles are released either by lysis of the host cell or by budding out through the host cell membrane, acquiring a new envelope in the process. This does not kill the host and so it continues to produce new viruses. Viruses account for a large number of infections and this can be manifested as a transient illness like the common cold or the virus may remain inside the cell, continuing to multiply as in chronic infection with **hepatitis** B virus, or in a latent state with the possibility of reactivation at a later stage. An example of this is the herpes zoster virus. This virus causes chickenpox and can enter the dorsal root ganglia and reactivate as shingles, a painful nerve and skin condition, years later (Brooks et al., 2013).

Fungal infection

There are over 100,000 species of fungi with around 200 being pathogenic to humans. Fungi are very diverse in shape and size, being microscopic and macroscopic. Fungi have a rigid cell wall containing a polysaccharide sugar known as **chitin** (Brooks et al., 2013). Fungal infections are known as **mycoses** and are classified according to the degree of tissue involved:

Superficial mycoses: occur in the epidermis, nails and hair (e.g. ringworm, athlete's foot).

Subcutaneous mycoses: confined to the dermis and subcutaneous tissue but may spread to underlying tissues. Caused by fungi that live in soil (e.g. sporotrichosis acquired by farmers and gardeners).

Systemic mycoses: deep, often life-threatening, infections of internal organs. Usually caused by inhalation of spores from infected soil into lungs which then spread via the circulation to other tissues (e.g. histoplasmosis, a chronic respiratory disease). Immunocompromised people are particularly at risk of fungal infection.

Parasitic infection

Parasitic disease is where the parasite, an organism living within another organism, benefits at the expense of the host species. Parasites vary from unicellular protozoa to multicellular worms. Of the many parasites, only a few cause diseases in humans and this is mainly in tropical climates. Parasites have a complex life cycle involving different hosts. Some can form protective coats called cysts that offer protection while outside the host. Parasites can enter the body in various ways, such as through contaminated food, insect bites or direct penetration of the skin.

Pathogenic protozoa include *Plasmodium falciparum* responsible for malaria. Malaria is one of the most common infections worldwide and the WHO estimates there were 216 million cases of malaria worldwide in 2016 with 445,000 deaths (WHO, 2017). The mosquito insect (arthropod) is a vector for *Plasmodium*. There are four different *Plasmodium* spp. but *P. falciparum* is the most fatal. Plasmodium has a complex life cycle involving sexual reproduction in the mosquito and asexual reproduction in the human liver and erythrocytes. Destruction of erythrocytes results in anaemia and tissue **hypoxia**.

Helminths or worms are not microorganisms but are parasites and cause disease in people throughout the world. Three types cause disease in humans: nematodes (or roundworms), cestodes (or tapeworms) and trematodes (or flukes). They have a complex life cycle and are often ingested as eggs or larvae in contaminated food or water, or they enter directly through the skin. They are often identified in the faeces of an infected person.

Stages in the development of disease

Infectious disease progression can be identified in three distinct phases:

- **Incubation period:** This is the period between introduction of the microbe to the host and the onset of the symptoms of the illness.
- Illness: During this phase the host experiences signs and symptoms of disease.
- **Convalescence:** This is the period of recuperation and recovery from disease.

The host can spread infection during all three stages.

SOME INFECTIOUS DISEASES

Sexually transmitted infections (STIs)

STIs are caused by a range of pathogens that can be acquired through sexual contact. They can lead to infertility, **pelvic inflammatory disease** and malignancy. A range of pathogens cause STIs – bacteria, viruses and fungi, protozoa and parasites (Table 7.7).

Table 7.7 Pathogens that cause STIs

Infection	Microorganism
BACTERIAL	
Chlamydia (urogenital infections)	Chlamydia trachomatis
Gonorrhea	Neisseria gonorrhoeae
Syphilis	Treponema pallidum
VIRAL	
Genital herpes	Herpes simplex virus (HSV)
Genital warts, cervical cancer	Human papilloma virus (HPV)
PROTOZOA	
Trichomoniasis	Trichomonas vaginalis

Sexually transmitted infections affect the external genitalia, the rectum and oral pharynx and/or produce systemic effects. The spread of STIs is a problem as frequently they are asymptomatic, so people are unaware that they have the infection and do not take adequate precautions or seek treatment. Other challenges include recurrent infections, more than one infection present at a time, the emergence of drug-resistant microorganisms and difficulty in notifying sexual partners who might have become infected.

Bacterial infections

Chlamydia

Chlamydia is one of the most common sexually transmitted infections and is caused by the bacterium *Chlamydia trachomatis*, a gram-negative obligate intracellular pathogen (Lehr et al., 2018). It is known as a polymicrobe because it behaves like both a virus and a bacterium. In the 'elementary' state the bacterium can survive outside the cell and when it attaches to the susceptible host cell it is ingested. Once inside the host cell it transforms into a larger reticulate body which takes over the metabolic machinery of the cell and reproduces by binary fission. New elementary bodies are formed and released from the infected host cell (Lehr et al., 2018).

Chlamydial infections are often asymptomatic but non-specific symptoms such as urinary frequency, **dysuria** and vaginal discharge, or muco**purulent** cervical discharge may be present. The cervix can become inflamed and more susceptible to further infection. The Fallopian tubes and **endometrium** can also become inflamed and there can be elements of inflammatory pelvic disease present. In men, chlamydial infection causes **urethritis** with symptoms of dysuria, itching and penile discharge. A painful, swollen scrotum and fever may indicate the presence of **epididymitis**.

Gonorrhoea

This is a sexually transmitted infection caused by *Neisseria gonorrhoeae*, a gram-negative diplococcus bacterium that is spread by direct contact with the mucosa of an infected individual. The portal of entry can be the genitourinary tract, eyes, oropharynx, rectum or skin. The bacteria attach to the mucosal epithelium and penetrate through to the deeper tissues, causing an inflammatory reaction (Sherrard, 2014). This is clinically manifested as dysuria with a purulent urethral discharge in males and, although often asymptomatic in females, dysuria can also occur with other features such as vaginal discharge, pelvic pain or tenderness and fever. Ascending infection can lead to acute **prostatitis** and epididymitis in males and infection of the uterus, fallopian tubes and ovaries in females.

Oro-genital contact may lead to **pharyngitis** or **tonsillitis**. Babies of infected mothers risk becoming infected during passage through the birth canal and can develop gonorrhoeal conjunctivitis which can lead to blindness if not treated. **Strain**s of resistant gonorrhoea have been reported recently by the European Centre for Disease Prevention and Control (ECDC, 2018b).

Syphilis

Syphilis is a sexually transmitted infection caused by the bacterium *Treponema pallidum*, an aerobic spirochete bacterium. *T. pallidum* is spread by direct contact with a skin or mucosal lesion through sexual activity. The microorganism gains entry through the mucosa or through breaks in the skin. The infection can also be transferred from infected mother to fetus through the placenta and this is referred to as congenital syphilis (Hook, 2017). Syphilis is a systemic infection with four clinically distinct stages (sometimes referred to as phases in other texts):

Primary: Occurs several weeks after infection and is characterised by a primary lesion (or lesions), called a chancre, at the point of contact on the skin or mucous. This is a painless, firm, ulcerated nodule. The immune response is initiated, and antibodies are formed at this stage. The infection is highly contagious and can often go unnoticed as the chancre heals spontaneously within 3–6 weeks.

Secondary: This stage, or secondary syphilis, occurs when the bacteria have already entered the general circulation and there is enlargement of the lymph nodes (lymphadenopathy). Highly infectious mucosal and cutaneous lesions full of bacteria develop and a widespread reddish **maculopapular rash** appears on the palms of the hands and the soles of the feet. Other general signs of infection, such as fever, sore throat, loss of appetite and inflamed eyes, are common.

Latent: After the second stage in an untreated infection, the person becomes asymptomatic for more than a year after the initial infection. This is known as the latent phase, which may last for many years.

Tertiary: If individuals become symptomatic, they enter the tertiary stage where the infection progresses and there is the formation of lesions known as **gummas**. These can occur anywhere in the body but are more common in the bone, skin and mucous membranes. Gummas are necrotic fibrous lesions caused by tissue necrosis which can lead to aneurysms in the aorta if formed in the cardiovascular system, bone destruction and damage to the central nervous system, leading to blindness, dementia and sensory/motor loss. This condition can lead to death.

Genital herpes

Herpes simplex virus (HSV) causes genital herpes and is a highly contagious infection. There are two types of herpes simplex virus that are associated with STIs: these are HSV-1, associated with blisters and cold sores, and HSV-2, which causes most cases of genital herpes. Both viruses are genetically similar, and both can cause genital and oropharyngeal herpes but it is now being seen more often in the genitalia due to the increase in frequency of oral sex. HSV-2 typically infects the genitalia (Garland and Steben, 2014).

HSV is transmitted by direct contact with infectious lesions and the incubation period is 2–12 days. Often the infected person is asymptomatic and viral shedding (expulsion and release of virus after successful reproduction within the host cell) can contribute to the spread of infection.

The initial symptoms include painful **vesicles** on the skin of the external genitalia with itching and pain in the genital area. The vesicles rupture and form wet ulcers that are associated with dysuria, urethral discharge and local lymph node enlargement. Systemic symptoms of fever, muscle ache, headache and regional lymph node enlargement are a feature. Vesicles are found on the cervix, vulva and urethra in women. In men, lesions form on the penis, scrotum and urethra. Rectal and perianal lesions may also occur. Following the acute stage, HSV migrates along the peripheral nerve to the dorsal root ganglia where it can remain dormant in the latent phase. Reactivation of the virus may be triggered by many factors such as **stress** and other infections and recurrent episodes are usually milder and of shorter duration than the primary episode.

The vesicles contain the virus and the infection can spread to the eyes or skin through hand contamination. Lesions of the cervix and vagina can transmit the infection to the baby during vaginal delivery. Neonatal herpes infection can be fatal.

Human papilloma virus (HPV)

HPV is a nonenveloped, double-stranded DNA virus that affects the genital tract. There are several types of HPV, some of which are associated with cervical cancer. HPV types 6 and 11 infect the squamous epithelial cells, causing genital warts, also known as condylomata acuminata. These lesions occur on the penis and scrotum as well as the female genitals, perineum and perianal skin. They may also affect the mucous membrane of the vagina, urethra, anus or mouth. They vary in appearance from soft fleshy projections to cauliflower-like masses. The incubation period is 2–3 months. Vaccination against HPV is one of the most effective ways of controlling HPV-related diseases (Maver and Poljak, 2017).

Protozoan infection

Trichomoniasis is an STI caused by the protozoan *Trichomonas vaginalis*, an anaerobic flagellated protozoan. It is associated with other STIs and resides in the urethra in men and in the vagina in women. These protozoa attach easily and feed off the mucosa they inhabit. Active infection causes a copious, malodourous yellow discharge with associated inflammation and itchiness of the mucosa. Systemic treatment with metronidazole or tinidazole is effective.

Other infectious diseases

Meningitis

Infectious agents can affect any part of the body including the nervous system. The coverings of the brain and spinal cord are susceptible to invasion by microorganisms that can access the nervous system in several ways. The most common means of access is via the arterial blood supply but direct invasion through open trauma or, rarely, by invasive **surgery** or diagnostic tests can also occur. Local extension from an infected nearby structure may also occur, for example infected sinuses, teeth or the middle ear.

Meningitis is inflammation of the **meninges**, usually as a result of infection. However, the meninges can become inflamed in response to a non-infectious cause such as carcinoma. Infectious meningitis can be caused by bacteria, often referred to as acute pyogenic meningitis, by viruses, referred to as aseptic meningitis, or by fungi and *Mycobacterium tuberculosis*. This last is usually a chronic form of the infection.

Bacterial meningitis (acute pyogenic meningitis)

Different bacteria cause bacterial meningitis, and this varies with age. *Escherichia coli* and group B streptococcal bacteria are the most common causative organisms in neonates. In adolescents and young adults *Neisseria meningitidis* (meningococcus) is the most common pathogen and in older adults *Streptococcus pneumoniae* (pneumococcus) and *Listeria monocytogenes* cause most cases (Kim, 2010). Risk factors associated with developing meningeal infection include base of skull **fractures**, **otitis media**, sinusitis neurosurgery, systemic **sepsis** and a compromised immune system.

N. meningitidis is often carried in the nasopharynx of an asymptomatic carrier and is spread by respiratory droplet transmission, through kissing, coughing, sneezing or sharing utensils, food and drink. It is often epidemic in environments where there is close contact between people, such as educational institutions or where young people reside together. Six subgroups of meningococcus have been identified – A, B, C, W-135, X and Y (Brooks et al., 2013).

Once the microorganism has crossed the **blood–brain barrier** it gains access to the cerebrospinal fluid (CSF), where it replicates and undergoes lysis. This releases toxins that cause alterations in cerebrovascular permeability, leading to oedema and inflammation of the pia and arachnoid maters. A purulent exudate is produced, and the meningeal vessels become engorged. Neutrophils can be found in the subarachnoid space and **phlebitis** can occur, leading to venous occlusion and **infarction** of the surrounding tissues. The meninges thicken and **adhesions** form which may obstruct the outflow of CSF, giving rise to **hydrocephalus** (obstructive hydrocephalus). Typical symptoms of acute bacterial meningitis result from meningeal irritation with sudden onset of headache, fever, irritability, neck stiffness, photophobia and altered mental state. Nausea, vomiting, **seizures** and reduced **consciousness** are an indication of raised intracranial pressure. A rose-coloured **petechial rash** with palpable **purpura** (bleeding into the skin) is a feature of meningococcal meningitis and can rapidly progress to haemorrhagic infarction of the skin, leading to systemic sepsis, shock and multiple organ failure.

Diagnosis is based on clinical signs and examination of CSF obtained by lumbar puncture and positive **Kernig sign** (resistance to knee extension in the supine position with the hips and knees flexed against the body) and **Brudzinski sign** (flexion of the knees and hips when the neck is flexed forward rapidly). Lumbar puncture reveals increased pressure and CSF examination shows neutrophils, increased protein and reduced glucose. Prompt treatment with antibiotics and supportive care increases chances of recovery and reduces risk of morbidity and mortality.

Aseptic meningitis (viral meningitis)

Viruses such as enterovirus (coxsackievirus, poliovirus, echovirus), herpes simplex virus (HSV) and Epstein–Barr and mumps virus can cause meningitis. The virus enters the nervous system by crossing the blood–brain barrier, by direct spread along peripheral nerves or through the **choroid plexus** epithelium (Doran et al., 2016). The inflammatory response is activated, and the clinical signs are similar to bacterial meningitis but milder and typically self-limiting. Lymphocytes rather than neutrophils are found in CSF, with moderate protein elevation and normal glucose levels. Viral meningitis is managed by treating symptoms and the administration of antiviral drugs.

Chronic meningitis

Chronic meningitis is defined as chronic inflammation in the cerebrospinal fluid, persisting for at least one month without spontaneous resolution (Baldwin and Zunt, 2014). *Mycobacterium tuberculosis* and *Cryptococcus* species are some of the most common causes of chronic meningitis.

Chronic meningitis is characterised by general symptoms of headache, **malaise**, mental confusion and vomiting. Protein levels in CSF are elevated and CSF glucose levels are normal or reduced. Infection with *M. tuberculosis* can lead to the development of a mass within the cerebral tissue that can block CSF resorption and lead to hydrocephalus. Cerebral vessels may be affected, causing **vasoconstriction** and eventually thrombosis with cerebral infarction (Baldwin and Zunt, 2014).

SEPSIS

It is estimated that sepsis affects more than 30 million people worldwide every year, potentially leading to around 6 million deaths (Fleischmann et al., 2016). One in ten deaths associated with pregnancy and childbirth is due to maternal sepsis (Say et al., 2014). In the UK, it is estimated that 46,000 people die from sepsis each year (Daniels and Nutbeam, 2017). Certain age groups are more at risk of developing sepsis such as the very young (under 1 year) and older people over 75 years. People who are immunocompromised because of drugs or illness or receiving **chemotherapy** for cancer or those that are taking immunosuppressant drugs are also at higher risk (NICE, 2016).

Severe microbial infections can lead to **bacteraemia** (bacteria in the blood) and this can trigger what is known as **systemic inflammatory response syndrome (SIRS)**. This is associated with a massive release of inflammatory mediators from the innate and adaptive immune cells which result in cardiovascular abnormalities, leading to shock and often progressing to **multiple organ dysfunction syndrome (MODS)**. SIRS was defined in the 1992 international consensus conference based on deranged clinical findings in temperature, respiratory rate, heart rate and white blood cell count (Bone et al., 1992). A diagnosis of SIRS was based on meeting two of the four criteria outlined in Table 7.8.

Table 7.8 SIRS diagnostic criteria: diagnosis is based on any two or more of the criteria

Parameter	SIRS (systemic inflammatory response syndrome)
Tachypnoea	Respiratory rate >20 breaths/min
Tachycardia	Heart rate >90 beats/min
Hyperpyrexia	Body temperature >38 °C or <36 °C
Leucocytosis	White blood cell count >12,000 cells/mm^3 or <4000/mm^3

The SIRS criteria have been used to identify the signs and symptoms of sepsis. However, the most recent definition of sepsis stems from the 2016 international consensus definition as 'life-threatening organ dysfunction caused by a dysregulated host response to infection' (Singer et al., 2016). Septic shock is defined as a subset of sepsis in which profound circulatory, cellular and metabolic abnormalities are associated with a greater risk of mortality than with sepsis alone (Singer et al., 2016). Adults with suspected infection can be rapidly identified if they have at least two of the following clinical criteria: respiratory rate of 22/min or greater, altered mentation, or systolic blood pressure of 100 mmHg or less (Singer et al., 2016).

Pathophysiology of sepsis and septic shock

Sepsis is the result of a complex sequence of cellular activation and inflammatory mediators, associated with infection. Gram-positive bacteria, gram-negative bacteria and fungal pathogens are all associated with sepsis. The most common gram-positive pathogens are *Staphylococcus aureus* and *Streptococcus pneumoniae*, while *Escherichia coli, Klebsiella species* and *Pseudomonas aeruginosa* are the most common gram-negative organisms. The bacterial cell wall releases endotoxins (gram-positive cells) and exotoxins (gram-negative cells) that engage receptors on the cells of the immune system (macrophages).

These receptors are called Toll-like receptors (TLRs) and they recognise the molecules on the bacterial cell called 'pathogen-associated-molecular patterns' (PAMPs). Once activated, the immune cells produce cytokines, including tumour necrosis factor (TNF), Interleukin 1 (IL-1), IL-12 and IL-18. Other mediators such as **platelet-activating factor (PAF), prostaglandin** and **nitric oxide (NO)** are also released. Complement and coagulation are activated (Deutschman and Tracey, 2014) (Table 7.9).

A significant feature of sepsis is this proinflammatory state, which is counteracted with anti-inflammatory responses at the same time (Hotchkiss et al., 2013). As sepsis progresses, there is widespread vasodilation caused partly by NO being further released from damaged endothelial cells. This leads to **hypotension**, and compensatory tachycardia with increased cardiac output; this is the early stage of septic shock. Endothelial cell activation leads to widespread vascular leakage and subsequent tissue oedema, reducing the circulating blood volume. Derangement in coagulation leads to a decrease in the production of

Table 7.9 Summary of mediators involved in sepsis

Mediator molecule	Function
Nitric oxide	Causes and maintains vasodilation. Contributes to increased permeability
Complement proteins	Neutralise pathogens, mobilise white blood cells and amplify the immune response
Thrombin	Promotes clot formation by changing fibrinogen into fibrin. Involved in nitric oxide production
Interleukins	Complex group of proteins which attract white blood cells to the area and modulate inflammation. Some cause inflammation and some suppress the inflammatory response
Tumour necrosis factor (TNF)	Pro-inflammatory cytokine

anti-coagulant factors and an increase in pro-coagulation factors. Tissue **perfusion** is reduced due to oedema and decreased blood volume and flow and this in turn leads to the systemic activation of thrombin and the formation of thrombi in the microcirculation. Coagulation factors and platelets are consumed, resulting in bleeding and haemorrhage. This derangement of coagulation is known as **disseminated intravascular coagulation (DIC)**. Poor tissue perfusion leads to cellular hypoxia, eventually progressing to septic shock (Hotchkiss et al., 2013).

Stress-induced hormones drive **gluconeogenesis** and proinflammatory cytokines promote **insulin** resistance, leading to hyperglycaemia (Kumar et al., 2018). Septic shock can progress to **multiple organ dysfunction syndrome (MODS)**, where two or more organ systems fail due to the overwhelming uncontrolled inflammatory response.

Sepsis and septic shock are manifested by hypotension and flushed skin due to vasodilation. Compensatory tachycardia with a strong pulse is present in the early stages and there is an increase in respiratory rate. Temperature may be high or low and there may be alteration in mental state. Sepsis can progress rapidly to septic shock unless it is recognised early and appropriate treatment commenced.

Treatment

Treatment is focused on finding the causative agent and treating it with targeted antimicrobials. Early fluid resuscitation and the use of **vasopressors** to support the circulation and optimise tissue perfusion and oxygen delivery to the cells are essential. Once sepsis is recognised, there are six steps that can be performed by health care professionals within the first hour to improve the person's chances of survival (Daniels and Nutbeam, 2017) (see Table 7.10).

Table 7.10 Sepsis 6 screening and action tool

Action complete within 1 hour	Why we do this
1. Administer oxygen	To improve oxygen content to the blood and therefore its delivery to the tissues
2. Take blood cultures	To help identify pathogens to determine likely source and guide antimicrobial therapy
3. Give IV antibiotics	To control underlying infection, removing the trigger for immune over-reaction

Action complete within 1 hour	Why we do this
4. Give IV fluids	To improve preload to the heart by correcting hypovolaemia, improving cardiac output and blood pressure
5. Check serial lactate	High lactate indicates hypoperfusion. Response of lactate helps guide resuscitation
6. Measure urine output	Urine output falls if the patient is hypovolaemic; also provides an indicator of adequate cardiac output

Source: Adapted from Daniels and Nutbeam, 2017

CHALLENGES OF MICROBIAL INFECTIONS

Antimicrobial resistance

Antimicrobial resistance is a growing problem worldwide in treating and controlling infections (Khabbaz et al., 2014). Some bacteria such as *Staphylococcus aureus* have developed resistance to **broad spectrum antibiotics** including methicillin-type antibiotics. Methicillin-resistant Staphylococcus aureus (MRSA) is the most important cause of health care-associated infections worldwide and use of antibiotics is the main driver for this (Boswihi and Udo, 2018; den Heijer et al., 2013). While the prevalence of MRSA has decreased significantly in Europe between 2013 and 2016, it still remains a public health priority. There have been significant increases in the percentages of other types of bacterial resistance such as *Enterococcus faecium*, resistant to vancomycin and also known as vancomycin-resistant enterococcus (VRE), and *Klebsiella pneumoniae*, resistant to third-generation cephalosporins and carbapenems (ECDC, 2018a).

Mechanism of bacterial resistance to drugs

There are several ways bacteria can develop resistance to antibiotics. Gram-negative bacteria produce enzymes that destroy the β-lactam component of penicillin-type antibiotics. A reduction in permeability, including closure of porin channels in the cell wall, prevents entry of the antibiotic into the cell and the creation of a modified target so that the antibiotic no longer recognises its target receptor. Bacteria also use an export mechanism to actively pump the antibiotic out of the cell. This mechanism leads to resistance to multiple classes of antibiotics (Karam et al., 2016).

Resistance can also occur as a result of genetic mutations in the microorganism with 'resistance' genes found on a **chromosome** or a plasmid. Plasmids are small pieces of extrachromosomal DNA that use cellular proteins to replicate. By a process of selection, the cells with resistance genes will not be killed by the antibiotic and are passed on to daughter cells, thus maintaining resistance. Bacteria that contain the resistance gene can transfer the gene to other bacteria in the population that are sensitive to the antibiotic. These bacteria then become resistant, thus contributing to the spread of resistance (Bhattacharjee, 2016). The widespread use and misuse of antibiotics has resulted in the development of resistance in microorganisms, including the use of antibiotics in animals that are part of the food chain. A global action plan has been agreed to address the problem of microbial resistance with a particular focus on the use of antibiotics (WHO, 2015). Prudent use of antimicrobials, for example avoidance of prescribing antibiotics for viral infection for which they have no effect, effective infection control measures to reduce spread, reduced use of antibiotics in farm animals, and screening and isolation of infected patients in hospitals are recommended (ECDC, 2018a).

ACTIVITY 7.3: UNDERSTAND

Antibiotic resistance

An interesting overview on antibiotic resistance has been produced by BBC Future Now. To read the article, type 'futurenow antibiotic resistance' into a search engine. If using the eBook click on the icon to the right.

ARTICLE: ANTIBIOTIC
RESISTANCE

CHAPTER SUMMARY

In this chapter you have studied how the immune system defends the body against threats to homeostasis and the consequences of a malfunctioning immune system. Inappropriate responses leading to hypersensitivity, misdirected responses of autoimmunity and alloimmunity, and inadequate response leading to immune deficiency disorders were examined. How microorganisms cause infectious diseases and how the immune system deals with them were also examined, along with some of the challenges we face in controlling the spread and treatment of infectious diseases. In considering these pathophysiological processes, it is essential to consider that people in your care can be vulnerable to such disorders of immunity, whether in a hospital situation or community setting. These disorders have the potential to make someone seriously ill, leave them with a lifelong illness and impact on their ability to function independently, have a family and may even result in death. As nurses, people in our care are often experiencing some form of illness that may lead them to be vulnerable to an immune disorder and we therefore need to ensure that we minimise such risks, particularly where our actions as health care professionals may be a link in the chain of infection; handwashing is one of the most important factors in preventing cross-contamination, as is the use of aseptic non-touch techniques when there is a risk of introducing/contamination with pathogens. Understanding the factors relating to disorders of immunity addressed in this chapter is central to your effectiveness as a person-centred practitioner.

KEY POINTS

- Disorders of the immune system result in homeostatic imbalances: hypersensitivity, where the immune system overreacts; autoimmunity, where the immune system attacks the body's own tissues; and immunodeficiency, where components of the immune system fail.

- Environmental and genetic factors play a role in immune system disorders.

- In autoimmune diseases the mechanism of self-tolerance is lost, and almost any cell or tissue in the body can be affected.

- Immune deficiency disorders occur when there is failure of the immune system to function normally, resulting in an increased susceptibility to infections. This is either genetically determined (primary) or an acquired (secondary) disorder.

- Bone marrow transplantation involves the transplantation of stem cells harvested from donor bone marrow or blood. Graft-versus-host disease (GVHD) is a condition where the donor T cells recognise the recipient tissue as foreign and react against it, involving CD4$^+$ cells and CD8$^+$ T cells.

- HIV is a retrovirus transmitted through body fluids that spread the virus via three major routes: sexual contact, inoculation with infected blood and mother to baby transmission.

- Infectious diseases are caused by microorganisms such as bacteria, viruses, fungi and protozoa.

- The spread of sexually transmitted infections (STIs) is aided by the fact that they are often asymptomatic, so people are unaware they have the infection and do not take adequate precautions or seek treatment.

- *Neisseria meningitidis* is the most common cause of bacterial meningitis in young adults. It is often carried in the nasopharynx of an asymptomatic carrier and is spread by respiratory droplet transmission through kissing, coughing, sneezing or sharing utensils, food and drink.

- Sepsis occurs through a complex sequence of cellular activation and inflammatory mediators and results in life-threatening organ dysfunction caused by a dysregulated host response to infection.

- Bacteria develop resistance to antibiotics in several ways:

  o production of enzymes that destroy the β-lactam component of penicillin-type antibiotics
  o reduction in permeability, including closure of porin channels in the cell wall, preventing entry of the antibiotic into the cell
  o creation of a modified target so that the antibiotic no longer recognises its target receptor
  o use of an export mechanism to actively pump the antibiotic out of the cell. This mechanism leads to resistance to multiple classes of antibiotics.

In this chapter you will have learned about disorders of immunity and their complexity. Use the questions below to check your knowledge and understanding.

Answers are available online. If you are using the eBook just click on the answers icon below. Alternatively go to **https://study.sagepub.com/essentialpatho/answers**

REVISE

TEST YOUR KNOWLEDGE

1 Explain the immunological mechanisms that are responsible for allergic reactions.

2 Explain why it is important that people with a known risk of anaphylactic shock need to carry an epinephrine 'pen' with them at all times.

3 Discuss the type of reaction triggered by a Mantoux test and why it is used.

4 Describe four clinical features of SLE.

5 Identify how HIV is transmitted.

6 Describe how HIV causes destruction of the immune system.

7 Outline the virulence factors that a microorganism needs to cause infectious disease.

8 Describe the stages of the sexually transmitted infection syphilis.

9 What are the risk factors for developing meningitis?

10 Outline the clinical signs of systemic inflammatory response syndrome (SIRS).

11 Explain how sepsis can lead to multiple organ dysfunction syndrome (MODS).

12 Explain the six steps of treatment once sepsis is suspected.

13 Explain how microorganisms become resistant to antimicrobial drugs.

14 Identify what steps can be taken to reduce microbial resistance.

REVISE

ACE YOUR ASSESSMENT

- Further revision and learning opportunities are available online

- Test yourself away from the book with **Extra multiple choice questions**

- Learn and revise terminology with **Interactive flashcards**

If you are using the eBook access each resource by clicking on the respective icon. Alternatively go to **https://study.sagepub.com/essentialpatho/chapter7**

CHAPTER 7
ANSWERS

EXTRA
QUESTIONS

FLASHCARDS

REFERENCES

Abbas, A.K., Lichtman, A.H. and Pillai, S. (2015) *Cellular and Molecular Immunology*, 8th edn. Philadelphia, PA: Elsevier Saunders.

Baldwin, K.J. and Zunt, J.R. (2014) Evaluation and treatment of chronic meningitis. *The Neurohospitalist, 4* (4): 185–95.

Battersby, A.C. and Cant, A.J. (2017) Advances in primary immunodeficiencies. *Paediatrics and Child Health, 27* (3): 116–20.

Bhattacharjee, M. (2016) *Chemistry of Antibiotics and Related Drugs*. Cham: Springer Nature.

Bone, R.C., Balk, R.A., Cerra, F.B. et al. (1992) American College of Chest Physicians/Society of Critical Care Medicine Consensus Conference: definitions for sepsis and organ failure and guidelines for the use of innovative therapies in sepsis. *Critical Care Medicine, 20* (6): 864–74.

Boore, J., Cook, N. and Shepherd, A. (2016) *Essentials of Anatomy and Physiology for Nursing Practice*. London: Sage.

Boswihi, S.S. and Udo, E.E. (2018) Methicillin-resistant Staphylococcus aureus: an update on the epidemiology, treatment options and infection control. *Current Medicine Research and Practice, 8* (1): 18–24.

Brooks, G.F., Carroll, K.C., Butel, S.B., Morse, S.A. and Mietzner, T.A. (2013) *Jawetz, Melnick & Adelberg's Medical Microbiology*, 26th edn. New York: McGraw-Hill.

Bufford, J.D. and Gern, J.E. (2005) The hygiene hypothesis revisited. *Immunology and Allergy Clinics of North America, 25*: 247–62.

Cant, A.J., Slatter, M. and Battersby, A. (2013) Advances in management of primary immunodeficiency. *Paediatrics and Child Health, 23* (3): 115–20.

Choi, S.W. and Reddy, P. (2014) Current and emerging strategies for the prevention of graft-versus-host disease. *Nature Reviews Clinical Oncology, 11*: 536–47.

Daniels, R. and Nutbeam, T. (2017) *The Sepsis Manual 2017–2018*, 4th edn. Birmingham: United Kingdom Sepsis Trust.

Deeks, S.G., Lewin, S.R. and Havlir, D.V. (2013) The end of AIDS: HIV infection as a chronic disease. *Lancet, 382* (9903): 1525–33.

den Heijer, C.D., van Bijnen, E.M., Paget, W.J., Pringle, M., Goossens, H., Bruggeman, C.A. et al. and APRES Study Team (2013) Prevalence and resistance of commensal *Staphylococcus aureus*, including meticillin-resistant S. aureus, in nine European countries: a cross-sectional study. *The Lancet Infectious Diseases, 13* (5): 409–15.

Deutschman, C.S. and Tracey, K.J. (2014) Sepsis: current dogma and new perspectives. *Immunity, 40* (4): 463–75.

Doran, K.S., Fulde, M., Gratz, N., Kim, B.J., Nau, R., Prasadarao, N. et al. (2016). Host–pathogen interactions in bacterial meningitis. *Acta Neuropathologica, 131* (2): 185–209.

European Centre for Disease Prevention and Control (ECDC) (2018a) Antimicrobial resistance (EARS-Net). In Annual Epidemiological Report for 2014. Stockholm: ECDC. Available at: https://ecdc.europa.eu/sites/portal/files/documents/AER_for_2014-AMR-EARSnet.pdf (accessed 1 August 2018).

European Centre for Disease Prevention and Control (ECDC) (2018b) Communicable disease threats report (CDTR_, Week 13, March 25–31. Stockholm: EDCD. Available at: www.ecdc. europa.eu/sites/portal/files/documents/Communicable-disease-threats-report-31-mar-2018.pdf (accessed 1 August 2018).

Farh, K.K.H., Marson, A., Zhu, J., Kleinewietfeld, M., Housley, W.J., Beik, S. et al. (2015) Genetic and epigenetic fine mapping of causal autoimmune disease variants. *Nature, 518* (7539): 337–43.

Fleischmann, C., Scherag, A., Adhikari, N.K., Hartog, C.S., Tsaganos, T., Schlattmann, P. et al. (2016) Assessment of global incidence and mortality of hospital-treated sepsis: current estimates and limitations. *American Journal of Respiratory and Critical Care Medicine, 193* (3): 259–72.

Frieri, M. and Stampfl, H. (2016) Systemic lupus erythematosus and atherosclerosis: review of the literature. *Autoimmunity Reviews, 15*: 16–21.

Gal, Y., Gilad, T., Ben-Ami Shor, D., Furer, A., Sherer, Y., Mozes, O. et al. (2015) A volcanic explosion of autoantibodies in systemic lupus erythematosus: a diversity of 180 different antibodies found in SLE patients. *Autoimmunity Reviews, 14* (1): 75–9.

Galli, S.J. and Tsai, M. (2012) IgE and mast cells in allergic disease. *Nature Medicine, 18*: 693–704.

Garland, S.M. and Steben, M. (2014) Genital herpes: best practice and research. *Clinical Obstetrics & Gynaecology, 28* (7): 1098–110.

Ghosn, J., Taiwo, B., Seedat, S. and Autran, B. (2018) HIV. *The Lancet* [online]. Available at: http://dx.doi.org/10.1016/S0140-6736(18)31311-4 (accessed 31 July 2018).

Global Health Estimates (2018) *Deaths by Cause, Age, Sex, by Country and by Region, 2000–2016*. Geneva: World Health Organisation.

Gordon, C., Amissah-Arthur, M.B., Gayed, M., Brown, S., Bruce, I.N., D'Cruz, D., et al. (2018) The British Society for Rheumatology guideline for the management of systemic lupus erythematosus in adults. *Rheumatology, 57* (1): e1–e45.

Gupta, R.K., Lucas, S.B., Fielding, K.L. and Lawn, S.D. (2015) Prevalence of tuberculosis in post-modern studies of HIV-infected adults and children in resource-limited settings: a systematic review and meta-analysis. *AIDS, 29* (15): 1987–2002.

Hook, E.W. (2017) Syphilis. *The Lancet, 389* (10078): 1550–57.

Hotchkiss, R.S., Monneret, G. and Payen, D. (2013) Sepsis-induced immunosuppression: from cellular dysfunctions to immunotherapy. *Nature Reviews Immunology, 13* (12): 862–74.

Johnson, C., Kennedy, C., Fonner, V., Siegfried, N., Figueroa, C., Dalal, S. et al. (2017) Examining the effects of HIV self-testing compared to standard HIV testing services: a systematic review and meta-analysis. *Journal of the International AIDS Society, 20*: 215–94.

Justiz Vaillant, A.A. and Zito, P.M. (2018) *Hypersensitivity Reactions, Immediate.* StatPearls [Internet]. Treasure Island, FL: StatPearls Publishing.

Karam, G., Chastre, J., Wilcox, M.H. and Vincent, J.L. (2016) Antibiotic strategies in the era of multidrug resistance. *Critical Care, 20* (1): 136.

Kaufmann, F. and Demenais, F. (2012) Gene–environment interactions in asthma and allergic diseases: challenges and perspectives. *Journal of Allergy and Clinical Immunology, 130*: 1229–40.

Khabbaz, R., Moseley, R., Steiner, R., Levitt, A.M. and Bell, B.P. (2014) Challenges of infectious diseases in the USA. *The Lancet, 384* (9937): 53–63.

Kim, K.S. (2010) Acute bacterial meningitis in infants and children. *The Lancet Infectious Diseases, 10* (1): 32–42.

Kumar, V., Abbas, A.K. and Aster, J.C. (2018) *Robbins Basic Pathology,* 10th edn. Philadelphia, PA: Elsevier Saunders.

Larsen, J.N., Broge, L. and Jacobi, H. (2016) Allergy immunotherapy: the future of allergy treatment. *Drug Discovery Today, 21* (1): 26–37.

Lehr, S., Vier, J., Hacker, G. and Kirschnek, S. (2018) Activation of neutrophils by *Chlamydia trachomatis*-infected epithelial cells is modulated by the chlamydial plasmid. *Microbes and Infection, 20* (5): 284–92.

Maver, P.J. and Poljak, M. (2017) Progress in prophylactic human papillomavirus (HPV) vaccination in 2016: a literature review. *Vaccine, 36* (36): 5416–23. Available at: https://doi. org/10.1016/j. vaccine.2017.07.113 (accessed 29 July 2018).

McInnes, I.B. and Schett, G. (2017) Pathogenetic insights from the treatment of rheumatoid arthritis. *The Lancet, 389* (10086): 2328–37.

NHS-RCP (National Health Service (NHS) Plus, Royal College of Physicians) (2008) Faculty of Occupational Medicine. Latex allergy: occupational aspects of management. A national guideline. London: RCP.

NICE (National Institute for Health and Care Excellence) (2016) Belimumab for treating active autoantibody-positive systemic lupus erythematosus. Technology appraisal guidance [TA397]. Available at: www.nice.org.uk/guidance/ta397/chapter/2-The-technology (accessed 1 August 2018).

Notarangelo, L.D. (2010) Primary immunodeficiencies. *Journal of Allergy and Clinical Immunology, 125* (2): S182–S194.

Payne, H., Mkhize, N., Otwombe, K., Lewis, J., Panchia, R., Callard, R. et al. (2015) Reactivity of routine HIV antibody tests in children who initiated antiretroviral therapy in early infancy as part of the Children with HIV Early Antiretroviral Therapy (CHER) trial: a retrospective analysis. *The Lancet Infectious Diseases, 15* (7): 803–9.

Perkey, E. and Maillard, I. (2018) New insights into graft-versus-host disease and graft rejection. *Annual Review of Pathology: Mechanisms of Disease, 13*: 219–45.

Reber, L.L., Hernandez, J.D. and Galli, S.J. (2017) The pathophysiology of anaphylaxis. *Journal of Allergy and Clinical Immunology, 140* (2): 335–48.

Rees, F., Doherty, M., Grainge, M., Davenport, G., Lanyon, P. and Zhang, W. (2016) The incidence and prevalence of systemic lupus erythematosus in the UK, 1999–2012. *Annals of the Rheumatic Diseases, 75*: 136–41.

Rees, F., Doherty, M., Grainge, M.J., Lanyon, P. and Zhang, W. (2017) The worldwide incidence and prevalence of systemic lupus erythematosus: a systematic review of epidemiological studies. *Rheumatology, 56* (11): 1945–61.

Rote, N. (2017) Infection and defects in mechanisms of defence. In Huether, S.E. and McCance, K.L. (eds), *Understanding Pathophysiology*, 6th edn. St Louis, MO: Elsevier Saunders.

Say, L., Chou, D., Gemmill, A. et al. (2014) Global causes of maternal death: a WHO systematic analysis. *The Lancet Global Health, 2* (6): e323–33.

Scherr, T.D., Hanke, M.L., Huang, O., James, D.B., Horswill, A.R., Bayles, K.W. et al. (2015) *Staphylococcus aureus* biofilms induce macrophage dysfunction through leukocidin AB and alpha-toxin. *MBio, 6* (4): e01021–15.

Schrijvers, R., Gilissen, L., Chiriac, A. and Demoly, P. (2015) Pathogenesis and diagnosis of delayed-type drug hypersensitivity reactions, from bedside to bench and back. *Clinical and Translational Allergy, 5*: 31.

Sherrard, J. (2014) Gonorrhoea. *Medicine, 42* (6): 323–6.

Shields, A.M. and Patel, S.Y. (2017) The primary immunodeficiency disorders. *Medicine, 45* (10): 597–604.

Sicherer, S.H. and Sampson, H.A. (2018) Food allergy: a review and update on epidemiology, pathogenesis, diagnosis, prevention and management. *Journal of Allergy and Clinical Immunology, 141* (1): 41–58.

Singer, M., Deutschman, C.S., Seymour, C.W., Shankar-Hari, M., Annane, D., Bauer, M. et al. (2016) The third international consensus definitions for sepsis and septic shock (Sepsis-3). *JAMA, 315* (8): 801–10.

Tanno, L.K., Calderon, M.A., Demoly, P. and Joint Allergy Academies (2016) New allergic and hypersensitivity conditions section in the International Classification of Diseases-11. *Allergy, Asthma & Immunology Research, 8* (4): 383–8.

Walker, B. and McMichael, A. (2012) The T-cell response to HIV. *Cold Spring Harbor Perspectives in Medicine, 2*: a007054.

World Health Organisation (WHO) (2015) *Global Action Plan on Antimicrobial Resistance*. Geneva: WHO.

World Health Organisation (WHO) (2016) *Consolidated Guidelines on the Use of Antiretroviral Drugs for Treating and Preventing HIV Infection. Recommendations for a Public Health Approach*, 2nd edn. Geneva: WHO.

World Health Organisation (WHO) (2017) *World Malaria Report 2017*. Geneva: WHO.

World Health Organisation (WHO) (2018) *HIV/AIDS (Fact Sheet)*. Geneva: WHO.

Young-Peterson, F. (2013) Alterations in immune function. In Copstead, L.E. and Banasik, J. (eds), *Pathophysiology*, 5th edn. St Louis, MO: Elsevier Saunders.

DISORDERS OF BLOOD AND BLOOD SUPPLY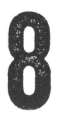

UNDERSTAND: CHAPTER VIDEOS

Watch the following videos to ease you into this chapter. If you are using the eBook just click on the play buttons. Alternatively go to **https://study.sagepub.com/essentialpatho/videos**

DEEP VEIN THROMBOSIS
(6:07)

PERIPHERAL VASCULAR
DISEASE (2:30)

LEARNING OUTCOMES

When you have finished studying this chapter you will be able to:

1. Describe the major effects of reduced blood flow on cell **metabolism**.
2. Identify major conditions which reduce blood flow to the tissues.
3. Recognise the effects, signs and symptoms of reduced blood supply on tissues.
4. Understand what happens in reduced blood flow to the major organs of the body.

INTRODUCTION

Blood circulation supplies all the different tissues and organs of the body with the requirements for life at the appropriate concentration, i.e. nutrients, oxygen, **electrolyte** and acid–base balance and hormones to regulate function. It also regulates waste products by picking up substances to be removed or maintained in balance and carries them to the relevant organs: carbon dioxide to the lungs, urea and electrolytes to the kidneys, and other substances to the liver. Anything affecting blood flow to tissues can cause a reduced supply of requirements for normal function and an enhanced accumulation of waste products, resulting in reduced homeostasis of the affected part. Various conditions can influence blood flow and result in disturbed function of different organs. Various causes and alterations in the blood vessels and blood supply to tissues are discussed.

We will begin by examining the effect of a reduced supply of blood on cell **metabolism** and then consider some of the different ways in which blood flow is altered. Later in the chapter we will look at some of the specific disturbances that can occur. Blood flows due to heart contraction, passing through blood vessels to supply tissues, all of which can be diminished. In addition, the nature of the blood itself can be altered.

PERSON-CENTRED CONTEXT: THE BODIE FAMILY

BODIE FAMILY CASE NOTES

The blood circulation plays a central role in maintaining the supply of necessary substances and removing waste products. Difficulties with the circulation result in disturbances in function of different organs in the body. The Bodie family contains members who have such conditions and have friends and colleagues who also have such conditions which affect their abilities. Maud and George belong to the local branch of U3A (University of the Third Age), an international movement which is run for and by retired people to provide a range of educational, social, creative and health-related activities, and provides opportunities to meet others with similar interests. Within these activities they have met numerous people with a range of conditions such as those discussed in this chapter.

Maud has mild **heart failure** in which contractility of her heart is limited and thus the volume of blood pumped out is reduced. In addition, her blood viscosity is increased. The effects of these changes are minimised by digoxin for the heart failure, and warfarin to thin her blood and make it flow more easily. Richard Jones has **diabetes mellitus** and is thus susceptible to disturbances in the structure of blood vessels, **atherosclerosis**, which can reduce blood flow.

EFFECTS OF REDUCED BLOOD FLOW

Circulatory disorders can be due to problems with the blood, the blood vessels or the heart.

Reduced blood flow to various tissues can occur for various reasons:

- Reduced blood volume due to:
  - loss from injury causing external or internal bleeding
  - limited coagulation through lack of coagulating proteins, e.g. **haemophilia**, leading to increased blood loss externally or into the tissues
  - reduced blood volume due to loss of fluid, i.e. **dehydration** due to high body or environmental temperature.
- Occlusion of the arteries carrying blood to be carried through the capillaries to the tissues, causing a reduced supply of blood to the tissues.

Metabolic changes and their effect

As blood volume decreases, the amount of blood circulating through the capillaries to supply the cell requirements also decreases. The metabolism within the cells necessary to carry out the range of activities normally performed is reduced and from this flows the other effects on the body. Maintenance of **homeostasis** requires normal cell metabolism to continue to manage the production and management of energy.

REVISE: A&P RECAP

Major nutrient and metabolic pathways

Changes in metabolism can be reviewed in Chapter 9, Figure 9.7, of *Essentials of Anatomy and Physiology for Nursing Practice* (Boore et al., 2016), which shows the major nutrient and metabolic pathways.

In the situation with reduced blood flow, oxygen and nutrient supply is reduced and the cells move from **aerobic metabolism** towards anaerobic metabolism, with increased **lactate** formation and a fall in pH resulting in acidosis (normal pH is 7.35–7.45); and this will also reduce metabolism. The amount of ATP (adenosine tri-phosphate, the energy store for cell function) created per glucose molecule is drastically reduced, as shown in Figure 8.1 which illustrates the metabolic changes and reduced ATP produced. What is clear is that the amount of ATP created is significantly reduced when oxygen supply is limited and, thus, there is reduced availability for all aspects of homeostasis.

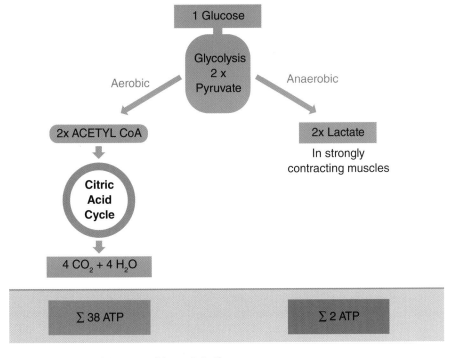

Figure 8.1   Fall in ATP with anaerobic metabolism

Many of the bodily effects of reduced blood flow and of **inflammation**, in which increased blood flow occurs, are opposite: reduced blood flow causes coldness of the part involved, pallor and/or **cyanosis** (blue discoloration), pain and reduced sensation. As the **haemoglobin** releases its oxygen (becoming deoxyhaemoglobin), the colour of the blood becomes bluish, and as the amount of blood in the tissues is reduced the skin appears pale. In addition, as blood carries heat from the core of the body to the peripheries, a reduction in flow results in a cooling of the tissues. Pain is variable, but if the blood flow to, for example, the legs is reduced and the person affected is walking he or she is likely to have pain in the muscle. Similarly, a **myocardial infarction** (heart attack) occurs when blood flow to the heart is reduced, the muscle of the heart receives inadequate oxygen and, as it is continually contracting, pain normally occurs. However, a **stroke** occurs as a result of reduced blood flow to the brain and generally leads to reduced function and weakness, but not pain (the brain itself has no nociceptors). Reduced blood flow to a specific part of the body can lead to numbness of that area (Lakhani et al., 2009). There are a number of different conditions due to reduced blood flow and a number of these will be considered.

BLOCKAGE OF BLOOD VESSELS

Blood flows through the arteries, capillaries and veins to deliver the nutrient requirements to body cells. Problems can occur at all stages in the pathway and some major issues will be considered.

Arterial disturbances

The blood flow through the arteries can be reduced in various ways. The major relevant condition is atherosclerosis, which is discussed below. In addition, there is a condition called **arteriosclerosis**. The terms atherosclerosis and arteriosclerosis are often used interchangeably but they are not the same.

–––––––––––––––––––––––– **UNDERSTAND** ––––––––––––––––––––––––

Arteriosclerosis vs. atherosclerosis

These two terms relate to different disturbances in the arterial walls:

Arteriosclerosis: the arterial walls become thickened and hardened as smooth muscle is replaced by **collagen** and hyaline cartilage. No lipid material is deposited. The blood vessel becomes less compliant and is associated with raised blood pressure.

Atherosclerosis: an arterial **disease** in which fatty material is deposited on the inner walls of the vessels. It is discussed below.

Atherosclerosis

Pathophysiological changes

In this chronic inflammatory disease, **atheroma** builds up in the arteries as plaque is laid down and this in time narrows the arteries and reduces the blood flow which normally supplies oxygen, nutrients and hormones to the different parts of the body. There are various systemic risk factors for atherosclerosis development, including: **obesity**, age, blood **cholesterol** levels and smoking.

Figure 8.2 illustrates how this plaque (also known as atheroma) builds up and narrows the arteries. Part A (the upper illustration) shows a normal artery with expected blood flow and a cross-section showing the smooth inner wall of the healthy artery. Part B (below) is an artery with considerable build-up of plaque with the limited blood flow, and the cross-section demonstrates the limited space for blood to pass.

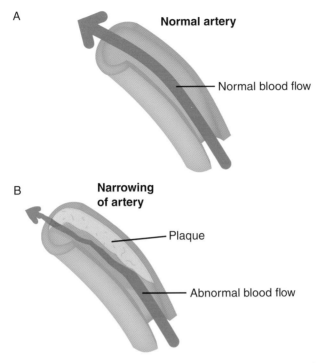

Illustrated by Shaun Mercier © SAGE Publications

Figure 8.2   Development of atheroma

However, the atheroma-creating plaque occurs mainly at specific parts of the arterial tree (i.e. within the branching pattern of the arteries). The **endothelial cells** lining the blood vessels are sensitive to the stress of the shearing force created by the blood flow against the cell wall. Regions of the arterial tree with bends and arterial branching are known as **atheroprone** (i.e. prone to development of atherosclerosis) where the blood flow is disturbed and there is low shear stress (Green et al., 2018). These are sites where atheroma development begins and is increased and atherosclerosis develops, as indicated in Figure 8.2.

The low shear stress and **oscillation** (i.e. regular fluctuation or vibration about a central point) are linked with increased levels of inflammatory molecules, including ATP signalling and increased specialised molecules that promote adhesion of **leucocytes** to the **endothelium** (Green et al., 2018). Plaque itself is composed of fat, cholesterol, calcium and other substances, largely derived from the diet, which pass through the **intima** and begin to cause dysfunction of the endothelium and deposition of **connective tissue**. Atheroma goes through several stages of development (Table 8.1). However, it is important to remember that for this to start, the lining of the blood vessel has to become eroded to some extent and while low shear stress is one factor, the other significant factor is sugar (sucrose). Sucrose is abrasive to the intima of blood vessels and once it causes erosion, cholesterol deposits are directed from the liver to patch and repair the damage. This cholesterol then becomes trapped in pockets of the inflamed vessel and begins to accumulate. While historically fat has been blamed as the cause for atherosclerosis, sucrose is the guilty party (Kearns et al., 2016).

Table 8.1 Stages of atheroma development

1	Early fatty streak development	Begins in childhood and adolescence. LDLs (**low density lipoproteins**) accumulate in the intima and are converted to pro-inflammatory particles. Fat droplets may accumulate in the cytoplasm of smooth muscle cells
		Activated endothelial cells initiate inflammation and secrete molecules which draw monocytes, **lymphocytes**, **mast cells** and **neutrophils** into the arterial wall. Intimal smooth muscle cells secrete various connective tissue cells
		Monocytes become **macrophages**, absorb lipids and become foam cells. Microscopic changes become visible
2	Early fibroatheroma	Appears in teens and 20s. Macrophage foam cells, other inflammatory cells and natural arterial cells accumulate
		Macrophages control plaque development, but inflammation may become excessive. Smooth muscle cells increase their lipid-binding capacity. Death of macrophages and smooth muscle cells occurs and necrotic debris provokes more inflammation and cell **necrosis**. Normal intima is distorted until completely disrupted. Lipid-rich necrotic cores dominate the central part of the intima, until it occupies 30–50% of arterial wall volume. Fibrous tissue forms a cap over lipid-rich necrotic cores and under the endothelium to form fibrous plaque that becomes the dominant **lesion**
3	Advancing atheroma: thin-cap fibroatheroma and its rupture	Occurs in persons aged ≥55 years. Thin-cap fibroatheroma (TCFA) develops and may rupture
		TCFA becomes thin and weakened by **proteolytic enzymes** dissolving fibrous tissue, making it liable to rupture, resulting in a thrombus extending into the arterial lumen. Called a vulnerable plaque, these appear at about 55 to 65 years, before the peak of myocardial infarction and **stroke**. TCFAs and ruptured plaques within coronary arteries are focal and limited in patients dying of cardiovascular causes, contrasting with extensive distribution in coronary arteries of all earlier grades. Plaque may grow into adjacent arterial walls and distort them; the local segment of arterial wall may enlarge its **calibre**. These may leak, producing haemorrhage and fibrous tissue
4	Complex lesion development	Many TCFA ruptures are clinically silent as they heal by fibrosis but may rupture again with thrombus formation. These cyclic changes of rupture, **thrombosis** and healing may recur up to four times at a single lesion, causing multiple layers of healed tissue. In 60% of **sudden cardiac death**s, cyclic healing of clinically silent ruptures has been reported. Calcium deposits in the wall occur throughout all these steps, as small aggregates, followed by large nodules. Plaques may rupture into the lumen and expose the nodules, which become sites for thrombosis. The increasing mass of some plaques may cause significant **stenosis** and cause lethal **ischaemia** by flow restriction. All of these changes may be significantly influenced by risk factors, notably the stresses of local haemodynamics and blood flow patterns

Source: Adapted from Insull, 2009; Sheppard and Herrington, 2014

There are a number of risk factors which increase the possibility of developing atherosclerosis. Genetic makeup is a key issue, with a high incidence in the family increasing the risk of its development in other family members. In addition, there are medical conditions such as **hypertension** (contributes to shear stress) and diabetes (too much sugar remaining in the blood and being corrosive), as well as lifestyle factors including smoking, lack of exercise, obesity and an unhealthy diet.

Complications of atherosclerosis

There are a number of conditions which can develop in those with atherosclerosis affecting mainly the aorta and those vessels supplying major organs – the brain, heart, gut and kidneys (Table 8.2).

Table 8.2 Complications of atherosclerosis

Organs affected	Conditions occurring
Aneurysm: major arteries	Abdominal aorta, iliac and popliteal, and cerebral arteries Can rupture and lead to haemorrhage and shock
Brain: cerebral arteries	Cerebrovascular disease: cerebral infarction (stroke); **transient ischaemic attack (TIA)** or mini-stroke; arteriopathic (vascular) dementia
Heart: coronary arteries	**Ischaemic heart disease**: can cause myocardial infarction (MI); heart failure; sudden death
Legs	Peripheral vascular disease. Intermittent claudication (exercise-induced cramping pain in calves of legs); **gangrene**
Gut: mesenteric arteries	Mesenteric claudication (severe abdominal pain after eating); intestinal infarction
Kidneys: renal arteries	Hypertension; **renal failure**

Source: Adapted from Sheppard and Herrington, 2014

Management of atherosclerosis

A major focus on treating those with atherosclerosis is enabling them to change their lifestyle to achieve appropriate lipoprotein levels. These changes include: dietary alterations to increase fibre intake through eating more fruit and vegetables; undertaking regular exercise; and stopping smoking. Medications may also be prescribed to treat conditions often associated with atherosclerosis, including **dyslipidaemia** (distorted lipoprotein cholesterol: high levels of **LDL (low density)** or low levels of **HDL (high density) lipoprotein** cholesterol); hypertension; and diabetes mellitus. There are a range of drugs which can be used to reduce inflammation and enhance endothelial function including: antiplatelet drugs, ACE inhibitors, **beta-blockers** and **statins** (Aziz and Yadav, 2016). In particular, statins are valuable in reducing the levels of **triglycerides** in the blood and limiting the cardiovascular risk (Bergheanu et al., 2017).

In some conditions, **surgery** may be required to enhance blood flow through blocked arteries. Methods used can include the following:

- **Angioplasty** and **stent** placement: a catheter, containing an additional catheter with a balloon on the end, is inserted into the relevant artery. The balloon is inflated and arterial contents are compressed. A stent (mesh tube) left in position keeps the blood vessel open.
- **Endarterectomy**: fatty deposits can be removed surgically from the walls of the diseased artery.
- Bypass surgery: a graft, synthetic or from another part of the body, can be inserted to bypass around a blocked or damaged artery.

Surgery may also be needed if necrotic tissue has developed when blood flow is completely cut off, most commonly in the toes, feet and lower legs. The dead tissue is removed: usually by amputation behind the point where blood flow is blocked.

Venous disturbances

Blood is returned to the heart via the veins so blockage of these does not limit blood flow to the tissues. However, any blockage may limit the movement of fluid back from the tissues, causing increased pressure in the tissues and the formation of **oedema** (Chapter 15), thus distorting the normal circulation. Blockage of the veins can be due to venous thrombosis, spasm, or external compression, with venous thrombosis being the commonest.

Venous thrombosis and embolism

Venous thrombosis usually occurs due to decelerated blood flow and most often in the legs, in the deep veins of the calf, but may spread upwards into the thigh (femoral or iliac veins or, even, the inferior vena cava). There are a range of risk factors for deep venous (or vein) thrombosis (DVT), including: surgery or trauma; immobilisation either by bed rest or long-haul flights; old age, obesity, heart failure; pregnancy and the puerperium, or the contraceptive pill; and familial thrombophilia (an increased level of blood coagulation).

The major health hazard associated with DVT is a pulmonary **embolus**, when part of the thrombus breaks off and is carried to the heart where it can become impacted in the right side of the heart or is carried in the pulmonary artery or arteries, occluding them and reducing blood supply to one or both lungs. Emboli can vary considerably in size: a large embolus will get stuck in the right ventricle or block the circulation to one of the lungs completely. On the other hand, a number of small emboli can enter the lungs and occlude a number of small blood vessels. The person affected will be short of breath, have pain on inspiration and **cough** up blood (Sheppard and Herrington, 2014).

FAILURE OF THE CIRCULATION

There are some disorders of the circulation which can lead to reduced delivery of the essential ingredients needed for normal cell metabolism. Some key ones are considered here.

Shock

Shock is a condition in which there is low **perfusion** of the tissues due to a fall in blood pressure and increased heart rate which is aiming to compensate for this drop in blood volume. The intention is to prevent collapse of the circulation. Other signs result from reduced blood flow to the organs normally supplied and include reduced urine output, disturbed **consciousness** (unconsciousness or confusion) and reduced **pulse pressure**. Shock is a medical emergency necessitating rapid treatment to permit survival. There are various causes but all affect the circulatory system and threaten life.

ACTIVITY 8.1: UNDERSTAND

Shock: Key facts

This video will help you grasp the key facts about shock. If you are using the eBook just click on the play button. Alternatively go to **https://study.sagepub.com/essentialpatho/videos**

▷

SHOCK (3:04)

Pathophysiology of shock

The primary disturbance is limited blood flow to the tissues which results in an oxygen supply to body cells that is not adequate for aerobic respiration. There will be a substantial shift towards anaerobic respiration and a considerable drop in the formation of ATP. Increased anaerobic respiration will also cause a rise in carbon dioxide and lactate formation, leading to a fall in tissue pH (i.e. acidosis, increased hydrogen ions). The adequacy of cell activity falls in this environment, and without rapid effective treatment, cell damage becomes irreversible and the person dies.

Early in shock, physiological mechanisms compensate for the fall in blood flow and maintain the blood flow to the most important organs of the body (the heart, nervous system and kidneys) but cause a further reduction in blood flow to other tissues and organs. The presentation of this state includes: pale, cold, sweaty skin (**diaphoresis**) (possibly with cyanosis of the extremities); confusion and restlessness; low blood pressure and fast, thready pulse; and increased respiratory rate and depth. This will often progress to **coma** and unless blood flow is restored, multi-organ failure will result in death (Sheppard and Herrington, 2014).

Although there are a number of different causes of shock, with some variation in presentation, most types will follow the description presented above, with some additional factors depending on the specific causes: for example, someone with **septic shock** may not be pale. There are several different classification systems for shock. The one we are using includes the main groups discussed below, but some of these also include sub-groups which some classifications present as separate entities.

Hypovolaemic shock

This is the condition which occurs as a result of a significant decrease in blood volume. The reduced venous return to the heart leads to reduced **cardiac output** to supply the organs of the body. Initially, this is compensated for by increasing the heart rate and blood pressure. Causes are indicated in Table 8.3.

Table 8.3 Causes of hypovolaemic shock

Bleeding	Internal or external: trauma, surgery, peptic **ulcer**, ruptured aortic aneurysm, **oesophageal varices**, **ectopic pregnancy**
Fluid loss: skin	Burns, excessive sweating due to exposure to heat
Fluid loss: GI tract	Diarrhoea, vomiting
Fluid loss: kidneys	Diabetes, diabetes insipidus, **adrenal insufficiency**, salt-losing nephritis, excessive diuretics, diuretic phase of acute renal failure
Fluid loss: to extravascular space	Increased capillary permeability due to inflammation, **anoxia**, sepsis and other conditions

Source: Procter, 2018

ACTIVITY 8.2: UNDERSTAND

Haemorrhagic shock

Watch this video to aid your understanding of this type of shock. If you are using the eBook just click on the play button. Alternatively go to

https://study.sagepub.com/essentialpatho/videos

HAEMORRHAGIC SHOCK
(2:33)

Hypovolaemic shock

A friend of Bodie family members Michelle and Kwame Zuma who also works in Brussels usually cycles to work. However, 6 months ago he was knocked off his bike by a car driver and sustained some injuries to his legs and body. An ambulance was swiftly on the scene and paramedics treated him. The most serious aspect was that he had developed **hypovolaemic shock**, becoming pale and with a low blood pressure (hypotension) and fast pulse rate (tachycardia). Intravenous (IV) fluids were started to enable maintenance of fluid volume. Oxygen was administered, open wounds covered rapidly and he was speedily transferred to hospital. He was diagnosed with a ruptured spleen and a splenectomy was performed. He has now made a good recovery.

Distributive shock

This type of shock develops when there is an imbalance between the circulatory volume and a dilated circulation, either arterial or venous division. While the blood volume may be normal or even raised, there are various ways in which the capillaries supplying the tissues are bypassed, including arteriovenous shunts or blood pooling in capillary beds. There are three main types of **distributive shock**, which are sometimes presented as distinct categories.

Septic shock

This form of shock is related to an inappropriate response to infection in which the tissue perfusion is reduced and results in failure of a number of bodily organs. It is a subset of **sepsis**, which itself has a varied mortality rate from moderate (e.g. 10%) to substantial (e.g. >40%) depending on the pathogenic organism, the status of the person infected and, crucially, the speed of diagnosis and initiation of treatment. Septic shock's mortality rate is decreasing, now averaging 30–40% (but individual characteristics result in a wider range of 10–90%) (Maggio, 2018).

Gram-negative bacilli, including *Escherichia coli*, *Pseudomonas*, *Klebsiella* and *Enterobacter*, are the commonest causes of septic shock which develops from a localised infection. If the infection is not restricted to its original site, inflammation and the action of **cytokines** (small proteins secreted by cells of the immune system) affect other cells of the body. Infection spreads, leading firstly to **bacteraemia** (bacteria in the blood but without major clinical disease) and then septicaemia (includes a state of shock). These bacteria create **endotoxins** which are **lipopolysaccharides** (a molecule consisting of combined lipid and polysaccharide (a carbohydrate) in the outer membrane of gram-negative bacteria) and stimulate the release of **tumour necrosis factor**-alpha (TNFα) from macrophages. These, and other cells, initiate a cascade of interleukin secretion produced by leucocytes which regulate the immune response and can activate the clotting system to start **disseminated intravascular coagulation** (DIC) (Angus and van der Poll, 2013; McConnell and Coopersmith, 2016).

DIC can present either with widespread blood clotting or with inadequate clotting, causing haemorrhage. It can occur suddenly (e.g. with complications of childbirth) followed by resolution, or as a chronic condition. Small clots develop throughout the circulation and mini-infarctions can occur and cause organ damage. In addition, these clots use up the coagulation factors in the circulation so bleeding becomes uncontrolled (Lakhani et al., 2009). DIC leads to cardiac failure, peripheral resistance falls, capillaries leak and the capillary–**epithelium** interface in the lung alveoli is damaged (Chetty and Lucas, 2014).

The physiological disturbances associated with septic shock can result in **multiple organ dysfunc-tion syndrome (MODS)** which is altered organ function in an acutely ill person requiring medical intervention to achieve homeostasis. This involves two or more organs, which can include the lungs, kidneys, heart, gastrointestinal tract and liver; MODS can be fatal.

Those affected with septic shock can present with a wide range of symptoms: fever, raised heart rate, sweating and rapid breathing. Initially, BP remains normal but as the condition worsens the BP falls. Although the skin is warm; confusion or reduced wakefulness occurs, particularly in the old and young. Later, coolness, paleness and cyanosis develop in the extremities (and can lead to gangrene and amputation) and indicators of specific organ damage develop: these include the brain, lungs, heart, kidneys, intestine and liver (Maggio, 2018). It is important to remember that someone in septic shock may also have a low or normal body temperature.

Early diagnosis and treatment have improved the mortality rate from septic shock. Diagnosis involves careful clinical examination, some physiological parameters (e.g. blood pressure, central venous pressure [pressure filling the right atrium], central venous oxygen saturation), a range of biochemical markers (e.g. full blood count, electrolyte levels, **creatinine**, lactate), and microbiological cultures of all possible sites of infection. The principles of treatment are indicated in Table 8.4.

Table 8.4 Principles of treatment of septic shock

Perfusion	IV fluids (largely isotonic saline) to restore tissue perfusion without **pulmonary oedema**
Oxygen	Mask or nasal prongs, possibly intubation and **ventilation** needed
Broad-spectrum antibiotics	After specimens taken, antibiotics started immediately. Selection depends on possible sources and educated guess. Broad-based gram-positive and -negative bacteria covered. Immunocompromised people, antifungal drugs administered
Source control	Sites of infection identified and controlled as soon as possible. Tubes removed or changed, **abscesses** drained, excision of necrotic tissue etc.
Other supportive measures	Maintenance of blood glucose, IV **insulin** titrated to maintain glucose level Corticosteroid therapy may be helpful

Source: Maggio, 2018

Anaphylactic shock

This is a reaction which can occur when an individual has developed a Type 1 or immediate **hyper-sensitivity** to a particular **antigen**, the pathophysiology of which is discussed in detail in Chapter 7. There are different types and severity of these reactions, but **anaphylactic shock** is the most severe, being extreme and often life-threatening in nature. The main mechanism for this type of shock is related to an abnormal immune reaction due to a minute amount of the relevant antigen which influences the function of a number of different cells of the immune response. The effects lead to **bronchospasm**, causing constriction of the airway and oedema of the respiratory tract, leading to difficulty with breathing (**dyspnoea**) (Reber et al., 2017).

Individuals with such hypersensitivity are usually prescribed, and always carry with them, an auto-injector (e.g. EpiPen) to enable rapid injection of adrenaline (epinephrine) to cut short the development of anaphylaxis.

ACTIVITY 8.3: UNDERSTAND

Anaphylactic shock

Watch this video to better understand the physiological changes that occur in this type of shock. If you are using the eBook just click on the play button. Alternatively go to
https://study.sagepub.com/essentialpatho/videos

ANAPHYLACTIC SHOCK (9:40)

Neurogenic shock

Neurogenic shock occurs when upper parts of the central nervous system (the brain, cervical spine or upper thoracic spine) are severely injured (Popa et al., 2010). The changes in neurogenic shock consist primarily of **hypotension, bradycardia** and loss of sympathetic nervous activity to the blood vessels (a triad – all three are necessary for this classification). The sympathetic nervous system emanates from thoracic spinal area T5/6 and damage from this point and above inhibits the normal vascular contraction and enables dilation of blood vessels and pooling of blood.

ACTIVITY 8.4: UNDERSTAND

Neurogenic shock

Watch this video to better understand the physiological changes that occur in this type of shock. If you are using the eBook just click on the play button. Alternatively go to
https://study.sagepub.com/essentialpatho/videos

NEUROGENIC SHOCK (8:18)

Cardiogenic shock

This type of shock occurs because the heart is no longer able to pump blood round the body adequately. The commonest cause is myocardial infarction (heart attack, MI) but there are other possible causes, including: mechanical disorders of the heart (ventricular septal or other cardiac wall rupture, papillary muscle rupture causing mitral valve regurgitation), acute **myocarditis** (inflammation of the **myocardium**), **cardiac tamponade** (fluid in the pericardium compressing the heart), arrhythmias, cardiac myopathies (enlargement of the heart muscle – thick, rigid), high-risk pulmonary **embolism**, and decompensation of chronic heart disease. **Cardiogenic shock** usually develops within 24 hours of an MI and often results in multi-organ failure and a mortality rate of 35–50% if not adequately treated (Kataja and Harjola, 2017). Often, the cause is unsuccessfully treated (e.g. severe damage to the myocardium) and treatment largely is to buy time and improve quality of life.

The fall in ventricular contraction leads to reduced cardiac output and **stroke volume**, resulting in hypotension and lowered perfusion of tissues. As the volume of blood leaving the heart is reduced, a backup of blood can occur in the venae cavae that can lead to oedema formation. Vasoconstriction occurs to aim to compensate for the fall in blood pressure but decreases still further the blood supply to tissues. Secretion of **catecholamines** and **cortisol** increase due to hypothalamic–pituitary activation, increasing muscle activity and tissue blood flow, but also raising oxygen requirements. The hypotension and hypoperfusion lead to enhanced inflammation and further tissue damage.

Cardiogenic shock can also include **hypothyroidism** and **thyrotoxicosis** (although these can be presented in a separate category – endocrine causes of shock). Hypothyroidism can lead to reduced cardiac output with hypotension and reduced respiration. Thyrotoxicosis can lead to enlarged cardiac muscle which may become rigid and thick.

Management of cardiogenic shock

Cardiogenic shock still results in a mortality rate of 40–50% (Thiele et al., 2015). However, a number of different approaches may be used in physiological support and repair, summarised in Table 8.5.

Table 8.5   Approaches to management of cardiogenic shock

Revascularisation techniques	Aiming to re-open blocked blood vessels in the heart, e.g. coronary artery bypass, insertion of stents
Anti-platelet and anti-thrombotic medication	During treatment: to enhance blood flow by reducing risk of blood clotting
Intensive care unit treatments	
Fluids, vasopressors, inotropes	Expansion of blood volume with fluids (not blood, which increases mortality rate)
	Catecholamines first choice to raise blood pressure for as short a time as possible. Inotropes improve contractility of heart
Hypothermia	Aims to reduce metabolic rate and minimise brain cell damage
	Studies still under way related to cardiogenic shock
Mechanical support	Left ventricular support devices used to enhance perfusion pressure
Intraaortic balloon pumping	Increases diastolic pressure and lowers end-systolic pressure without altering mean B/P
Extracorporeal life support systems	Include blood pump, heat exchanger and oxygenator
	Work still ongoing on development of these mechanisms

Source: Thiele et al., 2015

ACTIVITY 8.5: UNDERSTAND

Cardiogenic shock

Watch this video to better understand the physiological changes that occur in this type of shock. If you are using the eBook just click on the play button. Alternatively go to

https://study.sagepub.com/essentialpatho/videos

CARDIOGENIC SHOCK (5:30)

Obstructive shock

Obstructive shock is a form of shock that links with cardiogenic shock. It sometimes occurs when some physical obstruction prevents normal blood flow; the obstruction limits ventricular filling and thus diminishes cardiac output. It often presents with signs and symptoms similar to those of right-sided heart failure, depending on the site of the obstruction which may result in increased pressure in the cardiac chambers. The pressure to be exerted by the right ventricle in expelling blood to the lungs is raised and the right ventricle becomes enlarged, while the compression on the left ventricle leads to a decrease in size. The cardiac output and stroke volume are both reduced, leading to a fall in blood pressure which exacerbates the deterioration and can lead to death (Banasik and Copstead, 2018).

There are three main causes:

- Pulmonary embolism: pulmonary emboli usually arise from a thrombus in the veins of the legs, developed under conditions such as immobility, trauma or hypercoagulability. When part of this thrombus breaks off as an embolus, it is carried to the pulmonary circulation where it stops and prevents blood flowing normally. The degree of blockage can be small or large, determining the presentation. The person concerned will have sudden severe pain, dyspnoea and deteriorating blood gases.
- Cardiac tamponade: occurs when fluid accumulates in the pericardium surrounding the heart. This can be due to pericarditis (i.e. inflammation of the pericardium), blunt chest trauma or surgery (e.g. removal of pacing wires). Pressure is exerted on both right and left sides of the heart.
- **Tension pneumothorax**: this occurs when intrapleural air accumulates in the pleural cavity under pressure. This may be caused by spontaneous rupture of the pleural membrane covering the lungs which allows air to escape into the pleural cavity, or trauma. There will be dyspnoea, reduced air entry into the affected side (and eventually the opposite lung), and there will be asymmetrical rise of the chest during inhalation. The trachea may become deviated (as a late sign) and arterial PaO_2 blood gas levels fall rapidly. The increased and increasing pressure in the chest causes collapse of the lung on the affected side and a shifting and compression of the structures in the mediastinum. This includes pressure on the heart, limiting filling of the left ventricle. The person may deteriorate rapidly if the obstruction is not removed quickly (i.e. release of the air that is under pressure). Relief of the air pressure is necessary to restore cardiac output and prevent cardiovascular collapse. This is normally through a needle decompression, followed by insertion of a chest drain with an underwater seal. These measures are necessary to also prevent recollection of the air.

Management of shock

A person in shock is critically ill and treatment is started immediately, followed by admission to a critical care environment. Clinical management falls primarily into identifying and treating the cause (where possible), physiological support and monitoring, and the different aspects needing attention are initiated together.

Initially, first aid is provided with a focus on maintaining respiration, cerebral perfusion and control of intravascular volume. The individual affected is positioned so that the airway is patent and is intubated and ventilated (e.g. intermittent positive pressure ventilation) if necessary, controlling oxygen levels within defined parameters. Intravenous fluids are administered as necessary to maintain body fluid volume and blood pressure for vital organ perfusion. Additional treatment is administered as required and takes account of the type of shock and specific details about the individual.

Monitoring will include:

- Cardiovascular information: including ECG, blood pressure, pulse (rate, rhythm and amplitude), CVP (central venous pressure) and complex methods for cardiac output etc.

- Respiratory function: respiratory rate and depth, oxygen levels by pulse oximetry or more accurately through arterial blood gas analysis.
- General metabolism: body temperature, skin temperature, colour, blood sugar.
- Fluid balance: fluid intake including intravenous fluids, urinary output (by in-dwelling catheter, often measuring hourly with a urometer).
- Neurological: level of consciousness through examining defined performance based on specified stimuli in relation to eye opening, verbal response and motor response using the Glasgow Coma Scale (Procter, 2018), checking the pupils for equality and speed of constriction to light (and dilation afterwards) and monitoring limb strength.

ACTIVITY 8.6: UNDERSTAND

The Glasgow Coma Scale

This video clarifies the use of the Glasgow Coma Scale. If you are using the eBook just click on the play button. Alternatively go **https://study.sagepub.com/essentialpatho/videos**

GLASGOW COMA SCALE (7:55)

While the major focus in this section has been on physiological function, in providing person-centred care emotional support for the individual affected and their relatives is also crucially important.

DISORDERS OF BLOOD

Blood is composed of fluid (i.e. plasma), red blood cells and white blood cells. In this section we are primarily concerned with problems arising from disorders of the blood, which can involve the three types of blood cells: erythrocytes (red blood cells), leucocytes (white blood cells), or thrombocytes (platelets). Each can be increased or decreased in concentration for various reasons.

Erythrocytes

The main function of red blood cells is the carriage of oxygen to the tissues. There are two main types of disorders: inadequate or abnormal red blood cells or excessive red blood cells.

Anaemia

Anaemia is a group of disorders where erythrocyte numbers or haemoglobin and oxygen carrying capacity are reduced. This can result in various signs and symptoms:

- fatigue, weakness, may be breathless, lightheaded or dizzy
- the skin may be pale or yellowish, hands and feet may be cold
- irregular heart function and chest pain
- headache.

There are a number of different causes and types of anaemia, most of which are outlined in Table 8.6. There are also some other forms of anaemia, including **thalassaemia** and some others associated with malaria: the genes for these conditions protect against malaria when present in the heterozygote (Moore et al., 2016).

Table 8.6 Types of anaemia

Iron deficiency anaemia	Commonest type of anaemia worldwide, due to inadequate iron needed to form haemoglobin. Treatment is iron supplements Causes: pregnancy in some women; blood loss, e.g. from heavy menstrual bleeding, peptic ulcer, cancer, regular use of e.g. aspirin
Vitamin deficiency anaemia	Folate and vitamin B_{12} needed to form red blood cells. Lack of these can result in decreased red blood cell production Some people are unable to process vitamin B_{12}. Results in **pernicious anaemia**
Anaemia of chronic disease	Some diseases disrupt red cell formation: e.g. cancer, HIV/AIDS, rheumatoid arthritis, kidney disease, Crohn's disease, other chronic inflammatory diseases
Aplastic anaemia	Rare, life-threatening anaemia – body does not produce enough red blood cells Causes: infections, certain medicines, autoimmune diseases, toxic chemicals
Anaemias due to bone marrow disease	Certain diseases (cancer and cancer-like disorders), e.g. leukaemia and myelofibrosis, reduce bone marrow blood production Effects vary from mild to life-threatening
Haemolytic anaemias e.g. Sickle cell anaemia	Red blood cells are destroyed faster than replaced by bone marrow. Certain blood diseases increase red blood cell destruction This is an inherited haemolytic anaemia. The abnormal red cells form into a sickle shape, causing low number of red cells

Source: Mayo Clinic, 2017. Used with permission of Mayo Foundation for Medical Education and Research, all rights reserved

ACTIVITY 8.7: UNDERSTAND

Types of anaemia

Watch this video to understand the different types of anaemia that occur. If you are using the eBook just click on the play button. Alternatively go to

https://study.sagepub.com/essentialpatho/videos

TYPES OF ANAEMIA (6:33)

In the various types of anaemia there are lowered haemoglobin levels, either because of inadequate formation of erythrocytes or the haemoglobin in them, or excessive loss of the cells. Erythrocytes can vary in size and be: **microcytic** (smaller than normal), **normocytic** (normal in size), or **macrocytic** (larger than normal) volume. In general, anaemia results in a reduced oxygen-carrying capacity of the blood due to one of four main categories:

- Nutritional deficiencies
- Impaired red cell formation

- Increased red cell destruction
- Blood loss

Nutritional deficiencies

The principal deficiencies that occur are as follows:

- *Iron deficiency anaemia*: One of the main constituents of haemoglobin is iron and inadequate dietary iron intake or absorption, or increased loss results in lowered haemoglobin. Iron deficiency causes a microcytic, hypochromic (paler than normal red cells) anaemia, leading to tiredness, pallor, hair thinning and brittle nails (Hoffbrand and Moss, 2016). Treatment is iron supplementation and a balanced diet.
- *Macrocytic anaemias*: Folic acid or vitamin B_{12} deficiency – inadequate amounts of folate or vitamin B_{12} necessary for DNA synthesis in the formation of erythrocytes. Folic acid is particularly rich in leafy vegetables, but preparation (e.g. boiling vegetables to eat) reduces the amount absorbed and may result in an inadequate intake.

Vitamin B_{12} deficiency can result from lack of intrinsic factor in the stomach which combines with this vitamin and enables absorption in the last section of the small intestine. This results in pernicious anaemia with neurological disturbances, particularly, but not solely, damage to the dorsal column and corticospinal tract (subacute combined degeneration of the spinal cord). Regular intramuscular B_{12} injections are necessary (Hunt et al., 2014).

Impaired red cell formation

These are another group of disorders in which the formation of red cells is impaired in two sub-groups:

- *Bone marrow dysfunction*: Bone marrow failure can be inherited (e.g. Fanconi anaemia) or acquired, known as aplastic anaemia. This can occur due to a range of physical or chemical agents, certain drugs, infections, or an immune response. It may be treated with blood transfusion to correct the anaemia; antibiotics may also be used for infections. Stem-cell transplantation may be used in severe cases (Pallister and Watson, 2011).
- *Abnormal haemoglobin formation (haemoglobinopathies)*: There are two main groups of **haemoglobinopathies**, both caused by mutation or deletion of genes in the globin genes. The thalassaemias are conditions in which the rate of formation of haemoglobin is reduced but the structure is normal. Supportive treatment involves regular blood transfusions linked with the removal of excess iron from the bloodstream; **chelation therapy** is the use of drugs that bind iron with a substance that then can be excreted from the body, largely through the kidneys. In severe conditions, a donor is sought and stem-cell transplant performed.

Structural haemoglobinopathies are conditions in which the structure of the globin molecules is abnormal. They consist of a number of different variants, including sickle cell anaemia. In some of these conditions, haemolysis occurs due to the unstable structure of the haemoglobin while others have abnormal oxygen transportation (Kohne, 2011).

Increased red cell destruction

Haemolytic anaemia occurs when erythrocytes are broken down before their normal life span is ended. They fall into two main categories: healthy erythrocytes acted on by an external agent, and erythrocytes with some defect (Moore et al., 2016).

Extrinsic causes of haemolysis

Haemolysis occurs due to an immune response of one of two types:

* Alloantibodies, antibodies produced in alloimmunity, occur when the body's immune system recognises foreign blood cells that have been introduced as a blood transfusion or due to pregnancy when the fetal blood mixes into the maternal bloodstream.
* Autoantibodies develop when the individual's own immune system produces antibodies to their own erythrocytes which they recognise as foreign and cause their destruction.

Blood loss

Blood loss can be a cause of **anaemic hypoxia**, when the blood is unable to carry sufficient oxygen to the tissues, which has a number of direct effects including:

* skeletal muscle hypoxia, leading to fatigue and tiredness
* cardiac muscle hypoxia and weakness, causing reduced tolerance to exercise, fatigue, possibly angina
* gut hypoxia, producing anorexia and constipation
* liver hypoxia, reducing drug metabolism and resulting in increased drug effects
* nerve hypoxia, initiating reduced and slowed reflexes.

The normal response to blood loss involves a cardiovascular response that results in an increased heart rate and vasoconstriction occurs to redistribute blood flow. Hypovolaemic shock can also occur (see later in this chapter). The kidneys respond to the decreased haemoglobin level by increasing the secretion of erythropoietin which stimulates the formation of erythrocytes. In addition, there is a shift of the haemoglobin–oxygen dissociation curve to the right which increases the release of oxygen into the tissues (Hillman et al., 2010). Blood loss can be acute or chronic.

Acute blood loss

This is loss of a large volume of blood occurring rapidly. Loss of up to 30% of blood volume can be tolerated by young to middle-aged people, but older people have a lower tolerance. A greater volume loss than this often results in postural hypotension and possible hypovolaemic shock (see earlier in this chapter). It is the loss of blood volume rather than of red cells which is problematic and potentially life-threatening.

Compensatory mechanisms minimise the deleterious effects. The volume can be restored by IV colloid solutions which, with **vasoconstriction** as necessary, will maintain blood pressure. In response to the reduced oxygen in the tissues, the oxyhaemoglobin dissociation curve will shift to the right and, thus, release more oxygen to the tissues. It is the restoration of volume rather than haemoglobin which is most crucial (Pallister and Watson, 2011).

Chronic blood loss

Small volumes of blood lost over a longer period of timer (e.g. 200–300 ml daily) can be compensated for and blood volume maintained. However, anaemia will develop if red blood cells/haemoglobin are not replaced adequately. A fall of the haemoglobin to 80–90 g/L will result in signs and symptoms of anaemia (Hillman et al., 2005).

Management of anaemias

The primary aspect of management of anaemia is accurate diagnosis through undertaking a detailed personal and family history, including diet and drugs taken, and a range of laboratory tests. Initially, the various deficiencies are investigated and, if necessary, appropriate supplementation of iron, vitamin B_{12} or folic acid are prescribed. The various other potential causes are then considered, for example, infection, inflammation, **neoplasia**, a drug or exposure to a chemical or an autoimmune disorder. Having determined then cause of anaemia, treatment to deal with the specific pathology is then prescribed (Parker-Williams, 2009). Sometimes, this may require transfusion of blood products.

Polycythaemia

At the opposite end of the scale, **polycythaemia** (meaning many cells in blood) is a condition in which there is a raised level of red blood cells or haemoglobin. This can be due to increased synthesis of these elements or due to a fall in plasma volume without an alteration in cell mass (Hillman et al., 2005). This can result in increased blood viscosity and a risk of arterial or venous blood clotting which can lead to further disorders discussed later in this chapter, e.g. myocardial infarction (heart attack) or stroke. There are two main types of polycythaemia (Hoffbrand and Moss, 2016): **polycythaemia vera** and secondary polycythaemia.

Polycythaemia vera

This is a malignant disorder of haematopoietic stem cells, leading to raised red cells; the term **erythrocytosis** is often used but this refers to increased erythrocyte mass. Polycythaemia vera is often linked with raised leucocytes and platelets, causing hypervolaemia and hyperviscosity (Pallister and Watson, 2011). Signs and symptoms include:

* neurological disturbances, including headaches, dizziness, visual disturbances and cognitive disturbances
* engorged organs
* increased risk of arterial and/or venous thrombosis
* platelet changes which can lead to bruising and bleeding due to trauma.

There are also other, non-malignant types of polycythaemia.

Secondary polycythaemia

This is due to increased stimulation of erythropoiesis (red cell formation) in response to hypoxia or other stimulus of erythropoietin secretion.

Leucocytes

The range of different types of white cells can be reviewed in Boore et al. (2016, Chapters 2 and 12). Here we are outlining major disorders of leucocytes under two main groupings of proliferative disorders (excessive white cells), including malignancies, which are mainly grouped as leukaemias and lymphomas, and **leukopenias,** which are insufficient numbers of white cells. Each of these types of disorders can occur with each of the different white cells.

Proliferative disorders

Leucocytosis is an increase in white cells in the circulation, usually due to inflammation. The main changes leading to this increase are: increased formation or release of these cells from the bone marrow, and a decrease in attachment of these cells to blood vessels or uptake in tissues. It can affect different types of white cells.

Neutrophilia

Neutrophilia is a raised neutrophil count in the blood. Infection normally results in this condition but it can also occur due to other inflammatory states, destruction of tissue, haemorrhage and haemolysis, disorders of metabolism or certain drugs (Pallister and Watson, 2011).

Leukaemias and lymphomas

Leukaemias are malignant disorders of haematopoietic (blood-forming) tissue within the bone marrow or peripheral blood supply. They can be acute or chronic. Lymphoma is cancer occurring within lymphoid tissue, i.e. lymph nodes or the spleen (Moore et al., 2016). The development of oncogenes, i.e. genes that can cause cancer, is often a factor in the development of these conditions.

There are four main types of leukaemias:

Acute myeloid leukaemia (AML)

Acute myeloid leukaemia (AML) is a rapid-growing cancer of the blood and bone marrow and the most common form of leukaemia. It affects the myeloid stem cells which results in blast cells that do not differentiate into the types of leucocytes needed to fight off pathogens. In this form of leukaemia, erythrocytes and thrombocytes can also develop abnormally as a result of the myeloid cells being affected. Abnormal cells rapidly develop and become more dominant than healthy blood cells. There are many subsets of AML.

Acute lymphocytic leukaemia (ALL)

Also known as acute lymphoblastic leukaemia, **acute lymphocytic leukaemia (ALL)** arises from lymphoid stem cells. As abnormal cells accumulate in the bone marrow, they crowd out the bone marrow and this prevents the production of healthy cells further.

Chronic myeloid leukaemia (CML)

Similar to AML, the myeloid cells are affected in this form of leukaemia but it is slower in progression. Distinctly, **chronic myeloid leukaemia (CML)** is associated with an abnormal chromosome known as the Philadelphia chromosome, affecting chromosomes 22 and 9. In this form of leukaemia, there is an overproduction of granulocytes and their precursors. After a number of years, CML can become an acute form of leukaemia.

Chronic lymphocytic leukaemia (CLL)

CLL is a malignant disorder that originates with lymphoid stem cells and results in immature lymphocytes. It is more common in Western society; the cause is largely unknown and it occurs more commonly in those over 50 years of age.

APPLY

Treatment of leukaemias and lymphomas

The principles of treatment of these conditions falls into two groups (Pallister and Watson, 2011):

Destroying the malignant cells: This can involve chemotherapy, stem-cell transplantation and sometimes radiotherapy. As these treatments can be toxic to normal cells, the treatment is often administered in pulses, with gaps in treatment to permit recovery.

Supportive management: These forms of treatment aim to permit normal function to be supported. Approaches to care include transfusion of packed red cells for anaemia, concentrates of platelet to promote blood clotting and packages of white cells to control infections. Anti-emetic drugs help to control the nausea and vomiting which can result from the cytotoxic therapy.

Leukopenias

Leukopenias are conditions in which there is a reduction in the number of white blood cells (leucocytes). Various factors can cause a fall in one or another type of white blood cells, principally neutrophils or lymphocytes.

Neutropenia

Neutropenia is due to a fall in production or an increase in loss from the blood of neutrophils. There are a wide range of causes, for example: medications, toxins, immune disorders, some congenital conditions, and major infections. The major problem is that resistance to infection is decreased and, in severe conditions, mouth and throat infections are common, with skin and anal **ulcers** sometimes occurring.

Lymphocytopenia (lymphopenia)

Lymphocytopenia or **lymphopenia** can be classified according to the low levels of one or more of the three main types of lymphocytes: T lymphocytes, B lymphocytes or natural killer lymphocytes. There are a number of possible causes including infections such as **influenza** A, or physical disturbances such as **rheumatoid arthritis**, severe **stress**, **corticosteroid** administration, **chemotherapy** and radiation.

Treatment of leukopenias

Management of these conditions comes under a number of aspects:

Medications: to simulate formation of white blood cells or to treat any infections involved.

Reviewing treatments: some treatment may be causing leukopenia and needs to be stopped to allow time for recovery.

Growth factors: these can stimulate the formation of white blood cells.

Diet: a diet prepared in a way that will minimise microorganisms contaminating food.

Care at home: carry out the following principles – Eat well, Rest, Be very careful, Keep away from germs.

Thrombocytes

As with the other types of blood cells, excessive or inadequate numbers of thrombocytes can be produced.

Thrombocythaemia

Thrombocythaemia is a disorder in which excess platelets are produced, leading to abnormal blood clotting or bleeding. This can be due to a genetic mutation or some other cause of raised platelet count. Blood tests usually provide a diagnosis, but sometimes a bone marrow biopsy is needed. Arterial or venous thrombosis can occur.

Thrombocytopenia

This is when there is a reduced number of platelets being formed, resulting in a low level of platelets in the blood. It results in increased risk of bleeding. Skin **purpura** (red/purple spots) caused by subcutaneous bleeding due to platelet, vascular or coagulation disorders, or other causes can occur. Mucosal haemorrhage or significant bleeding after trauma can develop. Causes can include: failure of platelet formation due to bone marrow depression, increased use of platelets, abnormal platelet distribution (e.g. in splenomegaly), and/or excessive dilution due to the transfusion of stored blood. Some of these may be due to the side-effects of medication.

ORGAN DAMAGE DUE TO REDUCED BLOOD FLOW

The conditions already considered will affect numerous organs of the body, with the major organs disrupted being brain, heart and kidneys.

Brain

There are a number of different types of disease resulting in reduced oxygen supply to part of the brain.

Carotid artery disease

The two internal carotid arteries and the two vertebral arteries supply the brain with blood. The vertebral arteries join to form the basilar artery. These three arteries join the Circle of Willis which encircles the base of the brain and supplies blood to all parts of the brain. These arteries can become affected by atherosclerotic plaque and reduce or block the blood flow to the brain. There are two main conditions that can occur: a stroke and a transient ischaemic attack (TIA).

Stroke

A stroke occurs when there is a gradual or rapid, non-convulsive onset of neurological deficits that fit a known vascular territory and that last for 24 hours or more. There are two types: ischaemic (thrombo-embolic) and haemorrhagic: the second of these is significantly more severe than the first, with a much higher mortality rate. The effects of a stroke can vary considerably, depending on which blood vessels are affected and the size and location of the damage to the brain and the nervous supply to the body.

ACTIVITY 8.8: UNDERSTAND

Physiological changes in stroke

This video will help you to understand the physiological changes in a stroke. If you are using the eBook just click on the play button. Alternatively go to
https://study.sagepub.com/essentialpatho/videos

▷

STROKE (2:48)

ACTIVITY 8.9: APPLY

Life after stroke

Stroke can have a major impact on life and can occur across the life span. Watch this video to gain insight into the lives of two people after stroke. If you are using the eBook just click on the play button. Alternatively go to **https://study.sagepub.com/essentialpatho/videos**

▷

LIFE AFTER STROKE (2:50)

Ischaemic stroke

Ischaemic strokes are a result of inadequate blood flow to the brain secondary to a partial or complete occlusion of an artery. They make up around 85% of all strokes. Most people who develop an ischaemic stroke do not have a decreased level of consciousness in the first 24 hours. Rather, their symptoms often worsen during the first 72 hours due to **cerebral oedema**. Ischaemic strokes can be caused by a thrombus or embolus:

- *Thrombotic*: These are the most common form of ischaemic strokes. They develop slowly over minutes or hours and are commonly caused by thrombi occurring in atherosclerotic vessels. Remember, a thrombosis occurs in relation to injury to a blood vessel wall. Usually only one region supplied by a single cerebral artery is affected and the extent of the stroke depends on the **collateral** circulation in that affected area. Two-thirds of thrombotic ischaemic strokes are associated with hypertension and diabetes and they are often preceded by a TIA (see later in chapter).

- *Embolic*: This cause of ischaemic stroke is the result of a moving clot (embolus) that occludes a cerebral artery. This can occur in atherosclerosis. Embolic ischaemic strokes tend to occur suddenly and there is usually no collateral compensation available. As a result, the maximum deficit is present immediately and hypoxia is maximal, causing extensive tissue damage. This is because the embolus lodges in and occludes the cerebral artery. The result is a cerebral infarction and oedema in the region.

APPLY

Drug treatment in ischaemic stroke

Thrombolysis with alteplase

Thrombolysis is when the thrombosis is dissolved using medication. Alteplase is one such drug and it should be administered only within a well-organised stroke service where there are staff trained specifically in its use and monitoring, where there are nurses trained in acute stroke and thrombolysis to care for the person and where there is immediate access to neuroradiology for imaging purposes.

Aspirin and anticoagulant treatment

Aspirin and anticoagulant treatments are often used when a primary **intracerebral haemorrhage** has been excluded (as soon as possible but within 24 hours). Aspirin 300 mg is normally given (orally if the person is not dysphagic - otherwise it is given **enterally** or rectally). This 300 mg is usually continued until two weeks after onset and at that point the person is commenced on long-term antithrombotic treatment. Remember that a proton pump inhibitor is normally required if the person had previous dyspepsia associated with aspirin.

Haemorrhagic stroke

Haemorrhagic stroke is caused by a rupture of a blood vessel. This can cause an intraparenchymal haemorrhage where there is a clot formed in the tissue of the brain, or it can be a **subarachnoid haemorrhage** when there is an arterial rupture and blood flows into the **subarachnoid space** (and sometimes into the ventricles of the brain). A subarachnoid haemorrhage is usually from the rupture of a cerebral aneurysm. In haemorrhagic stroke, cerebral oedema and **hydrocephalus** can occur, the latter as a result of impairment of CSF reabsorption in the subarachnoid space (because of the presence of blood). Haemorrhagic stroke has the highest mortality and causes can include hypertension, aneurysmal rupture and trauma.

Stroke identification

In order to provide rapid treatment, it is important to identify what is happening and get medical treatment as soon as possible. Public Health England (PHE) has launched an Act FAST stroke campaign to encourage rapid action (Public Health England, 2018). FAST stands for:

- Face – has their face fallen on one side? Can they smile?
- Arms – can they raise both their arms and keep them there?
- Speech – is their speech slurred?
- Time – to call 999

Stroke is a major cause of mortality and **morbidity** in the UK, with 1 in 6 people having a stroke at some time in their lives. While the majority (59%) occur in the older population, the incidence among middle-aged adults (40–69 years) has increased to 38% of strokes in this group. The average ages for first-time strokes has declined (from 2007 to 2016) from 71 to 68 for men and 75 to 73 for women.

Deaths have declined in the last 15 years due, it is thought, to enhanced prevention, and earlier and more advanced treatment (Public Health England, 2018). The impact of a stroke on different sides of the brain is identified in Table 8.7.

Table 8.7 Effect of stroke on each side of the brain

Left hemisphere stroke	Right hemisphere stroke

• Good awareness
• Minimal cognitive impairment
• Better outlook for recovery
• Prone to depression
• Psychological disorders after stroke have been well documented
   o Depression: 35-50%%
   o Anxiety disorder: 25%
   o Apathy: 20%
   o Pathologic affect: 20%
   o Catastrophic reaction: 20%
   o Mania: rare
   o Bipolar disorder: rare
   o Psychosis: rare
	• Visio-spatial deficits
	• Lack of insight and awareness
	• Short attention span
	• Poor judgement
	• Neglect of affected side - risk of injury
	• Euphoric and optimistic
	• Rehabilitation compounded by these effects

Transient ischaemic attack (TIA)

A TIA is a temporary focal loss of neurological function (less than 24 hours) caused by ischemia, in the same way that angina affects the heart. Most TIAs resolve within 3 hours and they are often caused by micro-emboli that temporarily block blood flow within the brain. A TIA is a warning sign of progressive cerebrovascular disease.

APPLY

ABCD² tool

The ABCD² tool is a risk assessment tool designed to improve the prediction of short-term stroke risk after a transient ischemic attack (TIA) (Wardlaw et al., 2015). The tool is optimised to predict the risk of stroke within 2 days after a TIA and also predicts stroke risk within 90 days. The score is calculated by summing up points for five independent factors:

(Continued)

(Continued)

- Age
- Blood pressure
- Clinical features
- Duration
- Diabetes

To see and use the ABCD^2 tool search online for 'ABCD2 tool stroke'.

APPLY

Communication Loss – Aphasia

After stroke, the person may have profound difficulties in communicating. The group of disorders is called **aphasia** and there are different types of aphasia, depending on the exact nature of brain injury incurred:

Global aphasia

In this form, the person will produce few recognisable words and understand little or no spoken language. They can also neither read nor write.

Broca's aphasia ('non-fluent aphasia')

A person with **Broca's aphasia** has severely reduced speech output as Broca's area of the brain has been affected. Their speech is limited mainly to short utterances of fewer than four words and they have limited access to vocabulary. The formation of sounds is laborious and clumsy. However, they may be able to understand speech relatively well and be able to read, but be limited in writing ability.

Mixed non-fluent aphasia

People with this form of aphasia have sparse and effortful speech. This form can resemble severe Broca's aphasia but they have limited speech comprehension and they cannot read or write beyond a basic level.

Wernicke's aphasia ('fluent aphasia')

In **Wernicke's aphasia**, the ability to grasp the meaning of spoken words is primarily impaired. The person can usually produce connected speech well but sentences often do not connect well and there are usually irrelevant words intruding. Reading and writing are often severely impaired.

Anomic aphasia

This is the persistent inability to supply words for the things the person wants to say. Their speech is usually grammatically fluent but contains vague circumlocutions (the use of many words where fewer would do) and expressions of frustration. People with **anomic aphasia** understand speech well and usually read adequately. Their difficulty in finding words for speech is also evident in writing.

Primary progressive aphasia

This is a rare neurological **syndrome** where language capabilities become slowly and progressively impaired while other cognitive functions remain preserved.

=== ACTIVITY 8.10: APPLY ===

Aphasia etiquette

Having the skills to communicate sensitively with people with aphasia is important if we are to create a therapeutic relationship. Watch this short video to help you learn how you can enhance your communication skills. If you are using the eBook just click on the play button. Alternatively go to
https://study.sagepub.com/essentialpatho/videos

(▷)

APHASIA ETIQUETTE (2:12)

Heart

Coronary heart disease

Coronary artery disease (CAD) occurs when plaque develops in the coronary arteries which normally supply the heart with oxygen-rich blood. The developing plaque reduces blood flow to the myocardium and increases the risk of thrombosis occurring, which can result in complete or partial blood blockage. There are two main conditions that can occur: angina and myocardial infarction (heart attack).

Angina

Reduced blood flow provides less oxygen to the myocardium and, as the blood flow to the heart muscle is reduced or blocked, angina may occur with pain (which may be severe) in the chest, often radiating to the shoulders, neck and arm (the left one). Treatment usually relieves the pain within a short time (NHS Choices, 2018).

Unstable angina

As with angina, **unstable angina** also represents reduced blood flow to the coronary arteries secondary to unstable plaques that rupture or erode, exposing the plaque core to blood flow. This can occur as a result of coronary stenosis (narrowing), spasm and/or constriction. In unstable angina, the person will experience pain at rest as a result of myocardial ischaemia secondary to insufficient oxygen to meet myocardial tissues demands. Unstable angina is one of two conditions that make up acute coronary syndrome (myocardial infarction [MI] being the second) and is considered a medical emergency.

Acute myocardial infarction

Acute myocardial infarction (AMI) is a serious medical emergency where there is rupture or erosion of an atherosclerotic plaque with thrombotic occlusion of an epicardial coronary artery and ischaemia across the wall of the heart (myocardium) (Heusch and Gersh, 2016). The size of the resulting infarction depends on three factors (Heusch and Gersh, 2016):

1. Size of the ischaemic area at risk
2. Duration and intermittency of occlusion of the vessel
3. Extent of collateral blood flow and coronary microvascular dysfunction

It is important to note that 30–50% of the area at risk remains viable and salvageable by reperfusion between 4–6 hours from onset of chest pain. There are two divisions of MIs: STEMI (ST segment elevation MI) and non-STEMI (NSTEMI). In STEMI there is usually a complete obstruction of the coronary artery whereas in NSTEMI the vessel is normally only partially occluded. The ST segment is the component of the ECG that is elevated (Figure 8.3); the ST segment represents the interval between ventricular depolarisation and repolarisation. ST segment depression can indicate myocardial ischaemia as can T wave inversion.

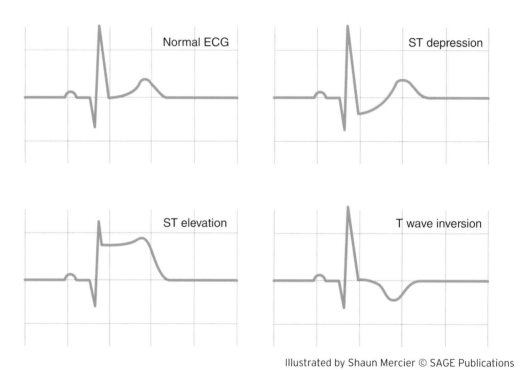

Illustrated by Shaun Mercier © SAGE Publications

Figure 8.3 ECG changes in acute MI

The signs and symptoms of acute MI are similar to those of angina but more severe and longer lasting. They consist of:

* chest pain, which can feel like a heavy object pressing on the chest and, as in angina, radiates from the chest to the jaw, neck, arms and perhaps the back
* feeling lightheaded or dizzy, sweating
* being short of breath, coughing or wheezing
* feeling nauseated or vomiting
* having an overwhelming sense of anxiety (similar to a panic attack).

However, while chest pain is usual, it is not always severe and sometimes not present at all. It can be mild and feel like indigestion (NHS Choices, 2016).

Treatment involves pain relief, drugs to break down blood clots, and possibly surgery to restore the blood flow through a coronary angioplasty or coronary artery bypass graft.

ACTIVITY 8.11: APPLY

The lived experience of a myocardial infarction

In order to have sympathetic presence and in striving to be empathetic, it is essential to understand the lived experience of illness. Watch this video on the lived experience of having a myocardial infarction and reflect on how well we consider the lived experience when there are many physiological priorities. If you are using the eBook just click on the play button. Alternatively go to

https://study.sagepub.com/essentialpatho/videos

SURVIVING HEART
ATTACK (2:38)

Biochemical markers in AMI

Biochemical markers are useful in confirming a diagnosis of MI, particularly if the person has a silent MI (where no pain is felt) or where there are subtle ECG changes. When an MI occurs, proteins (enzymes) are released into the circulation from the damaged **myocytes** (myocardial cells) and these proteins can therefore be specific biochemical markers that myocardial damage has occurred. Specifically, these are:

- troponins T and I
- creatinine-kinase myocardial band (CK-MB)

The plasma concentrations of these markers become elevated at different times after infarction and the degree of elevation indicates the extent of myocardial damage. The troponins are highly sensitive and specific for myocardial tissue damage. They are released into the circulation 6–8 hours after myocardial injury, peak at 12–24 hours and remain elevated for 7–10 days (Mythili and Malathi, 2015). CK indicates tissue damage and CK-MB is more specific to the myocardium. CK-MB levels rise in the circulation at 4–9 hours after the onset of chest pain, peak around 24 hours after and return to baseline between 48 and 72 hours (Mythili and Malathi, 2015).

Thrombolytic therapy in AMI

Thrombolytic therapy is one of the most common interventions in AMI; its intention is to salvage the myocardium by breaking down the obstruction in the coronary artery. Thrombolytic drugs dissolve blood clots by activating plasminogen to form plasmin. Plasmin is a proteolytic enzyme capable of breaking connections between **fibrin** molecules; these connections normally hold blood clots together. As a result of breaking down these connections, the clot dissolves and the circulation can be restored to the myocardium.

Legs

Peripheral artery disease

This occurs as plaque builds up in the major arteries that supply legs, arms and pelvis. If blood flow is reduced or blocked, then numbness, pain and, sometimes, infections can occur. Intermittent claudication is the term to describe pain in the calf muscle which occurs with relatively mild exercise, e.g. walking, and recovers with rest. Atherosclerosis can result in a virtually complete blockage of the blood flow to the legs, resulting in the development of gangrene and the necessity for amputation.

ACTIVITY 8.12: UNDERSTAND

Peripheral vascular disease

This video will help you to understand peripheral vascular disease (or **peripheral artery disease**). If you are using the eBook just click on the play button. Alternatively go to
https://study.sagepub.com/essentialpatho/videos

▷

PERIPHERAL VASCULAR
DISEASE (6:13)

Kidneys

Chronic kidney disease

Plaque can also develop in the renal arteries and result in **chronic kidney disease** (CKD) with a gradual loss of renal function. Renal transplant may be the only effective treatment (Chapter 11).

CHAPTER SUMMARY

In this chapter we have examined the effects of reduced blood flow on the cells and organs of the body, including alterations in metabolism. Some of the circumstances that reduce the blood's ability to supply the body cells with their requirements and remove waste products are considered. In particular, atherosclerosis and shock are considered in some detail, and the effect on certain organs of the body are reviewed.

KEY POINTS

- Reduced blood supply results in a fall in energy available for cell and body metabolism as the supply of oxygen to the tissues falls and cells move from aerobic metabolism (needing oxygen) to anaerobic metabolism (with reduced oxygen). The amount of ATP formed in anaerobic metabolism is reduced, resulting in less energy being available for cellular functioning.

- Atherosclerosis is the major factor reducing blood flow through the arteries. Plaque builds up and narrows the arteries, disturbing blood flow and resulting in complications affecting various organs of the body. Medications can limit the effect of complications related to atherosclerosis; surgical treatments may be used to improve blood flow through the arteries.

- Blockage of the veins can be due to venous thrombosis, spasm or external compression. An embolism can break off from a thrombosis and result in pulmonary embolus disrupting venous return from the lungs to the heart.

- Shock is a medical emergency in which the circulation fails and the body aims to compensate by an increased heart rate and a fall in blood pressure. There are various types of shock, with different causes and management. These include:
  ○ Hypovolaemic shock: decrease in blood volume
  ○ Distributive shock: including septic shock, anaphylactic shock and neurogenic shock: imbalance between circulatory volume and a dilated circulation
  ○ Cardiogenic shock: heart cannot pump blood round body adequately
  ○ Obstructive shock: obstruction limits ventricular filling and diminishes cardiac output.
- Anaemia is when there is a lack of red blood cells; there are a number of different causes which require a treatment specific to the cause.
- Different organs of the body can be affected by a lack of blood supply, including:
  ○ Brain: carotid artery disease; stroke (cerebrovascular accident); transient ischaemic attack (TIA)
  ○ Heart: coronary heart disease; angina; heart attack (myocardial infarction)
  ○ Legs: peripheral artery disease, gangrene
  ○ Kidneys: chronic renal disease.

REVISE

TEST YOUR KNOWLEDGE

The content of this chapter will help you understand the implications of the causes of disturbed blood flow. Revise the sections in turn. How well do you remember the different causes and effects of the conditions concerned? Then try to answer the questions below.

Answers are available online. If you are using the eBook just click on the answers icon below. Alternatively go to **https://study.sagepub.com/essentialpatho/answers**

1   What is the effect on metabolism of reduced blood supply to the tissues?

2   Describe how atherosclerosis develops and its effect on blood flow. What is the difference between atherosclerosis and arteriosclerosis?

3   Identify the causes of blockage of the veins and describe how an embolism occurs.

4   What is meant by 'shock' and what are the main changes that occur? Specify the different types of shock.

5   Clarify the changes that lead to hypovolaemic shock.

6   What is meant by distributive shock? Differentiate between the three categories of this type of shock.

7   Outline the physiological changes in cardiogenic shock and the main approaches to management.

8   What is meant by obstructive shock and what are the three main causes?

9   What are the main signs and symptoms of anaemia? Identify at least four types of anaemia.

10 What is a stroke and how does it differ from a TIA? Describe the items comprising the Public Health England (2018) scale for identifying the occurrence of a stroke.

11 Identify the effects on the heart of reduced blood supply.

REVISE

ACE YOUR ASSESSMENT

- Further revision and learning opportunities are available online
- Test yourself away from the book with **Extra multiple choice questions**
- Learn and revise terminology with **Interactive flashcards**

If you are using the eBook access each resource by clicking on the respective icon. Alternatively go to **https://study.sagepub.com/essentialpatho/chapter8**

CHAPTER 8 ANSWERS

EXTRA QUESTIONS

FLASHCARDS

REFERENCES

Angus, D.C. and van der Poll, T. (2013) Severe sepsis and septic shock. *New England Journal of Medicine, 369*: 840–51.

Aziz, M. and Yadav, K.S. (2016) Pathogenesis of atherosclerosis: a review. *Medical and Clinical Reviews, 2* (22). doi: 10.21767/2471-299X.1000031.

Banasik, J.L. and Copstead, L-E.C. (2018) Shock. In *Pathophysiology*, 6th edn. St Louis, MO: Elsevier Health Sciences. Ch. 20, p. 441.

Bergheanu, S.C., Bodds, M.C. and Jukema, J.W. (2017) Pathophysiology and treatment of atherosclerosis: current view and future perspective on lipoprotein modification treatment. *Netherlands Heart Journal, 25* (4): 231–42. doi: 10.1007/s12471-017-0959-2.

Boore, J., Cook, N. and Shepherd, A. (2016) *Essentials of Anatomy and Physiology for Nursing Practice*. London: Sage.

Chetty, R. and Lucas, S.B. (2014) Infections. In C.S. Herrington (ed.), *Muir's Textbook of Pathology*, 15th edn. London: CRC Press/Taylor and Francis. Ch. 19.

Green, J.P., Souilhol, C., Xanthis, I., Martinez-Campesino, L., Bowden, N.P., Evans, P.C. et al. (2018) Atheroprone flow activates inflammation via endothelial ATP-dependent P2X7-p38 signalling. *Cardiovascular Research, 114*: 324–35.

Heusch, G. and Gersh, B.J. (2016) The pathophysiology of acute myocardial infarction and strategies of protection beyond reperfusion: a continual challenge. *European Heart Journal, 38* (11): 774–84.

Hillman, R.S., Ault, K.A. and Rinder, H.M. (2005) *Haematology in Clinical Practice*, 4th edn. New York: Lange Medical, McGraw-Hill.

Hillman, R.S., Ault, K.A., Leporrier, M. and Rinder, H.M. (2010) *Haematology in Clinical Practice*, 5th edn. New York: Lange Medical, McGraw-Hill.

Hoffbrand, A.V. and Moss, P.A.H. (2016) *Hoffbrand's Essential Haematology*, 7th edn. Chichester: John Wiley.

Hunt, A., Harrington, D. and Robinson, S. (2014) Vitamin B12 deficiency. *British Medical Journal, 349*: g5226.

Insull, W. (2009) The pathology of atherosclerosis: plaque development and plaque responses to medical treatment. *American Journal of Medicine, 122* (1A): S3–S14.

Kataja, A. and Harjola, V.P. (2017) Cardiogenic shock: current epidemiology and management. *Continuing Cardiology Education, 3* (3): 121–24.

Kearns, C.E., Schmidt, L.A. and Glantz, S.A. (2016) Sugar industry and coronary heart disease research: a historical analysis of internal industry documents. *JAMA Internal Medicine, 176* (11): 1680–5.

Kohne, E. (2011) Hemoglobinopathies clinical manifestations, diagnosis, and treatment. *Deutsches Ärzteblatt International, 108* (31–32): 532–40.

Lakhani, S.R., Dilly, S.A. and Finlayson, C.J. (2009) *Basic Pathology: An Introduction to the Mechanisms of Disease,* 4th edn. London: Hodder Arnold, Hachette.

Maggio, P.M. (2018) Sepsis and septic shock. MSD Manual Professional Version/Critical Care Medicine [online]. Available at: www.msdmanuals.com/en-gb/professional/critical-care-medicine/sepsis-and-septic-shock/sepsis-and-septic-shock (accessed 4 May 2018).

Mayo Clinic (2017) Anemia. Mayo Foundation for Medical Education and Research [online]. Available at: www.mayoclinic.org/diseases-conditions/anemia/symptoms-causes/syc-20351360 (accessed 9 May 2018).

McConnell, K.W. and Coopersmith, C.M. (2016) Pathophysiology of septic shock: from bench to bedside. *La Presse Medicale, 45* (4, Pt 2): e93–e98 [online]. Available at: http://doi.org/10.1016/j.lpm.2016.03.003 (accessed 6 December 2018).

Moore, G., Knight, G. and Blann, A. (2016) *Haematology,* 2nd edn. Oxford: Oxford University Press.

Mythili, S. and Malathi, N. (2015) Diagnostic markers of acute myocardial infarction. *Biomedical Reports, 3* (6): 743–8.

NHS Choices (2016) Heart attack [online]. Available at: www.nhs.uk/conditions/heart-attack/symptoms/ (accessed 9 May 2018).

NHS Choices (2018) Angina [online]. Available at: www.nhs.uk/conditions/angina/ (accessed 9 May 2018).

Pallister, C.J. and Watson, M.S. (2011) *Haematology,* 2nd edn. Banbury: Scion Publishing.

Parker-Williams, E.J. (2009) Investigation and management of anaemia. *Medicine, 37* (3): 137–42. Available at: www.medicinejournal.co.uk/article/S1357-3039(09)00004-8/pdf (accessed 9 May 2018).

Popa, C., Popa, F., Grigorean, V.T., Onose, G., Sandu, A.M., Popescu M. et al. (2010) Vascular dysfunctions following spinal cord injury. *Journal of Medicine and Life, 3* (3): 275–85.

Procter, L.D. (2018) Shock. MSD Manual Professional Version/Critical Care Medicine/Shock and Fluid Resuscitation [online]. Available at: www.msdmanuals.com/en-gb/professional/critical-care-medicine/shock-and-fluid-resuscitation/shock#v928024 (accessed 2 May 2018).

Public Health England (2018) New figures show larger proportion of strokes in the middle aged. Public Health England: GOV.UK [online]. Available at: www.gov.uk/government/news/new-figures-show-larger-proportion-of-strokes-in-the-middle-aged (accessed 9 May 2018).

Reber, L.L., Hernandez, J.D. and Galli, S.J. (2017) The pathophysiology of anaphylaxis. *Journal of Allergy and Clinical Immunology, 140* (2): 335–48.

Sheppard, M.N. and Herrington, C.S. (2014) The cardiovascular system. In S.C. Herrington (ed.), *Muir's Textbook of Pathology,* 15th edn. London: CRC Press/Taylor and Francis. Ch. 6.

Thiele, H., Ohman, E.M., Steffen Desch, S., Eitel, I. and de Waha, S. (2015) Management of cardiogenic shock. *European Heart Journal, 36* (20): 1223–30.

Wardlaw, J.M., Brazzelli, M., Chappell, F.M., Miranda, H., Shuler, K., Sandercock, P.A. et al. (2015) ABCD² score and secondary stroke prevention: meta-analysis and effect per 1,000 patients triaged. *Neurology, 85* (4): 373–80.

CELLULAR ADAPTATION AND NEOPLASTIC DISORDERS

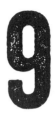

UNDERSTAND: CHAPTER VIDEOS

Watch the following videos to ease you into this chapter. If you are using the eBook just click on the play buttons. Alternatively go to **https://study.sagepub.com/essentialpatho/videos**

Cell cycle

The first video will remind you of the importance of the cell cycle in the maintenance of life. The second one is longer but reviews cell division in more depth.

Cell adaptation

The next two videos introduce the different forms of cell adaptation followed by an introduction to cancer.

CELL DIVISION AND CYCLE (5:34) CELL CYCLE (11:23) CELL ADAPTATION (3:40) CANCER BIOLOGY (12:07)

LEARNING OUTCOMES

When you have finished studying this chapter, you will be able to:

1. Explain how body cells divide through the cell cycle and outline the different types of cell adaptation.
2. Explain how altered physiology of the cell can lead to neoplasia and differentiate between benign and malignant (cancerous) tumours.
3. Identify the role of genes, microbial and environmental factors in the development of cancers and describe the staging of cancers and grading of tumours.
4. Identify methods of treatment for cancer.
5. Describe the epidemiology of cancer and strategies used for cancer prevention.
6. Discuss the importance of person-centred nursing in helping individuals affected, and their families cope with the pressures due to their condition and treatment.

INTRODUCTION

Cells within the body modify their structure and function in order to adapt to different conditions. Some of these are normal and an important example is the changes that occur during pregnancy in order to carry the fetus safely during development in the uterus, and in preparation for feeding the baby after delivery. Some alterations develop in response to endocrine activity or are due to environmental stimuli such as irritation or enhanced muscular activity through exercise and result in abnormal cells. Often these changes are reversible when the stimulus is removed. However, there are changes (including neoplastic changes) that result in permanent cell damage or death, and may have deleterious effects on the body's ability to maintain **homeostasis**.

In this chapter we will start by reviewing normal cell growth and division, then move on to consider the changes that occur in cell adaptation. A large component of this chapter examines how cancer develops, what influences its development, the treatment options available and the impact a cancer diagnosis has on the person, family and society.

Many of the **disease** conditions that people develop occur as a result of disturbed cell function, including changes in cell division, and response to endocrine regulation. These changes may be **benign** in nature as the cells adapt to the factors causing such changes and enable the tissue concerned to contribute (at least to some extent) to homeostasis. The range of adaptive changes is discussed below.

The World Health Organisation (WHO) defines cancer as a 'generic term for a large group of diseases characterised by the growth of abnormal cells beyond their usual boundaries that can then invade adjoining parts of the body and/or spread to other organs' (WHO, 2018a). Cancer is primarily a disease of the cell, where abnormal cell growth and division are uncontrolled, leading to altered function of cells and tissue. The process by which a normal cell becomes a cancer cell is a result of sustained genetic and epigenetic changes in the cellular DNA that change the way the cell behaves. Environmental and human behavioural factors influence the risk of developing cancer, and advances in our understanding of how this happens are influencing treatment and survival.

Finally, the chapter looks at the **epidemiology** of cancer. Cancer is a major cause of illness and death globally; in 2015 it was responsible for 1 in 6 deaths worldwide (WHO, 2018b) and had affected 1 in 2 people born after 1960 in the UK (Cancer Research UK, 2018a). Statistics show that about 14.1 million new cases of cancer were diagnosed worldwide in 2012 (Cancer Research UK, 2018b). A cancer diagnosis is a devastating event for a person, their family and friends and it can have a profound emotional and physical impact on their lives. Cancer is associated with significant **morbidity**, complicated treatment regimens and facing the possibility of death. Research has improved our understanding of how cancer develops and evolves, what causes it and how best to treat it. Many factors combine to increase the risk of developing cancer, including environmental, heredity and behavioural factors. Prevention strategies aim to reduce risk. Improvements in treatment and ongoing care have been effective at improving survival following a cancer diagnosis.

PERSON-CENTRED CONTEXT: THE BODIE FAMILY

BODIE FAMILY
CASE NOTES

A diagnosis of cancer has many implications for a person and their family, not only having to face pain and suffering as indicated above, but often this is a frightening experience and one where the person may feel isolated and lack control over events or decisions about treatment or care. Cancer affects a person physically, psychologically, socially and spiritually. A cancer diagnosis has an impact on independence, relationships and roles in society, and a person-centred approach involving a number of different professionals is essential in promoting quality of life and care.

Within the Bodie family there are numerous factors that might increase their risk of developing cancer. George and Maud are both at increased risk due to their age and both being **overweight**. Edward Bodie is overweight, which increases his risk, and Sarah Bodie and Hannah Jones are currently going through the menopause and their risk for breast cancer increases when post-menopausal. Hannah also has a history of smoking in her early 20s which would have put her at greater risk of developing lung cancer, but as she does not smoke now, she has reduced her risk. Jack Garcia has a family history of testicular cancer and this increases his risk of developing it, however as he regularly performs testicular self-examination he is increasing his chances of early detection and therefore early diagnosis and treatment. Other factors such as air pollution, UV exposure and exposure to chemical **carcinogens** may increase the risk for all Bodie family members for cancer development.

CELL GROWTH AND DIVISION

Normal cell growth and regulation of cell division

The cell is the functional and structural unit of the human body and its growth and function are tightly regulated to maintain a balance between cell growth and cell death. Cell division is vital for growth, development, tissue repair and renewal. Most cells in the body undergo cell division but the rate at which cells proliferate varies greatly. Cancer results from an inability of the cell to differentiate into the type of cell from which it is derived and grow as a normal process at the usual rate. Regulatory controls over cell growth are defective and cancer is a disease of abnormal cell growth. In order to understand how this occurs we need to review the regulation of cell growth and differentiation.

REVISE: A&P RECAP

The cell

Read Chapter 2 in *Essentials of Anatomy and Physiology for Nursing Practice* (Boore et al., 2016) to refresh your knowledge and understanding of the cell and cell division.

Cell **proliferation** is the process when cells increase in number through mitotic division. Cell **differentiation** is the process whereby proliferating cells (dividing cells) are transformed into different and more specialised cell types. This process leads to an adult cell with a specific set of structural, functional and life expectancy characteristics (Boore et al., 2016). Cell proliferation and differentiation are regulated by growth factors that accelerate or slow down the process, thus maintaining a balance between replacing damaged or worn cells and inhibiting the growth of unwanted cells. Defects in this process can lead to **neoplasia** (i.e. new growth which can be benign or **malignant**).

Cell cycle

When the cell is stimulated to proliferate, it proceeds through the stages of the cell cycle (Figure 9.1).

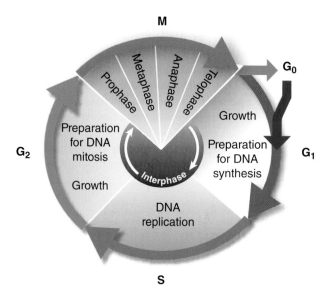

Figure 9.1 Normal cell cycle

The cell cycle consists of two main phases – **interphase** and cell division. Interphase is subdivided into G_1 (G = Gap), S (= Synthesis) and G_2 where growth and preparation for division take place. The M (= **Mitosis**) phase is the phase of nuclear division (Marieb and Hoehn, 2016). Each stage is controlled by enzymes and proteins known as **cyclins**.

Interphase allows the cell time to grow and duplicate its organelles and proteins through the different stages:

- G_1 is the phase between mitosis and DNA synthesis where the cell starts to prepare for DNA replication. Here the cell is functioning and growing and carrying out protein synthesis.
- S phase lasts for about 10–12 hours and DNA is duplicated during this phase.
- G_2 is the phase between the completion of DNA synthesis and the next phase, the M phase. During the G_2 phase RNA and other proteins required for cell division are synthesised.
- Mitosis results in cell division.

After each Gap (G) phase there is a checkpoint where DNA is checked for damage or incomplete replication. These checkpoints act as stop/go signals for the cell progressing through the cell cycle. The G_1/S checkpoint checks for DNA damage and the G_2/M checkpoint checks that DNA replication is complete. Some cells in the body do not move through the cycle and are in a non-dividing state called the G_0 stage. Muscle and nerve cells remain in this phase.

If DNA is damaged or replication is incomplete, **progression** through the cell cycle is inhibited until the DNA is repaired or replicated. This ensures that each daughter cell has the identical information as the parent cell. Cells that cannot be repaired undergo **apoptosis** which is programmed cell death.

Cyclins

Cyclins are proteins that control stimulation and progression through the cell cycle. They bind with enzymes called **cyclin-dependent kinases** to monitor and control different stages of the cell cycle including repair of DNA at the checkpoints. Errors in DNA can occur spontaneously or due to exposure to substances that damage DNA. Control of the cell cycle is maintained by balancing genes that inhibit or stimulate cell growth and division. If these genes are damaged there may be insufficient or excessive cellular growth or division. Where there is uncontrolled cell division and growth a **tumour** occurs.

Chemical signals known as growth factors stimulate or inhibit cell growth and division (Figure 9.2). Cells respond to these signals in one of two ways: by dividing and growing, or by apoptosis. This ensures that cell growth and division are kept in balance.

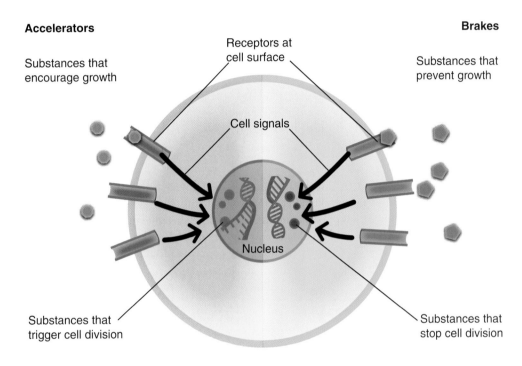

Illustrated by Shaun Mercier © SAGE Publications

Figure 9.2   Regulation of cell cycle

Characteristics of benign and malignant tumours

The process of cell proliferation and differentiation is carefully balanced by cellular signals that stimulate or inhibit cell development (Mader and Windelspecht, 2018). An undifferentiated cell no longer resembles its tissue of origin and the less differentiated a cell becomes the more malignant its behaviour, with growth being uncoordinated, uninhibited and lacking normal regulatory controls. Table 9.1 differentiates between benign and malignant tumours.

Cell adaptation

The cells of the body alter their rate and type of growth in response to changed conditions in the body. Some of these are normal effects of, for example, pregnancy during which uterine and breast tissue grow

Table 9.1 Characteristics of benign and malignant tumours

Characteristics	Benign	Malignant
Structure	Highly differentiated; structure typical of tissue of origin	Varying degrees of imperfect differentiation; structure often atypical
Mode of growth	Expansion, does not infiltrate surrounding normal tissue, encapsulated	Expansion, **infiltration** of surrounding tissue, not confined by capsule
Rate of growth	Usually slow and progressive	Erratic, mitosis frequently rapid and abnormal
Continuation of growth	Usually slow, may stop/progress	Continues to grow until death, very rare regression
Metastases	Never	Almost all if not treated, some local
Clinical results	Harmless except: Position (brain) Complication (infection, rupture) Hormone production (pituitary) Malignant changes (intestinal polyps)	As benign and cause death by invasiveness and ability to metastasise

in size and change in structure to be able to carry the fetus and provide its **nutrition** after birth. Often these normal adaptations will be reversed after the hormonal and other factors which stimulated the adaptation are removed. However, if the structure and function are altered to the extent that homeostasis is inhibited, then disease may develop (VanMeter and Hubert, 2014). If the changes are irreversible, the DNA structure or function is altered. These alterations may or may not lead to permanent tissue damage or neoplasia. The commonest adaptations that occur are discussed below.

Atrophy

This is when cells decrease in size, resulting in wasting part of the organ or structure of the body. The reduction in size means that the tissue will undertake less work, use less oxygen and undertake less synthesis of cell organelles and proteins. **Atrophy** may occur because of **mutation**s within the cell DNA which prevent normal activity and cells, tissues or organs shrink in size following normal maturation. Another term used is **hypoplasia** which refers to reduction in size before maturity.

There are a number of different causes of atrophy due to the decrease in work demands:

* Disuse or lack of exercise of part of the body can result in atrophy
* Decreased **nutrition** supply
* Reduced blood supply
* Decreased endocrine stimulation
* **Denervation**, i.e. loss of nerve supply to the organ concerned.

Hormonal and nerve inputs that maintain function of an organ or body part are said to have trophic effects and atrophy can occur as a diminished muscular trophic condition.

Hypertrophy

Essentially this is the reverse of atrophy. The cells increase in size, thus causing a comparable increase in tissue mass. It occurs because the cells have an increased workload. The tissue involved is commonly muscle, which is unable to increase the rate of cell division, but does increase the organelles within the cells in order to carry out the increased workload. Skeletal muscle cells in athletes who regularly carry out physical exercise have increased demand, resulting in enlarged muscle mass. As these muscle cells **hypertrophy**, additional actin and myosin, which form the muscle fibres to carry out the work of the cell, are produced, cell enzymes are formed and more ATP is synthesised.

Hypertrophy may be a normal physiological response but it can also occur under abnormal pathological situations which place an increased workload on a particular organ. An example of pathological hypertrophy is ventricular hypertrophy that sometimes develops in individuals with **hypertension** or cardiac valve disorder, placing increased demands on the cardiac muscle.

Hyperplasia

This is when cell division multiplies, resulting in an increasing number of cells in the organ or tissue affected. It happens in tissues that are able to undertake mitosis for cell division, such as the epidermis, glandular tissue or **connective tissue** in wound healing when fibrous tissue is produced. The stimulation leading to **hyperplasia** may be the result of genetic disturbance or because of abnormalities in endocrine secretion. As cell division is central to this adaptation, it is not surprising that hyperplasia can lead to the development of cancer.

Metaplasia

This condition usually develops with chronic irritation and **inflammation** and appears to be an adaptation to enhance the response to the irritation/inflammation. One type of mature cell becomes converted into another that is better able to deal with the conditions causing the change. However, the change occurs within the basic tissue type, for example, in smokers the columnar **epithelium** in the respiratory tract may convert into stratified squamous epithelium (Kumar et al., 2018).

Dysplasia

This is a condition in which the cells of a particular tissue vary in size and shape, mitosis is increased and large cell nuclei are seen. Epithelial cells often show such changes in, for example, the cervix, bronchi and liver. Dysplasia may be due to infection, inflammation or can be a precursor of cancerous changes. However, often cancer does not develop and the abnormal changes revert to normal after the irritating cause is removed (VanMeter and Hubert, 2014).

Anaplasia

These cells are undifferentiated, i.e. they do not resemble in structure or form the normal mature cell from which they are derived. They show variation in nuclei and cell structures, and are undergoing mitosis. They are characteristic of cancer cells.

Neoplasm

This term is used widely and means 'new growth'; it is also called a **tumour**, which may be benign or malignant (i.e. cancer). The characteristics of tumours are related to the cells from which they are derived, but the more malignant ones are less similar (see later in this chapter).

Causes of cell injury

Porth (2015) identifies a number of cell injury causes in five groups: physical agents, radiation, chemical injury, biological agents and nutritional factors. Some details of these groups are shown in Table 9.2.

Mechanisms of cell injury

The alterations which can result in cell damage include changes in **metabolism**, reduced ATP formation, altered cell pH, and cell membrane and receptor damage (VanMeter and Hubert, 2014). There are various types of cell injury; the two main areas being considered here are apoptosis and **necrosis**.

Table 9.2 Causes of cell injury

Physical agents	Mechanical forces	Body impact with another object. Tissue torn or split, bone **fractures**, injured blood vessels, disrupted blood flow
	Extremes of temperature	Damage to cell, organelles, enzyme systems
		Low-intensity heat: 43–46° C (partial thickness burns/heat stroke) vascular injury, cell **metabolism** raised, inactivated enzymes, cell membrane damage
		Higher temperature: coagulation of blood and tissue proteins
		Cold: increased blood **viscosity**, **vasoconstriction**, hypoxic injury, freezing (ice crystal formed); blood stasis, **thrombosis**, **oedema**
	Electrical forces	Body acts as conductor of electrical current. Tissue injury, disruption of neural and cardiac impulses
Radiation injury	Ionising radiation	Above UV range: produces free radicals – can kill cells, disrupt cell division, cause mutations
	Ultraviolet radiation	UV – energetic rays can: damage intracellular bonds and DNA, cause sunburn, increase the risk of skin cancer
	Nonionising radiation	i.e. infrared light, ultrasound, microwaves, laser beams. Causes vibration and rotation of molecules and atoms, leading to heat injuries to skin and subcutaneous tissues
Chemical injury	Drugs	Many drugs damage cells
	Lead toxicity	Particularly toxic: range of biochemical effects on organs of body
	Mercury toxicity	Mercury in various forms is toxic to central nervous system and kidneys
Biological agents	Viruses	Enter cells and integrate into cellular DNA – new viruses formed
	Gram-negative bacteria	Release **endotoxins**, causing injury to cells and increased permeability of capillaries
	Exotoxins from bacteria	Exotoxins can interfere with the synthesis of cellular proteins
Nutritional imbalances	Dietary excess – **obesity**	High levels of saturated fats increase risk of **atherosclerosis**
	Starvation	Lack of calories and protein leads to extensive tissue damage
	Selective deficiencies	Deficiency of specific vitamins or minerals can lead to specific disorders, e.g. iron-deficiency **anaemia**, scurvy

Source: Adapted from Porth, 2015

ACTIVITY 9.1: UNDERSTAND

Necrosis vs. apoptosis

Watch this video for a better understanding of necrosis vs. apoptosis. If you are using the eBook just click on the play button. Alternatively go to
https://study.sagepub.com/essentialpatho/videos

NECROSIS VS. APOPTOSIS (4:43)

Types of adaptive change

Apoptosis

Apoptosis is the most extreme of these adaptive changes and is also known as programmed cell death. It plays an important role in maintaining the balance between growth and death of tissues. In health it plays an important role in maintaining overall body structure, including cell turnover, normal embryonic development and appropriate functioning of the immune system. Pathological apoptosis (excessive or too little) is involved in many disorders, including neurodegenerative ones, ischaemic damage, autoimmune diseases and many cancers (Elmore, 2007).

There are two pathways leading to apoptosis. The extrinsic pathway is initiated by extracellular proteins binding to cell membrane receptors called *death* receptors and activating the pathway leading to apoptosis. The intrinsic pathway is independent of the death receptors and is initiated by a number of conditions that cause physiological stress and impact on the **mitochondrial** membrane. The resulting changes lead to a fall in ATP production and other changes that also lead to apoptosis (Favaloro et al., 2012).

Necrosis

Adigun and Bhimji (2018) describe cell necrosis as injury leading to cell death caused by the action of one of various external stimuli, including infectious agents, hypoxia, or extreme environmental conditions. It differs from apoptosis which is organised programmed cell death through the pathways indicated above.

These authors describe two major types of necrosis: liquefactive and coagulative. In addition, they specify four visually different types. Table 9.3 provides some details.

Management of necrosis

There are two main areas of management of necrosis, namely antibiotic treatment and **surgery**, but some other therapies are available. Antibiotic treatment is important in treating infections associated with the condition and is determined by the susceptibility of the particular organism to different antibiotics. Caseous necrosis requires treatment for the TB mycobacterium. Surgery may involve drainage of an **abscess**, debriding the wound (removal of dead, damaged, or infected tissue to improve healing of the remaining healthy tissue), or amputation.

Table 9.3 Necrosis: main types and morphological patterns

Major types of necrosis

Coagulative	Due to **ischaemia** or hypoxia in all organs except the brain	Tissue remains firm with clear structure (including cell outline) for days
Liquefactive	Due to infection, or following ischaemia in the brain	Tissue becomes liquid and may be creamy yellow due to pus. Inflammatory cells with **neutrophils**
Morphological patterns of necrosis		
Caseous	Unique to tuberculosis	White, soft, cheesy-looking **Lymphocytes** and **macrophages** known as a **granuloma** attempt to wall off foreign substances
Fat	**Adipocytes** in tissues: enzymes digest lipids to free fatty acids	Whitish deposits because of formation of calcium soaps
Fibrinoid	Vascular damage: **autoimmunity**, immune complex, infections	**Fibrin** deposited in blood vessels
Gangrenous	Ischaemic necrosis of peripheral tissue	Black skin with varying putrefaction Coagulative - ischaemia (dry **gangrene**) or coagulative (wet gangrene) if infected as well

Source: Adigun and Bhimji, 2018

Some of the methods of treatment can be distressing for the person and one of these is medicinal larvae therapy, used to debride and promote the healing of necrotic wounds. The use of larvae to promote would healing is associated with maggot–host interactions, some of which are physical and some chemical. Larvae perform three main functions:

- **Debridement**: during which the maggots crawl over the wound and remove dead tissue with small spines. They produce digestive enzymes which liquefy the necrotic tissue and then ingest it.
- Disinfection: the gut **microbiome** produces substances that kill the ingested bacteria, and external secretions of anti-microbial substances also reduce the bacterial levels.
- Speeding tissue growth: ASE (alimentary secretions and **excretions**) stimulate the division and growth of **fibroblasts** and endothelial tissue, and enhance angiogenesis, leading to improved blood flow and oxygenation of tissues (Sherman, 2014).

Larvae therapy has been effective in wound debridement while promoting wound healing and has been used to treat multiple types of wounds (Jordan et al., 2018). The effects on wound healing last for a few weeks after the treatment ends, but maintenance larvae therapy is helpful (Sherman, 2014).

The nurse caring for a person with a necrotic wound will need to provide reassurance, information and support as they progress through treatment that may cause anxiety and fear.

CANCER – MALIGNANT DISORDERS

Terminology and characteristics of cancer

Several terms are associated with **cancer** and often describe the origin, tissue type and progression of the cancer. This assists in the identification and classification of cancer and avoids confusion. A tumour

ACTIVITY 9.2: UNDERSTAND

Larvae therapy

Watch these two short videos for an understanding of maggot therapy for severe wounds. If you are using the eBook just click on the play button. Alternatively go to

https://study.sagepub.com/essentialpatho/videos

MAGGOT DEBRIDEMENT
THERAPY (2:48)

MAGGOT
THERAPY (2:19)

is a swelling that can result from various conditions, including inflammation and trauma. **Neoplasm**, meaning new growth, is growth that is no longer responding to the body's normal regulatory controls, and can be benign or malignant. The terms tumour and neoplasm are used interchangeably (Porth, 2015). Neoplasms with well-differentiated cells clustered together in a single mass surrounded by a capsule are considered benign. Neoplasms with cells with the ability to break loose and enter the lymphatic or circulatory systems and form secondary tumours are considered to be malignant. Malignant tumours lack a capsule and have a rapid growth rate and loss of differentiation, resulting in the absence of normal tissue organisation. Benign tumours are named after the tissue they originate from, whereas malignant neoplasms are named according to the cell type of origin (Heuther and McCance, 2017). Table 9.4 provides an overview of tumour nomenclature.

Table 9.4 Nomenclature of benign and malignant tumours

Tissue/cell of origin	Malignant	Benign
Epithelial tissue	Carcinoma	-oma
Glandular epithelium	Papillary adenocarcinoma Adenocarcinoma	Papilloma Adenoma
Squamous epithelium	Squamous cell carcinoma	Squamous cell papilloma
Connective tissue	Sarcoma	
Lymphatic tissue	Lymphomas	
Blood cells	Leukaemias	
Glial cells	Glioma	
Bone	Osteogenic sarcoma	Osteoma
Cartilage	Chondrosarcoma	Chondroma
Fibrous tissue	Fibrosarcoma	Fibroma
Fat	Liposarcoma	Lipoma

Genetic mechanisms of cancer

Genes control the chemical signals that induce or inhibit cell growth and stimulate apoptosis (programmed cell death). **Carcinogenesis** is when a normal cell is changed into a malignant cell through changes in its genetic structure. These changes can occur by mutational or epigenetic mechanisms. A mutation often involves changes in the DNA which in turn affect the functioning of the gene. **Epigenetics** is the external modifications that switch genes on or off so that they are expressed, or silenced. The modifications do not alter DNA sequence but instead they affect how the cell reads the gene.

Oncogenes

Genes that usually protect the cell from abnormal growth can be inactivated by some mutations and other mutations can actively stimulate cell growth. Gene overactivity involves **proto-oncogenes** which are normal genes that code for proteins that stimulate cell growth (growth factors) and differentiation. Normally, these growth factors bind to receptors on the cell surface and stimulate a cascade of reactions that result in cell proliferation. A proto-oncogene that is overactive or overexpressed is a mutated form of the gene and is known as an **oncogene** (Heuther and McCance, 2017). An oncogene is independent of normal regulatory mechanisms and it can affect growth factor pathways, thus stimulating cellular proliferation and avoiding growth-inhibiting signals, leading to uncontrolled cell growth. Oncogenes do this in the following ways:

* Overproduction of growth factors
* Overexpression of growth factor cell receptors such as human epidermal growth factor receptor-2 (HER-2) which is amplified in 25–30% of breast cancers (Kumar et al., 2018)
* Excessive cytoplasmic signalling such as overactivation of the *RAS* gene, causing increased cell proliferation
* Activation of transcription factors which affect genes in the nucleus that stimulate unchecked growth.

Tumour suppressor genes

Growth inhibitory signals are controlled by genes known as **tumour suppressor genes (TSG)** that normally control the cell cycle. Mutations can also occur in these genes which can lead to inactivation and loss of the inhibitory mechanisms that control cell growth. Epigenetic influences can silence or switch off these genes. Therefore, it is the inactivation of the TSG that can lead to a cell becoming cancerous. One such TSG is the *Retinoblastoma (Rb)* gene, so called as it was first discovered in relation to retinoblastoma, a tumour of the eye. This gene is often referred to as the 'master brake' of the cell cycle which restrains cell division by inhibiting transcription factors that initiate the cell cycle (Copstead and Banasik, 2013). When the *Rb* gene is mutated it is inactivated, leading to unregulated cellular proliferation and growth. *Rb* mutation causes a number of different cancers not just retinoblastoma, but lung, breast and bone cancers (Kumar et al., 2018).

Another significant tumour suppressor gene is *Tumour Protein P53 (TP53)*. This gene codes for the protein p53 and is located on the short arm of **chromosome** 17. Mutations in *TP53* are found in all cancer types and it is the most frequently mutated gene in most cancers (Olivier et al., 2010). *TP53* supresses the cell cycle, particularly in response to cellular **stress**, and activates caretaker genes to repair damaged DNA. If not repaired, *TP53* may signal the cell to initiate apoptosis, thus preventing further mutations. Inactivation of *TP53* allows mutated and damaged cells to survive and replicate, thus increasing the rate of mutation and enhancing the risk of malignant behaviour.

Mutations in tumour suppressor genes can be transmitted from one generation to the next. In the hereditary form of retinoblastoma, which accounts for about 40% of cases, the mutated *Rb* gene is inherited from a parent, thus increasing the person's risk for developing retinoblastoma. Where a second mutation occurs in a **somatic cell** that already carries the inherited mutation, both **alleles** then carry the defective *Rb* gene and the risk of retinoblastoma occurring increases (Kumar et al., 2018). Inherited mutations in other tumour suppressor genes have been identified, such as *BRCA1* and *BRCA2* in the development of breast cancer. These genes repair breaks in DNA strands, and inherited mutations on either of these genes greatly increase the risk of breast, ovarian and **prostate cancer** development (Table 9.5).

Table 9.5 Inherited mutations in tumour suppressor genes which increase risk of cancer

Gene	Cancer
TP53	50% of all cancers
Rb	Retinoblastoma
BRCA1	Breast, ovarian
BRCA2	Breast, ovarian, prostate

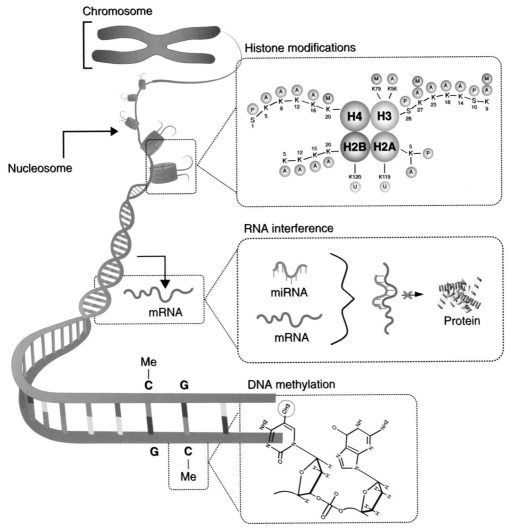

Illustrated by Shaun Mercier © SAGE Publications

Figure 9.3 Types of epigenetic mechanisms – DNA methylation, histone modifications and RNA-mediated gene silencing

Epigenetics

Epigenetic regulation of **gene expression** is a part of normal cell development and function (Figure 9.3). Epigenetic processes that involve changes in gene expression without changing the DNA can silence or activate genes. Disordered epigenetic gene regulation can lead to cancer development where tumour suppressor genes are silenced, such that although the gene is present it does not function to code for proteins that will suppress tumour development. The mechanisms by which epigenetics can happen are methylation, **histone modification** and through micro RNA mechanisms.

DNA methylation

This mechanism is a controlled process to regulate gene expression. Methylation of DNA renders genes silent by blocking access to transcription factors. The methylation of DNA means the addition of a methyl group (CH3) to the base cytosine (C) in the DNA nucleotide. In the DNA double helix, cytosine and guanine (G) form a link between the two DNA strands, in the same way that adenine and thymine form a link. However, C and G can be next to each other (with a phosphate group between them) on the same DNA strand, known as CpG, and cytosine methylation can occur in this structure. CpGs are distributed throughout the genome except where CpG clusters are found in the promoter regions of the gene (Bird, 2002). Here they are typically not methylated so that transcription can occur. Aberrant **DNA methylation** of these sequences can lead to inappropriate gene silencing and loss of tumour suppressor gene expression, leading to the formation of cancer cells.

Histone modification

The histone is like a protein spool that the DNA strand wraps around. Genes are transcribed when chromatin (DNA and its histone) is modified by the addition of acetyl to lysine in the histone, known as histone acetylation. This is initiated by an enzyme called histone acetyltransferase (HAT). This leads to uncoiling of the DNA from around the histone, opening it up to transcription factors to express (switch on) the gene. The gene can be switched off when the acetyl group is removed by the enzyme histone deacetylase (HDAC), thus preventing the expression of the gene.

RNA-induced

Micro RNA (miRNA) is a non-coding small RNA which modulates gene expression by pairing with **messenger RNA (mRNA)**, mediating post-transcriptional gene silencing. They have an important role in controlling cell growth, differentiation and survival. Abnormal expression of miRNA alters the activity of oncogenes and tumour suppressor genes and decreases stability, either by increasing the expression of oncogenes or decreasing the expression of tumour suppressor genes. The miRNAs associated with cancer are termed oncomirs and they play a critical role in its development.

Development and progression of malignant cells

There are several steps that must happen for a normal cell to become a malignant cell and it takes more than one mutation in a gene. The cell has multiple checkpoints to prevent mutant genes from inducing the cell to become malignant. The development of a malignant cell is a complex multi-step process which the cell must go through. This involves the stages of initiation, **promotion** and progression to **metastasis** with development of a blood supply (angiogenesis) and avoidance of the immune system.

Initiation

The mutation of a gene is the first stage in the development of a tumour cell and often several mutations may be necessary for a cell to become malignant. Substances capable of inducing cancer are known as carcinogens and these can initiate the genetic damage that can lead to cancer. Examples of such substances are ultra-violet and ionising radiation, certain viruses and chemicals. Once initiated, cancers continue to undergo changes that enable them to grow excessively and survive.

Promotion

Promotion is the proliferation of the mutant cell and several factors can contribute to this, such as nutritional factors, infection and hormonal influences as well as the cells' ability to avoid DNA repair mechanisms and evade apoptosis. This allows the mutation to be passed on to the daughter cells and proliferation to continue unchecked, leading to highly evolved tumour cells.

Progression

Progression is the stage where the mutant dividing cells begin to exhibit malignant properties. These cells have a growth advantage and proliferate easily with an unstable genetic structure that allows more mutations to occur. The tumour cell has characteristics that are different from the cell of origin, such as the ability to invade surrounding tissue and metastasise.

Metastasis

This is the process whereby cancer cells spread from their original site and proliferate in distant sites. Once tumour cells have metastasised, cancer becomes more difficult to treat and chances of survival are reduced. The process of metastasis is a key characteristic of cancer. It involves the cells detaching from the basement membrane in the tissue of origin and travelling in the blood and/or lymphatic systems, eventually colonising in distant tissue. For a cancer cell to become established in distant sites, it must acquire oxygen and nutrition and therefore needs a blood supply, a process known as angiogenesis. It also needs to evade the immune destruction and develop the ability to invade and metastasise.

Angiogenesis

Without a blood supply, tumour cells could not continue to grow and spread. Angiogenesis is the process of forming new blood vessels, and cancer cells produce factors that stimulate the growth of new blood vessels in response to hypoxia. Inactivation of tumour suppressor genes and increased expression of oncogenes lead to stimulation of an angiogenic regulator known as hypoxic inducible factor-1α (HIF-1α). This induces angiogenic factors such as **vascular endothelial growth factor**

(VEGF) which stimulates the proliferation of vascular **endothelial cells**, contributing to blood vessel development.

Evasion of body's immune system

Tumour cells have antigens on their cell surface and should be recognised as foreign by the host immune system. Immune cells such as **cytotoxic T cells** and natural killer cells normally recognise altered cell

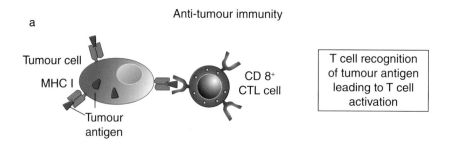

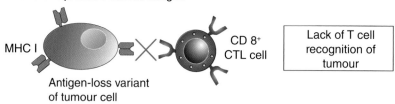

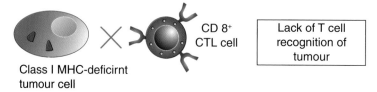

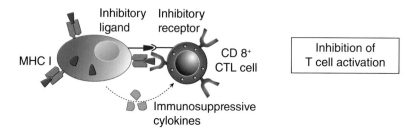

Figure 9.4 Mechanisms by which tumour cells evade the immune system

Source: Abbas et al. (2015) *Cellular and Molecular Immunology*, 8th edn. Philadelphia, PA: Elsevier Saunders, p. 390. Reproduced with permission.

surface proteins and antigens. Tumour cells develop mechanisms that allow them to evade the immune system and these can be intrinsic to the tumour cell or mediated by other cells. Intrinsic mechanisms include the loss of tumour-specific antigens or mutations in the **major histocompatibility complex (MHC)**, leading to decreased synthesis of antigens which causes a lack of recognition of the antigen by cytotoxic T lymphocytes (Figure 9.4). Tumour cells may produce substances that reduce T cell activity. One such substance is interleukin-10 (IL-10), an immunosuppressive cytokine that decreases T-helper cell activity and suppresses the capacity of cytotoxic cells to recognise and kill tumour cells. TGF-β (transforming growth factor-beta), a cytokine, is secreted by many tumour cells to inhibit the activity of lymphocytes and macrophages (Abbas et al., 2015).

ACTIVITY 9.3: APPLY

Immunotherapy for the treatment of cancer

Immunotherapy has been the subject of cancer research for many years, but only relatively recently have tumour-specific treatments been devised which are showing promising results and making headline news. For an example published in *The Guardian* newspaper in June 2018, search online for 'Guardian + Immunotherapy + prostate cancer'. If you are using the eBook just click on the icon.

The person's immune system is stimulated to react to cancer cell antigens and thus stop cancer progression. Watch this video for information on immunotherapy. If you are using the eBook just click on the play button. Alternatively go to

https://study.sagepub.com/essentialpatho/videos

ARTICLE: IMMUNOTHERAPY   IMMUNOTHERAPY (3:27)

Ability to invade and metastasise

For cells to separate from the primary tumour and colonise in a distant secondary environment (metastases) they first must invade the surrounding tissue. Invasion of surrounding tissues involves reduced cell-to-cell adhesion and destruction of the extracellular matrix by **proteases** to allow the cell to detach and have increased motility. Mobile cancer cells invade and gain access to the venous and lymphatic circulations and must withstand the forces of the blood and lymphatic flows and avoid further exposure to immune cells. The circulatory network of vessels to which the cancer cells have gained access can determine the pattern of spread of the cancer. Regional lymph nodes which drain the tumour area are often the first site of metastases through the lymphatic system, while spread to distant sites is often through the venous circulation. Once in a distant site the cancer cells must be able to establish themselves by adhering to the tissue, establish a surrounding micro environment and proliferate (Figures 9.5 and 9.6).

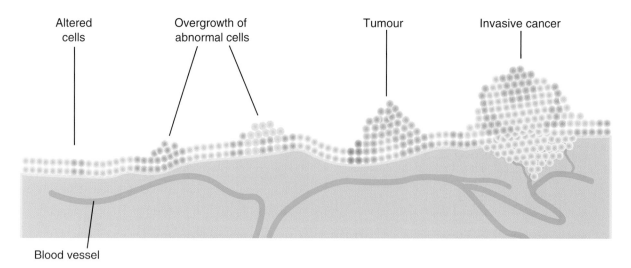

Illustrated by Shaun Mercier © SAGE Publications

Figure 9.5 Initiation, promotion, progression and metastases

How cancer affects the person

A number of factors will have an impact on how cancer affects the body, such as the stage and the location of the cancer. Early stages of cancer may not exhibit any signs or symptoms but as the tumour grows and begins to press on and then invade surrounding tissues, symptoms may start to appear. The location of the tumour will have specific symptoms related to the organ or tissue affected, e.g. a tumour in the lungs may result in a persistent **cough** or shortness of breath or chest pain. A tumour in the bowel may cause a change in bowel pattern, altered stools and/or rectal bleeding. Systemic manifestations of cancer include pain, **cachexia**, fatigue, **anaemia** and infections.

Pain

Often occurring in the more advanced stages of cancer, pain may be local at the site of the primary tumour or referred away from the original site. Pain is due to the invasion of a surrounding tissue with a stretching of visceral surfaces and increased pressure on sensory nerves due to the growth of the tumour. Inflammation and infection will also stimulate pain receptors.

Cachexia

This is weight loss and muscle wasting due to a loss of appetite (**anorexia**) and a high metabolic rate. This is thought to occur when the cancer cells produce specific catabolic factors and **cytokines** that suppress appetite and cause abnormal protein metabolism in muscles. Adipose tissue breakdown is also increased. **Nausea** and **vomiting** can be symptoms of cancer.

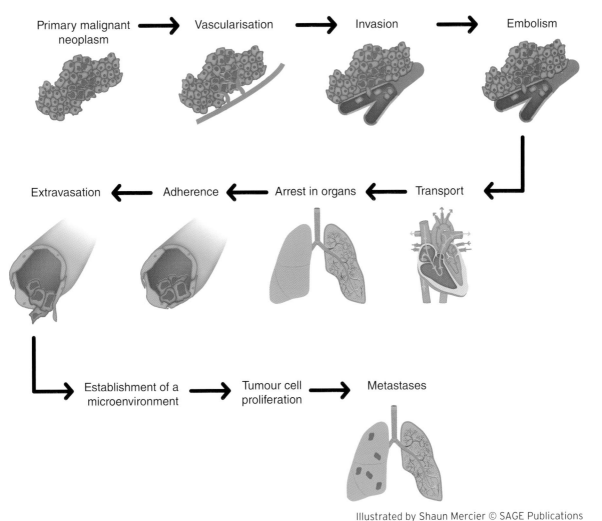

Illustrated by Shaun Mercier © SAGE Publications

Figure 9.6 Pathogenesis of metastasis

Anaemia

This is a deficiency in circulating red blood cells and may be as a result of the reduced production of erythrocytes due to bone marrow suppression or because of chronic bleeding that can occur in some cancers such as colon cancer. Malnutrition and dysregulation of iron metabolism can lead to iron deficiency. Signs and symptoms include fatigue, breathlessness and increased heart rate.

Fatigue

Severe fatigue is described as lack of energy and weakness distinct from normal tiredness. It is associated with cachexia and anaemia and inflammatory changes. Physiological and psychological factors are both involved in cancer-related fatigue.

Paraneoplastic syndromes

As the tumour progresses and malignancy develops, the intensity and variety of symptoms can increase. However, in addition to the specific symptoms other symptoms can occur that appear to be unrelated to the primary or metastatic disease (Table 9.6). These symptoms are referred to as **paraneoplastic syndromes** and are often caused by substances that are produced by the tumour, such as hormones. For example, small cell carcinoma of the lung can produce excess adrenocorticotropic hormone (ACTH), leading to symptoms of **Cushing's syndrome** (see Chapter 7, Boore et al., 2016). **Hypercalcaemia** is associated with abnormal production of a protein linked to parathyroid hormone by tumour cells. Such syndromes are significant as they may be the first unexplained symptoms that a person presents with and could confuse the diagnosis of cancer.

Table 9.6 Effects of tumour on the body

Overall effect	Related tumour action
Altered function of the involved tissue, bleeding, haemorrhage	Destruction of normal tissue, compression of blood vessels, ischaemia
Ulceration, necrosis, infection, obstruction, swelling	Expansive growth of tumour, compression and invasion of surrounding tissues
Anaemia, hypercalcaemia	Bleeding, depression of red blood cell production, invasion of bone
Pain	Liberation of pain mediators from tumour compression, ischaemia of structures
Weakness, wasting, cachexia	Catabolic effect of tumour on metabolism, rapidly dividing and growing cells
Inappropriate hormone production	Production of hormones by tumour and lack of normal control mechanisms

Diagnosis

A diagnosis of cancer is life-changing and can have a profound effect on the person. Consider someone in the Bodie family and the implications this diagnosis has on that individual and the whole family.

Diagnosis is based on a combination of factors such as the history behind the presenting signs and symptoms, the person's health history and their family health history. Symptoms of cancer are varied and diverse and depend on the location of the cancer. Diagnostic tests can provide information that can contribute to definitive diagnosis and include blood tests, screening for **tumour markers**, imaging tests such as X-ray, CT scans, MRI scans and histological staging from a tissue biopsy of the tumour.

Blood tests

These can reveal abnormalities associated with cancer such as anaemia or abnormal blood cells. In blood cancers such as leukaemia the abnormal cell characteristics can be detected through blood samples.

Tumour markers

These are biochemical substances produced by some cancer cells and are found in the blood, urine or spinal fluid. These tumour markers may be enzymes, antigens, **antibodies** or hormones and can be used to aid diagnosis (Table 9.7). Many of these substances are also produced by non-cancerous cells and are associated with other diseases, and therefore their presence cannot be used alone as a diagnosis for cancer. Tumour markers can be used to screen individuals at high risk of cancer and to monitor the activity of a tumour.

Table 9.7   Examples of tumour markers

Marker	Type	Associated tumour
Adrenocorticotrophic hormone (ACTH)	Hormone	Pituitary adenomas
Human chorionic gonadotrophin (hCG)	Hormone	Testicular tumours
Oncofetal antigens (α-fetoprotein)	Fetal yolk sac and gastrointestinal structures early in life	Liver cancer, germ cell cancer of the testes
Immunoglobulins	Protein	Multiple myeloma
Prostate-specific antigen (PSA)	Protein	Prostate cancer

Tumour tissue biopsy

Once a diagnosis of cancer is suspected and a tumour identified then a biopsy of the tumour tissue should be evaluated for histologic and cytologic examination. These are tests that examine the tissues and cells for abnormalities. Samples of tissue are obtained in a number of ways, including:

* surgical excision, where the entire tumour is removed
* laparoscopic and endoscopic methods
* needle biopsy, which involves withdrawing cells and fluid from a palpable tumour
* exfoliative cytology, where cells shed from the surface are collected for examination, for example a cervical smear test.

Early detection and definitive diagnosis of cancer can influence treatment options and often improve treatment outcomes. It is a priority in cancer management and has led to national screening programmes (discussed later).

Staging and grading of tumours

Once cancer has been diagnosed it is then critical to identify the behaviour of the tumour and ascertain if it has spread. Determining the severity of the disease and the extent of spread helps to select the appropriate treatment. Tumours are classified according to their cellular characteristics and extent of spread and this is known as **staging**. The international Tumour Nodes Metastasis (TNM) system has been established to standardise the way cancers are classified (AJCC, 2018) (Table 9.8). This not only helps to provide an indication of prognosis and plan treatment, but can also help in evaluating the results of treatment. The standardisation of the classification system also facilitates information exchange between centres and contributes to international research. T describes the tumour size, N identifies and classifies lymph node involvement and M identifies if there is metastasis and the extent of spread. Each TNM category is assigned a number to indicate the stage, and the higher the number the more advanced the cancer.

Table 9.8   Classification of tumours - TNM system (AJCC, 2018)

T (Tumour)	
Tx	Primary tumour cannot be adequately assessed
To	No evidence of primary tumour
Tis	Carcinoma in situ
T1-4	Size and/or extent of primary tumour
N (Nodes)	
Nx	Regional lymph nodes cannot be assessed
No	No evidence of regional lymph node involvement
N1-3	Involvement of regional lymph nodes (number and/or extent of spread)
M (Metastasis)	
Mo	No distant metastasis
M1	Distant metastasis (cancer has spread to distant parts of the body)

Source: Adapted from AJCC (American Joint Committee on Cancer), 2018

The calculations of TNM are put into a stage category identified by Roman numerals and which relates to prognosis. The higher the number, the greater the extent of spread and the more aggressive the tumour.

Stage I – no spread from the original site
Stage II – spread to neighbouring tissues
Stage III – spread to regional structures, e.g. lymph nodes
Stage IV – spread to distant sites

This is a broad staging system and many types of cancers have more specific staging and classification systems, for example colon cancer.

ACTIVITY 9.4: APPLY

Living with familial bowel cancer

Read about one man's experience of living with familial bowel cancer.

If you are using the eBook just click on the icon. Alternatively go to www.tellingstories.nhs.uk/ and search for 'Paul's story - How genetic information can help reduce the risk'.

ARTICLE: BOWEL
CANCER

Treatment of cancer

The goals of cancer care and treatment fall into three broad categories – cure, control and palliation. Cure implies the eradication of all cancer cells in the body. Control is when treatment is aimed at inducing **remission** and is used to prevent growth and spread. Where there are widespread metastases and a poor prognosis, palliation aims to reduce the size of the tumour and ease pain and other symptoms.

Treatments for cancer are evolving, with immunotherapy, epigenetic therapies and genetic therapies showing promising results (Zhang and Chen, 2018). A number of the relevant treatments are discussed in Chapter 3 and should be studied alongside the information here.

Surgery

Surgical intervention is effective in the removal of solid tumours with well-defined margins that have not spread. The tissue around the tumour is also removed to ensure complete removal of cancerous cells. Surgery enables tissue samples to be taken for examination. The type of surgery is determined by the location of the tumour and other structures involved. Surgery is not without risks as there is a risk of spread of cancer cells during surgical procedures.

Radiation therapy

Radiation can be used alone or in combination with surgery or with **chemotherapy** to kill cancer cells and shrink the size of the tumour. Ionising radiation damages the DNA of the cancer cell or can delay cell cycle progression, resulting in apoptosis. It is most effective where cells are undergoing mitosis. Radiation is delivered in multiple small doses so that damage to normal tissue is minimised. Radiation is suitable for localised areas of cancerous growth and areas that are difficult to access surgically. Side-effects of radiation therapy include bone marrow depression, epithelial cell damage of the skin and blood vessels and damage of the ovaries and testes, leading to a risk of sterility.

Chemotherapy

Chemotherapy is the use of drugs to treat cancer and it can be used alone or in combination with other therapies and other anticancer drugs. Most chemotherapeutic agents are cytotoxic and act on a specific phase of the cell cycle (cell division). Rapidly dividing cells are more vulnerable to the effects of chemotherapeutic agents but the diverse nature of tumours means that cells divide at different rates and are in different stages of the cell cycle. This is why several courses of chemotherapy are required to have maximum effect. Chemotherapeutic agents are not specific to cancerous cells and will therefore damage healthy dividing cells. Although cancer cells behave very differently from normal cells the targets are mostly the same, i.e. the proteins on the cell surface-receptors, enzymes, ion channels and carriers.

Tumour cells can become refractory to chemotherapeutic drugs through several mechanisms such as drug inactivation, epigenetic mechanisms and DNA damage repair (Housmann et al., 2014). This presents a problem in cancer chemotherapy and it is recommended that combination drug therapy using multiple drugs that act at different stages of the cell cycle will prevent the development of resistance.

Chemotherapeutic agents and mechanism of action

- **Alkylating agents** change the shape of DNA through formation of bonds with the DNA (alkylation), thus inducing cell death or slowing the replication of tumour cells, e.g. cyclophosphamide. Side-effects include bone marrow suppression with a reduction in erythrocyte, leucocyte and platelet numbers and can lead to acute non-lymphocytic leukaemia. Epithelial cells lining the GI tract are damaged, resulting in nausea and vomiting and diarrhoea.

- **Antimetabolites** disrupt metabolic pathways of the cell and interfere with nucleic acid metabolism, preventing normal cell division. An example of this is methotrexate. Side-effects include bone marrow toxicity and gastrointestinal toxicity.
- **Anti-tumour antibiotics/cytotoxic antibiotics** affect the function of DNA by binding to DNA and preventing normal synthesis, affecting its function, e.g. doxorubicin (Adriamycin). Side-effects include myelosuppression, nausea and vomiting, cardiac arrythmias and **heart failure**.
- Hormones/**hormone antagonists** slow the growth of hormone-dependent tumours, for example breast tumours or prostate tumours. **Oestrogens** (Stilboestrol) are used in post-menopausal breast cancer, progestogens (Megestrol) are used to treat endometrial cancer and **corticosteroids** (dexamethasone, prednisone) are used in the treatment of lymphomas, Hodgkin's lymphoma and leukaemia. Hormone **antagonists** (oestrogen antagonist tamoxifen) is an oestrogen receptor antagonist used in the treatment of breast cancer.

ACTIVITY 9.5: APPLY

The side-effects of chemotherapy

Watch this short video to learn about the acute side-effects of chemotherapeutic agents. If you are using the eBook just click on the play button. Alternatively go to
https://study.sagepub.com/essentialpatho/videos

CHEMOTHERAPY
SIDE EFFECTS (7:30)

Immunotherapy

Immunotherapy can be specific for particular tumour cells and aims to strengthen the immune response to the tumour. Tumour cells express antigens on their cell surface that should activate an immune response. Tumour immunotherapy includes the use of pro-inflammatory therapies, cytokines, antibodies, T cell transfer and vaccines. **Monoclonal antibodies** (mAbs) help activate T cells to control tumour progression (Whiteside et al., 2016). Administration of tumour-specific antibodies or T-cells is a form of passive immunity designed to stimulate the immune system to destroy cancer cells.

Epigenetic therapy

Epigenetic therapy has been used in the treatment of some cancers to reverse DNA methylation, for example some haematological disorders. Histone deacetylation inhibitors are used to reverse histone acetylation in the treatment of lymphoma. Epigenetic drug therapy requires low doses over a long term. Continued research into epigenetics will provide more targets for the development of cancer treatments in the future (Dawson and Kouzarides, 2012).

Gene and molecular therapy

Gene therapy may be used to suppress overactive oncogenes or activate tumour suppressor genes. Gene therapy can be used to alter the genetic behaviour of the tumour cell and make it more susceptible to cytotoxic drugs. However, there are still limitations in delivering genes to targets.

Stem cell transplantation

Haematological stem cells can be transplanted in malignant disorders such as leukaemia and lymphoma where stem cells are harvested from a healthy donor and infused into the new host where they begin to proliferate and become established as new healthy blood cells. It is important that all the cancerous cells are eliminated from the host prior to transplantation so intensive chemotherapy is used to achieve this. It is also necessary to suppress the host's immune system so that it is not activated by foreign transplanted cells and therefore rejects them. The person requires intensive monitoring during this time. Stem cell transplantation can also be used in other cancers such as breast cancer.

Epidemiology of cancer

Malignant disease is one of the major causes of morbidity (illness) and mortality (death) in developed countries: 8.8 million people worldwide died from cancer in 2015, almost 1 in 6 of all global deaths (WHO, 2018b). The global health burden of cancer has prompted efforts to understand the causes of cancer and identify risk factors, particularly those that can be modified to reduce risk and enhance primary cancer prevention. Cancer is a complex disease that results from the interaction of multiple causes related to genetics, behavioural or lifestyle factors, environmental influences, socio-economic factors and underlying diseases associated with increased risk of developing cancer.

Global impact of cancer

The collection of global data on cancer incidence and mortality is vital to help plan for and manage the disease and to inform preventative strategies. It is used to identify differences across populations and the impact of socioeconomic factors on cancer. Worldwide the most common causes of death due to cancer are lung cancer and liver cancer.

Globally, lung cancer is the most common type of cancer among men with prostate cancer second most common. In women breast cancer is the most common. Generally, the highest incidence rates of cancer are in economically developed countries such as North America and Western Europe, Japan, Australia and New Zealand. Lowest incidence rates occur in Africa and west and south Asia. Relatively more cancer deaths occur in low-income countries; this is partly explained by the significantly poor prognosis of the common types of cancers occurring in these areas, mostly liver, stomach and oesophageal cancer. Figure 9.7 illustrates the estimated world cancer incidence and mortality rates in 2012 for both sexes combined in the major world regions (IARC, 2014). Figure 9.8 provides information about the estimated prevalence of cancer affecting different sites.

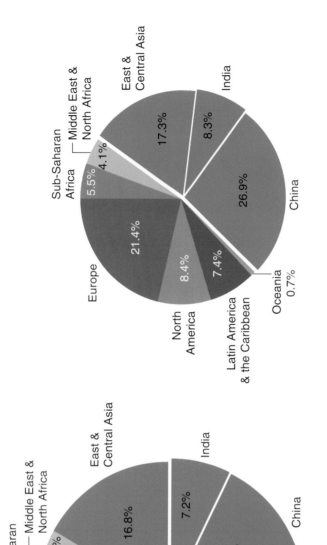

Figure 9.7 Estimated world cancer incidence and mortality in 2012 for both sexes combined in the major world regions (IARC, World Cancer Report 2014)

Source: Reproduced with permission from Stewart B.W. and Wild C.P. (eds) (2014) World Cancer Report 2014. Lyon, France: International Agency for Research on Cancer; compiled from Ferlay J., Soerjomataram I., Ervik M., Dikshit R., Eser S., Mathers C., Rebelo M., Parkin D.M., Forman D., Bray, F. GLOBOCAN 2012 v1.0, Cancer Incidence and Mortality Worldwide: IARC CancerBase No. 11 [Internet]. Lyon, France: International Agency for Research on Cancer; 2013. Available from http://globocan.iarc.fr.

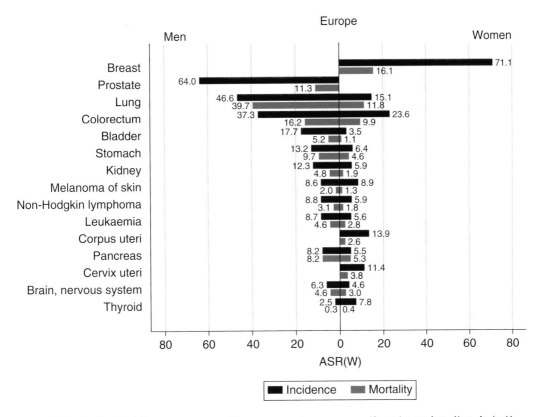

Figure 9.8 Estimated European cancer 5-year prevalence proportions by major sites, in both sexes combined, 2012

Source: Reproduced with permission from Stewart B.W. and Wild C.P. (eds) (2014) World Cancer Report 2014. Lyon, France: International Agency for Research on Cancer; compiled from Ferlay J., Soerjomataram I., Ervik M., Dikshit R., Eser S., Mathers C., Rebelo M., Parkin D.M., Forman D., Bray, F. GLOBOCAN 2012 v1.0, Cancer Incidence and Mortality Worldwide: IARC CancerBase No. 11 [Internet]. Lyon, France: International Agency for Research on Cancer; 2013. Available from http://globocan.iarc.fr.

Statistics for UK and Ireland show that by 2020 one in two people will develop cancer during their lifetime (Cancer Research UK, 2018b). Cancer incidence rates have increased by 13% since the early 1990s in the UK, but cancer survival has improved, with 67% of men and 74% of women surviving at one year post diagnosis. Although cancer accounts for 28% of all deaths in the UK, mortality rates have reduced by 16% over a 40-year period (Cancer Research UK, 2018c).

Aetiology

Several factors act together to produce the genetic abnormalities characteristic of cancer cells. Between 30% and 50% of cancers can be prevented by mitigating the risk factors associated with lifestyle, behaviour and environmental factors (IARC World Cancer Report, 2014) (Figure 9.9).

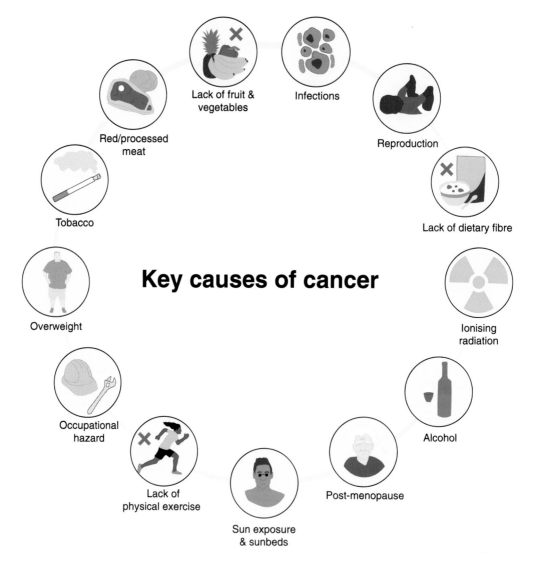

Illustrated by Shaun Mercier © SAGE Publications

Figure 9.9 Key associations and causes of cancer

Tobacco

Tobacco use is the leading cause of avoidable premature death worldwide and is responsible for 22% of all cancer-related deaths. Tobacco is a carcinogen (cancer-causing agent) in both the smoking and non-smoking form. More than 7000 chemicals have been found in tobacco smoke and 3000 chemicals in smokeless tobacco (Secretan et al., 2009). Many of these chemicals are known carcinogens, causing DNA mutations and epigenetic changes and inflammation. Smoking is the cause of many types of cancer in areas where smoke is directly deposited, i.e. the lung and oropharynx, to more disparate areas to where the carcinogens are carried in the circulation, for example the pancreas, stomach or urinary bladder. Chewing tobacco is known to cause cancer in the oral cavity and pancreas.

Alcohol consumption

Alcohol consumption causes cancers of the mouth, pharynx, larynx, oesphagus, liver, colorectum and breast. In 2010, 337,400 cancer deaths were attributable to alcohol worldwide (IARC, 2014). Ethanol is recognised as the most important carcinogen in alcohol and its metabolism to acetyaldehyde contributes to enzyme and metabolic dysfunction and changes in DNA repair. The amount of alcohol consumed is directly proportional to the increased risk of developing cancer, so the greater the inake of alcohol the greater the risk of cancer developing. Reducing alcohol intake is beneficial for health.

Nutrition, obesity and physical activity

The association between diet and cancer is difficult to measure as, by its very nature, diet is complex and it is a challenge to identify specific factors that cause, or indeed protect a person from, cancer. However, the incidence of different types of cancer across the world has led to its asssociation with diet.

Dietary fibre has been associated with reduced risk of colorectal cancer by adding bulk and inactivating carcinogens by altering the biochemical environment (Murphy et al., 2012). **Vitamin D** has been associated with lower risk of colorectal cancer and folate is a dietary source of methyl group and is important for DNA methylation, repair and synthesis. Diets high in processed meats, particularly those containing nitrates, nitrites or other preservatives that damage DNA, are associated with an increased risk of colorectal cancer (Oostindjer et al., 2014).

Obesity and overweight are increasing in developed countries and are linked to several health disorders. Body fat is assessed using body mass index (BMI) and cancer mortality increases with increasing BMI (IARC, 2014). Obesity is a risk factor for cancer of the oesophagus, colon, pancreas, breast (postmenopausal), **endometrium** and kidney. The mechanism by which obesity causes cancer is not fully understood but it is thought to be linked to metabolic dysregulation and altered signalling of adipose tissue that leads to **insulin** resistance, hyperglycaemia, hypoxia and chronic inflammation. These mechanisms increase the risk of cancer development.

Physical activity contributes to prevention of weight gain and obesity and therefore reduces the risk of cancer. There is evidence that it reduces the risk of breast and colon cancer, irrespective of its effects on BMI, by decreasing levels of sex hormones, altering inflammatory mediators and improving immune functions.

Infections and inflammation

Infections are high-risk factors for cancer development and human papilloma **virus** (HPV), *Helicobacter pylori* (*H. pylori*), **hepatitis** B virus and hepatitis C virus are the most common sources responsible for new cancer cases worldwide (IARC, 2014). Human papilloma viruses (HPV) have been identified as carcinogens for cervical cancer and persistence of infection is necessary for the development of cervical cancer. Infection with this group of viruses is also associated with vaginal, penile and anal cancers. The incidence of HPV infection linked with oropharyngeal cancer is increasing in developed countries (IARC, 2014). Chronic infection of the liver with hepatitis B or hepatitis C viruses is associated with liver cancer. *H. pylori* infection of the stomach increases the risk of gastric **adenocarcinoma**.

Other infectious agents, such as Epstein–Barr virus (EBV), are linked to the development of cancers of the nasopharynx, Burkitt's lymphoma, which is a B-cell non-Hodgkin lymphoma, and Hodgkin disease. Herpes virus causes the development of **Kaposi sarcoma**, a rare type of soft tissue sarcoma most common on the skin, but it can also affect the lymph nodes, lung, bowel, liver and spleen (Cancer Research UK, 2018d).

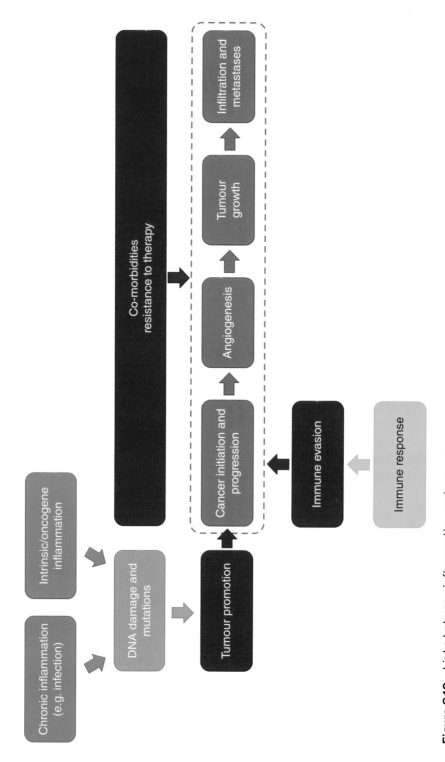

Figure 9.10 Links between inflammation and cancer

Chronic inflammation has long been recognised as a risk factor in the development of cancer due to genetic and epigenetic changes that lead to cancer. The microenvironment of the tumour is altered by macrophages and inflammatory mediators to favour tumour development and spread. The production of free radicals in chronic inflammation causes DNA damage and mutations in oncogenes and tumour suppressor genes (Figure 9.10).

Radiation

The risk of developing cancer is increased with exposure to ultraviolet (UV) and ionising radiation. UV radiation comes from sunlight and man-made sources, include tanning lights and sun beds. UV radiation is classified according to wavelength into three types – UVA, UVB and UVC. Most of the UV radiation that reaches the earth is UVA (95%) and only 5% is UVB. Exposure to sunlight is the main cause of skin cancers, including melanoma which affects the melanocytes (pigment cells), basal cell carcinoma affecting the stratum basale of the epidermis, and squamous cell carcinoma affecting the **keratinocytes** in the stratum spinosum of the skin surface. Melanoma is associated with a higher mortality rate because it tends to metastasise, while basal cell carcinoma and squamous call carcinoma are more common due to long-term exposure to sunlight. UV radiation causes gene mutations and DNA damage. People with fair hair and skin and who freckle and sunburn are at higher risk of melanoma. Ionising radiation causes ionisation in cells and tissues, which is the removal of an electron from the atom, leading to cell damage and tumour development. Sources of ionising radiation are X-rays, computed tomography (CT), exposure to medical radiation and radon gas.

Prevention of cancer

Advances in knowledge and understanding of the causes of cancer allow for more effective prevention by removing or avoiding exposure to known carcinognes (Golemis et al., 2018). For many this involves changes in high-risk behaviour and lifestyle. Education is an important aspect of this and campaigns often aim to inform people about the risks of specific behaviours and lifestyle choices. Healthy diet, increased physical activity and weight loss are key interventions that are associated with reducing risk of cancer. Weight management programmes are offered as part of **health promotion** strategies and increasing a person's physical activity is part of this. Government-supported policies and regulation can act as incentives to change behaviours, one such example being government influence on tobacco use, particularly cigarette smoking, where policies aim at prevention of initiation and promotion of cessation through measures such as pricing and taxes, restrictions on where smoking can take place, regulation of marketing by the tobacco companies and providing support for cessation. Avoidance of exposure to UV radiation is the most effective way to reduce the risk of skin cancer. This is determined by behaviour – keeping the skin covered in sunlight, regular use of sunscreen with high SPF and UV protection, and avoidance of tanning lights and sunbeds.

Vaccination

Sixteen per cent of cancers are caused by infections, and **vaccination** has a role in the primary prevention of infection-associated cancers. Vaccination has been effective against hepatitis B virus and liver cancer and most countries include this in their childhood immunisation programmes. A vaccine for human papilloma virus (HPV) has been effective in preventing cervical cancer in women not previously infected and is recommended in adolescent girls and is now being considered for boys of the same age group.

Screening

Screening programmes aim to detect cancer in its early stages so that treatment can be instigated promptly and chances of survival improved. The person very often may be asymptomatic and cervical cancer, breast cancer and bowel cancer have established screening programmes (Table 9.9). Cervical screening includes obtaining a sample of cervical cells for cytological examination, also known as a **Papanicolaou smear** (or Pap smear) test, testing for HPV infection and visual inspection. Breast cancer screening uses X-ray mammography through which small tumours can be detected. Bowel cancer screening involves obtaining a sample of faeces and testing it for occult blood. The sample can be obtained in the person's home at their own convenience by using a kit. Visual inspection and tissue sampling can be obtained through flexible sigmoidoscopy or colonoscopy.

Table 9.9 Evidence-based screening methods

Cancer	Screening method
Breast	Mammography
Cervical	Cytology, HPV testing, visual inspection
Colorectal	Faecal occult blood
	Flexible sigmoidoscopy
	Colonscopy

Source: American Joint Committee on Cancer (AJCC), downloaded 2018

CHAPTER SUMMARY

In this chapter you have studied ways in which cells and body tissues adapt to different stimuli through changes in cell growth and division. The stages of cell division and growth were examined, leading on to differentiation between benign and malignant growths. The different methods of cell adaptation were then examined, some of which can lead to neoplastic change. The major section of this chapter is about cancer: the causes, changes in cells, epidemiology, treatment and prevention.

KEY POINTS

- Cell division and growth through the cell cycle are essential for normal bodily structure and function.

- Various stimuli result in adaptive changes of cells of various types, including: atrophy, hypertrophy, **metaplasia**, **dysplasia**, **anaplasia**, neoplasia. They vary between being benign and malignant in nature.

- Apoptosis and necrosis are the two major mechanisms of cell injury. Apoptosis is planned cell death and plays an important role in maintaining the balance between oncogenes, growth and death of tissues. Necrosis occurs due to the effect of one of various stimuli leading to cell death.

- Cancer is the general name for malignant tumours.

- Genetic mechanisms are important in the development of cancer and can involve oncogenes, tumour suppressor genes and epigenetics. Epigenetics involves changes in gene expression without altering the DNA; there are a number of ways this can occur.

- There are a number of stages in the development and progression of malignant cells: initiation, promotion, progression, metastasis, angiogenesis, evasion of the immune system. In order to spread throughout the body, malignant cells must be able to invade and metastasise.

- One of the major symptoms of cancer is pain. As the tumour grows it will result in various signs and symptoms depending on which organs of the body are affected. These can include: cachexia, anaemia, fatigue, paraneoplastic syndromes.

- Diagnosis is based on a number of factors including: individual and family health history, signs and symptoms, blood tests, tumour markers, tumour tissue biopsy. Staging and grading of the tumour is based on the TNM system: **T**umour size, lymph **N**ode involvement and **M**etastases and their extent.

- Treatment of cancer can involve a number of different approaches: surgery, radiation therapy, chemotherapy, immunotherapy. These may be applied singly or in combinations.

- Cancer epidemiology examines the causes of morbidity and mortality and considers the global impact of cancer. It also assists in understanding the aetiology (i.e. specific causes of the condition). It provides the knowledge base for screening and prevention of cancer.

The content of this chapter has helped you to understand how cell function and structure change under different circumstances. Revise the different sections in turn then try to answer the questions below to challenge your knowledge.

REVISE
TEST YOUR KNOWLEDGE

Answers are available online. If you are using the eBook just click on the answers icon below. Alternatively go to **https://study.sagepub.com/essentialpatho/answers**

1 Outline the phases and stages of the cell cycle.

2 Differentiate between benign and maligant tumours.

3 Identify the different types of adaptive change and the main groups of causes of cell injury.

4 Describe what is meant by apoptosis and how this differs from necrosis.

5 What are the main methods of treatment of necrosis?

6 List four ways an oncogene influences cell growth.

7 Discuss how a cell becomes malignant.

8 Describe how a cancerous cell metastasises.

9   What is epigenetics?

10   Identify four general symptoms of cancer.

11   What diagnostic tests are used to test for cancer?

12   Name three types of carcinogens.

13   Discuss the classification of tumours.

14   Discuss three types of therapy used in cancer treatment.

15   What are the five most common types of cancer in men and in women worldwide?

16   Identify three screening methods that are used to detect cancer.

REVISE

ACE YOUR ASSESSMENT

- Further revision and learning opportunities are available online

- Test yourself away from the book with **Extra multiple choice questions**

- Learn and revise terminology with **Interactive flashcards**

If you are using the eBook access each resource by clicking on the respective icon. Alternatively go to **https://study.sagepub.com/essentialpatho/chapter9**

CHAPTER 9
ANSWERS

EXTRA
QUESTIONS

FLASHCARDS

REFERENCES

Abbas A.K.. Lichtman A.H. and Pillai S. (2015) *Cellular and Molecular Immunology*, 8th edn. Philadelphia, PA: Elsevier Saunders.

Adigun, R. and Bhimji, S.S. (2018) Necrosis, Cell (Liquefactive, Coagulative, Caseous, Fat, Fibrinoid, and Gangrenous). *StatPearls [Internet]*. Treasure Island, FL: StatPearls Publishing.

AJCC (American Joint Committee on Cancer) (2018) Cancer Staging System. Chicago: AJCC. Available at: https://cancerstaging.org/references-tools/Pages/What-is-Cancer-Staging.aspx (accessed 1 August 2018).

Bird, A. (2002) DNA patterns and epigenetic memory. *Genes and Development*, 16 (1): 2–21.

Boore, J., Cook, N. and Shepherd, A. (2016) *Essentials of Anatomy and Physiology for Nursing Practice*. London: Sage.

Cancer Research UK (2018a) Worldwide cancer statistics [online]. Available at: www.cancerresearchuk. org/health-professional/cancer-statistics/worldwide-cancer (accessed 1 August 2018).

Cancer Research UK (2018b) Cancer risk statistics [online]. Available at: www.cancerresearchuk.org/ health-professional/cancer-statistics/risk (accessed 1 August 2018).

Cancer Research UK (2018c) Cancer mortality statistics [online]. Available at: www.cancerresearchuk. org/health-professional/cancer-statistics/mortality#heading-Zero (accessed 1 August 2018).

Cancer Research UK (2018d) Kaposi's sarcoma [online]. Available at: www.cancerresearchuk. org/about-cancer/soft-tissue-sarcoma/types/which-treatments-are-used-for-kaposis-sarcoma) (accessed 26 July 2018).

Copstead, L.E. and Banasik, J. (2013) *Pathophysiology*, 5th edn. St Louis, MO: Elsevier Saunders.

Dawson, M.A. and Kouzarides, T. (2012) Cancer epigenetics: from mechanism to therapy. *Cell*, *150*: 12–17.

Elmore, S. (2007) Apoptosis: a review of programmed cell death. *Toxicologic Pathology*, *35* (4): 495–516.

Favaloro, B., Allocati, N., Graziano, V., Di Ilio, C. and De Laurenzi, V. (2012) Role of apoptosis in disease. *Aging*, *4* (5): 330–49.

Golemis, E.A., Scheet, P., Beck, T.N., Scolnick, E., Hunter, D.J., Hawk, E., et al. (2018) Molecular mechanisms of the preventable causes of cancer in the United States. *Genes and Development*, *32* (13–14): 868–902.

Heuther, S.E. and McCance, K.L. (2017) *Understanding Pathophysiology*, 6th edn. St Louis, MO: Elsevier Suanders.

Housmann, G., Byler, S., Heerboth, S., Lapinska, K., McKenna, L., Snyder, N. et al. (2014) Drug resistance in cancer: an overview. *Cancers*, *6* (3): 1769–92.

IARC (International Agency for Research on Cancer) (2014) *World Cancer Report 2014*. Lyon, France: IARC.

Jordan, A., Khiyani, N., Bowers, S.R., Lukaszczyk, J.J. and Stawicki, S.P. (2018) Maggot debridement therapy: a practical review. *International Journal of Academic Medicine*, *4*: 21–34.

Kumar, V., Abas, A.K. and Aster, J.C. (2018) *Robbins and Cotran Pathologic Basis of Disease*, 10th edn. Philadelphia, PA: Elsevier Saunders.

Mader, S. and Windelspecht, M. (2018) *Human Biology*, 15th edn. New York: McGraw-Hill Education.

Marieb, E.N. and Hoehn, K. (2016) *Human Anatomy and Physiology*, 10th edn. San Francisco, CA: Pearson.

Murphy, N., Norat, T., Ferrari, P., Jenab, M., Bueno-de-Mesquita, B., Skeie, G., Dahm, C.C., Overvad, K., Olsen, A., Tjønneland, A. and Clavel-Chapelon, F. (2012) Dietary fibre intake and risks of cancers of the colon and rectum in the European prospective investigation into cancer and nutrition (EPIC). *PloS ONE*, *7* (6): e39361.

Olivier, M., Hollstein, M. and Hainaut, P. (2010) TP53 mutations in human cancers: origins, consequences, and clinical use. *Cold Spring Harbor Perspectives in Biology*, *2* (1): a001008.

Oostindjer, M. et al. (2014) The role of red and processed meat in colorectal cancer development: a perspective. *Meat Science*, *97* (4): 583–96.

Porth, C.M. (2015) *Essentials of Pathophysiology*, 4th edn. Philadelphia, PA: Wolters Kluwer.

Secretan, B., Straif, K., Baan, R., Grosse, Y., El Ghissassi, F., Bouvard, V., et al. (2009). A review of human carcinogens – Part E: tobacco, areca nut, alcohol, coal smoke, and salted fish. *The Lancet Oncology*, *10* (11): 1033–4.

Sherman, R.A. (2014) Mechanisms of maggot-induced wound healing: what do we know, and where do we go from here? *Evidence-Based Complementary and Alternative Medicine*. eCAM, *2014*: 592419. http://doi.org/10.1155/2014/592419.

VanMeter, K.C. and Hubert, R.J. (2014) *Gould's Pathophysiology for the Health Professions*, 5th edn. St Louis, MO: Elsevier.

Whiteside, T.L., Demaria, S., Rodriguez-Ruiz, M.E., Zarour, H.M. and Melero, I. (2016) Emerging opportunities and challenges in cancer immunotherapy. *Clinical Cancer Research*, *22* (8): 1845–55.

World Health Organisation (WHO) (2018a) Cancer [online]. Available at: www.who.int/cancer/en/ (accessed 1 August 2018).

World Health Organisation (WHO) (2018b) Cancer: Fact sheet [online]. Available at: www.who.int/news-room/fact-sheets/detail/cancer (accessed 1 August 2018).

Zhang, H. and Chen, J. (2018) Current status and future directions of cancer immunotherapy. *Journal of Cancer*, *9* (10): 1773–81.

DISORDERS OF SUPPORT AND PROTECTION

UNDERSTAND: CHAPTER VIDEOS

Watch the following videos to ease you into this chapter. If you are using the eBook just click on the play buttons. Alternatively go to **https://study.sagepub.com/essentialpatho/videos**

PSORIASIS (1:17)   IMPETIGO (11:03)   ACNE (6:57)

LEARNING OUTCOMES

When you have finished studying this chapter you will be able to:

1. Describe the pathophysiology underpinning common disorders of the skin, including psoriasis, eczema, alopecia and pressure ulcers.
2. Reflect on the psychosocial implications of living with a skin disorder and how this may impact on self-esteem, self-image and psychosocial development.
3. Outline the systemic response to thermal injuries.
4. Describe the role of inflammation and autoimmunity in disorders of the skin.
5. Describe the pathophysiology underpinning disorders that affect bones, muscles, tendons, ligaments and joints.

INTRODUCTION

In this chapter, you will consider disorders of systems involved with support of the body and protection from the external environment. This will build on earlier chapters in this book and will examine the causes and effects of the major disorders of the musculoskeletal system and skin. Additionally, you will also consider the emotional/psychological and social implications of such pathophysiological changes, a central element of person-centred nursing.

The skin and musculoskeletal systems are vital to survival. The skin is our primary defence against pathogens, while the musculoskeletal system provides protection for organs and enables us to be independent and to respond physically to the environment. The musculoskeletal system comprises 70% of the human body and can be affected by many disorders, regardless of age, that may cause pain and disability. In considering this, it is clear that disorders in these systems can lead to reduced safety alongside a reduced health-related quality of life. Additionally, how we look and feel play a major part in how we interact with society and how we view ourselves. Youthful healthy skin can make you feel attractive and young, and being able to move with ease gives you vitality and independence. When these begin to erode, at whatever stage in life, people can become psychosocially withdrawn and have reduced self-confidence and self-esteem. How we see ourselves begins to alter and this can be devastating for some individuals. How we look and move are part of our signature, our identity.

——— PERSON-CENTRED CONTEXT: THE BODIE FAMILY ———

BODIE FAMILY
CASE NOTES

For example, Edward Bodie suffers from chronic lower back pain, primarily a musculoskeletal disorder with neurological involvement (pain). This may be one reason for his weight gain as it may impair his ability to mobilise and socialise. Michelle Zuma fractured her ankle when she was 22 and this may have implications for her in later life. Maud and George Bodie both have older, frailer skin and may be more at risk of developing a pressure sore or skin infection than their younger family members as a result of the skin being less able to deal with trauma, heal quickly and prevent pathogens invading. Into this mix, all the family members may have a genetic predisposition to an autoimmune condition that leads to one of many skin disorders; they may just be fortunate to not have encountered the trigger for such a disorder. The female members of the family are at risk of developing osteoporosis as they age, particularly after the menopause when they lose the protective effect of **oestrogen**. When reading this chapter, be aware of how the lives of people may be affected by these disorders and what the implications may be for them and their family. You will see from reading this chapter that disorders in these systems can extend across the life span.

——— REVISE: A&P RECAP ———

The skin and musculoskeletal system

Before reading this chapter you may want to revise Chapters 14 and 15 in *Essentials of Anatomy and Physiology for Nursing Practice* (Boore et al., 2016). The videos below may also help with revision. If you are using the eBook just click on the play button. Alternatively go to

https://study.sagepub.com/essentialpatho/videos

THE SKIN (11:59)

MUSCULOSKELETAL
SYSTEM (6:12)

SKELETAL STRUCTURE AND
FUNCTION (6:51)

SKIN DISORDERS

Psoriasis

Psoriasis vulgaris is a T-lymphocyte-mediated autoimmune skin disorder that affects 2–3% of the Caucasian population (Coimbra et al., 2010). It has a defined set of characteristics that include focal formation of inflamed, raised skin plaques that constantly **desquamate** scales as a result of excessive epithelial cell growth (Krueger and Bowcock, 2005) (Figure 10.1). In psoriasis, a number of linked cellular changes occur:

- Leucocyte skin **infiltration**, primarily by T lymphocytes and neutrophils:
  After antigen stimulation, T lymphocytes move into the circulatory system and migrate to inflamed skin (Coimbra et al., 2012). Additionally, intraepidermal T lymphocytes are found interspersed between **keratinocytes** throughout the epidermis and more so in the dermis. These T cells are largely memory cells that express the cutaneous lymphocyte antigen (CLA). Psoriasis is often referred to as the product of a cytokine storm as the levels of **cytokines** are high at the site of **lesions**. These cytokines are produced by the T cells and they trigger the **hyperplasia** of keratinocytes.
- Hyperplasia of keratinocytes occurs in the epidermis in a pattern termed 'psoriasiform' hyperplasia:
  This is secondary to keratinocytes proliferating and maturing rapidly which prevents terminal differentiation of the cell. As a result, these squamous keratinocytes retain their nuclei and do not secrete extracellular lipids that enable them to adhere to the skin layer below them and are easily shed. This process gives rise to the elongated raised, reddened **plaques** covered by silvery white scales and **acanthosis** (thickening) of the affected skin (Coimbra et al., 2010).
- Vascular hyperplasia and ectasia (vascular dilation or distension):
  Although the mechanism is not fully understood, activated **macrophages** have been identified as having a role in the inflammatory process of psoriasis; they are thought to stimulate **angiogenesis** through the release of **proteases**, growth factors and other cytokines (Coimbra et al., 2012).

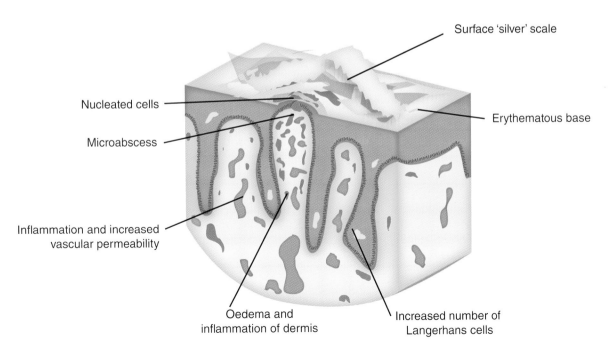

Illustrated by Shaun Mercier © SAGE Publications

Figure 10.1   Cellular changes in psoriasis

Around 10–30% of people with psoriasis go on to develop **psoriatic arthritis (PsA)** (Krueger and Bowcock, 2005). PsA is a chronic inflammatory joint **disease** that is primarily preceded by psoriasis in 60–70% of people (Kerschbaumer et al., 2016). A triad of pathophysiological processes occurs at the joint, namely flexor tenosynovitis, joint effusion and subcutaneous **oedema**. The synovium is infiltrated with T cells, B cells and macrophages, similar to what is seen in the skin in psoriasis. Cytokines are released by these cells and result in the inflammatory response. As with psoriasis, there is ongoing research into the genetic causes of both PsA and psoriasis; to date, there is evidence of genetic **polymorphisms** that give rise to both conditions (Kerschbaumer et al., 2016; Mease and Armstrong, 2014).

ACTIVITY 10.1: APPLY

Lived experience of psoriasis

Go to this website to watch a variety of videos that will give you insight into how young people experience living with psoriasis. If you are using the eBook just click on the play button. Alternatively go to **https://study.sagepub.com/essentialpatho/videos**

LIVING WITH PSORIASIS

Dermatitis/Eczema

The terms dermatitis and eczema are often used interchangeably to describe an inflammatory condition of the skin associated with epidermal barrier dysfunction. Eczema can affect people across the life span and is most commonly diagnosed before the age of 5. Genetic predisposition is complex and polygenic. Eczema can be endogenous or exogenous, with the latter being caused by contact with a substance external to the body and the former being caused by internal factors that are largely unknown; this is referred to as atopic eczema (Peacock, 2016). Atopic eczema is thought to occur as a result of a genetic predisposition and an environmental trigger typical of allergens. The result is a loss of natural moisturisers in the epidermis, most notably to the corneocytes whereby the lipid layer is lost, leading to cellular **dehydration** and subsequent shrinking and cracking of the cell. This change in cellular structure interrupts the protective layer of the epidermis, allowing pathogens access through the gaps and cracks that occur. These pathogens are then detected, triggering the inflammatory response. This response is primarily a T-helper cell (type 2 or Th2) dominated immune response both in skin and in circulation, with high amounts of cytokines; the Th2 cells induce IgE **antibodies** production by plasma cells. This results in an inhibition of the innate immune response of epithelial cells, resulting in lower amounts of antimicrobial peptides in the skin. This further allows pathogen colonisation.

Stevens–Johnson Syndrome/toxic epidermal necrolysis

Stevens–Johnson syndrome (SJS)/toxic epidermal necrolysis (TEN) is a rare, often fatal (10–30% mortality) range of mucocutaneous diseases usually attributable to severe adverse drug reactions (Table 10.1). The percentage of body surface area (BSA) affected denotes the naming of the disorder (Lim et al., 2016):

- SJS is characterised by >10% BSA affected
- SJS–TEN overlap is between 10 and 30% BSA
- TEN is >30% BSA affected

Table 10.1 Common drug causes of SJS/TEN

Allopurinol
Sulfonamides
Anticonvulsants
Nonsteroidal anti-inflammatory drugs

In SJS/TEN, there is widespread **inflammation** of the epidermis that results in necrosis and sloughing of tissue. Early stages of the disease are marked by fatigue, mucosal lesions, headache and bleeding whereas progressive stages are associated with marked erythema of the skin with **papules, vesicles** and **necrosis** present (Klein, 2016). The condition is not limited to the skin, and ocular, genitourinary, gastrointestinal and respiratory tract mucosal lesions can occur; oral mucosal involvement is most common (Schneider and Cohen, 2017).

People who develop SJS/TEN are genetically predisposed to the condition (**HLA**-linked) whereby a combination of **alleles** and medication result in a complex reaction. This includes a vitamin A toxicity as a result of liver dysfunction. Additionally, there appears to be an immune element. Drug or drug-peptide complexes are recognised by T-cell receptors and there is a resultant CD8$^+$ cytotoxic T-cell and natural killer cell-mediated cytotoxicity and cytokine expression that result in a cytokine storm of **granulysin** (Schneider and Cohen, 2017). In other words, there is a large T-cell response to drugs or their components that leads to a mass of cytokines (granulysin) being released. Granulysin is a cytokine that is identified as the key mediator of keratinocyte destruction through apoptosis (Schneider and Cohen, 2017), possibly due to excess retinoic acid (Klein, 2016). It is thought that this apoptosis results in the epidermis and dermis separating (referred to as a positive Nikolsky sign), leading to sloughing (Schneider and Cohen, 2017). Considering this complex reaction process, it is essential to remove the drug that has triggered the event as soon as possible. Administration of **tumour necrosis factor** has been shown in early studies to cease keratinocyte apoptosis and subsequently halt epidermal–dermal separation (Zarate-Correa et al., 2013).

Epidermolysis bullosa acquisita (EBA)

Epidermolysis bullosa acquisita (EBA) is a heterogeneous organ-specific autoimmune disease that occurs when autoantibodies to type VII collagen are induced, causing mucocutaneous blisters (Kasperkiewicz et al., 2016) (Table 10.2). Type VII collagen is a component of the anchoring fibrils of the dermal–epidermal junction. The blisters that occur in EBA are primarily of the mucous membranes and the skin. There are two primary variants of EBA (Kasperkiewicz et al., 2016):

Mechanobullous: In this variant, there is skin fragility, blisters form and result in scarring and there are dystrophic changes. Additionally, there is minimal inflammation (Table 10.2).

Inflammatory: This variant resembles other autoimmune bullous diseases whereby there is a distinct inflammatory process (Table 10.2). This is because people with this variant have IgG autoantibodies against type VII collagen.

Ultimately, as EBA advances, the integrity of the dermal–epidermal junction is compromised.

Table 10.2 Presentations of EBA

Mechanobullous presentation	Inflammatory presentation
Lesions affecting every region of skin and mucous membranes with predisposition to trauma-prone areas:	Blisters
	Erosions on inflamed or otherwise unaffected skin
Elbows	Crust formations
Knees	Urticarial-like erythema
Hands	Pruritus
Feet	
Knuckles	
Toes	
Sacral area	

Impetigo vulgaris

Impetigo is a common infection of the superficial layers of the epidermis. It is commonly caused by gram-positive bacteria and is highly contagious. Erythematous plaques with a yellow crust are the most common presentation and the area may be itchy or painful to touch. Impetigo is common in children, with around 10% incidence. There are two forms (Ghazvini et al., 2017) (Figure 10.2):

- *Bullous*: This form is almost exclusively caused by strains of *Staphylococcus aureus* that yield exfoliative toxins (exfoliative toxin A), impairing cell adhesion in the superficial epidermis. Approximately 10% is caused by Group A beta-haemolytic *Streptococcus* and another 10% by a combination of both. Increasingly, Methicillin-resistant Staphylococcus aureus (MRSA) is becoming more common. In this form, small vesicles become localised flaccid blisters that contain a clear serous fluid. These do not rupture as easily as the non-bullous form and so may be present longer. Once they rupture, the wet, erythematous base is visible.
- *Non-bullous*: This form is mostly caused by *Staphylococcus aureus*. Other causes are mixed infections of staphylococci and streptococci, or streptococci alone. This form occurs from direct bacterial invasion of intact healthy skin but may also occur as secondary infection when skin integrity has been compromised. Maculopapular lesions are present that become thin-walled vesicles which rupture and cause superficial ulceration. Exudate is yellow and dries to a crust. Exposed areas are most prone (e.g. face) and small areas of satellite infections occur from self-inoculation.

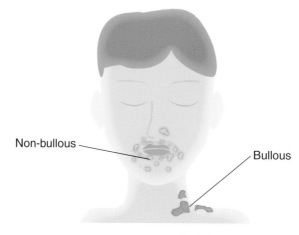

Non-bullous

Bullous

Illustrated by Shaun Mercier © SAGE Publications

Figure 10.2 Forms of impetigo: non-bullous and bullous

Additionally, impetigo can be classified as primary, when healthy skin is infected by bacteria, and secondary when there is recurrent infection at a skin site.

Impetigo occurs as a result of any disturbance in the protective layer of the epidermis that allows pathogens to infiltrate and access fibronectin receptors which the pathogens need to bind to. This can include trauma, insect bites and burns. Immunosuppression can also make someone more susceptible, such as in malnutrition. Impetigo therefore occurs largely as a result of three factors: bacterial adherence to host cells, invasion of tissue with evasion of the person's host defences and the distribution of toxins (Ghazvini et al., 2017).

Vitiligo

Vitiligo is a skin depigmentation condition where patches of skin progressively lose pigmentation, characterised by white skin with sharp, distinct margins (Sarkar et al., 2017). Depigmentation of the hair may also occur in that skin patch. The cause of vitiligo is multifactorial and is thought to be an autoimmune condition in which there is a genetic predisposition and an environmental trigger.

There are two primary types of vitiligo (Sarkar et al., 2017; Speeckaert and van Geel, 2017) (Figure 10.3 shows five types):

* *Non-segmental vitiligo*: This is the most common form, occurring in 90% of people with the condition. In this form, depigmentation occurs on both sides of the body. The condition takes a chronic trajectory and tends to progress over time.
* *Segmental vitiligo*: In this form, there is unilateral pigmentation that does not cross the midline of the body. It normally occurs on the face and trunk. This form of the condition tends to be rapid in onset and can last for up to two years, at which point it stabilises.

Further classifications of presentation are possible whereby there is minimal focal depigmentation, acrofacial presentation (lower legs and face), and universalis whereby most of the body is affected (Figure 10.3).

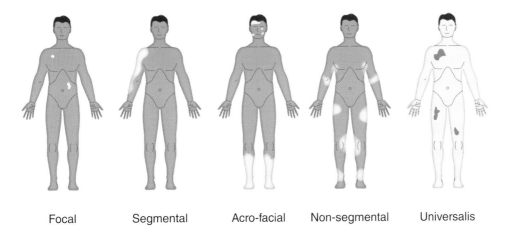

| Focal | Segmental | Acro-facial | Non-segmental | Universalis |

Illustrated by Shaun Mercier © SAGE Publications

Figure 10.3 Types of vitiligo presentation

Vitiligo is a complex multi-genetic disorder. It is a HLA-linked autoimmune disorder whereby there is development of autoreactive T cells and/or inefficient regulatory T-cell function. Additionally, there is development of an anti-melanocyte immune response as part of the condition (Sarkar et al., 2017;

Speeckaert and van Geel, 2017). Destruction of melanocytes leads to the depigmentation. First-grade relatives have a 6–8% risk of developing vitiligo; this increases to 23% in monozygotic twins (Speeckaert and van Geel, 2017).

APPLY

The psychological burden of vitiligo

The impact of skin disorders on health-related quality of life is well documented. Such is the impact that certain conditions have led to the development of assessment tools/scales to document this in order that it can be recognised and addressed. One example is the impact of vitiligo on self-esteem and self-image. The Vitiligo Impact Patient Scale (VIPS) (Salzes et al., 2016) has been developed to determine the psychological burden of vitiligo; more than one-third of people with the condition have depressive symptoms (Speeckaert and van Geel, 2017). The use of such tools is necessary if we are to advocate for people in our care and use signposting to ensure timely, proactive referrals. Only through recognising such impact will we be able to claim to be person-centred and compassionate in our approach to care.

ACTIVITY 10.2: APPLY

Living with vitiligo

Living with vitiligo can be challenging. Listen to this person's story and how they are reminded daily of their condition by society's reactions. If you are using the eBook just click on the play button. Alternatively go to

https://study.sagepub.com/essentialpatho/videos

'LIVING WITH VITILIGO' (2:48)

Acne vulgaris

Acne is a chronic condition affecting the pilosebaceous unit, with an 85% prevalence in the 12- to 24-year-old age group (Masterson, 2018). This chronic inflammatory dermatosis leads to open or closed comedones (blackheads and whiteheads), which are non-inflammatory lesions, and inflammatory lesions (e.g. papules, pustules and nodules) (Zaenglein et al., 2016) (Figure 10.4). These largely occur on the face but can occur on the back and chest. While acne usually becomes supressed in adulthood, it may persist for some. Although a common condition, the pathophysiology of acne is not fully understood due to its multifactorial nature. There are four recognised processes that contribute to acne occurrence (Figure 10.5), with the interplay between these being quite complex. Current treatment is to focus on these four processes and therefore the aim is to restore the homeostatic microbiome of the skin, usually through re-establishing the natural skin barrier, preventing **proliferation** of *Proprionibacterium acnes* (*P. acnes*) as much as possible using **topical** antibacterials and regulating the quantity and quality of sebum (Dréno, 2017).

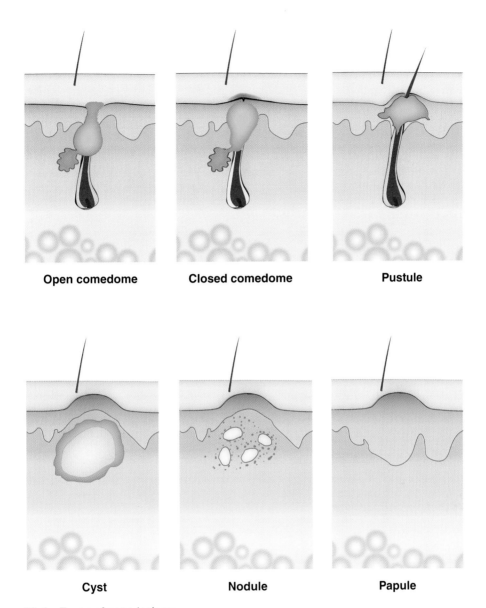

Open comedome **Closed comedome** **Pustule**

Cyst **Nodule** **Papule**

Figure 10.4 Types of acne lesions

ACTIVITY 10.3: APPLY

Acne and self-esteem

Consider that acnegenesis tends to occur in the early teenage years. What impact could this condition have on self-image and self-esteem at this important stage of development? It is important to recognise that acnegenesis is a complex pathophysiological process with factors that may not be under the person's control in the absence of specialist dermatological intervention. Even with such

(Continued)

(Continued)

intervention, we must consider the psychosocial impact of the condition and how that may impact upon mental health and development.

Listen to Chris' story to learn of his experience. If you are using the eBook just click on the play button. Alternatively go to **https://study.sagepub.com/essentialpatho/videos**

ACNE AND SELF-ESTEEM (1:22)

Propionibacterium acnes (*P. acnes*) proliferation

P. acnes is a bacterial flora normally found in the follicular unit and it contributes to lowering skin pH, making it more difficult for bacteria to survive. However, it is thought by some that it can stimulate the release of proinflammatory cytokines that lead to an inflammatory process (Dréno, 2017). However, recent opinion is that the microbiome itself is disturbed, rather than P. acnes being responsible for this cytokine release (Masterson, 2018).

Keratinocyte hyperproliferation in the follicle

Disrupted follicular keratinisation is a key component of pore blockage in acne. Hyperproliferation of keratinocytes can occur when there are changes in sebum production.

Processes involved in acnegenesis

Androgen-mediated increase in sebum production

Sebum production is triggered by androgen activity in the pilosebaceous unit. In acne, it is thought that excess androgens or a hypersensitivity to normal androgen levels may result in the increase in sebum production seen. Additionally, increased activity of 5α-dihydrotestosterone (5α-DHT) in the skin may also cause this increase in sebum production; this is key as testosterone is converted to 5α-DHT in the sebaceous gland (Masterson, 2018) which places it in an ideal location to increase sebum production.

Inflammation

Inflammation is thought to occur as a result of one of two processes. Either follicular hyperkeratinisation triggers an inflammatory process, or inflammation itself triggers an increased proliferation of keratinocytes (Masterson, 2018). However, the process of inflammation is more complex and involves cyclooxygenase upregulation and the production of a variety of substances that trigger inflammatory processes, such as leukotrienes and prostaglandins (Masterson, 2018). This component of acnegenesis is the subject of significant research.

Figure 10.5 Processes involved in acnegenesis

Epidermoid cysts

Epidermoid cysts, or sebaceous/keratin cysts, are dome-shaped lesions of the pilosebaceous follicle. They largely form as a result of infection around pilosebaceous follicles and are **benign** encapsulated, sub-epidermal nodules filled with keratin. Disruption to the follicle results in hyperkeratinisation that results in an accumulation of keratin within the sub-epidermal layer or dermis, giving rise to a blockage of the opening of a hair follicle on the skin surface and a proliferation of cells below. These cysts may also be congenital in origin whereby ectodermal material becomes entrapped (Baisakhiya and Deshmukh, 2011). While they are more commonly found on the face, neck, shoulders and back, they can occur anywhere that there is a sebaceous gland. These cysts are normally slow-growing, painless and generally present no issues. However, should the cyst wall rupture, the contents leak out and this triggers an inflammatory process (Jun et al., 2010). At this point, they are symptomatic and become painful and potentially infected. The site becomes tender with **hyperaemia** of the skin being evident.

Classification of the cyst depends on its make-up (Baisakhiya and Deshmukh, 2011; Sunil et al., 2014):

* *Epidermoid*: When the lining presents only stratified squamous epithelium and contains keratin debris
* *Dermoid*: When skin appendages are found
* *Teratoid*: When other tissue (muscle, cartilage and bone) is present

Once infected and inflamed, these cysts largely have to be excised and drained. The capsule must usually be removed to prevent reoccurrence but this can be unsuccessful if there is an attempt to remove it while infected.

Alopecia

Alopecia is typically referred to as hair loss. It may be focal or diffuse and when referring to the scalp, it is subdivided into **noncicatricial** and **cicatricial** (scarring). In the former, the hair follicle stays intact and therefore has the potential to regenerate hair (Beigi, 2018). It is important to remember that in cicatricial alopecias, the inflammatory infiltrate targets the bulge stem cells whereas in non-scarring alopecias the inflammatory cell attack occurs around the bulb which is why hair growth may be restored (Al-Makhzangy et al., 2015). In this chapter we are going to look at three types of alopecia: **areata, androgenic** and cicatricial.

Alopecia areata

Alopecia areata is noncicatricial and the pathophysiology is not fully understood. It is thought that it involves a T-cell-mediated autoimmune process that targets **anagen** stage follicles, disrupting the growth of hair (Beigi, 2018). The anagen phase of hair growth is the first phase and so targeting these follicles will disable the initial phases of hair growth. Hair follicles are immune-privileged as they lack major histocompatibility complex (MHC) class I expression (Hordinsky and Junqueira, 2015). This means there is no signal for an immune response to occur. However, in alopecia areata, this immune privilege is lost; both MHC class I and II antigens are expressed on the hair follicle and this triggers a T-cell response. Initially there are perifollicular infiltrates surrounding the anagen follicles and this progresses to follicular oedema, cellular necrosis, infiltration of pigmentation to surrounding tissues and microvesiculation (extracellular vesicles associated with pathophysiological processes). Hair follicles progressively pass through a **catagen** (second phase of hair growth) and **telogen** phase (final phase of hair growth) (Beigi, 2018).

Alopecia areata has a genetic component in that it is HLA-linked; familial incidence is between 10% and 50% (Hordinsky and Junqueira, 2015).

Androgenic alopecia

Androgenic alopecia is a genetic form of hair loss also referred to *as male pattern baldness* or *female pattern hair loss*. Androgenic alopecia is polygenetic in nature and therefore genetically susceptible hair follicles in androgen-dependent areas are affected (Lolli et al., 2017). Two major genetic risk loci have been identified: ARÆDA2R locus on the X-**chromosome** and chromosome 20p11 locus (Lolli et al., 2017). There is a gradual loss of hair in genetically predisposed people with men more affected than women. In this form of alopecia, there is miniaturisation of the hair follicle and alteration to the normal hair cycle; the anagen phase is reduced and the telogen phase unaffected or prolonged (Patel et al., 2017). Additionally, the follicular apparatus is gradually miniaturised, resulting in a global diffuse reduction in hair density. People with androgenic alopecia have high levels of androgen receptors in the hair follicles and also high levels of dihydrotestosterone (DHT). When DHT binds to the androgen receptors, there is a release of mediators from dermal papillae that reduce the presence of factors necessary to sustain the anagen phase (Patel et al., 2017). Thus, the anagen phase ends prematurely and the catagen phase begins early. Secondly, there is an activated T-cell infiltration of the follicle that results in micro-inflammation of the follicular apparatus (Patel et al., 2017). Thirdly, prostaglandins are thought to have a role in triggering follicle miniaturisation through disrupting stem cell maturation, interfering with hair development processes (Patel et al., 2017).

Cicatricial alopecia

Cicatricial alopecia is a form of hair loss where there is progressive and permanent destruction of hair follicles that is followed by replacement with fibrous tissue. It occurs mainly on the vertex of the scalp and expands centrifugally. Primary cicatricial alopecias (PCA) can be categorised into four groups according to their prominent inflammatory infiltrate (Kanti et al., 2018):

* Lymphocytic
* Neutrophilic
* Mixed
* Non-specific cell inflammation pattern

In the primary form, the hair follicle is directly affected, most notably affecting the bulge stem cells (Al-Makhzangy et al., 2015). In secondary cicatricial alopecia, the surrounding tissue is affected which then extends to the hair follicle and also the stem cells of the bulge. The secondary form is seen in trauma, burns, radiation side-effects, infections and in some chronic inflammatory diseases (Kanti et al., 2018). PCA is largely non-genetic in origin and the pathophysiological mechanism is largely not fully understood. Bacterial invasion and an excessive inflammatory response is one primary cause that has been identified, while other forms of this type of alopecia are thought to be caused by activated T-cells infiltrating the follicle in response to an unknown androgen (Wolff et al., 2016). These T-cells destroy the bulge stem cells. This is followed by hyperkeratinisation.

Burns (thermal injury)

Burns occur frequently in society; many do not require hospitalisation but those that do may have challenging pathophysiological processes at play at a cellular and systemic level. Burns have three zones of injury (Nielson et al., 2017) (Figure 10.6 and Table 10.3):

ACTIVITY 10.4: APPLY

The personal impact of alopecia

The psychological impact of alopecia should not be underestimated. It can lead to feelings of **depression** and social isolation (Rajabi et al., 2018). Reflect on how this condition and its variants can impact on someone's identify, self-image and self-esteem and consider the implications this has for nursing within a person-centred context. How can you help someone to adapt to life with alopecia and how can you help them to address any maladaptive responses? Consider the Person-Centred Nursing Framework – 2019 and how to work relationally with the person, their family and other professionals.

Go to the Healthtalk website in order to hear the experiences of young people with alopecia. If you are using the eBook just click on the play button. Alternatively go to

https://study.sagepub.com/essentialpatho/videos

ALOPECIA (0.49)

Table 10.3 Zones of thermal injury

Coagulation	Stasis	Hyperaemia
Tissue that was destroyed at the time of injury. It is irreversibly damaged	Area around the zone of coagulation where there is inflammation and low levels of perfusion. This area may progressively deteriorate and become necrotic in 48 hours	Area around the zone of stasis where microvascular perfusion is preserved

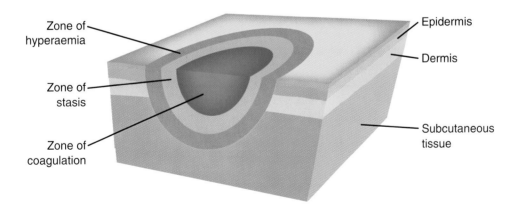

Illustrated by Shaun Mercier © SAGE Publications

Figure 10.6 Zones of thermal injury

With a burn, there is ultimately microvascular dysfunction. This is brought about by vesicular thrombosis as a result of vascular damage, upregulation of inflammatory mediators in response to the trauma, and proapoptotic factors that trigger programmed cell death (Nielson et al., 2017).

Severe burns trigger the immediate release of nuclear factor kappa-B (NF-κB), a transcription activator protein, which triggers a number of inflammatory mediators (e.g. tumour necrosis factor). These mediators trigger a biphasic response (Nielson et al., 2017).

Systemic inflammatory response syndrome (SIRS)

The first phase is characterised by the systemic inflammatory response syndrome, with profound hypermetabolism in response to the thermal injury. This hypermetabolism results in the release of cytokines and the formation of **reactive oxygen species**. These factors trigger a systemic inflammatory process that triggers apoptosis of cells not just at the location of injury but potentially in other organs of the body. As **neutrophils** and macrophages are activated in this process, they can themselves heighten the response by inducing the secretion of other proinflammatory mediators. Vascular dilation is also triggered by these mediators, increasing vascular hydrostatic pressure and resulting in systemic microvascular leakage secondary to widened **endothelial cell** junctions. The totality of this first phase can result in early organ failure in severe cases.

Counter anti-inflammatory response syndrome (CARS)

This second phase is characterised by **the counter anti-inflammatory response syndrome**. In this phase a systemic deactivation of the immune system occurs with the aim of restoring homeostasis from an inflammatory state; primarily it is countering SIRS but it can exist in isolation of SIRS in other disorders. In CARS, monocytes secrete far fewer cytokines. However, some cytokines are known to downregulate the inflammatory response; IL-10 is a cytokine that is known to have a role in **immunosuppression**, reducing the amount of TNF (Ward et al., 2008). In addition, the uptake of apoptotic cells by macrophages and **dendritic** cells triggers immune tolerance by stimulating the release of anti-inflammatory cytokines and suppressing the release of proinflammatory cytokines (Ward et al., 2008).

Systemic impact of burns

Thermal injury triggers inflammation, hypermetabolism, muscle wasting and insulin resistance. In the acute period following a burn, the increased vascular permeability can result in fluid shifts, oedema formation and intravascular **hypovolaemia**. Plasma proteins can move out of the vascular space and they draw fluid with them. This can also lead to hypoproteinaemia. Intravascular volume must be restored in order to prevent ischaemia and cellular shock. Cardiac output increases to compensate and a hypermetabolic response follows to maintain this and to respond to the mass inflammatory response within the body. This process is largely referred to as burn shock and represents the complex circulatory and microcirculatory impairment that occurs as a result of these changes, including oedema formation (Kaddoura et al., 2017). The net effect of this is insufficient delivery of oxygen and nutrients to cells coupled with inadequate removal of waste products, all exacerbating the inflammatory response. The hypermetabolic response compromises all systems in the body and is triggered by a sustained rise in release of catecholamines, cortisol, glucagon and dopamine. These in turn contribute to the development of insulin resistance in the presence of high blood glucose levels.

Muscle wasting occurs as muscle becomes a source of protein in the body which is needed due to the acute loss experienced due to increased vascular permeability. Renal impairment can occur in the form of **acute kidney injury** (Chapter 11); this can be as a result of hypoperfusion secondary to vascular hypovolaemia but is more commonly secondary to septic shock (Nielson et al., 2017). Should the person have had smoke inhalation, an inflammatory response may occur in the lungs which contributes to **pulmonary oedema** and potential airway obstruction. Additionally, wound healing is impaired as a result of impaired vascular permeability and hypoperfusion, increasing the risk of infection and subsequent sepsis (Kaddoura et al., 2017). Multiple organ failure is possible, depending on the severity of the burns, which organs have been affected and how their deterioration impacts on other systems in the body.

Pressure ulcers (decubitus ulcers)

Pressure necrosis, pressures sores or **decubitus ulcers** are primarily a result of immobility and multiple morbidities. They primarily occur as a result of hypoperfusion of tissues and are complicated by the presence of cognitive impairment. Technically, a pressure sore is a wound that occurs in the upper layers of the skin secondary to sustained, externally applied pressure that causes localised **ischaemia** and an inflammatory response. This wound then enlarges radially and deeper into tissue layers unless the underlying causes are addressed to counteract the course of events (Anders et al., 2010). Other factors such as **malnutrition**, shearing forces and moisture will all contribute to how rapidly a pressure ulcer will develop.

Grades of pressure ulcers

In the initial phases, hypoperfusion and pressure injury of the upper layers of the skin occur when sustained pressure prevents sufficient circulation of nutrients and removal of waste products. Erythema, superficial reddening of the skin, occurs in response to this hypoperfusion, and **induration**, localised hardening of tissues, can also develop. This is a grade 1 pressure ulcer (Figure 10.7). Removal of pressure can reverse this process if initiated early enough.

Should pressure not be relieved, hypoperfusion will result in cell death in the basal layer, causing these basal cells to detach. Necrosis can then spread deeper into tissues beyond the basal membrane. This is a grade 2 pressure ulcer (Figure 10.7). The stratum corneum is lost and an open wound now exists; this presents a risk of infection. Cell death will trigger an inflammatory response that will give rise to pain, localised oedema and exudate formation.

A grade 3 pressure ulcer occurs when the ulcer has extended further through to the subcutaneous tissue but not through the **fascia** (Figure 10.7). When it penetrates the fascia through to bone and muscle, this is a grade 4 pressure ulcer (Figure 10.7). There is a high risk of an accompanying **osteomyelitis** at this stage.

ACTIVITY 10.5: APPLY

Grading/staging pressure injury

Watch the following video to help you to stage/grade pressure injury. If you are using the eBook just click on the play button. Alternatively go to
https://study.sagepub.com/essentialpatho/videos

PRESSURE INJURY
STAGING (4:04)

INJURY AND TRAUMA

There are a wide range of musculoskeletal injuries, e.g. **fractures**, **sprains** and **strains** that result from a variety of physical forces common to a particular age group, activity or environmental setting. Childhood injuries commonly result from falls or sport-related injuries whereas trauma from road traffic collisions is a causative factor for adults. In people aged over 65 the most common cause of injury is falling, frequently causing fractures of the femur, humerus or radius/ulna.

Grade 1

Skin is unbroken but inflamed

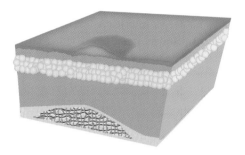

Grade 2

Skin damage is through to the epidermis and possibly the dermis. The stratum corneum is lost and an open wound now exists

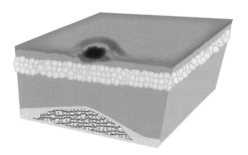

Grade 3

Ulcer has extended further through to the subcutaneous tissue but not through the fascia

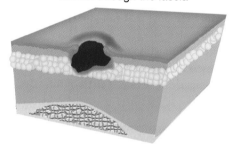

Grade 4

Ulcer penetrates the fascia through to bone and muscle

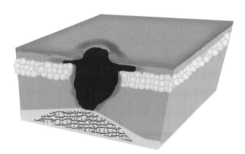

Illustrated by Shaun Mercier © SAGE Publications

Figure 10.7 Pressure ulcer grades

Soft tissue injuries

A soft tissue injury involving muscles, tendons or ligaments may occur independently or may accompany a skeletal injury. Injuries to soft tissue include **contusions**, **haematomas**, strains and sprains.

- *Contusion*: a bruise resulting from direct trauma, e.g. where a hard object strikes a body part. The skin remains intact but the injured tissues undergo a sequence of events including microscopic rupture of blood vessels, damage to muscle cells, swelling and inflammation. The local bleeding causes the area to become **ecchymotic** (black and blue); as the blood is reabsorbed the colour will change to brown and then yellow. Whilst the damage caused is usually minor, many contusions can be very painful.
- *Haematoma*: a large area of local haemorrhage. As blood accumulates in the tissue, pressure is exerted on the nerve endings, causing considerable pain. The pain, inflammation and oedema associated with a haematoma will take longer to reduce than that related to a contusion.

• *Strains and sprains*: Both are musculoskeletal injuries, however they differ in relation to the tissues affected. Strains involve damage to tendons (tissue that joins muscle to bone) whereas sprains involve damage to ligaments (tissue that joins bone to bone). A strain or sprain may result in haematoma formation, leading to tenderness, pain, oedema (swelling) and discolouration. Following injury to either a tendon or ligament, an inflammatory response is initiated; this is followed by the development of granulation tissue. Collagen fibre bundles develop within the first two weeks and create links with the remaining tendon/ligament. Tensile strength will continue to increase thereafter, however it may take six to eight weeks to restore the original tensile strength. Strains and sprains can be graded according to their severity and range from Grade 1 to Grade 3 (Table 10.4).

Table 10.4 Sprains and strains: grades of severity

Grade	Damage	Symptoms	Recovery time
1 - Mild	Possible minor microscopic tearing of fibres	Mild tenderness Minimal swelling	1-2 weeks
2 - Moderate	Partial tear of fibres	Moderate pain, tenderness and swelling Unable to apply load to injured area without pain	3-4 weeks
3 - Severe	Partial tear of fibres	Moderate pain, tenderness and swelling Unable to apply load to injured area without pain	3-4 weeks

APPLY

Treatment of soft tissue injury

Treatment of a soft tissue injury will require pain relief and involves: Rest, Ice, Compression and Elevation (RICE).

• Rest - try to avoid using or applying load to the injured structure
• Ice - apply an ice pack to the injured site for 15-20 minutes every 2-3 hours when awake
• Compression - wrap/apply a firm bandage, ensuring that it does not restrict circulation or cause additional pain. The bandage should cover the whole joint
• Elevation - raising the injured part reduces swelling

Pain relief is also a significant factor in the treatment of soft tissue injury. Analgesics used include: non-steroidal anti-inflammatory drugs (NSAIDs), paracetamol or opioid (codeine). However, Jones et al. (2015) found that there was no clinically important difference in analgesic efficacy between NSAIDs or any other analgesics. These findings are further supported by Hung et al. (2018), who found that there was no difference in analgesic effects or side-effects observed using oral paracetamol, ibuprofen or a combination of both in those attending emergency departments with mild to moderate pain after soft tissue injuries.

It may also be necessary to immobilise the injured joint for a few weeks. Following immobilisation, graded active exercises will be introduced and increase in intensity until full tensile strength has been regained.

Muscle tears

Muscle tears occur within the muscle itself or at points of attachment. They often result from overstretching or overexertion of the muscle or from direct trauma. Muscle tears can be graded as first-, second- or third-degree tears with significant degrees of contrast between each grade (Table 10.5).

Table 10.5 Degree of muscle tear

	First degree	Second degree	Third degree
Amount of muscle involved	Small % of muscle involved	Large % of muscle involved	Complete tear across the muscle
Pain	Mild	Severe	Severe
Contraction	None	Partially contracted	Unable to contract
Loss of strength movement	None	Substantial	Substantial
Internal bleeding	No	No	Yes

Dislocations

A **dislocation** occurs when there is loss of contact between the articulating surfaces of two bones at a joint. A partial dislocation (subluxation) occurs when the bone ends in the joint are still in partial contact. Table 10.6 identifies the types, causes and main sites of/for dislocations.

Table 10.6 Dislocation types, causes and sites

Type	Cause	Site
Congenital	Abnormal formation of hip joint during early fetal development	Hip
Trauma	Fall, abnormal rotation of joint	Hip, shoulder, knee, wrist
Pathological	Infection, **rheumatoid arthritis**, paralysis, neuromuscular disease	Hip

Fractures

A fracture refers to a break or disruption in the continuity of a bone. A fracture occurs when the stress placed on the bone is greater than it can absorb. It can be caused by: sudden injury, fatigue, stress and pathology (i.e. due to the presence of disease). In the United Kingdom (UK) there are approximately 536,000 fractures occurring every year (79,000 hip; 66,000 vertebral; 69,000 forearm and 322,000 other, e.g. pelvis, rib, humerus, tibia, fibula, clavicle, scapula, sternum and other femoral fractures) (NOGG (National Osteoporosis Guideline Group), 2017). Fractures are usually classified according to their: location (e.g. proximal, distal); type (e.g. **comminuted, impacted**); or direction (e.g. **transverse, oblique**). Fractures can also be classified by their communication to the external environment: closed (skin remains intact) or open/compound (bone fragments have broken through the skin) (Table 10.7).

Table 10.7   Classification of fractures

Classification	Image	Description
TYPE		
Proximal, distal or midshaft	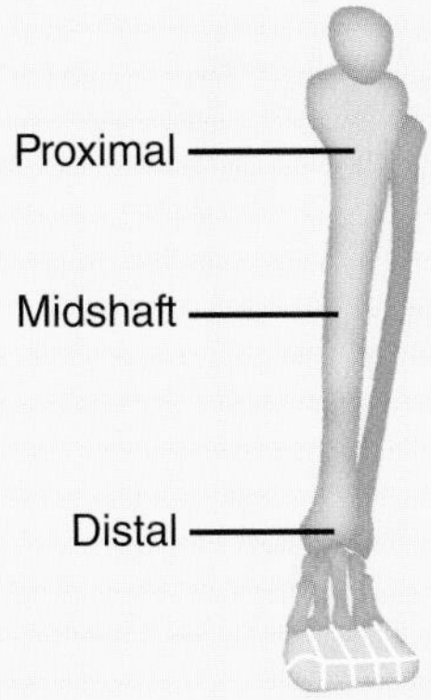 **Figure 10.8a** Proximal, distal or midshaft	Described in relation to the position the fracture occurs in the bone
TYPE Comminuted	**Figure 10.8b** Comminuted	Two or more pieces
Compression	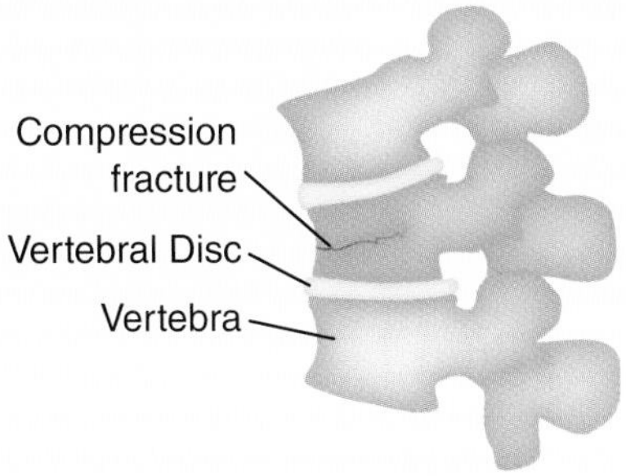 **Figure 10.8c** Compression	Two bones crushed together

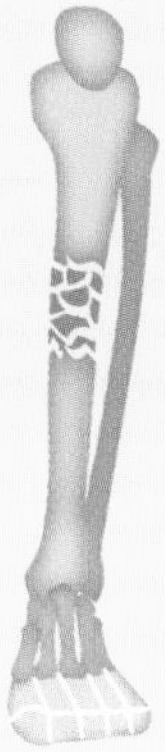

(Continued)

Table 10.7 (Continued)

Classification	Image	Description
TYPE		
Segmental	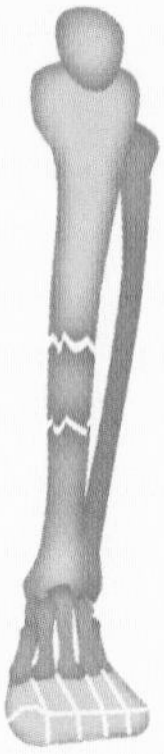 **Figure 10.8d** Segmental	At least two fracture lines that isolate a segment of bone
Impacted	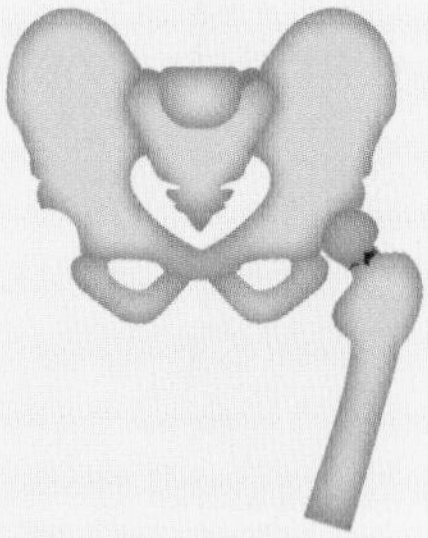 **Figure 10.8e** Impacted	Fracture fragments wedged together
Butterfly	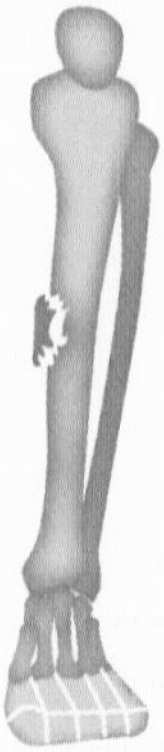 **Figure 10.8f** Butterfly	Two oblique fracture lines meet to form a wedge-shaped fragment

Classification	Image	Description
DIRECTION		
Transverse	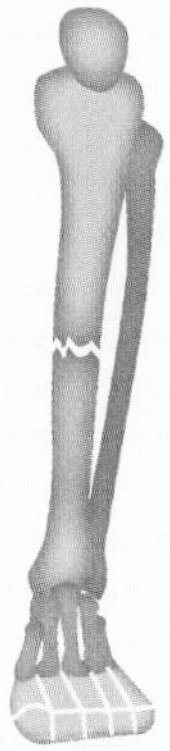 **Figure 10.8g** Transverse	Fracture line is perpendicular to the shaft of bone
Oblique	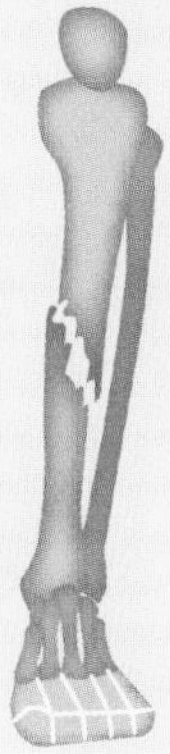 **Figure 10.8h** Oblique	At an angle through the bone
Spiral (torsion)	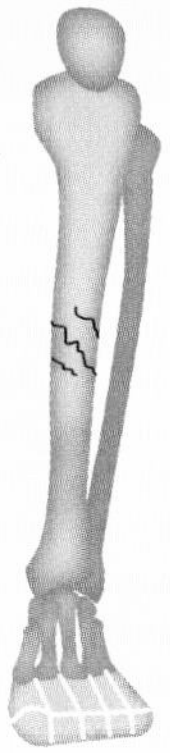 **Figure 10.8i** Spiral (torsion)	Rotating force/applied along the axis

Illustrated by Shaun Mercier © SAGE Publications

Signs and symptoms

The main features associated with a fracture are: pain, swelling, tenderness at site, loss of function, abnormal movement and deformity. A grating sound (**crepitus**) may be heard if the bone fragments rub against each other. If a long bone, e.g. femur, is fractured there will be angulation (bone fragments may push against soft tissue and cause the skin to tent), shortening and rotation (Figure 10.9).

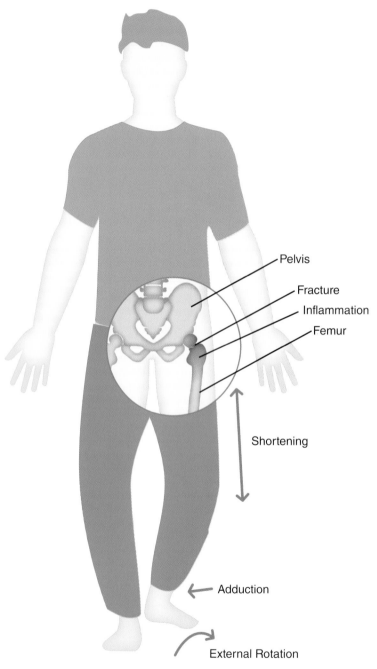

Illustrated by Shaun Mercier © SAGE Publications

Figure 10.9   Femur fracture

Bone repair

Healing of a fracture is a complex process and may occur through direct or indirect healing. Direct healing usually occurs when surgical fixation is required, adjacent bone cortices are in contact with each other and intramembranous **ossification** occurs. Indirect healing involves both intramembranous and endochondral ossification. The process of indirect bone healing takes place in four key steps:

1. *Formation of fracture haematoma*: blood vessels woven throughout the bone are damaged due to the break, blood leaks out of the vessels and a blood clot forms approximately 6–8 hours after the fracture. This haematoma destroys nearby bone cells. These dead cells attract macrophages and **osteoclasts** to the site to remove the dead bone, causing localised swelling and inflammation. Capillaries begin to grow into the haematoma to re-establish a blood supply to the bone; this may take several weeks.
2. *Formation of fibrocartilaginous **callus***: a **procallus** is formed when new blood vessels growing into the haematoma start to organise it into granulation tissue. **Fibroblasts** from the periosteum with **osteogenic** cells start to enter the procallus, develop into **chondroblasts** and start producing fibrocartilage. A fibrocartilaginous callus of collagen fibres and cartilage closes the gap between the two ends of the broken bone (taking up to three weeks). During the first four to six weeks of fracture healing, the fibrocartilaginous callus is very soft and a cast or other support is needed until the callus begins to ossify.
3. *Formation of the bony callus*: osteogenic cells between dead and new bone regions develop into **osteoblasts** and begin secreting extracellular matrix. They form spongy bone **trabeculae** which join the living tissue on either side of the fracture and the callus is now a bony callus which will last 3–4 months.
4. *Bone remodelling*: osteoclasts resorb the dead portions of the original fracture. The spongy bone around the periphery of the fracture is replaced by **compact bone**. Healing of the fracture can sometimes be so good that the original fracture line is undetectable by X-ray; however, there is usually evidence of a thickened area on the bone surface that identifies a healed fracture.

—————————— **REVISE: A&P RECAP** ——————————

Fractures

There is a useful activity on bones, fractures and repair in Activity 15.2 (page 412) of *Essentials of Anatomy and Physiology for Nursing Practice* (Boore et al., 2016).

DISORDERS OF BONES

Metabolic bone disease

Metabolic bone disease represents disorders of bone **metabolism** resulting in structural effects on the skeleton; this includes a decrease in bone density and a reduction in bone strength that may occur due to alterations in genes, diet or hormones.

Osteopenia

Osteopenia is common to all metabolic bone diseases; it is not a diagnosis but rather it is used to describe bone density loss that is seen on X-ray. The reduction in bone density is greater than would be expected for age, gender or race. It may be caused by a number of factors, including a decrease in bone formation, inadequate bone mineralisation or excessive deossification. The major causes of osteopenia include: **osteomalacia, osteoporosis, hyperthyroidism** and **hyperparathyroidism**.

Osteoporosis

Osteoporosis is the most common disease affecting bone but is not always a consequence of the ageing process as many older people retain strong, healthy bone. It is a complex, chronic, progressive metabolic bone disease, multifactorial in nature, characterised by a decrease in bone mineral density (BMD), leading to an increased risk of fractures.

The skeleton is constantly changing; throughout a person's life old bone is removed (resorption) and new bone is added (formation). During childhood and young adulthood, the rate of bone formation exceeds that of bone resorption, hence bones are larger, heavier and denser. Until the age of 30, the rate of bone formation is faster than resorption; at this point peak bone mass (maximum bone density and strength) is achieved. Peak BMD is determined by genetic factors, hormone levels, calcium levels, exercise and environmental factors. After the age of 30, bone resorption slowly starts to exceed the rate of bone formation.

In osteoporosis there is an imbalance between the rate at which old bone is being resorbed and the production of new bone, leading to a decrease in bone density; bones thereby become thinner and more porous. Bone density is based on the number of standard deviations that differ from the mean bone density of a young adult reference known as a T-score (Table 10.8). This was initially used solely to make a diagnosis of osteoporosis, however a revised description of osteopenia and assessment of osteoporosis was released by the World Health Organisation (WHO, 2018).

Table 10.8 WHO diagnosis of bone density and T-score

T-Score	Diagnosis
0 to -0.99 standard deviations	Normal bone mineral density
-1.0 to -2.49 standard deviations	Osteopenia
< -2.5 standard deviations	Osteoporosis
< -2.5 standard deviations with any fracture	Severe osteoporosis

The revised assessment includes BMD with selected risk factors for fracture along with height and weight. A fracture risk score, called FRAX, is calculated to determine the person's 10-year probability of fracture (Kanis et al., 2008). Progressive loss of bone density may continue until the skeleton is no longer able to support itself due to inadequate strength, leading to an increased risk of spontaneous fractures. Over time bones become more fragile and **fragility fractures** can occur, i.e. a fracture of a bone from a fall or bump that would not ordinarily have caused a bone to break. The most common sites for osteoporotic fractures are the vertebrae, neck of femur and wrist.

Osteoporosis can be either primary osteoporosis (postmenopausal osteoporosis) or secondary. Primary osteoporosis has an unknown aetiology but is thought to occur with ageing and is accelerated at menopause, whereas secondary osteoporosis is due to an underlying condition, e.g. Cushing's syndrome. There are a number of factors that may predispose a person to osteoporosis, and these include: ageing, hormonal imbalances/endocrine dysfunction, other medical conditions, insufficient intake or malabsorption of vitamins and minerals, excessive intake of alcohol, caffeine and nicotine, a decrease in activity or weight-bearing activities and certain drugs.

- *Ageing*: osteoblastic activity is less effective and there is a reduction in sex hormones. Sex hormones (in particular oestrogen) are major determinants of bone density in both males and females, and **androgens** (testosterone and dihydrotestosterone) are known to stimulate bone formation. As we age, the amount of oestrogen and androgens decrease, thereby leading to a decrease in BMD.
- *Endocrine dysfunction*: serum plasma levels of calcium and phosphate are maintained within a narrow range in order to maintain skeletal homeostasis; therefore endocrine dysfunction can lead to the development of metabolic bone disease. Imbalances of sex hormones, thyroid hormones, parathyroid hormones, growth hormone and cortisol are thought to be most commonly associated with osteoporosis.
- *Insufficient intake/malabsorption of dietary vitamins and minerals*: calcium absorption from the gastrointestinal tract is decreased with age. Deficiencies in calcium, magnesium and vitamin D can contribute to loss of bone density.
- *Decreased levels of trace elements* such as iron, copper, manganese and zinc have been linked with lower peak bone density and strength in developing bone and development of osteoporosis later in life (Zofková et al., 2013).
- *Excessive intake of alcohol, caffeine and nicotine* is known to lower bone density. Alcohol directly inhibits the activity of osteoblasts and may inhibit calcium absorption (Hallström et al., 2013).
- *Decreased physical activity or weight-bearing exercise* leads to a reduction in mechanical stress on the bone by muscle activity that is needed for osteoblastic activity and bone remodelling. Decreased mobility is related to ageing and may also be a contributing factor to decreased BMD in the older person.
- *Drugs* such as **glucocorticoids**, **proton pump inhibitors**, **selective serotonin reuptake inhibitors (SSRIs)** and anticoagulants can adversely affect normal bone homeostasis.

Osteomalacia and rickets

In contrast to osteoporosis which results in brittle bones due to loss of bone mass, osteomalacia leads to a softening of bones due to the inadequate and slowed mineralisation of osteoid in mature bone. Osteomalacia refers to the condition in adults, whereas rickets refers to the condition in children. In osteomalacia, the process of bone remodelling continues as normal through osteoid formation, however mineral calcification and deposition do not happen. Whilst the amount of bone formed remains the same, it consists of soft osteoid instead of rigid bone. In children this results in changes to bone growth, producing skeletal abnormalities such as genu varum (bow legs) or genu valgum (knock knees) (Figure 10.10). Adequate concentrations of calcium and phosphate are needed for the crystallisation of minerals in osteoid. When calcium and phosphate concentrations are too low, mineralisation and therefore ossification cannot proceed as normal. Vitamin D is responsible for regulating and enhancing the absorption of calcium from the intestine, therefore when there is a deficiency in vitamin D, mineralisation is disrupted. The list below identifies causes of vitamin D deficiency:

- Diet deficits
- Decreased endogenous production
- Intestinal malabsorption
- Renal tubular disease
- Tumours
- Anticonvulsant medication

A deficit in vitamin D will cause plasma calcium levels to fall; in turn this stimulates increased synthesis and secretion of parathyroid hormone. Whilst this may increase the concentration of calcium, it also stimulates the renal system to increase its clearance of phosphate. The resultant loss of phosphate ions means the concentration of bone phosphate is below the required level for mineralisation to proceed as normal.

Changes in mineralisation will occur in both spongy and compact bone. Haversian systems within compact bone become irregular and develop large channels; trabeculae in spongy bone will thin and lessen. Abnormal amounts of unmineralised osteoid will accumulate and subsequently will coat the

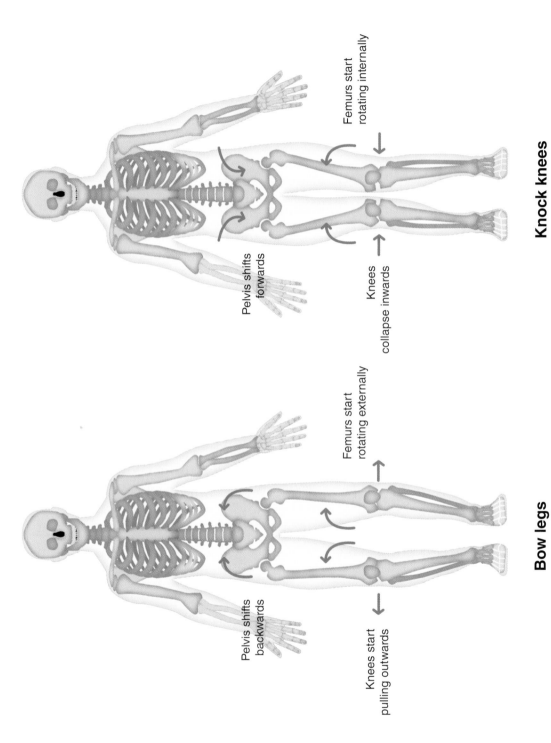

Knock knees

Femurs start
rotating internally

Pelvis shifts
forwards

Knees
collapse inwards

Illustrated by Shaun Mercier © SAGE Publications

Bow legs

Femurs start
rotating externally

Pelvis shifts
backwards

Knees start
pulling outwards

Figure 10.10 Bow legs and knock knees

lining of the Haversian canals and trabeculae. An increase in the amount of osteoid may also accumulate in areas under the periosteum. This excess osteoid will eventually lead to deformities of the skull, spine, pelvis, femur and humerus.

Signs and symptoms

- Varying degrees of widespread skeletal and muscular tenderness accompanied by pain.
- Facial deformities.
- Genu varum (bow leg) or genu valgum (knock knees) may be present.
- Vertebral collapse.
- Fractures or fragility fractures.

Paget disease of bone (osteitis deformans)

Paget disease of bone (PDB) is the second most common bone disease following osteoporosis. It is a progressive bone disease occurring in adults over the age of 40. There is an increased rate of metabolic activity in bone, leading to localised, abnormal and excessive remodelling of bone. It mostly affects bones in the skull, vertebrae, sacrum, pelvis, sternum and femur. The accelerated rate of remodelling leads to enlargement and softening of the affected bones, resulting in bowing deformity, fractures or neurological difficulties.

Whilst the cause of PDB remains largely unknown, it is purported that both environmental and genetic factors are involved. **Mutations** of a specific gene – $SQSTM_1$ – are implicated in susceptibility to PDB. It is estimated that approximately 40% of people with a family history of PDB and 10% of sporadic PDB carry this gene (Tan and Ralston, 2014). Environmental factors that predispose a person to PDB include viral infection, in particular the paramyxovirus family, e.g. mumps, measles, parainfluenza viruses, but no definite pathogen has been identified. Tan and Ralston (2014) also identify a dietary deficiency of calcium in childhood, rickets, vitamin deficiency, excessive mechanical force on the skeleton and pollutants as other environmental triggers that may predispose someone to PDB.

Signs and symptoms

- Skull deformities due to abnormal bone remodelling, causing thickening and asymmetry in shape. Initially frontal and occipital regions are involved but spreads to outer and inner surfaces of the entire skull.
- Altered mental state due to thickened regions of skull compressing the brain.
- Sensory abnormalities and impaired motor function, deafness, blindness (optic nerve **atrophy**), headache due to impingement on cranial nerves by newly formed bone.
- Malocclusion, tooth displacement due to thickening and sclerosis of mandible and maxilla.
- Exaggerated curvature of femur or tibia.
- Stress fractures.

Osteomyelitis

Osteomyelitis refers to infection of the bone and is most frequently caused by bacteria; however, other pathogens including fungi, parasites and viruses may also cause infection. Osteomyelitis may be classified as **haematogenous** or contiguous:

- Haematogenous osteomyelitis: caused when pathogens are carried through the bloodstream.
- Contiguous osteomyelitis: occurs when infection spreads to an adjacent bone. It is most commonly caused by fractures, surgical procedures or penetrating injuries. Metabolic and vascular disease, e.g. diabetes, peripheral vascular disease; lifestyle factors such as smoking, alcohol or drug use and ageing may also increase the risk of osteomyelitis.

—————————————— **GO DEEPER** ——————————————

Chronic non-bacterial osteomyelitis / chronic recurrent multifocal osteomyelitis

Chronic non-bacterial osteomyelitis (CNO) or chronic recurrent multifocal osteomyelitis (CRMO) is an auto-inflammatory bone disease of unknown aetiology thought to have a genetic component to disease susceptibility (Ferguson, 2018) with osteomyelitis occurring in more than one site. It results in persistent bone pain, bone destruction, functional disability and pathological fractures. It is associated with either a family or personal history of other inflammatory disease such as psoriasis or Crohn's disease (Ferguson, 2018).

Administration of antibiotics typically does not demonstrate any improvement, therefore initial treatment includes the administration of non-steroidal anti-inflammatory drugs (NSAIDs). For those who failed NSAID therapy, methotrexate, tumour necrosis factor inhibitors and bisphosphonates are commonly used to treat the condition (Zhao et al., 2017).

DISORDERS OF JOINTS

Osteoarthritis

Osteoarthritis (OA) is the most common joint disease and is associated with ageing. OA affects the entire joint and is characterised by the loss of and damage to **articular cartilage**, inflammation, **osteophytosis** (new bone formation of joint margins, leading to osteophytes [bone spurs]) and thickening of subchondral bone. Alongside these changes people may experience joint pain and stiffness, a decreased range of motion and, on occasion, joint instability and deformity. OA can affect both central and peripheral joints and is commonly found in the knees, hips, shoulder, spine (lower cervical, lumbosacral vertebrae), hands and wrists but may occur in any synovial joint. OA is thought to have both genetic and environmental risk factors although the exact cause remains unknown.

Box 10.1   Risk factors for osteoarthritis

- Age
- Gender - women > men
- Ethnicity, e.g. hand OA more prevalent in white women, whereas knee OA more prevalent in black women
- Congenital skeletal deformities
- Obesity
- Trauma - sprains, strains, fractures
- Long-term mechanical stress, e.g. athletics, ballet
- Decreased pain or proprioceptive reflexes due to neurological disorders, e.g. diabetic **neuropathy**
- Haematological disorders, e.g. haemophilia causing increased bleeding into joints
- Endocrine disorders, e.g. hyperparathyroidism leading to loss of bone calcium
- Drugs that stimulate collagen-digesting enzymes in **synovial membrane**, e.g. steroids, indomethacin

---

In OA there are significant changes in the composition and mechanical properties of the articular cartilage. Injury to the articular cartilage is thought to be caused by injury to the **chondrocyte** and release of cytokines including interleukin-1 (IL-1) and tumour necrosis factor (TNF) (Figure 10.11). The release of cytokines subsequently stimulates the release of proteases that destroy the joint structure, resulting in further chondrocyte injury and an impaired ability to maintain cartilage synthesis or to repair any damage.

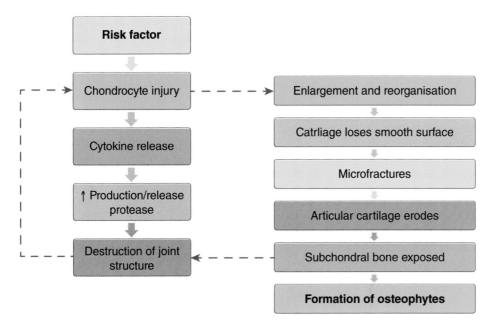

Figure 10.11   Disease process in osteoarthritis

In the early stages of the disease, chondrocytes in the superficial aspect of the articular cartilage undergo enlargement and reorganisation alongside oedematous changes in the cartilaginous matrix (Van der Kraan and Van den Berg, 2012). Subsequently, the cartilage loses its smooth surface and microfractures occur that facilitate the entry of synovial fluid and widen the crack. Vertical clefts form as the cracks get deeper, eventually extending through the full thickness of the articular surface into the subchondral bone. Over time, parts of the articular cartilage are completely eroded and subchondral bone that is now exposed becomes eburnated (ivory-like). Fragments of cartilage and bone may become dislodged and float freely as osteocartilaginous bodies. Cysts can form within the bone as a result of synovial fluid leaking through the defects in the remaining cartilage (Figure 10.12). As the condition progresses, the joint becomes less effective as a shock absorber due to thickening and sclerosis of the underlying subchondral bone. Osteophytosis occurs at the joint margins forming osteophytes (bone spurs) (Figure 10.11). Trauma to the synovial membrane, caused by the joint losing integrity, initiates a non-specific inflammatory response.

Signs and symptoms

* May not appear until the fifth or sixth decade of life.
* Depends on the bones involved.
* Pain with weight-bearing or use of the joint is usually the first symptom.

- Possibility of referred pain, e.g. OA in lower cervical spine may cause arm pain (brachial neuralgia); OA in hip may cause pain in knee or lower thigh.
- Stiffness and/or decreased range of movement.
- Swelling of joint.
- Tenderness.
- Muscle wasting.
- Deformity.
- Kyphosis and reduction in height (vertebral collapse).
- Fractures, especially of the distal radius, femur, vertebrae or ribs.

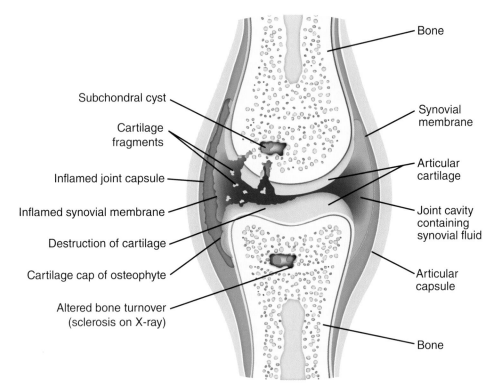

Illustrated by Shaun Mercier © SAGE Publications

Figure 10.12 Joint changes in osteoarthritis

ACTIVITY 10.6: APPLY

Living with osteoarthritis

The following video will give you an insight into the lived experience of osteoarthritis. Think about how it can affect those who are considered active and healthy. If you are using the eBook just click on the play button. Alternatively go to

https://study.sagepub.com/essentialpatho/videos

▷

LIVING WITH
OSTEOARTHRITIS (3:08)

Rheumatoid arthritis

Rheumatoid arthritis (RA) is a chronic, progressive, systemic autoimmune disease with periods of remission and exacerbation. It is characterised by tenderness and swelling which eventually destroy the synovial joint, resulting in disability. There is a strong genetic predisposition to developing the disease. It is thought that its development is a combination of genetic influences interacting with an immunological trigger, e.g. a microbial agent that causes a T-cell-mediated response. The genetic element is associated with the human leucocyte antigen (HLA) area of the **major histocompatibility complex (MHC)**. It is thought that specific amino acid malpositions in the HLA molecule associated with a HLA-DR allele, is a major factor in developing rheumatic disorders. It is also believed that the presence of T-cell abnormalities may relate to a deficit in **telomere** repair, resulting in the faster ageing of telomeres and less efficient immune function (Huether and McCance, 2017).

The first joint tissue to be affected is the synovial membrane, whereby fibroblast-like synovial cells and macrophage-like synovial cells line the joint cavity. A triggering factor activates synovial fibroblasts (SFs) that then undergo significant change, an exaggerated immune response and altered signalling pathways for immune reactions. Long-term exposure to the antigen causes normal antibodies (**immunoglobulins**, Ig) to become autoantibodies that attack **self-antigens** (host tissues). Altered antibodies found in those with RA are known as rheumatoid factors (RFs) and consist of two classes of immunoglobulin antibodies for IgG and IgM, and on occasion antibodies for IgA may also be involved; portions of immunoglobulin are the main antigenic target for these. Immune complexes are formed when RFs bind with their target self-antigens in synovial membrane and blood. Associated environmental factors are detailed below.

Box 10.2 Environmental risk factors for rheumatoid arthritis

- Geographical area of birth
- Diet
- Socioeconomic status
- Smoking – especially those with shared epitope HLA-DR4 marker (Klein and Gay, 2015; Putrik et al., 2016)

Cartilage damage in RA occurs as a result of a number of processes (Figure 10.11) which include the following:

1. Neutrophils and other cells in synovial fluid become activated and subsequently degrade the articular cartilage and surface layer.
2. Inflammatory cytokines, e.g. tumour necrosis factor-alpha (TNFα), interleukin-1beta (IL-1β) and interleukin-6 (IL-6) promote the breakdown of cartilage due to the release of enzymes including metalloproteinase, collagenase, elastase and PGE$_2$.
3. T-cells interact with SFs and convert the synovium into pannus (a thick, abnormal layer of granulation tissue).
4. Macrophages (from within the pannus) stimulate the release of IL-1, platelet-derived growth factor (PDGF) and fibronectin, and B-lymphocytes produce more RFs. Self-antigens are in constant supply and sustain the inflammatory response and unlimited generation of immune complexes.
5. Angiogenesis leads to increased opportunity for active SFs to enter the bloodstream and affect other joints.

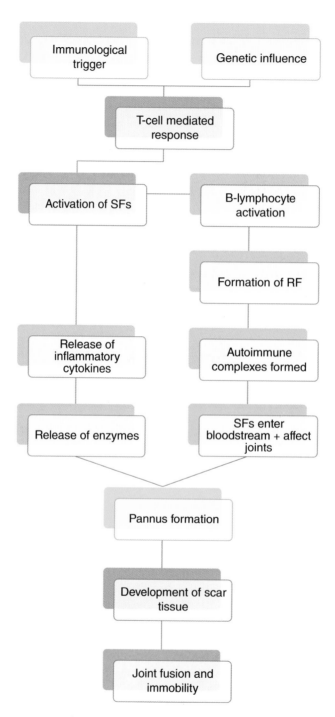

Figure 10.13 Disease process in rheumatoid arthritis

Note: SFs = synovial fibroblasts; RF = rheumatoid factors

There are numerous irreversible damaging effects and destructive changes of the synovial membrane, including:

- Oedema, caused by leucocyte infiltration.
- Proliferation and abnormal enlargement of cells cause hyperplastic thickening of the synovial membrane.
- Hypertrophied endothelial cells, fibrin and platelets occlude smaller venules, causing a reduction in vascular flow to synovial fluid.
- **Hypertrophy** and hyperplasia of cells increase the metabolic demands alongside a compromised circulation, resulting in **hypoxia** and **metabolic acidosis**.
- **Hydrolytic enzymes** are released into surrounding tissues from synovial cells as a consequence of metabolic acidosis and initiate erosion of the articular cartilage and surrounding supporting structures.
- Pannus formation leads to the development of scar tissue that subsequently immobilises the joint with possible joint fusion (**ankylosis**) over time.

Signs and symptoms

Signs and symptoms associated with RA can be related to articular changes and systemic effects and have an insidious onset. They include:

- Mild, general aching and stiffness – pain and stiffness last for 30 minutes but may extend to several hours.
- Inflammation may be apparent in metacarpophalangeal (MCP) joint, thumb joints, proximal interphalangeal (PIP) joints of fingers and metatarsophalangeal (MTP) joints. Joints are affected bilaterally/symmetrically.
- Joints appear red, swollen, painful and sensitive to the touch.
- Joint stiffness following rest. May be eased with mild activity.
- Impaired joint movement due to swelling and pain.
- Daily activities become more difficult.
- Mobility greatly impaired as joints become damaged/deformed. If knees/ankles are involved, walking may become difficult.
- Development of rheumatic nodules which may be: tender/non-tender; movable/immovable; small/ large. They are usually found over pressure points, e.g. extensor surface of ulna; they can also affect lungs (pulmonary fibrosis), heart (pericarditis) or eyes (episcleritis, scleritis and scleromalacia: inflammatory disorders of the eye between conjunctiva and connective tissue of white of eye, serious inflammatory disease of white of eye, rare form of necrotising scleritis).
- Malocclusion of teeth may develop if there is temporomandibular joint (TMJ) involvement.
- Systemic signs include: fatigue, weakness, **anorexia**, weight loss, mild fever, generalised lymphad-enopathy and iron deficiency **anaemia** with low serum iron levels.

ACTIVITY 10.7: APPLY

Living with rheumatoid arthritis

RA can impact on everyday life. Listen to Rachel's story and reflect on what you can do as a person-centred practitioner to support someone like Rachel. If you are using the eBook just click on the play button. Alternatively go to

https://study.sagepub.com/essentialpatho/videos

RHEUMATOID ARTHRITIS (5:01)

Gout

Gout is considered the most prevalent inflammatory arthritis worldwide. It is a syndrome that results in hyperuricaemia, caused by either increased uric acid production or decreased uric acid **excretion** by the kidneys and includes gouty arthritis, **tophi** (Figure 10.14) and kidney stones. Approximately 90% of cases of hyperuricaemia are attributed to decreased uric acid excretion and it is reported to have a strong genetic link. It is referred to in terms of primary or secondary gout:

- *Primary gout*: designates cases where the aetiology is unknown, may be linked to a congenital error in metabolism, leading to enzyme defects, decreased urinary excretion or both.
- *Secondary gout*: occurs when gout is not the primary disorder and the reason for hyperuricaemia is known. It may be attributable to chronic kidney disease, increased breakdown of nucleic acid, e.g. during treatment for **leukaemia** or **lymphoma** (rapid tumour cell lysis), or the use of some thiazide diuretics.

Gout is a disease linked to purine metabolism and kidney function. Uric acid is produced as a metabolite of purine nucleotides (used to synthesise nucleic acids), most of which is subsequently excreted by the kidneys. Uric acid crystallises when specific concentration levels are reached. This crystallisation leads to the formulation of monosodium urate crystals (insoluble precipitates) that are subsequently deposited in connective tissue throughout the body. Monosodium urate crystals become more insoluble at temperatures below 37°C, hence are usually deposited in the peripheries, e.g. great toe. Deposits of monosodium urate crystals in the synovial fluid trigger a proinflammatory response with the release of powerful proinflammatory mediators such as TNF-α, interleukins and **complement**. Neutrophils are chemotactically attracted by the presence of crystals and **phagocytosis** of these crystals leads to polymorphonuclear cell death and the release of lysosomal enzymes. The resultant inflammation in the joint is known as gouty arthritis. Prolonged exposure to inflammatory mediators and inflammation leads to the destruction of the cartilage and subchondral bone.

Over time, with repeated attacks of gouty arthritis, the deposition of crystals in the subcutaneous tissue leads to the development of tophi (hard white nodules) that may be visible through the skin (Figure 10.14). Tophi are most often found in the calcaneal (Achilles) tendon, the extensor surface of the forearm, the olecranon bursa, fingers, hands, knees and feet. Tophi do not usually appear until approximately ten years after the initial gout attack. They are usually painless but can lead to stiffness and aching of the affected joint. If tophi develop in the extremities they can cause carpal tunnel syndrome or tarsal tunnel syndrome due to nerve compression. Renal stones (the development of uric acid stones – staghorn calculi – is discussed in Chapter 11) are prevalent in those with gout.

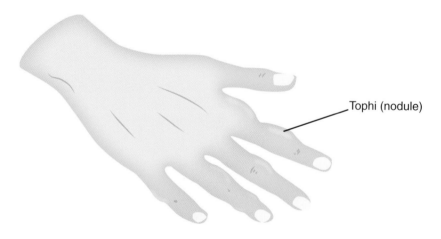

Tophi (nodule)

Illustrated by Shaun Mercier © SAGE Publications

Figure 10.14 Tophi in the fingers/hand

Signs and symptoms

- Initial attack is usually monoarticular, affecting the first MTP joint of the big toe. May also affect elbows, ankles, fingers or wrists.
- Usually begins at night and may be precipitated by certain foods, alcohol, exercise, medications.
- Abrupt onset of pain in affected joint.
- Redness and swelling of affected joint.
- Person may be asymptomatic and may not have another attack for months or years. Recurrence of frequent attacks leads to joint changes that may become permanent.

DISORDERS OF MUSCLES

Fibromyalgia

Fibromyalgia (FM) is a chronic syndrome affecting the musculoskeletal system that is characterised by widespread pain and increased sensitivity to touch, however there are no signs of systemic or localised inflammation. It is also associated with fatigue, non-restorative sleep, anxiety and depression. FM and its accompanying symptoms are thought to result from the amplification of pain transmission and interpretation due to central nervous system dysfunction (Huether and McCance, 2017).

It is increasingly believed that genetic factors may be involved in the development of the syndrome. Whilst the role of genetic factors has not been fully identified, studies suggest alterations in genes that affect the production/secretion of dopamine, serotonin and catecholamines may be involved (Arnold et al., 2013; Docamp et al., 2014). Environmental factors including infection, trauma, physical and/or emotional stress and psychosocial stress may also play a significant role in the development of FM. It affects seven times more women than men and usually occurs between the ages of 30 and 50, although it may also affect children and the elderly.

Signs and symptoms

- Widespread pain that is present for more than 3 months.
- Pain may begin in one area, e.g. shoulder and/or neck, and then become more localised.
- Tenderness in 11 of 18 specific points.
- Fatigue.
- Headaches.
- Memory loss.
- Anxiety and depression.

APPLY

Education and treatment for those with fibromyalgia

- It is important to reassure the person that the illness is real and not imagined.
- Drug therapy may include **analgesia**, anticonvulsants and antidepressants:
  - analgesia - paracetamol, codeine, tramadol
  - anticonvulsants - pregabalin
  - antidepressants - tricyclic, SSRIs or SNRIs.

(Continued)

(Continued)

- Psychological support:
  - cognitive behavioural therapy
  - psychotherapy
  - counselling
  - relaxation techniques.
- Alternative therapies:
  - acupuncture
  - massage
  - aromatherapy.
- Exercise:
  - aerobic exercise helps relieve pain and improves endurance - walking, cycling or swimming
  - resistance and strength training improve muscle strength and may make carrying out daily activities easier.
- Improve sleeping habits:
  - get up at the same time each morning
  - create a bedtime routine
  - avoid eating large meals and ingesting caffeine, alcohol and nicotine before bed
  - make sure the bedroom is quiet, dark and at a comfortable temperature.

Muscular dystrophies

Muscular dystrophies refer to a group of genetic disorders that lead to progressive loss of muscle fibres, resulting in weakness of voluntary muscles (mostly but not exclusively). Muscular dystrophies have different inheritance patterns and varying biochemical changes that are responsible for the specific type. Muscular dystrophies can cause disease across the life span; some cause disease in infancy, some in childhood and others in adulthood.

Duchenne muscular dystrophy (DMD)

Duchenne muscular dystrophy (DMD) is an inherited X-linked recessive trait and is considered the most severe form; it is present in 1 in 3600–6000 live male births (Bushby et al., 2010). Whilst it is X-linked it is thought that in up to 30% of cases the mother is not the carrier and it is the result of a new mutation (Sarnat, 2015). It affects primarily boys, but affected girls are encountered occasionally; female carriers are unaffected.

DMD is caused by a mutation in the Dystrophin or DMD gene (located on the short arm of the X chromosome). Dystrophin is a large protein responsible for attaching portions of the muscle **sarcomere** to the cell membrane, ensuring the structural integrity of both skeletal and cardiac muscle. Lack of dystrophin leads to fibres tearing, free calcium enters the muscle cells causing degeneration and necrosis, and the skeletal muscle fibres are replaced with fat and connective tissue, causing the muscle to increase in size (pseudohypertrophy) with a subsequent reduction in muscle strength.

As the muscle fibres become replaced with fat and connective tissue boys will present in their pre-school years, usually around the age of 2 or 3, with muscle weakness, pseudohypertrophy of the calves and walking difficulties. Weakness usually starts in the pelvic girdle, leading to difficulties in rising from the floor, climbing stairs and the development of a waddling gait. Development of joint immobility, contractures and scoliosis (abnormal curvature of the spine) occur due to imbalances in agonist and antagonist muscles over the next few years, and by the age of 7–12 use of a wheelchair may be necessary. Distal, extraocular and those muscles controlling urination and defaecation are usually well preserved.

As the child ages, progressive muscle weakness results in respiratory muscle involvement, leading to breathing difficulties, especially when sleeping, and an ineffective **cough**, resulting in frequent chest infections. **Cardiomyopathy** may also occur although the degree of cardiac muscle involvement does not correlate with the degree of skeletal muscle involvement. Death usually occurs in young adulthood due to cardiac and respiratory muscle involvement/failure. Appreciating the effects of this condition and how it affects both the individual concerned and the rest of the family is essential to be able to provide effective person-centred care.

Becker muscular dystrophy (BMD)

Becker muscular dystrophy (BMD) shares the same genetic locus as DMD, however, those with BMD present later in childhood and their progression is usually slower and less severe, with muscle weakness becoming noticeable between the ages of 5 and 15. The life expectancy of someone with BMD is longer than that of DMD, possibly into their 40s (GARD, 2016).

Facioscapulohumeral muscular dystrophy (FSHD)

Facioscapulohumeral muscular dystrophy (FSHD) is an autosomal dominant inherited disorder and is one of the most common muscular dystrophies. FSHD occurs due to a deletion on chromosome 4, however the precise mechanism that causes the disease is unclear as it is not associated with a particular gene. Someone with FSHD usually presents later in childhood with asymmetric muscle weakness that tends to start in the face and extends to the shoulders and legs. Shoulder and arm pain are commonly reported. Disease progression is usually slow and life expectancy is normal.

Myotonic muscular dystrophy (MMD)

Myotonic muscular dystrophy (MMD) occurs due to mutations in either of two genes, causing type 1 (*DMPK*) and type 2 (*CNBP*) MMD. It is a multisystem disease affecting the brain, smooth muscle, skeletal muscle, heart and endocrine system. It presents with distal muscle weakness, learning difficulties or intellectual disability or both. The **congenital** form of the disease is the most severe and can be present from birth or become apparent in the first few years of life. Those with the mild disease may not develop symptoms until adolescence or later and display mild muscle weakness, especially in distal muscles, cataracts and myotonia, and tend to have a normal life span. Those with the more classic form of MMD present in their teenage years with progressive muscle weakness, abnormalities related to cardiac conduction and cataracts, and their life expectancy is shortened.

CHAPTER SUMMARY

In this chapter you will have learned about skin and musculoskeletal disorders across the life span and how they impact not only physiologically but also how they influence health-related quality of life. These disorders can alter identity and significantly reduce independence and social integration. To be an effective person-centred practitioner, you need to be relational when considering these disorders; being compassionate and working with someone's belief system and values will enable you to care for them within the context of their culture and social structure.

- Musculoskeletal and skin disorders can negatively impact on body image, self-esteem and psychosocial development.

- Inflammatory and autoimmune processes play a significant role in a number of skin and musculoskeletal disorders.

- Many skin disorders are HLA-linked with largely unknown triggers that initiate the pathophysiological response.

- Thermal injuries have the potential to have a systemic wide inflammatory and immune response that can lead to multiple organ failure.

- Disorders of the musculoskeletal system can affect bones, joints and muscles and be debilitating and life-limiting.

- Osteoarthritis (OA) is the most common joint disease and is associated with ageing.

- Rheumatoid arthritis (RA) is a chronic, progressive, systemic autoimmune disease with periods of remission and exacerbation. There is a strong genetic predisposition to developing the disease. It is thought that the development of the disease is a combination of genetic influences interacting with immunological activities which causes a T-cell mediated response.

- Gout is the most common form of inflammatory arthritis.

- Duchenne muscular dystrophy (DMD) is an inherited X-linked recessive trait and is considered the most severe form, whereas facioscapulohumeral (FSH) muscular dystrophy is an autosomal dominant inherited disorder and is one of the most common muscular dystrophies.

REVISE

TEST YOUR KNOWLEDGE

The content of this chapter has helped you to understand how cell function and structure change under different circumstances. Revise the different sections in turn then try to answer the questions below.

Answers are available online. If you are using the eBook just click on the answers icon below. Alternatively go to **https://study.sagepub.com/essentialpatho/answers**

1 What is psoriasis and what causes it?

2 What is eczema and when is it most commonly diagnosed?

3 What causes atopic eczema?

4 What triggers Stevens–Johnson syndrome and toxic epidermal necrolysis and what is the first line of treatment?

5 Which cytokine is the most prominent mediator of keratinocyte destruction in Stevens–Johnson syndrome and toxic epidermal necrolysis?

6 Which component of the skin is targeted in epidermolysis bullosa acquisita (EBA) and what is the result?

7   What is impetigo and which age group is commonly affected?

8   What are the three key factors that cause impetigo?

9   What are the causes of vitiligo?

10   What are the four processes involved in acnegenesis?

11   Which stage of hair growth is targeted in most cases of alopecia?

12   What is a pressure ulcer?

13   What is the difference between a sprain and a strain?

14   What is osteopenia and what are the major causes of it?

15   Explain the different classifications of osteoporosis.

16   Identify the risk factors that predispose someone to osteoporosis.

17   Osteomalacia is caused by a lack of what vitamin?

18   Identify the joints most commonly affected by osteoarthritis (OA).

19   Identify the inflammatory mediators and enzymes involved in cartilage damage associated with rheumatoid arthritis.

20   Briefly explain the different types of muscular dystrophy.

REFERENCES

Al-Makhzangy, E.M., Elsayed, M.M., Assaf, M.I. and Esawy, A.M. (2015) Hair follicle stem cells in the pathogenesis of primary cicatricial alopecia. *Zagazig University Medical Journal*, 21 (2): 139–50.

Anders, J., Heinemann, A., Leffmann, C., Leutenegger, M., Pröfener, F. and von Renteln-Kruse, W. (2010) Decubitus ulcers: pathophysiology and primary prevention. *Deutsches Ärzteblatt International*, 107 (21): 371.

Arnold, L.M., Fan, J., Russell, I.J., Yunus, M.B., Khan, M.A., Kushner, I. et al. (2013) The fibromyalgia family study: a genome-wide linkage scan study. *Arthritis and Rheumatism*, 65 (4): 1122–8.

Baisakhiya, N. and Deshmukh, P. (2011) Unusual sites of epidermoid cyst. *Indian Journal of Otolaryngology and Head & Neck Surgery*, 63 (1): 149–51.

Beigi, P.K.M. (2018) *Alopecia Areata: A Clinician's Guide*. Cham: Springer Nature.

Boore, J., Cook, N. and Shepherd, A. (2016) *Essentials of Anatomy and Physiology for Nursing Practice*. London: Sage.

Bushby, K., Finkel, R., Birnkrant, D.J., Case, L.E., Clemens, P.R., Cripe, L., et al. (DMD Care Considerations Working Group) (2010) Diagnosis and management of Duchenne muscular dystrophy part 1: diagnosis and pharmacological and psychosocial management. *The Lancet Neurology*, 9 (1): 77–93.

Coimbra, S., Figueiredo, A., Castro, E., Rocha-Pereira, P. and Santos-Silva, A. (2012) The roles of cells and cytokines in the pathogenesis of psoriasis. *International Journal of Dermatology*, 51 (4): 389–98.

Coimbra, S., Oliveira, H., Reis, F., Belo, L., Rocha, S., Quintanilha, A. et al. (2010) C-reactive protein and leucocyte activation in psoriasis vulgaris according to severity and therapy. *Journal of the European Academy of Dermatology and Venereology*, 24 (7): 789–96.

Docamp, E., Escaramís, G., Gratacòs, M., Villatoro, S., Puig, A., Kogevinas, M., et al. (2014) Genome-wide analysis of single nucleotide polymorphisms and copy number variants in fibromyalgia suggest a role for the central nervous system. *Pain*, 155 (6): 1102–9.

Dréno, B. (2017) What is new in the pathophysiology of acne, an overview. *Journal of the European Academy of Dermatology and Venereology*, 31: 8–12.

Ferguson, P.J. (2018) Chronic recurrent multifocal osteomyelitis (CRMO). In G. Ragab, T. Atkinson and M. Stoll (eds), *The Microbiome in Rheumatic Disease and Infection*. Cham: Springer Nature.

GARD (Genetic and Rare Diseases Information Center) (2016) Becker muscular dystrophy. National Center for Advancing Translational Sciences (NCATS) [online]. Available at: https://rarediseases.info. nih.gov/diseases/5900/becker-muscular-dystrophy (accessed 5 August 2018).

Ghazvini, P., Treadwell, P., Woodberry, K., Nerette Jr, E. and Powery II, H. (2017) Impetigo in the pediatric population. *Journal of Dermatology and Clinical Research*, 5 (1): 1092.

Hallström, H., Byberg, L., Glynn, A., Lemming, E.W., Wolk, A. and Michaëlsson, K. (2013) Long-term coffee consumption in relation to fracture risk and bone mineral density in women. *American Journal of Epidemiology*, 178 (8): 898–909.

Hordinsky, M. and Junqueira, A.L. (2015) Alopecia areata update. *Seminars in Cutaneous Medicine and Surgery*, 34 (2): 72–5.

Huether, S.E. and McCance, K.L. (2017) *Understanding Pathophysiology*, 6th edn. St Louis, MO: Elsevier Saunders.

Hung, K.K.C., Graham, C.A., Lo R.S.L., Leung, Y.K., Leung, L.Y., Man, S.Y. et al. (2018) Oral paracetamol and/or ibuprofen for treating pain after soft tissue injuries: single centre double-blind, randomised controlled clinical trial. *PLoS ONE*, 13 (2): e0192043. Available at: https://doi.org/10.1371/journal. pone.0192043 (accessed 5 July 2018).

Jones, P., Dalziel S.R., Lamdin, R., Miles-Chan, J.L. and Frampton, C. (2015) Oral non-steroidal anti-inflammatory drugs compared with other oral pain killers for sprains, strains and bruises. Cochrane

Library [online]. Available at: www.cochrane.org/CD007789/MUSKINJ_oral-non-steroidal-anti-inflammatory-drugs-compared-other-oral-pain-killers-sprains-strains-and (accessed 5 July 2018).

Jun, G.B., Qi, H. and Golap, C. (2010) One-stage excision of inflamed sebaceous cyst versus the conventional method. *South African Journal of Surgery*, *48* (4): 116–18.

Kaddoura, I., Abu-Sittah, G., Ibrahim, A., Karamanoukian, R. and Papazian, N. (2017) Burn injury: review of pathophysiology and therapeutic modalities in major burns. *Annals of Burns and Fire Disasters*, *30* (2): 95–102.

Kanis, J.A., Johnell, O., Odén, A., Johansson, H. and McCloskey, E. (2008) FRAX™ and the assessment of fracture probability in men and women from the UK. *Osteoporosis International*, *19* (4): 385–97.

Kanti, V., Röwert-Huber, J., Vogt, A. and Blume-Peytavi, U. (2018) Cicatricial alopecia. *JDDG: Journal der Deutschen Dermatologischen Gesellschaft*, *16* (4): 435–61.

Kasperkiewicz, M., Sadik, C.D., Bieber, K., Ibrahim, S.M., Manz, R.A., Schmidt, E. et al. (2016) Epidermolysis bullosa acquisita: from pathophysiology to novel therapeutic options. *Journal of Investigative Dermatology*, *136* (1): 24–33.

Kerschbaumer, A., Fenzl, K. H., Erlacher, L. and Aletaha, D. (2016) An overview of psoriatic arthritis – epidemiology, clinical features, pathophysiology and novel treatment targets. *Wiener Klinische Wochenschrift*, *128* (21–22): 791–5.

Klein, D. (2016) *Stevens–Johnson Syndrome and Toxic Epidermal Necrolysis*. Westerville: Otterbein University.

Klein, K. and Gay, S. (2015) Epigentics and rheumatoid arthritis. *Current Opinion in Rheumatology*, *27* (1): 76–82.

Krueger, J.G. and Bowcock, A. (2005) Psoriasis pathophysiology: current concepts of pathogenesis. *Annals of the Rheumatic Diseases*, *64* (Suppl 2): ii30–ii36.

Lim, V.M., Do, A., Berger, T.G., Nguyen, A.H., DeWeese, J., Malone, J.D. et al. (2016) A decade of burn unit experience with Stevens–Johnson syndrome/toxic epidermal necrolysis: clinical pathological diagnosis and risk factor awareness. *Burns*, *42* (4): 836–43.

Lolli, F., Pallotti, F., Rossi, A., Fortuna, M.C., Caro, G., Lenzi, A. et al. (2017) Androgenetic alopecia: a review. *Endocrine*, *57* (1): 9–17.

Masterson, K.N. (2018) Acne basics: pathophysiology, assessment, and standard treatment options. *Journal of the Dermatology Nurses' Association*, *10* (1S): S2–S10.

Mease, P.J. and Armstrong, A.W. (2014) Managing patients with psoriatic disease: the diagnosis and pharmacologic treatment of psoriatic arthritis in patients with psoriasis. *Drugs*, *74* (4): 423–41.

Nielson, C.B., Duethman, N.C., Howard, J.M., Moncure, M. and Wood, J.G. (2017) Burns: pathophysiology of systemic complications and current management. *Journal of Burn Care & Research*, *38* (1): e469–e481.

NOGG (2017) Clinical guideline for the prevention and treatment of osteoporosis. National Osteoporosis Guideline Group [online]. Available at: www.sheffield.ac.uk/NOGG/NOGG%20Guideline%202017.pdf (accessed 5 August 2018).

Patel, B., Velasco, M.A.M., Gutierrez, F.T. and Khesin, D. (2017) Addressing androgenetic alopecia: a complex disorder – with a multilateral treatment strategy. *MOJ Bioequivalence & Bioavailability*, *3* (1): 00025.

Peacock, S. (2016) Use of emollients in management of atopic eczema. *Independent Nurse*, *2016* (4): 26–30.

Putrik, P., Ramiro, S., Keszei, A.P., Hmamouchi, I., Dougados, M.,Uhlig, T., et al. (2016) Lower education and living in countries with lower wealth are associated with higher disease activity in rheumatoid arthritis: results from the multinational COMORA study. *Annals of the Rheumatic Diseases*, *75* (3): 540–6.

Rajabi, F., Drake, L.A., Senna, M.M. and Rezaei, N. (2018) Alopecia areata: a review of disease pathogenesis. *British Journal of Dermatology*. Epub ahead of print. doi: 10.1111/bjd.16808.

Salzes, C., Abadie, S., Seneschal, J., Whitton, M., Meurant, J.M., Jouary, T. et al. (2016) The Vitiligo Impact Patient Scale (VIPs): development and validation of a vitiligo burden assessment tool. *Journal of Investigative Dermatology, 136* (1): 52–8.

Sarkar, R., Sethi, S. and Madan, A. (2017) Pathogenesis of vitiligo. In *Melasma and Vitiligo in Brown Skin*. New Delhi: Springer. pp. 191–6.

Sarnat, H.B. (2015) Muscular dystrophies In R.M Kliegman, B.M. Stanton, J.W. St.Geme. and N.F. Schor (eds), *Nelson Textbook of Pediatrics*, 17th edn. Philadelphia, PA: Elsevier Saunders.

Schneider, J.A. and Cohen, P.R. (2017) Stevens–Johnson syndrome and toxic epidermal necrolysis: a concise review with a comprehensive summary of therapeutic interventions emphasizing supportive measures. *Advances in Therapy, 34*: 1235–44.

Speeckaert, R. and van Geel, N. (2017) Vitiligo: an update on pathophysiology and treatment options. *American Journal of Clinical Dermatology, 18* (6): 733–44.

Sunil, S., Oommen, N., Rathy, R., Rekha, V.R., Raj, D. and Sruthy, V.K. (2014) Epidermoid cysts of head and neck region: case series and review of literature. *International Journal of Odontostomatology, 8* (2): 165–9.

Tan, A. and Ralston, S.H. (2014) Paget's disease of bone. *OJM: An International Journal of Medicine, 107* (11): 865–9.

Van der Kraan, P.M. and Van den Berg, W.B. (2012) Chondrocyte hypertrophy and osteoarthritis: role in initiation and progression of cartilage degeneration? *Osteoarthritis and Cartilage, 20* (3): 223–32.

Ward, N.S., Casserly, B. and Ayala, A. (2008) The compensatory anti-inflammatory response syndrome (CARS) in critically ill patients. *Clinics in Chest Medicine, 29* (4): 617–25.

Wolff, H., Fischer, T.W. and Blume-Peytavi, U. (2016) The diagnosis and treatment of hair and scalp diseases. *Deutsches Ärzteblatt International, 113* (21): 377–86.

World Health Organisation (WHO) (2018) *World Health Organization – WHO Criteria for Diagnosis of Osteoporosis*. Available at: www.4bonehealth.org/ededications, acknowledgements and bios ducation/world-health-organization-criteria-diagnosis-osteoporosis/ (accessed 6 July 2018).

Zaenglein, A.L., Pathy, A.L., Schlosser, B.J., Alikhan, A., Baldwin, H.E., Berson, D.S. et al. (2016) Guidelines of care for the management of acne vulgaris. *Journal of the American Academy of Dermatology, 74* (5): 945.e33–973.

Zarate-Correa, L.C., Carrillo-Gomez, D.C., Ramirez-Escobar, A.F. and Serrano-Reyes, C. (2013) Toxic epidermal necrolysis successfully treated with infliximab. *Journal of Investigational Allergology & Clinical Immunology, 23* (1): 61–3.

Zhao, Y., Dedeoglu, F., Ferguson, P.J.. Lapidus, S.K., Laxer, R.M., Bradford, M.C. et al. (2017) Physician's perspectives on the diagnosis and treatment of chronic nonbacterial osteomyelitis. *International Journal of Rheumatology*. Epub ahead of print. doi: 10.1155/2017/7694942.

Zofková, I., Nemcikova, P. and Matucha, P. (2013) Trace elements and bone health. *Clinical Chemistry and Laboratory Medicine, 51* (8): 1555–61.

SECTION 3
DISORDERS OF HOMEOSTASIS

The primary function of physiology is to maintain homeostasis and in this section we examine disorders of those systems of the body that have a major function in this area and endeavour to apply this knowledge to person-centred practice. This section examines the following disorders of homeostasis within the context of person-centred nursing:

Chapter 11: Disorders of Renal Function and Fluid Balance. Here we are examining the causes of disturbances in these functions and the implications of the disturbed homeostasis for the person affected and their family. This includes disorders of renal function, fluid and electrolyte regulation and disorders of urinary continence. Approaches to person-centred care to minimise the functional disturbances are considered.

Chapter 12: Disorders of Nutrient Supply and Faecal Elimination. The disturbed functions considered here involve the gastrointestinal tract (GIT) and accessory organs. Normal function is dependent at least partly on the human microbiome considered in the previous text. The emotional/psychological and social implications of the pathophysiological changes (central to person-centred nursing) due to disorders of the digestive system and accessory organs are considered.

Chapter 13: Disorders of Metabolism. This chapter builds on the chapter on metabolism in Boore et al. (2016) and examines some of the key disorders of metabolism, including diabetes types 1 and 2 and a sample of other disorders, including some associated with learning disorders. The impact on the people concerned and their families is central and the implications are considerable.

Chapter 14: Disorders of Oxygenation and Carbon Dioxide Elimination. Disorders of the respiratory system are relatively common. The physiological effects of the five main groups of disorders are examined: disturbed ventilation/perfusion relationships, failure of pulmonary perfusion, failure of ventilation, obstructive airways disease, and restrictive pulmonary disease. The signs and symptoms of respiratory failure are explored and the emotional and social implications for the person concerned and their family are considered.

Chapter 15: Disorders of the Cardiovascular System. This chapter builds on the content of Chapter 8. Factors influencing blood pressure are considered and the physiological changes in heart failure and the effect on homeostasis are examined. The five main causes of heart failure are discussed: increased workload in a healthy heart; increased pressure against which the heart must work; anatomical abnormalities causing ineffective pumping; myocardial hypoxia causing ineffective pumping; and cardiac irregularities causing ineffective pumping.

DISORDERS OF RENAL FUNCTION AND FLUID BALANCE

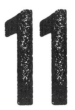

11

UNDERSTAND: CHAPTER VIDEOS

Watch the following videos to ease you into this chapter. If you are using the eBook just click on the play buttons. Alternatively go to **https://study.sagepub.com/essentialpatho/videos**

| CHRONIC KIDNEY DISEASE (15:50) | ACUTE RENAL INJURY/FAILURE (10:11) | URINARY STONES (14:59) | URINARY TRACT INFECTION (13:26) | GLOMERULONEPHRITIS (11:28) |

LEARNING OUTCOMES

When you have finished studying this chapter you will be able to:

1. Describe the types of acute kidney injury (AKI) and the associated pathophysiology.
2. Review a variety of disorders of fluid and electrolyte imbalance and the associated disordered physiology.
3. Identify the different forms of urinary incontinence and their pathophysiological basis.
4. Describe the pathophysiology of upper and lower urinary tract infections.
5. Outline the pathogenesis of urinary stones.
6. Outline the disordered physiology of chronic kidney disease (CKD).

INTRODUCTION

In this chapter, you will examine the main causes of disturbances in fluid, electrolytes and acid–base balance and how the associated homeostatic disturbance impacts upon the person and their family.

The renal system plays a key role in maintaining **homeostasis** for a number of key functions within the body; many of these functions are interlinked with other body systems. As a result, when the renal system does not function optimally, or when another system triggers the renal system incorrectly, disordered homeostasis can occur. This can result in an imbalance in fluid and electrolytes within the body, affecting almost all other systems. From a global perspective, end-stage renal **disease** (ESRD), also referred to as end-stage kidney disease (ESKD), incidence has stabilised in developed countries in the last decade. However, in developing countries, incidence appears to be on the rise (Wetmore and Collins, 2016). Simultaneously, improvements in management of renal disease have resulted in an increase in the number of people receiving dialysis as more people are surviving longer (Wetmore and Collins, 2016). The global burden of renal disease is increasing and this requires health care practitioners to understand the pathophysiological basis of the main forms of renal disease in order to prevent it, recognise it early and contribute to treating it proactively and effectively.

--- **REVISE: A&P RECAP** ---

Fluid and electrolyte homeostasis

As preparation for reading this chapter, we recommend that you read Chapter 11 in *Essentials of Anatomy and Physiology for Nursing Practice* (Boore et al., 2016) to refresh your knowledge on the fluid and electrolyte homeostasis (including the renin-angiotensin-aldosterone system [RAAS]) and the structure and functions of the renal system.

--- **PERSON-CENTRED CONTEXT: THE BODIE FAMILY** ---

BODIE FAMILY
CASE NOTES

If we consider the Bodie family, the older adult family members will have a decline in renal function as they age with an associated increased susceptibility to renal diseases (Esposito et al., 2007). If we take Maud Bodie, we need to consider that she takes digoxin since she developed right ventricular failure; the body requires effective renal function in order to eliminate digoxin from the body and therefore the dosage would have to be adjusted should any renal impairment be detected over time (Faull and Lee, 2007).

Similarly, many medications for treating type 2 **diabetes** (e.g. metformin, glibenclamide, glimepiride, **insulin**), which Richard Jones has been diagnosed with, also require effective renal function for them to be effectively cleared from the body (Faull and Lee, 2007). A number of antibiotics also require effective renal function for elimination, e.g. ciprofloxacin, fluconazole, which can affect any family member at any stage of their life when accessing such treatment.

DISORDERS OF FLUID AND ELECTROLYTE BALANCE

Disorders of fluid and electrolytes have the potential to impact significantly on people; water is the medium for all biochemical reactions to occur within the body and blood volume is central to enabling nutrients and waste products to be circulated around the body with sufficient pressure to perfuse all the tissues of the body. Electrolytes are essential for the functioning of the nervous system and in regulating where and how water moves between fluid compartments within the body as a result of their osmotic potential. It is worth remembering that sodium is the most abundant electrolyte in the extracellular fluid and potassium the most abundant in the intracellular fluid. As a result, disorders that affect these and water balance tend to have the most significant impact on the body. As the renal system is largely under neuroendocrine control in relation to fluid and electrolyte balance, the origins of most fluid and electrolyte disorders are within the renal system or in the processes that govern the neuroendocrine control (i.e. the nervous and endocrine systems – largely the hypothalamus and pituitary gland). Changes in fluid and electrolyte balance can be more detrimental in older age as renal and neuroendocrine function deteriorate as a part of the ageing process. Additionally, **acute** changes in fluid and electrolytes can have more immediate negative effects on the very young, as their ability to compensate can also be diminished.

Disorders of fluid and electrolyte balance are prevalent issues in practice. El-Sharkawy et al. (2015) found 37% of 200 older people in their study to be dehydrated on admission; after two days, 62% of these continued to be dehydrated, illustrating that the importance of hydration is not understood, and **dehydration** can go unidentified and poorly treated.

ACTIVITY 11.1: APPLY

Dehydration

As a person-centred practitioner, think of the factors that may result in older people being dehydrated and how you could identify and treat dehydration.

Fluid imbalance

Fluid imbalances are largely categorised as being **hypovolaemic** (low volume) or **hypervolaemic** (excess volume). Additionally, you can have normovolaemia with an altered distribution of fluid amongst the fluid compartments of the body. In this chapter, we will consider disorders that include the renal system as a key component of the fluid and electrolyte disorders. A number of conditions exist that have a rapid and profound effect on fluid and electrolyte balance; it is important to remember that electrolytes like sodium and potassium have a high osmotic potential and therefore bring water with them wherever they go. It is important to be able to identify these disorders and understand their treatments if you, as a nurse, are to be able to intervene with the interprofessional team to restore homeostasis.

APPLY

Electrolyte values in practice

Do you know the correct values for the electrolytes in the blood? Review Table 11.1 so you can ensure you detect results that are outside of homeostatic ranges. Signs, symptoms and causes are not exhaustive.

(Continued)

(Continued)

Table 11.1 Electrolyte values

Component	Homeostatic range*	Low	High	Symptoms and signs of imbalance
Na⁺	133-146 mmol/l	Vomiting Diarrhoea Cardiac/renal failure (water retention) Psychogenic polydipsia Syndrome of inappropriate ADH secretion (SIADH)	Vomiting Diarrhoea Dehydration	Confusion Agitation Nausea Vomiting Muscle weakness, spasms, cramps Arrhythmias
K⁺	3.5-5.3 mmol/l	↓ dietary intake Renal or GI loss	↑ intake Thermal injury Renal failure	Constipation Muscle weakness Hypotension Arrhythmias
Mg²⁺	0.70-0.95 mmol/l	↓ dietary intake ↑ loss	Rare ↓ loss ↑ intake	Confusion Agitation Nausea Vomiting Muscle weakness, spasms, cramps Arrhythmias
Ca²⁺	2.10-2.55 mmol/l	Parathyroid disease **Vitamin D** deficiency Sepsis Acute pancreatitis	Parathyroid disease	Impaired cognition and cardiac function
Phosphate	0.8-1.5 mmol/l (adults) 1.3-2.3 mmol/l (children)	Vitamin D deficiency Hyperparathyroidism Alcoholism	Renal disease Parathyroid disease Metabolic or respiratory **acidosis**	Impaired consciousness Impaired cardiac function Muscle weakness
Urea	2.9-8.2 mmol/l	Hypoproteinaemia Liver disease	↓ renal clearance (renal disease)↑ protein catabolism (infection, **stress**)	Weakness Confusion Nausea Vomiting Loss of appetite
Creatinine	50-110 µmol/l	Liver disease	↓ renal clearance (renal disease)	Fatigue Oedema Dyspnoea
Haematocrit / Packed Cell Volume	0.35-0.49 (children) 0.40-0.54 (men) 0.37-0.47 (women)	Anaemia ↓ iron, B₁₂ and folate Malnutrition Overhydration/ haemodilution	Overhydration Erythrocytosis	Dyspnoea Fatigue

*Homeostatic ranges vary from country to country; you should check your national values. Most ranges are for adults (except where indicated otherwise)

There are three key disorders that are neuroendocrine and renal in origin that impact on fluid and electrolyte imbalance (John and Day, 2012):

- **Central neurogenic diabetes insipidus (CNDI)** – results in **hypernatraemia** and hypovolaemia
- **Syndrome of inappropriate secretion of antidiuretic hormone** (SIADH) – results in hyponatraemia and hypervolaemia
- **Cerebral salt-wasting syndrome (CSWS)** – results in **hyponatraemia** and hypovolaemia

These largely occur as a result of injury to the hypothalamus and the pituitary gland which work together in regulating fluid and electrolyte homeostasis through the release of ADH. Alternatively, they represent a lack of response in the kidney to normal homeostatic mechanisms.

Diabetes insipidus

Diabetes insipidus (DI) is a condition where there is insufficient secretion of or a lack of response to ADH. In DI, there is an excess amount of urine production (**polyuria**), an accompanying excessive thirst in order to attempt to replace this lost fluid volume (**polydipsia**) and an absence of glucosuria, distinguishing it from diabetes mellitus. The preservation of thirst sensation enables the person to replace fluid as it is lost. However, when someone is unable to drink independently and replace this fluid, then they are at risk of significant hypovolaemia. DI is considered to have primarily two branches: nephrogenic DI (NDI) and central neurogenic DI (CNDI). Gestational DI can also occur. In order to identify which form of DI is present, there is a 24-hour urine volume, **osmolarity** and glucose sample collected. During this period, the person continues to eat and drink as normal without being administered any medication that would affect diuresis (Robertson, 2016). Beyond infancy, the following criteria indicate DI:

- urine volume >40 ml/kg body weight
- urine osmolarity <300 mOsm/kg
- negative test for glucose.

Nephrogenic diabetes insipidus (NDI)

In **nephrogenic diabetes insipidus (NDI)**, the renal tubule fails to respond to the presence of ADH. In other words, the kidney is not able to concentrate urine and fails to reabsorb water back into the intravascular space. There are two main forms of NDI:

- *Primary*: Mostly seen in children, this form of NDI is inherited. It is an X-linked condition where there is a **mutation** in the *AVPR2* gene. In its autosomal recessive form, there is a mutation in the *AQP2* gene on **chromosome** 12 (Bockenhauer and Bichet, 2015). In most people with **congenital** NDI, mutations are found in either of these genes with 90% occurring in the *AVPR2* gene. This means that men are largely affected by this X-linked form but it can also occur in women due to gene mutations. Babies born with congenital NDI often present with a failure to thrive alongside polydipsia and polyuria.
- *Secondary*: Mostly seen in adults, this form of NDI is acquired and is largely attributed to lithium treatment (Bockenhauer and Bichet, 2015). While discontinuing lithium can often resolve this form of NDI, the primary disorder for which the lithium was prescribed is adversely affected and so discontinuation is often not a viable option. People with acquired NDI largely present with polyuria and polydipsia.

When a person presents with signs of DI, the desmopressin test (or DDAVP test [vasopressin analogue 1desamino8-D-arginine vasopressin]) is administered. Following administration, urine osmolarity is checked and a result of >800 mOsm/kg is within normal parameters (not NDI) whereas a urine osmolarity below plasma osmolarity indicates *AQP2* deficiency (primary/congenital NDI).

Central neurogenic diabetes insipidus (CNDI)

In central neurogenic diabetes insipidus (CNDI), there is a deficit in the production and secretion of ADH as a result of injury or genetic defect to the neurohypophysis[1] and therefore there is insufficient amounts to stimulate the renal tubule to reabsorb water and concentrate the urine. Primarily, the neurohypophysis is damaged from a traumatic brain injury or from a **tumour**. A variant of CNDI is **primary polydipsia** whereby an excessive intake of water suppresses the secretion of ADH, resulting in the same effect. This is referred to either as dipsogenic polydipsia when the person has an excessive thirst and psychogenic polydipsia when this abnormal thirst is secondary to cognitive impairment (Robertson, 2016).

In CNDI, the person experiences an abnormally high urinary output with an associated thirst. While there is some electrolyte content in this urine, it is largely a renal **excretion** of water and so results in a drop in extracellular fluid volume, particularly if the person is not replacing the fluid whilst drinking. This dehydration will result in a loss of intracellular water content as water will move through all three fluid compartments of the body by osmosis. This process can result in significant dehydration and all the contents of the plasma, interstitial fluid and intracellular fluid become more concentrated. CNDI occurs as a result of damage to the posterior pituitary gland and usually has three phases (John and Day, 2012):

1. *Polyuria*: There is a high urinary output (>250 ml/hr) due to a lack of ADH secretion; ADH is needed to reabsorb water back into the vascular space.
2. *Normouria*: After approximately 5 days, stored ADH is released and urinary output largely returns to normal.
3. *Polyuria*: After around 7 days from onset, urinary output increases significantly again as the ADH stores become depleted. This can be transient or permanent, depending on the exact cause of CNDI.

The person with CNDI will have the following signs:

* High urinary output, usually >250 ml/h
* Urine specific gravity <1.005
* Urine osmolarity <200 mOsm/kg
* Serum osmolarity >295 mOsm/kg
* Elevated serum sodium >145 mmol/l
* There may be low or normal urinary sodium levels but high urinary potassium and magnesium levels
* 3–5% loss of body weight
* Person may become confused
* Signs of dehydration (poor skin turgor, dry mucous membranes, hypotension, tachycardia)

In CNDI, fluid must be replaced alongside replenishing any lost electrolytes such as sodium, potassium and magnesium. Fluids are replaced according to the volume lost, either orally or intravenously. As serum sodium levels may have risen beyond homeostatic parameters, hypotonic solutions are often administered in order to lower the sodium levels to within normal limits. For example, 0.45% sodium chloride (NaCl) is often the fluid of choice, or 0.18% with 4% dextrose. Using 5% dextrose can result in cerebral oedema due to its lack of electrolyte content, allowing water to flow freely into all cells. However, in order to prevent continued loss of fluids and disordered electrolyte balance, ADH availability must be restored. In this situation, synthetic ADH (desmopressin) is administered through a nasal spray. Alternatively, thiazide diuretics can be administered; these increase renal sodium excretion and thus stimulate further excretion of water.

---

[1]The posterior lobe of the pituitary gland

Syndrome of inappropriate secretion of ADH (SIADH)

In SIADH, people develop high levels of, or continuously secrete, ADH; the negative feedback loop that normally controls the amount of ADH secretion fails. As a result, there is increased renal reabsorption of water, resulting in a hypervolaemic, haemodilutional state. As a result, electrolytes are diluted in the blood and their levels read as low. The most common electrolyte affected is sodium as it is the most abundant electrolyte in the extracellular fluid. Damage to the hypothalamic–neurohypophyseal system will result in SIADH, as can subarachnoid haemorrhage and certain medications (e.g. chlorpromazine, chlorpropamide, chlorothiazide, carbamazepine) (John and Day, 2012). Factors that raise intrathoracic pressure can also bring about SIADH; this is thought to occur due to the stimulation of baroreceptors.

When someone develops SIADH, they present with a low urinary output as a result of water retention. The signs of SIADH include:

* Serum sodium <135 mmol/l
* Serum osmolarity <275 mOsm/Kg
* Urinary sodium >25 mmol/l
* Urine osmolarity greater than serum osmolarity
* Seizures (when serum sodium is <120 mmol/l)
* Reduced haematocrit

As SIADH results in water retention, hyponatraemia occurs, in part, from water dilution. However, there can also be high renal losses of sodium too. As a result, restoring electrolyte homeostasis is largely achieved through restoring water excretion, or restricting water intake, and replacing sodium. Therefore, people with SIADH often have a fluid restriction of less than one litre in 24 hours and hypertonic saline (3%) is administered. Diuretics can also be administered but they can deplete sodium levels further and so are administered with caution. Raising sodium levels must be done with extreme caution to prevent **central pontine myelinolysis**, an irreversible demyelination of neurons in the pons which occurs from too rapid serum sodium level correction. As a result, sodium is replaced at no more than 0.5 mmol/l/h. In recent years, **vaptans** (or **aquaretics**), which are oral vasopressin antagonists, have emerged as the most effective form of treatment. One such medication, tolvaptan, is a non-peptide vasopressin V2 receptor antagonist; it prevents arginine vasopressin (ADH) from binding with receptors in the distal nephron. This results in water being excreted without depleting serum electrolytes (Chen et al., 2014).

APPLY

Diuretics

Table 11.2 gives examples of the types of diuretics used in practice and their actions.

Table 11.2 Diuretics and their actions

Classification of diuretic	Example	Location of action	Effect
Osmotic	Mannitol	Extracellular space	↓ intracellular volume
	Urea		↑ ECF volume
	Isosorbide		↓ H_2O renal reabsorption

(Continued)

Table 11.2 (Continued)

Classification of diuretic	Example	Location of action	Effect
Loop	Frusemide Bumetanide Torasemide	Loop of Henle	↓ Na^+, Cl^-, Ca^{2+} and Mg^{2+} reabsorption
Thiazide/thiazide like	Bendroflumethiazide Chlortalidone Metolazone	Distal convoluted tubule	↓ Na^+ reabsorption
Sodium channel antagonist	Amiloride hydrochloride Triamterene (both are K^+ sparing)	Collecting duct	↓ Na^+ reabsorption ↓ K^+ and H^+ secretion
Aldosterone antagonist	Spironolactone Eplerenone	Collecting duct	↓ Na^+ reabsorption ↓ K^+ and H^+ secretion

Cerebral salt wasting syndrome (CSWS)

In CSWS, there is a loss of both sodium and water from the extracellular space as a result of a renal loss of sodium which takes water with it. ADH levels are often elevated in CSWS in an attempt to reabsorb water back into the extracellular fluid compartment. This can result in the condition being mistaken for SIADH. However, in CSWS, the primary cause of water depletion is sodium excretion, which is why it is called a salt wasting syndrome; the rise in ADH is a compensation to try to correct the water loss and so is not an inappropriate secretion of it. CSWS largely occurs in those with traumatic brain injury and subarachnoid haemorrhage. Release of natriuretic peptides is largely considered to be the cause of CSWS, most notably brain natriuretic peptide (BNP) as well as atrial natriuretic peptide (ANP) and C-type natriuretic peptide (Dholke et al., 2016). These are released from the damaged brain and cause vasodilation, inhibiting renin release from the kidneys. This prevents the renin angiotensin aldosterone system (RAAS) from intervening to restore water and sodium balance through reabsorption of both in the renal tubule under the influences of ADH and aldosterone. Hyponatraemia results, causing a secondary affect across the blood–brain barrier that can lead to cerebral oedema. In SIADH, intravascular volume is increased whereas in CSWS, intravascular volume is low. This is often the distinguishing feature. Signs of CSWS are:

- Serum osmolarity normal or decreased (<285 mOsm/kg)
- Urine osmolarity high
- High urinary output
- Signs of intravascular volume depletion (dehydration, raised heart rate, lowered blood pressure)
- Serum sodium <135 mmol/l

The primary treatment for CSWS is to replace lost water volume, largely through administering **crystalloid solutions**. In cases where hyponatraemia is mild, normal saline (0.9% sodium chloride) is administered and in cases where hyponatraemia is severe, hypertonic saline solutions (3% sodium chloride) are often used. Sodium is replaced at no more than 0.5 mmol/l/h in order to prevent central pontine myelinolysis, **metabolic acidosis**, intravascular volume overload and **pulmonary oedema** (Dholke et al., 2016).

Renal dysregulation of electrolytes

Electrolytes can be excreted in the urine or reabsorbed in the renal tubule. Through these processes, the balance of electrolytes can be moderated in the body by the kidney. However, other factors can impair these homeostatic mechanisms.

Osmotic diuresis

The two primary causes of **osmotic diuresis** are glucosuria and the use of osmotic diuretics.

Glucosuria

Hyperglycaemia can result in the renal threshold for glucose being exceeded. As the proximal tubule can only reabsorb a finite amount of glucose, once that level has been exceeded glucose becomes excreted in the urine (glucosuria or glycosuria). This threshold level is theoretically 11 mmol/l but is not an abrupt point of change; it is gradual and glucose can begin to fail to be reabsorbed from around 10 mmol/l upwards. The higher the blood glucose levels, the greater the reabsorption deficit. In those with diabetes mellitus, the renal threshold is substantially higher than 11 mmol/l and varies significantly from person to person (Poudel, 2013). Glucose has osmotic potential and so it draws water with it, resulting in a high urinary output that causes hypovolaemia. Diabetes mellitus is the primary cause of glucosuria but it can be renal in origin and is termed renal glucosuria. In this form, there is no elevated serum glucose level but a failure of the renal tubule to reabsorb it. This is primarily caused by an inherited disorder called familial renal glucosuria (FRG). In FRG, the person has a mutation in the sodium–glucose cotransporter *SGLT2* coding gene, *SLC5A2*, of which there are up to 21 mutations isolated (Lee et al., 2012).

Diuretics

Osmotic diuretics can result in potassium wasting and are thus a common cause of renally mediated hypokalaemia. The effect is dose-dependent and can often require diuretics to be changed over to potassium-sparing diuretics. Diuretics can also result in sodium loss in the urine.

Hyperaldosteronism

Hyperaldosteronism, an excessive secretion of aldosterone, disrupts electrolyte homeostasis as it results in an increase in sodium reabsorption in the renal tubule and promotes the loss of potassium and hydrogen. Pathophysiologically, hyperaldosteronism is part of complex mineralocorticoid disorders that influence aldosterone's effects on its target tissues. Aldosterone-producing adenomas are the most common causes of primary hyperaldosteronism. Secondary hyperaldosteronism is largely as a result of excess production and release of aldosterone through the RAAS and one of the main causes is **hypertension**.

Renal tubular acidosis (RTA)

There are three categories of **renal tubular acidosis (RTA)**, a condition where there is impaired renal hydrogen ion excretion (type 1), impaired bicarbonate reabsorption (type 2), or abnormal aldosterone production or response (type 4). In type 1 there is a failure of the α-intercalated cells (cells in the distal renal tubule that regulate acid–base homeostasis) to secrete hydrogen ions and reabsorb potassium, resulting in hypokalaemia. In type 2 there is a failure to reabsorb bicarbonate ions in the proximal renal tubule, which also results in hypokalaemia and there is a stimulated release of aldosterone, resulting in hyperaldosteronism. Type 4 is as a result of a deficiency of aldosterone, or a resistance to its effects, causing hyperkalaemia. Type 3 is no longer included in classifications.

Polydipsia

Polydipsia refers to increased thirst sensation and can result in a high water intake. In most cases, this can be regulated through normal homeostatic mechanisms. However, in excessive amounts, it results in a suppression of ADH release and can then result in a high urinary output that can result in sodium and potassium wastage in the urine, leading to hyponatraemia and **hypokalaemia**. In non-psychogenic forms, polydipsia is primarily as a result of a disorder of the hypothalamus, e.g. head injury.

URINARY TRACT INFECTIONS

A urinary tract infection (UTI) is caused by bacteria (usually gut flora) which rapidly reproduce and overwhelm the defence mechanisms of the host. Most infections are ascending, i.e. organisms in the perianal area travel along the continuous **mucosa** of the urinary tract, causing **inflammation** of the urinary **epithelium**. A UTI may occur at any point throughout the urinary tract, including the bladder, urethra, ureter or kidney. Whilst most UTIs are ascending, on occasion **pyelonephritis** may be caused by a blood-borne infection (**haematogenous spread**).

Escherichia coli (E. coli) (usually found in the intestine) is the most common causative organism and is responsible for up to 85% of all UTIs. Other organisms that cause UTIs include: Staphylococcus saprophyticus, Klebsiella pneumoniae, Proteus mirabilis, Enterococcus faecalis, Enterobacter, Pseudomonas, Chlamydia and Mycoplasma.

Aetiological factors

There are a number of factors that may increase the likelihood of a person developing a UTI. These include: urinary tract obstruction, reflux or **neurogenic bladder** dysfunction. These lead to organism growth as they are not flushed out of the bladder during micturition. Catheterisation can lead to the introduction of bacteria directly into the bladder; it can also traumatise the bladder wall, thereby breaking the barrier to infection. People who have been diagnosed with diabetes mellitus are also at an increased risk of UTIs due to vascular impairment and glucosuria. The older members of the Bodie family, i.e. Maud and George, are at increased risk of developing a UTI as there is a tendency towards incomplete emptying of the bladder, decreased fluid intake, impaired blood supply to the bladder and immobility.

Women are more likely to develop UTIs due to anatomically having a short, straight urethra and the proximity of the urinary meatus to the vagina and anus. Sexually active women are also more predisposed due to irritation of the epithelium. Antibiotic therapy can alter the flora of the vagina; this change in ratio may increase bacteria numbers, causing a UTI.

An infection of the male reproductive tract (which shares some of the structures of the urinary tract) may lead to a UTI. Older men with a diagnosis of prostatic **hypertrophy**, which leads to urinary retention or frequency, are more likely to develop a UTI.

Types of urinary tract infections

UTIs can be divided into:

* lower urinary tract infections – cystitis
* upper urinary tract infections – pyelonephritis.

Cystitis

Cystitis is inflammation of the bladder and is the most common site for a UTI. Cystitis can range in severity: mild inflammation, whereby the bladder mucosa has an increased blood supply and is hyperaemic; in more severe infection, the epithelial surface of the bladder may suppurate (formation of pus). Untreated or prolonged infection may lead to the bladder mucosa sloughing and the development of an **ulcer**.

The distal section of the urethra may contain some pathogenic microorganisms, however urine is usually sterile or bacteria-free (due to the washout phenomenon, i.e. the bacteria is washed out of the urethra during micturition). Contamination of urine occurs due to the retrograde movement of a pathogen into the urethra and bladder with subsequent movement to the ureter and eventually the kidney.

APPLY

Cystitis in practice

Signs and symptoms

Infection initiates an inflammatory response and causes the clinical manifestations associated with cystitis:

* Urgency and frequency – oedema in the wall of the bladder stimulates stretch receptors causing a sensation of fullness, however only small amounts of urine are voided.
* Dysuria – burning sensation and pain on urination due to the acidic urine irritating the wall of the bladder or urethra.
* Pyuria and foul odour – the inflammatory response causes the bladder mucous to suppurate; sloughing of the dead cells occurs and causes cloudy appearance of urine.
* Haematuria – mucosa becomes hyperaemic and may haemorrhage.
* Suprapubic pain – caused primarily by distension of the bladder and increased pressure within the urinary tract.
* Systemic signs of infection (present in some cases) – raised temperature/fever, increased C-reactive protein (CRP), leucocytosis (elevated white blood cell count).

Diagnosis and treatment

Diagnosis of a UTI is usually based on the presenting signs, symptoms and examination of the urine for microorganisms. If the infection is thought to be of an obstructive pathology then X-ray, ultrasound and/or computerised tomography (CT) may be required.

Urinalysis (urine dipstick) for markers of infection, e.g. presence of leucocytes, nitrate or blood, provides useful information and may be used for the diagnosis of an uncomplicated UTI. However, it

(Continued)

(Continued)

may also be necessary to perform a urine culture to identify the specific microorganism that is causing the infection and determine the sensitivity to specific antibiotics.

Antibacterial drugs such as fluoroquinolones, e.g. ciprofloxacin, or sulfonamides, e.g. co-trimoxazole, are used to treat UTIs; a urinary antiseptic, e.g. nitrofurantoin, may also be used. As an adjunct to antimicrobial therapy, an increased fluid intake is encouraged to help relieve signs and symptoms. Cranberry juice or blueberry juice may also be encouraged as a preventative measure for those with recurrent UTIs (see Apply box).

ACTIVITY 11.2: APPLY

Urinalysis

Read the following article to learn about undertaking urinalysis and interpreting the results:

Yates, A. (2016) Urinalysis: how to interpret results. *Nursing Times*, Online issue 2, 1-3.

ARTICLE:
URINALYSIS

APPLY

Urinary tract infections and cranberry products

Products derived from cranberry have been used as a complementary, non-antibiotic therapy for the treatment and prevention of UTIs for decades. Blatherwick and Long (1923) identified that the acidity of urine increased following large amounts of cranberry juice being ingested. However, subsequent research to support this assumption has failed to do so (Liu et al., 2006).

Whilst the exact mechanism of action in relation to prophylaxis of UTIs is unknown, it is purported that the compounds contained in cranberries prevent bacteria (in particular *E. coli*) adhering to the urinary epithelium, thereby preventing colonisation.

How much and what type of product is required?

Numerous studies have been conducted relating to types of cranberry products, however evidence to support its use is inconclusive. Wang et al. (2012) conducted a systematic literature review and meta-analysis of random controlled trials using cranberry-containing products for the prevention of UTIs in susceptible populations. They concluded that consumption of cranberry-containing products may protect against UTIs in certain populations and are more effective in children and women with recurrent infections. They also noted that taking cranberry products at least once a day was more effective as the anti-adhesion properties of cranberry juice on *E. coli* lasts for approximately eight hours. Whereas a literature review by Wang (2013) reported that there is no clear consensus on the use of cranberry products (juice or capsules) for the prevention of UTI. Wang (2013) concluded that whilst cranberry juice or products may be used as a supplement or prophylaxis, it should not be prescribed in the place of anti-microbial therapy.

Pyelonephritis

Pyelonephritis is an infection of the upper urinary tract affecting the renal parenchyma, i.e. renal pelvis and medulla (tubules and interstitial tissue). It can be acute or **chronic**; acute pyelonephritis is caused by bacterial infection whereas chronic pyelonephritis is more complex as it is not only due to bacterial infection but also other contributing factors such as reflux or **renal calculi** (kidney stones). Common contributing factors to pyelonephritis are listed in Table 11.3.

Table 11.3 Contributing factors to pyelonephritis

Contributing factor	Pathophysiology
Urinary tract obstruction: calculi, scarring and **stricture**, tumours, congenital defects	Bacteriuria and hydronephrosis due to obstruction and urinary stasis; epithelial irritation with entrapment of bacteria
Neurogenic bladder	Caused by neurological damage, e.g. stroke, spinal injury, MS, tumour that interferes with normal bladder contraction
Vesicoureteral reflux	Retrograde flow of urine caused by ureter entering the bladder at a right angle, therefore one-way valve is not formed to prevent backflow
Catheterisation	Introduction of bacteria into bladder and urethra
Sexual intercourse	Bacteria enter the bladder through the urethra. Some women lack a normally protective mucosal enzyme and have decreased levels of cervicovaginal **antibodies** to enterobacteria
Pregnancy	Increased levels of progesterone leading to ureteral relaxation and enlarged uterus leads to obstruction

Acute pyelonephritis

This is a bacterial infection (usually *E. coli*) that causes a suppurative (pus-forming) inflammation of one or both kidneys. It can be uncomplicated, commonly occurring in young females with no history of structural or urinary tract obstruction, or complicated, occurring in children or adults with a history of structural or functional urinary tract abnormalities.

Bacteria can gain access to the kidney via two routes:

1. Ascending infection from the lower urinary tract (this is the most common route).
2. Haematogenous spread (via the bloodstream), seeding of the kidney by bacteria from a distant location due to septicaemia or infective endocarditis. It is more likely to occur in those with a long-term condition or those receiving immunosuppressant therapy.

The inflammatory process primarily affects the renal pelvis, calyces and medulla and is focal and irregular in nature. The infection leads to the **infiltration** of white blood cells, renal inflammation, oedema and purulent urine. In severe cases, abscesses may form in the medulla and become necrotic, and may extend to the **renal cortex**.

APPLY

Acute pyelonephritis in practice

Signs and symptoms

- Abrupt onset associated with fever, shaking and chills
- Pain/constant ache in loin area (side of body from below the ribcage to above the pelvis) caused by stretching of renal capsule due to inflammation
- Tenderness over costovertebral angle on affected side
- Nausea, vomiting and malaise associated with abdominal pain
- Symptoms associated with lower UTI (discussed previously) may also be present.

Diagnosis and treatment

It may be difficult to differentiate between the symptoms of cystitis and pyelonephritis; diagnosis is determined by presenting signs and symptoms, urinalysis and urine culture. It may be necessary to perform urinary tract X-ray, ultrasound or CT in complicated cases.

The mainstay of treatment depends on the isolated causative microorganism; once this is identified, specific antimicrobial therapy will be administered for 2-3 weeks. As with cystitis, the person will be encouraged to increase their fluid intake substantially.

Chronic pyelonephritis

Chronic pyelonephritis may occur in one or both kidneys. It is a progressive process due to recurring or persistent bacterial infections associated with acute pyelonephritis or an obstructive pathological condition such as obstruction or reflux or in many cases due to both. Persistent inflammation leads to scarring and deformation of renal calyces and pelvis, destruction of renal tubules and **atrophy** and thinning of the renal cortex, leading to loss of tubular function and the ability to concentrate urine, resulting in: polyuria, nocturia and proteinuria. Chronic pyelonephritis is a significant cause of **chronic kidney disease (CKD)** (discussed later in the chapter).

APPLY

Chronic pyelonephritis in practice

Signs and symptoms

In the early stages of chronic pyelonephritis the symptoms are usually minimal, however they can include: hypertension, **dysuria**, frequency and urgency. There may also be associated flank pain (pain in upper abdomen, back or sides, may also be referred to as loin pain).

Diagnosis and treatment

It will be essential to find the underlying cause and treat accordingly. Urinalysis and radiological imaging of the urinary tract will be necessary to ascertain this. Antimicrobial therapy may be used to treat prolonged/recurrent infection but ultimately the obstruction must be relieved.

APPLY

Antibiotic resistance

Urinary tract infections (UTIs) are the second most commonly diagnosed infectious illness worldwide with *E. coli* (gram-negative bacilli) accounting for 75–90 % of cases (Aboumarzouk, 2014). Recurrent UTIs require repeated prescription of antibiotics as both curative and preventative measures. Antibiotic therapy includes the use of β-lactams, β-lactam/β-lactamase inhibitory flouroquinolones and carbapenems. Recently, however, **pathogen**s are developing and becoming increasingly resistant to the use of most of these antibiotics. One particular example of this is extended spectrum β-lactamase (ESBL), an enzyme produced by gram-negative bacilli. ESBL is contributing to increasing worldwide antibiotic resistance. Aboumarzouk (2014) indicates that ESBL organisms tend to be multidrug-resistant and UTIs complicated by ESBL may lead to uncertain outcomes and may prolong hospitalisation. The World Health Organisation (WHO) (2018) indicates that there are countries in many parts of the world where antibiotic treatment is now ineffective in more than half of patients. Frieri et al. (2017) have indicated that antimicrobial resistance is increasing at an alarming rate and is a challenge associated with high morbidity and mortality. WHO (2014) reported approximately 25,000 deaths in the European Union associated with antibiotic-resistant organisms, whilst the Center for Disease Control (CDC) and Prevention estimates 2 million cases of antibiotic-resistant bacteria, resulting in 23,000 deaths per year in the United States of America (CDC, 2018).

So what can be done?

Antibiotic stewardship (AS)

AS indicates approaches to help limit the use of antibiotics to the least length of time possible, and ensure that the appropriate antimicrobial therapy is used for the specific **strain**, thereby reducing antibiotic resistance and improving patient outcomes (MacGowan and Macnaughton, 2017; Sumner et al., 2018). As nurses we are ideally placed to play a significant role in AS. As nurses we are targeted with promoting the responsible use of antimicrobial therapy based on verification of organism sensitivity, e.g. ensuring that cultures are obtained as quickly as possible from the person and sent to the laboratory for testing. It is also essential that we ensure a multidisciplinary approach, i.e. working alongside doctors and pharmacists to ensure that the appropriate antimicrobial therapy is being used for the appropriate time. Patient education is vital in the prevention of antibiotic resistance; it is imperative that as nurses we provide those in our care with the information they need on the use of antimicrobial therapy.

Calcium

Calcium kidney stones are formed from calcium and may be due to hypercalcaemia, hyercalcuria, excessive bone resorption caused by hyperparathyroidism, vitamin D intoxication or renal tubule acidosis. Calcium stones are the most common type of kidney stones accounting for 70%–80%.

Magnesium Ammonium Phosphate (Struvite stones)

These types of stones are formed in alkaline urine in the presence of bacteria that possess urase (an enzyme that splits urea in the urine into ammonium and carbon dioxide) (urea splitting UTI). The ammonia ion picks up a hydrogen ion now ammonium, thereby increasing the pH and alkalinity of the urine. Magnesium is always present in urine, however, due to increased alkalinity, phosphate levels in the urine increase. Together magnesium and phosphate combine to form struvite stones. Bacterial growth results in the stone continuing to increase in size and due to its shape they can eventually be known as Staghorn stones.

Types of Kidney Stone

Uric Acid

These stones are formed due to high concentrations of uric acid in urine and gout. They form most readily when the pH of urine ranges from 5.1 to 5.9.

Cystine

Due to an inherited disorder of amino acid metabolism called cystinuria (genetic defect in renal transport of cystine). Whilst they cause less than one percent of all kidney stones they account for a high proportion of calculi in childhood.

Figure 11.1 Types of kidney stones

RENAL CALCULI (KIDNEY STONES) (UROLITHIASIS)

Kidney stones are the most common cause of upper urinary tract obstruction. They can form in any part of the urinary system but mostly in the kidney; they are polycrystalline aggregates composed of materials that the kidney normally excretes. Development of kidney stones is a complex process involving a number of factors:

- Increase in blood and urinary levels of stone components and the interaction of these components
- Anatomical changes in urinary tract structures
- Endocrine and/or metabolic influences
- Factors related to diet and intestinal **absorption**
- Urinary tract infections.

Factors that may contribute to the development of kidney stones are **supersaturation of urine** and a specific environment that allows the stone to grow.

Supersaturation of urine refers to the increased presence of stone components, e.g. calcium salts, uric acid, magnesium ammonium phosphate and cystine. It depends on urinary pH, concentration of solutes, strength of ions and complexation (combination of individual molecules to form a large molecule). Precipitation is more likely to occur when the concentration of two ions is high.

A nucleus or nidus that facilitates crystal aggregation is also required for stone formation to occur. The presence of small clusters of crystals such as calcium oxalate in supersaturated urine can lead to the formation of stones. Small clusters of ions are unstable and tend to disperse as the forces holding them together are too weak; however, large clusters of ions form nuclei and therefore remain stable due to increased forces that hold them together. Once stable these nuclei can continue to grow at levels of supersaturation much lower than was necessary for their original formation. Deficiency of stone inhibitors, i.e. magnesium, citrate and the Tamm–Horsfall mucoprotein, can also promote the formation of kidney stones.

There are four types of kidney stones: calcium (oxalate, phosphate or a combination of both), magnesium ammonium phosphate, uric acid and cystine (Figure 11.1).

APPLY

Kidney stones in practice

Signs and symptoms

Kidney stones can be asymptomatic, unless recurrent infections prompt investigations. Pain associated with renal calculi is due to the ureter contraction vigorously in an attempt to force the stone out. It can be classified as:

- Renal colic – acute intermittent and excruciating pain in flank and upper outer quadrant of abdomen on the affected side that accompanies stretching of the collecting system or ureter. The pain can be accompanied by cool and clammy skin, nausea and vomiting.
- Non-renal colic – caused by stones that produce distension of renal calyces or renal pelvis that is usually a dull, deep ache in the flank or back that can vary in intensity from mild to severe.

Diagnosis and treatment

Diagnosis of kidney stones is based on presenting symptoms and diagnostic tests including: urinalysis, X-ray (plain film), intravenous pyelogram (IVP) and abdominal ultrasound.

Kidney stones that are small enough will eventually pass over time. Urine should be strained to identify the presence of the stone. Larger stones may require to be broken down (fragmentation) using extracorporeal shock-wave lithotripsy or laser lithotripsy.

(Continued)

(Continued)

Treatment of kidney stones is also aimed at preventing recurrence; it is therefore essential that the underlying cause is treated, e.g. hyperparathyroidism. It is also necessary to increase fluid intake as this will help reduce the concentration of stone-forming crystals in the urine.

Depending on the type of stone that has formed, it may be necessary to change the concentration of the elements that are responsible for forming the stone. This may include dietary changes, medication or both. It may be necessary for those who form calcium oxalate stones to reduce the amount of oxalate in their diet, e.g. reduce their intake of spinach, peanuts, pecans, cocoa and chocolate. Alpha-adrenergic blockers, e.g. tamsulosin, and calcium-channel blockers, e.g. nifidipine, may be used as they relax ureteral muscle and promote passage of the stone. Table 11.4 indicates the types of treatments for each type of stone.

Table 11.4 Types and treatment of kidney stones

Type of stone	Treatment
Calcium	Treat underlying condition, increase fluid intake, thiazide diuretic (decreases urinary calcium excretion, thereby preventing further stones), decrease foods high in oxalate, e.g. spinach, peanuts, pecans, cocoa and chocolate
Magnesium ammonium phosphate (struvite stones)	Treat underlying UTI, acidification of urine, increase fluid intake
Uric acid	Alkalinisation of urine with potassium citrate
Cystine	Alkalinisation of urine with potassium citrate, increase fluid intake

KIDNEY DYSFUNCTION

Kidney injury can range from acute and rapidly progressive (hours to days) to chronic. Damage occurring from **acute kidney injury** (AKI) may be reversible in most cases, whereas over months or years **chronic kidney disease** (CKD) will progress to end-stage kidney failure.

Terms associated with kidney disease and decreasing renal function include:

- **Renal insufficiency**: a decline to about 25% of normal renal function; **glomerular filtration rate (GFR)** is approximately 25–30 ml/minute (normal GFR is 90 ml/minute). There is slight elevation in serum urea and creatinine.
- **Renal failure**: represents significant loss of renal function; end-stage kidney disease is said to occur when less than 10% of normal kidney function remains.
- **Azotaemia**: refers to an increased blood serum level of urea and frequently increased levels of creatinine. Azotaemia is caused by both renal insufficiency and renal failure.
- **Uraemic syndrome**: a syndrome related to renal failure, characterised by increased blood serum levels of urea and creatinine alongside neurological changes, nausea, vomiting, **anorexia** and fatigue. Consequences of uraemia and renal failure include the retention of nitrogenous toxic waste, electrolyte imbalances and activation of the immune system, promoting a pro-inflammatory state.

Acute kidney injury (AKI)

Acute kidney injury (AKI) is one of a number of conditions that acutely affects the structure and function of the kidney; these conditions are referred to as acute kidney diseases and disorders (AKD) (Kidney Disease: Improving Global Outcomes, 2013). The definition of AKI is ever changing and the concept of AKD is new and requires further refining. As AKI is a subset of AKD it is imperative that the definition of AKD includes the definition of AKI. Furthermore, AKI and AKD can occur in those already diagnosed with CKD. Figure 11.2 illustrates the relationship between AKD, AKI and CKD.

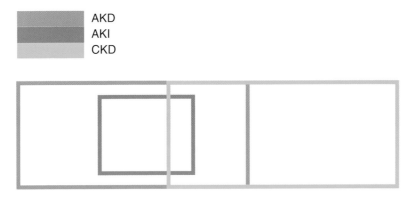

Figure 11.2 Relationship between AKD, AKI and CKD

AKI can be described as a rapid decline in kidney function occurring over hours to days, resulting in the inability to maintain fluid, electrolyte and acid–base balances, evidenced by a decrease in glomerular filtration rate and urine output and an increase in nitrogenous waste, leading to azotaemia and/or uraemia. AKI can range from very subtle/minimal changes in renal function to complete failure that may require renal replacement therapy. AKI is preferred to acute renal failure as it more fully represents the diversity of the condition; Figure 11.3 illustrates a model for kidney disease. Kidney Disease: Improving Global Outcomes – 2012 (2013) identified three stages of AKI severity; the diagnosing and staging of AKI are based on Risk, Injury, Failure, Loss and End-stage (commonly referred to as RIFLE). RIFLE indicates the increasing severity of classes of AKI (Figure 11.3).

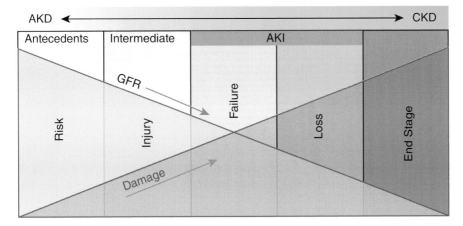

Figure 11.3 RIFLE criteria and kidney disease

AKI results from **ischaemia** of kidney tissue caused by a decrease in blood volume, decreased renal blood flow, toxins or **sepsis**. The injury starts an inflammatory response, vascular responses and cell death. AKI can be classified as: **volume-responsive** (prerenal), **intrinsic** (intrarenal) or **postrenal**. Causes of the different types of AKI are identified in Table 11.5.

Table 11.5 Causes of acute kidney injury (AKI)

Type of AKI	Causes
Volume-responsive AKI	Resulting from decreased blood supply to the kidneys (glomeruli and renal tubule undamaged)
Intrinsic AKI	Resulting from abnormalities within the kidney, including damage to the blood vessels, glomeruli and tubules
Postrenal AKI	Resulting from an obstruction in the urinary collection system; may arise anywhere from renal pelvis to urethra

Volume-responsive (prerenal) AKI results from decreased blood supply to the kidneys (glomeruli and renal tubule undamaged). It is the most common cause of AKI – failure to treat with early and adequate volume almost inevitably causes **acute tubular necrosis (ATN)**. If treated promptly, the damage done by the initial insult is immediately reversible.

Intrinsic AKI results from abnormalities within the kidney, including damage to the blood vessels, glomeruli and tubules and may be caused by: ischaemia, inflammation, nephrotoxicity and acute tubular necrosis (ATN).

Acute tubular necrosis (ATN) is the main cause of intrinsic AKI and may occur due to many causative factors. Severe ischaemia, with an inadequate supply of oxygen and nutrients to tubular epithelial cells, occurs most often following surgery (approximately 40–50%), however it can be due to sepsis, haemorrhagic trauma or burns. Hypovolaemia-induced hypotension leads to ischaemia and initiation of an inflammatory response that promotes the production of toxic oxygen-free radicals leading to oedema, injury and necrosis. As a result of injury and ischaemia, vasoconstriction of the intrarenal microvasculature occurs. Necrosis can be distributed along any part of the nephron and is patch in nature.

Nephrotoxic ATN can be caused by poisons, toxins or medications that destroy the tubular epithelial cells, including some antibiotics, various insecticides and heavy metals (e.g. mercury, lead). Intratubular obstruction caused by **myoglobinuria** or **haemoglobinuria** may also contribute to the development of nephrotoxic ATN. Necrosis tends to be confined to the proximal tubule and is uniform in nature.

Postrenal AKI results from an obstruction in the urinary collection system and may arise anywhere from renal pelvis to urethra, usually affecting both kidneys. The obstruction can cause an increase in intraluminal pressure, leading to a subsequent decrease in GFR.

Oliguria (<400 ml/24 hours) may occur in AKI; it is thought that three mechanisms contributing in varying degrees and combination throughout the trajectory of the disease may cause a decrease in urine output:

1. Alteration in renal blood flow – vasoconstriction of the efferent arteriole caused by the release of intrarenal angiotensin II or due to blood flow from the renal medulla to the renal cortex being redistributed. Impaired autoregulation of blood flow may lead to a decrease in GFR. Ischaemia may also be responsible for changes in glomerular permeability and reduction in GFR.
2. Tubular obstruction – sloughing of cells, causes formation of ischaemic oedema in necrotic tubules and may result in obstruction; subsequently a retrograde increase in pressure occurs, leading to a reduction in GFR.
3. Tubular backleak – tubular reabsorption is accelerated due to changes in permeability caused by ischaemia and increased tubular pressure from obstruction. However, GFR will remain normal.

AKI can be classified into three stages:

- *Initiation*: Initially volume-responsive AKI causes ischaemia and hypoxic damage causes intracellular oedema and, if unreversed, cell death. Oliguria usually occurs within 2 days and may last up to 2 weeks. As renal function declines (decreased GFR), urine output decreases, and serum urea and creatinine levels rise.
- *Established or maintenance (oliguric)*: Cell damage releases vasoactive **cytokines**, leading to further intrarenal vasoconstriction. Preglomerular vasoconstriction reduces glomerular **perfusion** and thus glomerular filtration. Widespread intracellular oedema physically compresses lumens, obstructing flow of the filtrate produced. Medullary damage reduces sodium reabsorption in the loop of Henle (urinary sodium is high). Serum urea and creatinine levels continue to rise. **Oliguria** and **anuria** persist throughout the established phase. There is a marked decrease in GFR metabolites, e.g. urea, potassium and creatinine are now retained. Urinary output is at its lowest point and results in oedema, water intoxication and pulmonary congestion. If oliguria persists, it will result in hypertension and uraemia.
- *Recovery or diuretic*: Tubular cells readily regenerate and the recovery phase begins as they do. As damaged tubules recover function and new (immature) tubule cells grow, filtration improves but tubular reabsorption and solute exchange remain poor. Large quantities of poor-quality urine are produced; serum urea and creatinine remain high although they start to decrease. When tubular cells mature, normal function is recovered; urine volumes return to normal and electrolyte balance is restored. Return to normal renal function can take from 3 to 12 months. However, in some cases, full recovery of GFR or tubular function may not occur.

APPLY

AKI - diagnosis and treatment

Early detection and treatment of AKI will improve outcomes. Diagnosis of AKI is related to the cause; it is therefore imperative that the aetiology is evaluated and reversible causes are identified or corrected. It is acknowledged that GFR is the most valuable index of renal function in both health and disease, however measuring urine output and serum creatinine are suitable alternatives. An abrupt decline in GFR will manifest in a rise in serum creatinine or oliguria. Investigations should include: careful monitoring of urine output; urinalysis, biochemistry to check for blood serum levels of urea, creatinine, potassium, phosphate and estimated GFR (eGFR) and urinary electrolytes to determine urine osmolarity and urine sodium concentrations. Differentiation between prerenal AKI and intrinsic AKI may be difficult, however this may be achieved by measuring serum urea and creatinine levels, urine sodium levels, urine osmolarity and urine specific gravity (Table 11.6). It may also be necessary to have an ultrasound of the renal tract and a kidney biopsy.

The main goal of treatment is to maintain the person's life, preventing complications and deterioration until renal function returns. Treatment is aimed at managing the physiological alterations caused by AKI and includes:

- maintaining blood pressure
- correction of fluid and electrolyte imbalances, especially hyperkalaemia
- ensuring that the person is receiving appropriate **nutrition**
- prevention of and, if necessary, treatment of infection
- manipulation of drug therapy, particularly those that are nephrotoxic
- initiation of renal replacement therapy (RRT) in cases of severe hyperkalaemia, fluid overload or acidosis. RIFLE criteria can also be used to determine if RRT is required.

(Continued)

(Continued)

Table 11.6 Differentiation between volume-responsive and intrinsic AKI

Type of AKI	Urine volume	Urea creatinine ratio	Urine sodium levels	Urine osmolarity	Urine specific gravity
Volume-responsive	<400 ml/24 h	>15:1	<10 mmol/l	>500 mOsm	1.016–1.020
Intrinsic	<400 ml/24 h	<15:1	>30 mmol/l	<400 mOsm	1.010–1.012

Chronic kidney disease (CKD)

CKD is a slow, progressive and irreversible pathophysiological process with multiple aetiologies, including the following:

- Hypertension
- Diabetes mellitus
- Glomerulonephritis
- Chronic pyelonephritis
- Systemic lupus erythematosus (SLE)
- Obstructive uropathies
- Vascular disorders.

Regardless of cause, CKD results in the permanent loss of nephrons, tubular absorptive capacity, decline in renal function and loss of endocrine functions; it frequently leads to kidney failure. The definition of CKD is based upon a decrease in GFR (usually less than 60 millilitre per minute per 1.73m²), increased excretion of urinary albumin (**albuminuria**) or both for three or more months, regardless of clinical diagnosis (Jha et al., 2013; Levey and Coresh, 2012). The prevalence of CKD is estimated to be 8–16% worldwide and it is becoming an increasing public health issue (Jha et al., 2013).

As already mentioned, there are a number of causes for CKD, however it is thought the two most common causes are diabetes (Jha et al., 2013) and hypertension (Levey and Coresh, 2012). Hyperglycaemia due to diabetes can cause changes in the microvasculature of the kidney, whilst the afferent and efferent arterioles and glomerular capillaries are affected. These changes lead to glomerular thickening, deposits of **immunoglobulin** G (IgG) and albumin, resulting in diffuse **glomerulosclerosis**. Late **nephropathy**, tubular **atrophy** and interstitial **fibrosis** also occur. Hypertensive **nephrosclerosis** involves the development of sclerotic **lesions** in the renal arterioles and glomerular capillaries, causing them to become thickened and narrowed; this eventually causes the capillaries to become necrotic.

The kidneys have the ability to adapt to the decline in the number of functioning nephrons. Signs and symptoms related to decreased renal function do not become evident until late because of the kidneys' ability to compensate. It is postulated that the intact nephron theory is the reason for this compensation. It proposes that as nephrons are destroyed, the remaining nephrons undergo structural and functional hypertrophy, thereby increasing renal function and thus maintaining excretory and homeostatic mechanisms even when up to 70% of nephrons are damaged. However, intact nephrons will reach a point of maximal filtration and any further loss of glomerular mass will be accompanied by an incremental loss in GFR and the subsequent accumulation of filterable toxins. Mechanisms involved in the progressive destruction of nephrons depend upon the primary cause of renal failure. Secondary insults, e.g. alteration in renal perfusion, nephrotoxic drugs, urinary obstruction and infections, can rapidly accelerate the process of further loss of nephrons. The urine produced by a person with CKD may contain abnormal amounts of red blood cells, casts or protein but the end products of excretion will remain similar to those of normal functioning kidneys until the advanced stages of renal failure. The advancement of renal disease is closely related to albuminuria and the activity of **angiotensin II**. Albuminuria results from increased glomerular permeability and hyperfiltration, leading to loss of negative charge. Albuminuria subsequently accumulates in the interstitial space of the renal tubules, and **macrophage**s and complement proteins are activated, promoting inflammation and progressive fibrosis, further contributing to tubulointerstitial injury. Vasoconstriction of efferent arterioles following the release of angiotensin II causes glomerular hypertension and hyperfiltration alongside an increase in systemic hypertension. Increased glomerular pressure increases glomerular permeability, further contributing to the presence of albuminuria. Inflammatory cells and growth factors may also be activated by angiotensin II, thereby causing further tubulointerstitial fibrosis and scarring.

Classification and stages of CKD are based on the reduction of GFR and the complications associated with this decline (Table 11.7).

Table 11.7   Stages of chronic kidney disease (CKD)

Stage	Description	GFR level and associated complications
Normal kidney function	Healthy kidneys	90 ml/min or more
Stage 1	Kidney damage with normal or high GFR	90 ml/min or more - persistent microalbuminuria, persistent proteinuria, persistent haematuria, structural abnormalities, biopsy proven glomerulonephritis, hypertension is common
Stage 2	Kidney damage with mild decrease in GFR	60-89 ml/min - characterised by 40-50% loss of renal function. Kidneys still able to maintain excretory and regulatory functions, patients typically asymptomatic. Early signs of renal failure, e.g. increased BUN/creatinine levels only evident after 50-60% loss. Proteinuria or haematuria evident, hypertension
Stage 3	Moderate decrease in GFR	30-59 ml/min - residual function is only 20-40% of normal, by this time solute clearance ability to concentrate urine and hormone secretion are compromised. Signs of renal failure start to manifest, e.g. hypertension, fatigue, polyuria and nocturia
Stage 4	Severe decrease in GFR	15-29 ml/min - characterised by residual renal function of <15% of normal. Normal regulatory, excretory and hormonal functions are severely impaired. ESRD/ESKD evidenced by marked increases in blood urea, decreased creatinine clearance, anaemia, electrolyte imbalances, metabolic acidosis, hyperphosphataemia and fluid overload
Stage 5	End-stage kidney failure (Established renal failure)	<15 ml/min or on dialysis - as per stage 4

APPLY

CKD in practice

Signs and symptoms

Signs and symptoms occur gradually and usually do not become evident until the disease is far advanced. Uraemia and azotaemia are the cause of many of the clinical signs and symptoms associated with CKD.

(Continued)

(Continued)

Diagnosis and treatment of CKD

Diagnosis of CKD is based upon the person's medical history, risk factors, signs and symptoms and diagnostic tests, e.g. eGFR, serum urea and creatinine and electrolytes, urine albumin:creatinine ratio, urinalysis to identify proteinuria. It may also be necessary to perform radiological imaging, e.g. magnetic resonance imaging (MRI), an ultrasound scan of the renal tract or a kidney biopsy.

Management of CKD is aimed at preventing **progression** and limiting complications associated with the disease. Regardless of which stage of CKD the person is diagnosed with, treatment will include: regular measurement of kidney function; blood pressure monitoring; and general health advice, aimed at smoking cessation, weight loss, aerobic exercise, limiting alcohol intake, and dietary advice regarding potassium, phosphate, calorie and salt intake appropriate to the severity or stage of CKD. It is important that people with CKD are not offered low-protein diets, i.e. a dietary protein intake of less than 0.6–0.8 g/kg/day.

Treatment at all stages of CKD also includes cardiovascular prophylaxis. In a person with a 10-year risk of cardiovascular disease of >20% consider antiplatelet and lipid-lowering drug therapy, control of hypertension with use of an **ACE inhibitor** or angiotensin receptor blocker and avoidance of nephrotoxins, e.g. intravenous radiocontrast agents, NSAIDs (e.g. ibuprofen, aspirin, diclofenac) and aminoglycosides (e.g. gentamicin, tobramycin).

Additional management for stage 3 includes a review of all prescribed medication regularly to ensure appropriate doses and immunisation against **influenza** and pneumococcus; and annual measurement of haemoglobin, creatinine and potassium. If Hb <110 g/L this must be treated with erythropoiesis-stimulating agents to maintain Hb 110–120 g/L.

Additional management for stage 4 and 5 includes: three-monthly tests for serum creatinine (eGFR), Hb, calcium, phosphate, bicarbonate and parathyroid hormone; dietary assessment; correction of acidosis; immunisation against hepatitis B; and early referral to a nephrologist and initiation of renal replacement therapy as necessary.

ESRD/ESKD and renal replacement therapy (RRT)

It is estimated that more than two million people worldwide are being treated for ESRD/ESKD (Robinson et al., 2016). In young people, a lower quality of life, limited employment, independence and relationships are associated with established kidney failure compared with healthy peers (Hamilton et al., 2017). For many older adults with a new diagnosis of ESRD, the question of whether the treatment would be of benefit or, more importantly, would improve their quality of life (QOL) sits at the forefront of their mind.

There are a wide range of treatment modalities available, including: home dialysis options, i.e. peritoneal dialysis or home haemodialysis; in-hospital haemodialysis and kidney transplantation (Balogun et al., 2017). Regardless of the treatment option chosen, ESRD and RRT have a significant impact on the person's ability to carry out their daily activities. Bailey et al. (2018) found that across different countries and different health care settings, young adults on RRT experience difference and liminality, even after transplantation. It is therefore imperative that tailored social and psychological support is provided to ensure that young adults experience wellness while in receipt of RRT, and not have their life on hold. Balogun et al. (2017) identified that 47% of older people undergoing RRT showed improved overall health-related QOL and mental component summary QOL, which therefore indicates that RRT should not be excluded as a treatment option in the older population.

URINARY INCONTINENCE

Urinary incontinence is the loss of voluntary control of the bladder, resulting in involuntary leakage of urine. Normal urinary elimination is dependent on coordination between the bladder and the urethra, known as the vesico-urethral unit. Incontinence will result where there is a change in the structure of the muscle of the bladder or the urethra, or where the nerves coordinating the vesico-urethral unit are affected. The ageing process, neurological conditions including spinal lesions, chronic conditions such as diabetes, trauma and childbirth can all lead to incontinence.

There are several types of urinary incontinence which result from a number of different conditions, leading to decreased muscle tone and sphincter weakness. The three main types of urinary incontinence are: **stress incontinence**, **urge incontinence** and overflow incontinence.

Stress incontinence

Stress incontinence is defined as the involuntary loss of urine on effort, physical exertion, coughing or sneezing (Haylen et al., 2010). The increased intra-abdominal pressure associated with these activities exceeds urethral pressure, thus preventing closure of the external sphincter. Urethral closure pressure is the pressure difference between the urethra and the bladder and this is decreased where there is weakness of the pelvic floor muscles.

Reduced muscle tone associated with normal ageing, childbirth or surgical procedures can weaken the urogenital diaphragm and result in stress incontinence. Stress incontinence is a common problem in women as a result of weakness of the pelvic floor muscles and inadequate support of the vesico-urethral sphincters. It is uncommon in men and when present is usually associated with prostate surgery.

Urge incontinence

Urge incontinence is the involuntary loss of urine that is accompanied by or immediately preceded by urgency (Haylen et al., 2010). It is often associated with **overactive bladder syndrome**, which is a syndrome characterised by increased urinary frequency, nocturia and urgency with or without urge incontinence in the absence of infection. Overactive bladder syndrome is associated with detrusor muscle overactivity, causing increased bladder contractions while the bladder is filling (Figure 11.4). In conditions such as stroke, **Parkinson's disease** and **multiple sclerosis**, nerve impulses to the bladder are affected, leading to increased sensitivity to bladder filling or increased excitability of the nerves that control bladder emptying. The ageing process alters detrusor muscle structure and diminishes its strength, leading to urge incontinence. Some chronic conditions that affect nerves, such as diabetes and alcoholism, are associated with urgency and frequency.

Stress incontinence and urge incontinence often coexist and this is known as **mixed urinary incontinence**.

Overflow incontinence

This occurs due to bladder distension in the absence of detrusor muscle activity. Obstruction to the outflow of urine can lead to dribbling, a weak urinary stream, frequency and nocturia. Uterine prolapse in women and enlargement of the prostate gland in men are common causes of obstruction to outflow. Incontinence due to neurological causes is known as neurogenic bladder (Chapter 16). This can be due to overactivity of the detrusor muscle often associated with stroke or spinal cord injury. Detrusor hypocontractility leads to overflow incontinence and is associated with lower spinal cord lesions.

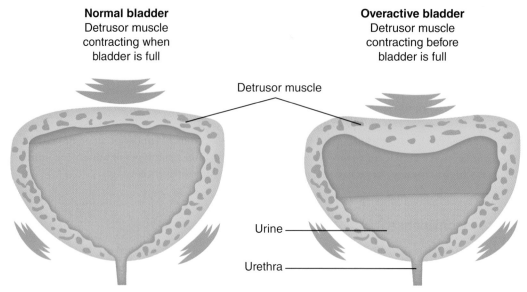

Normal bladder
Detrusor muscle
contracting when
bladder is full

Overactive bladder
Detrusor muscle
contracting before
bladder is full

Detrusor muscle

Urine

Urethra

Illustrated by Shaun Mercier © SAGE Publications

Figure 11.4   Detrusor muscle activity in overactive bladder syndrome, leading to urge incontinence

APPLY

Urinary incontinence - diagnosis and treatment

Assessment begins with a detailed history of the severity and frequency of the person's symptoms, including any triggers or relieving factors. It is important to establish the impact of the symptoms on the person's quality of life and social circumstances. A diary is a useful tool for the person to record data about their symptoms. A physical examination, urine analysis and blood tests will help exclude or identify any underlying cause.

Depending on the cause, treatment can include lifestyle modification, pelvic floor muscle strengthening and bladder training. Lifestyle modifications include reducing caffeine and alcohol intake and maintaining a healthy weight and altering fluid intake. Bladder training teaches a person how to hold more urine in the bladder and so reduce the number of times a person needs to pass urine. This is recommended as the first-line management of urge and stress incontinence (NICE, 2015).

Pelvic floor muscle strengthening exercises involve at least eight contractions performed three times per day and should continue for at least three months (NICE, 2015).

Pharmacological management includes drugs that affect myogenic causes such as antimuscarinic medications for overactive bladder or alpha-receptor antagonists for outflow obstruction. More complex dysfunction that does not respond to treatments will require further assessment through urodynamic studies, endoscopy and imaging.

Absorbent products and toileting aids can be practical as an adjunct to ongoing therapy and can help manage the day-to-day practicalities of incontinence.

There are some useful information leaflets on pelvic floor exercises for women and men available at:

www.baus.org.uk (search the website for 'pelvic floor exercises')

Information and support for incontinence can be found at the following links:

www.bladderandbowel.org

www.bbuk.org.uk

Age and incontinence

The incidence of urinary incontinence increases with age and it can lead to social isolation and skin breakdown and infections. Physiological changes in ageing such as diminished detrusor muscle strength and muscle mass, reduced blood flow and alterations in nervous control contribute to the development of incontinence. Added to this, reduced mobility and comorbidities such as dementia, constipation and infections and medications can all precipitate incontinence. The person's needs and preferences must be taken into account when caring for and managing incontinence and the nurse must support the person to make informed choices about their care and treatment.

CONCLUSION

Having worked through this chapter, you will now be aware of the complexity of many of the disorders associated with kidney injury and disease and indeed disorders of fluid, electrolyte and bladder control. Renal dysfunction is potentially life-limiting and has the ability to significantly reduce health-related quality of life. As a person-centred practitioner, it is important to remember that such disorders may occur acutely but have long-term consequences, altering the life of a person and their family significantly and often for life. Understanding the conditions leads to better insights into appropriate care and such informed practice on your part will positively impact on the care received in such challenging times.

KEY POINTS

- The origins of most fluid and electrolyte disorders are within the renal system or in the processes that govern the neuroendocrine control (i.e. the nervous and endocrine systems).

- There are three key disorders that are neuroendocrine and renal in origin that impact on fluid and electrolyte imbalance:
  - Central neurogenic diabetes insipidus (CNDI) – results in hypernatraemia and hypovolaemia
  - Syndrome of inappropriate secretion of antidiuretic hormone (SIADH) – results in hyponatraemia and hypervolaemia
  - Cerebral salt-wasting syndrome (CSWS) – results in hyponatraemia and hypovolaemia

- Diabetes Insipidus (DI) is a condition where there is insufficient secretion of, or a lack of response to, ADH. There are two main forms:
  - NDI: when the renal tubule fails to respond to the presence of ADH and the kidney is unable to concentrate urine, failing to reabsorb water back into the intravascular space.
  - CNDI: when there is a deficit in the production and secretion of ADH as a result of injury or genetic defect to the neurohypophysis; leads to insufficient ADH to stimulate the renal tubule to reabsorb water and concentrate the urine.

- In SIADH, people develop high levels of, or continuously secrete, ADH, leading to increased renal reabsorption of water and a resultant hypervolaemic, haemodilutional state.

- CSWS is a loss of both sodium and water from the extracellular space as a result of a renal loss of sodium which takes water with it. The release of natriuretic peptides causes vasodilation, inhibiting renin release from the kidneys. This prevents the RAAS from reabsorbing water and sodium in the renal tubule under the influences of ADH and aldosterone.

- Cystitis is inflammation of the bladder from pathogenic invasion.

- Pyelonephritis is an infection of the upper urinary tract affecting the renal parenchyma. It can be acute or chronic; acute pyelonephritis is caused by bacterial infection whereas chronic pyelonephritis is due to bacterial infection and other contributing factors.

- Kidney stones form in any part of the urinary system as a result of polycrystalline aggregates composed of materials that the kidney normally excretes.

- AKI, a subset of AKD, is a rapid decline in kidney function occurring over hours to days, resulting in the inability to maintain fluid, electrolyte and acid–base balances, evidenced by a decrease in glomerular filtration rate and urine output and an increase in nitrogenous waste, leading to azotaemia and uraemia.

- CKD is a slow, progressive and irreversible pathophysiological process with multiple aetiologies that results in the permanent loss of nephrons, tubular absorptive capacity, a decline in renal function and loss of endocrine functions; it frequently leads to kidney failure.

REVISE

TEST YOUR KNOWLEDGE

In this chapter you will have learned about disorders of fluid and electrolyte homeostasis and disorders that affect renal function and urinary continence. Test your knowledge by answering the questions below.

Answers are available online. If you are using the eBook just click on the answers icon below. Alternatively go to **https://study.sagepub.com/essentialpatho/answers**

1 What drug is normally used to treat diabetes insipidus and what is it a synthetic form of?

2 What levels are raised in SIADH?

3 What substances are lost from the extracellular compartment in CSWS?

4 What are the two main causes of osmotic diuresis?

5 Differentiate between upper and lower urinary tract infection (UTI) and identify the relative signs and symptoms.

6 Identify the common microorganisms that cause UTIs.

7 What are the risk factors associated with UTIs?

8 Identify the different types of kidney stones and explain how they are formed.

9 Identify the different types and causes of acute kidney injury (AKI).

10 Explain the three stages of AKI.

11 Explain how hypertension and diabetes mellitus can cause chronic kidney disease. Explain the pathophysiology of the signs and symptoms.

12 Identify and briefly explain the stages of CKD.

13 Identify the different types of urinary incontinence.

14 Explain the changes that occur with ageing that increase the incidence of urinary incontinence.

- Further revision and learning opportunities are available online

- Test yourself away from the book with **Extra multiple choice questions**

- Learn and revise terminology with **Interactive flashcards**

REVISE

ACE YOUR ASSESSMENT

If you are using the eBook access each resource by clicking on the respective icon. Alternatively go to **https://study.sagepub.com/essentialpatho/chapter11**

CHAPTER 11 ANSWERS

EXTRA QUESTIONS

FLASHCARDS

REFERENCES

Aboumarzouk, O.M. (2014) Extended spectrum beta-lactamase urinary tract infections. *Urology Annals*, 6 (2): 114–15.

Bailey, P.K., Hamilton, A.J., Clissold, R.L., Inward, C.D., Caskey, F.J., Ben-Shlomo, Y. et al. (2018) Young adults' perspectives on living with kidney failure: a systematic review and thematic synthesis of qualitative studies. *BMJ Open*, 8 (1): e019926.

Balogun, S.A., Balogun, R., Philbrick, J. and Abdel-Rahman, E. (2017) Quality of life, perceptions and health satisfaction of older adults with end-stage renal disease: a systematic review. *Journal of the American Geriatrics Society*, 65 (4): 777–85.

Blatherwick, N. and Long, M. (1923) Studies of urinary acidity, II: the increased acidity produced by eating prunes and cranberries. *Journal of Biological Chemistry*, 57: 815–18.

Bockenhauer, D. and Bichet, D.G. (2015) Pathophysiology, diagnosis and management of nephrogenic diabetes insipidus. *Nature Reviews Nephrology*, 11: 576–88.

Boore, J., Cook, N. and Shepherd, A. (2016) *Essentials of Anatomy and Physiology for Nursing Practice.* London: Sage.

Centers for Disease Control and Prevention (CDC) (2018) *Antibiotic Resistance: A Global Threat.* Available at: www.cdc.gov/features/antibiotic-resistance-global/index.html (accessed 6 July 2018).

Chen, S., Zhao, J., Tong, N., Guo, X., Qiu, M., Yang, G. et al. (2014) Randomized, double blinded, placebo-controlled trial to evaluate the efficacy and safety of tolvaptan in Chinese patients with hyponatremia caused by SIADH. *Journal of Clinical Pharmacology, 54* (12): 1362–7.

Dholke, H., Campos, A., Reddy, C.K. and Panigrahi, M.K. (2016) Cerebral salt wasting syndrome. *Journal of Neuroanaesthesiology & Critical Care, 3* (3): 205–10.

El-Sharkawy, A.M., Watson, P., Neal, K.R., Ljungqvist, O., Maughan, R.J., Sahota, O. et al. (2015) Hydration and outcome in older patients admitted to hospital (The HOOP prospective cohort study). *Age and Ageing, 44* (6): 943–7.

Esposito, C., Plati, A., Mazzullo, T., Fasoli, G., De Mauri, A., Grosjean, F. et al. (2007) Renal function and functional reserve in healthy elderly individuals. *Journal of Nephrology, 20* (5): 617–25.

Faull, R. and Lee, L. (2007) Prescribing in renal disease. *Australian Prescriber, 30* (1), doi: 10.18773/austprescr.2007.008.

Frieri, M., Kumar, K. and Boutin, A. (2017) Antibiotic resistance. *Journal of Infection and Public Health, 10*: 369–78.

Hamilton, A.J., Clissold, R.L., Inward, C.D., Caskey, F.J. and Ben-Shlomo, Y. (2017) Sociodemographic, psychological health and lifestyle outcomes in young adults on renal replacement therapy. *Clinical Journal of the American Society of Nephrology: CJASN, 12* (12): 1951–61.

Haylen, B.T., de Ridder, D., Freeman, R.M., Swift, S.E., Berghams, B., Lee, J. et al. (2010) An International Urogynecological Association (IUGA)/International Continence Society (ICS) joint report on the terminology for female pelvic floor dysfunction. *Neurourology and Urodynamics, 29* (1): 4–20.

Jha, V., Garcia-Garcia, G., Iseki, K., Li, Z., Naicker, S., Plattner, B. et al. (2013) Chronic kidney disease: global dimension and perspectives. *The Lancet, 382* (9888): 260–72.

John, C.A. and Day, M.W. (2012) Central neurogenic diabetes insipidus, syndrome of inappropriate secretion of antidiuretic hormone, and cerebral salt-wasting syndrome in traumatic brain injury. *Critical Care Nurse, 32* (2): e1–e8.

Kidney Disease: Improving Global Outcomes (KDIGO) CKD Work Group (2013) KDIGO 2012 Clinical Practice Guideline for the Evaluation and Management of Chronic Kidney Disease. *Kidney Int* (Suppl. 3): 1–150.

Lee, H., Han, K., Park, H., Shin, J., Kim, C., Namgung, M. et al. (2012) Familial renal glucosuria: a clinicogenetic study of 23 additional cases. *Pediatric Nephrology, 27* (7): 1091–5.

Levey, A.S. and Coresh, J. (2012) Chronic kidney disease. *The Lancet, 379* (9811): 165–80.

Liu, Y., Black, M.A., Caron, L. and Camesano, T. (2006) Role of cranberry juice on molecular-surface characteristics and adhesion behavior of *Escherichia coli. Biotechnology and Bioengeneering, 93* (2): 297–305.

MacGowan, A. and Macnaughton, E. (2017) Antibiotic resistance. *Medicine, 45* (10): 622–8.

NICE (2015) Urinary incontinence in women: management. Clinical guideline [CG171]. National Institute for Health and Care Excellence. Available at: www.nice.org.uk/guidance/cg171 (accessed 9 October 2018).

Poudel, R.R. (2013) Renal glucose handling in diabetes and sodium glucose cotransporter 2 inhibition. *Indian Journal of Endocrinology and Metabolism, 17* (4): 588–93.

Robertson, G.L. (2016) Diabetes insipidus: differential diagnosis and management. *Best Practice & Research: Clinical Endocrinology & Metabolism, 30*: 205–18.

Robinson, B.M., Akizawa, T., Jager, K.J., Kerr, P.G., Saran, R. and Pisoni, R.L. (2016) Factors affecting outcomes in patients reaching end-stage kidney disease worldwide: differences in access to renal replacement therapy, modality use, and haemodialysis practices. *The Lancet*, *388* (10041): 294–306.

Sumner, S., Forsyth, S., Collette-Merrill, K., Taylor, C., Vento, T., Veillette, J. et al. (2018) Antibiotic stewardship: the role of the clinical nurses and nurse educators. *Nurse Education Today*, *60*: 157–60.

Wang, C-H., Fang, C-C., Chen, N-C., Liu, S. S-H., Yu, P-H., Wu, T-Y. et al. (2012) Cranberry-containing products for prevention of urinary tract infections in susceptible populations. *Archives of Internal Medicine*, *172* (13): 988–96

Wang, P. (2013) The effectiveness of cranberry products to reduce urinary tract infections in females: a literature review. *Urological Nursing*, *33* (1): 38–45.

Wetmore, J.B. and Collins, A.J. (2016) Global challenges posed by the growth of end-stage renal disease. *Renal Replacement Therapy*, *2* (1): 15.

World Health Organisation (WHO) (2014) WHO's first global report on antibiotic resistance reveals serious, worldwide threat to public health. [online]. Available at: www.who.int/mediacentre/news/releases/2014/amr-report/en/ (accessed 6 July 2018).

World Health Organisation (WHO) (2018) Antimicrobial resistance. [online]. Available at: www.who.int/news-room/fact-sheets/detail/antimicrobial-resistance (accessed 6 July 2018).

DISORDERS OF NUTRIENT SUPPLY AND FAECAL ELIMINATION

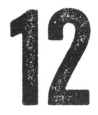

UNDERSTAND: CHAPTER VIDEOS

Watch the following videos to ease you into this chapter. If you are using the eBook just click on the play buttons. Alternatively go to **https://study.sagepub.com/essentialpatho/videos**

VOMITING (7:42)

COELIAC DISEASE (14:19)

INFLAMMATORY BOWEL DISEASE (8:58)

LEARNING OUTCOMES

When you have finished studying this chapter you will be able to:

1. Identify general disturbances of gastrointestinal function.
2. Describe the pathophysiology underpinning disorders of the upper gastrointestinal tract including: hiatal (or hiatus) hernia, gastroesophageal reflux, peptic ulcer disease and gastritis.
3. Outline conditions that affect the ability to meet nutritional requirements of the body.
4. Describe the pathophysiology underpinning disorders that affect the small and large intestine.
5. Outline the processes involved in inflammatory bowel disease.
6. Describe the pathophysiology of disorders that affect the accessory organs of digestion.

INTRODUCTION

In this chapter, you will consider disorders of the digestive system and accessory organs, nutrient supply and faecal elimination. As you do this, you will also consider the emotional/psychological and social implications of such pathophysiological changes, a central element of person-centred nursing.

The digestive system (gastrointestinal tract [GIT] and accessory organs) contributes to **homeostasis** by ensuring that the cells of the body receive the nutrients they require through digestion and **absorption** of the food we eat. The GIT is essentially external to the body; it is a continuous hollow organ that extends from the mouth to the anus and functions with the accessory organs including salivary glands, liver, gall bladder and pancreas. Disorders of the digestive system may disrupt one or more of its functions and can alter a person's self-image, their self-esteem and significantly reduce independence and social integration.

REVISE: A&P RECAP

The digestive system

Before reading this chapter, you may want to revise the digestive system. A full summary can be found in Chapter 8 of *Essentials of Anatomy and Physiology for Nursing Practice* (Boore et al., 2016).

This video on the digestive system may also help with revision. If you are using the eBook just click on the play button. Alternatively go to **https://study.sagepub.com/essentialpatho/videos**

DIGESTIVE SYSTEM (10:31)

PERSON-CENTRED CONTEXT: THE BODIE FAMILY

BODIE FAMILY
CASE NOTES

Each of the Bodie family is active in their own way and needs energy to be able to function socially and to have a sense of wellness. Gaining adequate **nutrition** is vital for them to function and so any disruption to the successful ingestion, digestion and absorption of nutrients would impact on such independence and their social role. Without adequate nutrients, the body cannot heal or fight off any **pathogen**s that may invade.

DISTURBANCES OF GASTROINTESTINAL FUNCTION

Constipation

Constipation refers to infrequent or difficult defaecation and usually indicates a decrease in the number of bowel movements per week and hard stools that are difficult to pass. Bowel habits may range from one to three times per day to once per week based on the person's activity levels and diet. It is important to note that what may constitute constipation for one person may well be normal for someone else. Box 12.1 presents the indicators for constipation.

Box 12.1   Indicators for constipation

Constipation is constituted by the presence of at least two of the following for a period of at least three months (Lacy et al., 2012):

- Straining to defaecate at least 25% of the time
- Lumpy/hard stools at least 25% of the time
- Sensation of incomplete emptying at least 25% of the time
- Manual evacuation of stools for at least 25% of defaecations
- Fewer than three bowel movements per week

Constipation can occur as a primary or secondary condition (Costilla and Foxx-Orenstein, 2014). Primary constipation can be classified into three categories:

1. *Normal transit constipation*: also known as functional constipation and involves a normal frequency of passing stools but evacuation is difficult. It is linked to a sedentary lifestyle, a low residue diet (limited intake of high fibre foods) or low fluid intake.
2. *Slow transit constipation*: involves infrequent bowel movements, straining to pass stools and mild abdominal distension caused by impaired colonic activity.
3. *Pelvic floor/outlet dysfunction*: dysfunction of the pelvic floor muscles or anal sphincter leads to difficulty or inability to defaecate.

Secondary constipation is related to disruption in neural pathways, **neurotransmitters** and a delay in transit time through the colon (see Chapter 16, **neurogenic bowel**). It may be caused by drugs, neurological disorders, e.g. **Parkinson's disease, multiple sclerosis** or **stroke**. Opiates, **diabetes mellitus, hypothyroidism, irritable bowel syndrome (IBS)** and pregnancy are also contributory factors. Ageing is inextricably linked with constipation and may be caused by a decrease in activity levels, mobility, comorbidities and concomitant drug use. Constipation is not usually considered significant unless it impairs quality of life; it may also be an indicator of colorectal **cancer** (Guérin et al., 2014).

Diarrhoea

Diarrhoea is the excessive passage of loose, watery stools. It can be **acute**, persistent or **chronic**. Acute diarrhoea occurs when three or more loose stools develop within 24 hours and can last up to 14 days. It can be divided into large volume (non-inflammatory) and small volume (inflammatory). Table 12.1 identifies the characteristics of both types of acute diarrhoea.

Persistent diarrhoea refers to diarrhoea that lasts longer than 14 days and up to 30 days. Chronic diarrhoea refers to diarrhoea that persists for 3 or 4 weeks. It is associated with **malabsorption syndrome, inflammatory bowel disease (IBD)** (both discussed later in the chapter), **hyperthyroidism** or **diabetic autonomic neuropathy** (a complication associated with diabetes, it is a form of peripheral **neuropathy**, i.e. damage to either parasympathetic or sympathetic nerves or both) (Vuckovic-Rebrina et al., 2013). There are three primary categories of diarrhoea:

- *Osmotic diarrhoea*: nonabsorbable substances are hyperosmotic and excess water is pulled into the bowel and increases the volume and weight of stools. It can be due to **lactose intolerance**, excessive use of antacids and osmotic laxatives or decreased transit time.

- *Secretory diarrhoea*: occurs due to increased mucosal secretions of fluid and **electrolytes**. It can be caused by infectious agents, e.g. **viruses**, bacteria, excess bile agents or overgrowth of small bowel **microbiome**, and leads to large volume diarrhoea. Small volume diarrhoea is commonly caused by acute or chronic inflammation of the colon.
- *Motility diarrhoea*: occurs when there is a decrease in transit time, meaning that fluid absorption is decreased. It can be caused by short bowel syndrome (resection of the small intestine), fistula formation, irritable bowel syndrome (IBS) or laxative abuse.

Table 12.1 Characteristics of large and small volume diarrhoea

Large volume (non-inflammatory)	Small volume (inflammatory)
Volume increased	Volume not increased
Watery, non-bloody stools	Bloody stools
Periumbilical cramps	Lower abdominal pain
Bloating	Urgent desire to defecate
Nausea and vomiting	No nausea or vomiting
Caused by toxin-producing bacteria, e.g. *Escherichia coli (E. coli)*, *Staphylococcus aureus*	Caused by bacterial invasion of intestinal cells, e.g. *Shigella, Salmonella*
Hypokalaemia, metabolic acidosis	
No tissue invasion or inflammation	

Vomiting

Vomiting or **emesis** is the forceful expulsion of **chyme** (stomach and/or intestinal contents) through the mouth (Babic and Browning, 2014). Nausea or 'feeling sick' is a subjective experience that is related to a number of conditions, e.g. pain, hypersalivation or 'water brash' (regurgitated excessive saliva from the lower part of the oesophagus, often with some acid from stomach). **Retching** is the muscular event that occurs but it does not expel stomach contents. Both nausea and retching may precede vomiting, however spontaneous vomiting that is not preceded by nausea or retching is known as projectile vomiting and is caused by direct stimulation of the vomiting centre, e.g. raised intracranial pressure (ICP).

The vomiting centre is located in the medulla oblongata and is responsible for co-ordinating activities associated with vomiting. It can be activated by numerous stimuli including: irritation/distension of the stomach/duodenum, severe pain, **stress**, unpleasant sights or smells, raised ICP, motion sickness and the side-effects of drugs. A number of involuntary activities are involved in the vomiting reflex, including the relaxation of oesophageal sphincters, raising of intrathoracic pressure, the contraction of abdominal muscles and activation of the autonomic nervous system (Figure 12.1).

DISORDERS OF NUTRITION

Anorexia

In **anorexia** the normal physiological stimuli that produce hunger remain intact, however there is a lack of desire to eat. It is usually associated with nausea, diarrhoea and abdominal pain. It can also be caused by psychological stress, as a side-effect of drugs and diseases of other organs/systems, e.g. kidney disease, cancer. Anorexia is different from anorexia nervosa, a mental ill-health disorder that is related to restricting the amount of food consumed coupled with excessive exercise. With anorexia nervosa, the way the person sees themselves is usually at odds with how others see them.

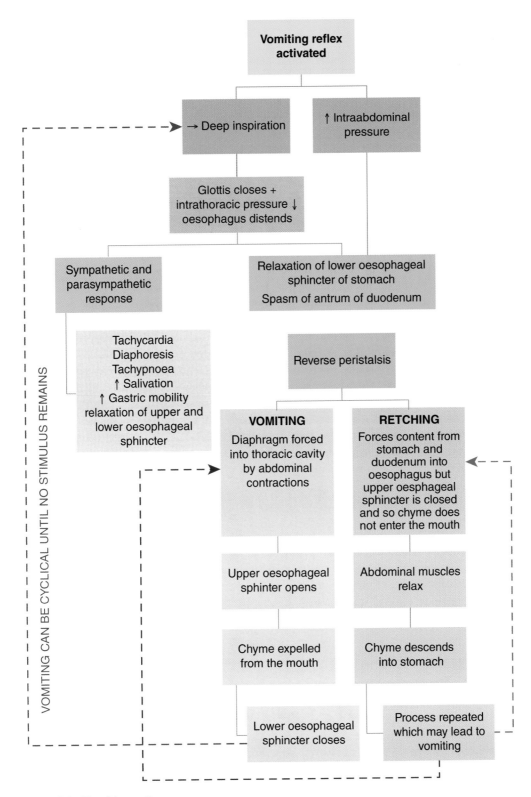

Figure 12.1 Vomiting reflex

Malnutrition

Malnutrition refers to a lack of nourishment due to inadequate/inappropriate amounts of calories, macronutrients (fat, protein and carbohydrates) and micronutrients (vitamins and minerals). It is due to improper diet, changes in digestion and absorption, long-term disease or a combination of one or more of these factors. Whilst malnutrition usually implies someone is underweight, it is important to remember that someone who is **overweight**/obese can also be malnourished.

Starvation

Starvation refers to a decrease in energy intake that can be considered in relation to short-term or long-term starvation; ultimately both lead to weight loss.

Short-term starvation refers to a period of time, usually several days, where there is total dietary deprivation or abstinence. **Glycogenolysis**, the conversion of **glycogen** to glucose, is the process that occurs when all available energy has been absorbed by the intestine. After 4–8 hours the process of **gluconeogenesis**, i.e. the production of glucose from **lactate**, amino acids and the glycerol component of fat, begins. Both glycogenolysis and gluconeogenesis deplete the body's stored nutrients; over time, the energy demands of the body will no longer be able to be met. Despite this depletion, proteins are catabolised to a minimal degree and provide the carbon that is needed to generate glucose required by the brain.

Long-term starvation begins after several days of not ingesting nutrients; eventually it will lead to death. Long-term starvation is related to a reduction in energy expenditure and increased use of **ketones** as a source for cellular energy. There is increased **lipolysis** (breakdown of fats/lipids into fatty acids) due to reduced levels of **insulin** and **glucagon**. Lipolysis provides a supply of fatty acids that can be used as energy by skeletal and cardiac muscle and ketone bodies that can be used by the brain to maintain function. **Proteolysis** (breakdown of proteins) is initiated once adipose tissue is depleted. Breakdown of muscle protein is the last energy source the body can use. Electrolyte abnormalities, loss of kidney, respiratory and cardiac function will eventually lead to death.

CACHEXIA

Cachexia refers to weight loss, muscle atrophy, fatigue and weakness that are associated with physical wasting. It is caused by the release of inflammatory **cytokines** that decrease the body's response to **ghrelin** and starts wasting of skeletal muscle. Cachexia is usually seen in relation to many end-of-life long-term conditions, e.g. end-stage **chronic obstructive pulmonary disease (COPD)**, cancer or **acquired immunodeficiency syndrome (AIDS)**.

APPLY

Refeeding syndrome

Refeeding syndrome (RFS) is a syndrome that consists of metabolic disturbances following reinstitution of nutrition to people who are severely malnourished, starved or metabolically stressed due to severe illness, e.g. **sepsis**, major **surgery** or critical illness. RFS is potentially fatal and there is limited knowledge regarding its management. Increased knowledge and understanding of the nutritional needs of the critically ill will prevent illness associated with RFS and over time this will contribute to reducing the **morbidity** and mortality associated with FRS (Nasir et al., 2018).

RFS occurs when too much food and/or liquid nutrition (**enteral** or **parenteral**) is consumed within the first few days of refeeding. Refeeding triggers the synthesis of glycogen, fat and protein in cells to the detriment of serum concentrations of potassium, magnesium and phosphorous. A potentially fatal shift in fluid occurs that results from hormonal and metabolic changes; the hallmark of RFS is **hypophosphataemia** (Mehanna et al., 2009), although deranged sodium and fluid balance, thiamine deficiency, hypomagnesaemia and hypokalaemia may also be present. The formation of phosphyrolated carbohydrate compounds in the liver and skeletal muscle leads to the depletion of **adenosine triphosphate (ATP)** and 2-3 diphosphoglycerate in red blood cells that leads to cellular dysfunction and inadequate oxygen supply to body cells and tissues. Symptoms of refeeding include neurological deficits and alterations in cardiac and pulmonary function. Whilst RFS is recognised as a life-threatening condition, Matthews et al. (2018) identified that RFS was a rare underlying cause of death. Tables 12.2 and 12.3 will help you identify those at risk of RFS and the associated criteria for risk of refeeding problems.

Table 12.2 Risk factors for developing refeeding syndrome (RFS)

AIDS	Chronic malnutrition, e.g. morbid obesity with profound weight loss, IBD, **cystic fibrosis**, high stress unfed for >7days
Alcohol dependency	
Anorexia nervosa	
Oncology patients	Chronic pancreatitis
Postoperative patients	Elderly persons with comorbidities and decreased physiological reserve
Uncontrolled diabetes mellitus	Long-term use of antacids or diuretics

Source: National Institute for Health and Care Excellence (NICE), 2017

Table 12.3 Criteria for identifying people at high risk of refeeding problems

One or more of the following:	Two or more of the following:
BMI <16	BMI <18.5
Unintentional weight loss >15% in 3-6 months	Unintentional weight loss >10% in 3-6 months
Little or no nutritional intake >10 days	Little or no nutritional intake >15 days
Decreased levels of potassium, phosphate or magnesium before feeding	History of alcohol/drug misuse including insulin, chemotherapy, antacids, diuretics

Source: National Institute for Health and Care Excellence (NICE), 2017

Overweight and obesity

Overweight and obesity can be defined as the abnormal or excessive fat accumulation that may impair health and is one of the greatest public health challenges of the twenty-first century (World Health Organisation (WHO), 2018). Regulation of appetite, energy **metabolism**, eating behaviours and body fat mass is under neuroendocrine control. Signalling mediators, including insulin, ghrelin, **leptin**, **adiponectin**, glucagon-like peptide-1 and peptide YY from the peripheries, act centrally on the **hypothalamus** and brain stem to regulate hunger and satiety (Scerif et al., 2011). Food intake and energy expenditure are controlled by the interaction of these mediators and hypothalamic **neurons**, orexigenic (appetite stimulating) neurons that increase food intake, and decrease metabolism or anorexigenic neurons that decrease food intake and increase metabolism. The limbic system is responsible for the reward/pleasure experience of food. The rewarding nature of food, i.e. palatability and pleasure, is capable of overriding the homeostatic mechanism response (act as a stimulus in energy deficit absence) due to opioid and cannabinoid receptors that stimulate hypothalamic beta-endorphin release; food intake is thereby increased due to palatability as opposed to hunger.

The development of obesity therefore involves the interaction of both central and peripheral pathways and the release of hormones and neurotransmitters (Dickson et al., 2011). White **adipocytes** (in peripheries) are responsible for the storage of **triglycerides** and the secretion of **adipokines**, e.g. leptin, adiponectin and other hormones. They have the ability to undergo **hypertrophy** and hyperplasia, depending on the amount of triglyceride to be stored. An increase in visceral fats leads to a dysfunction/dysregulation of cytokines and hormones and the interaction with hypothalamic neurons responsible for increased fat mass associated with obesity (Scerif et al., 2011).

Leptin is known as the 'satiety hormone' and is released from adipocytes and functions alongside the hypothalamus to maintain body weight within a narrow range. Leptin production increases with an increased number of adipocytes. However, increased leptin levels are ineffective at reducing appetite and energy; this condition is known as leptin resistance (Sáinz et al., 2015). Orexigenic neurons are not inhibited and this leads to a promotion of overeating and weight gain. As leptin levels rise there is a simultaneous increase in ghrelin 'hunger hormone' that consequently stimulates orexigenic neurons to increase appetite, leading to further food consumption. Scerif et al. (2011), however, have identified that ghrelin levels are actually reduced in people with obesity. A further decrease in anorexigenic stimulation occurs due to reduced levels of peptide YY (reduces appetite) and adiponectin (insulin-sensitising and increases glucose uptake). Insulin resistance develops as levels of adiponectin decrease.

Hyperplastic adipocytes increase the rate of lipolysis and the secretion of proinflammatory adipokines from T-lymphocytes and activated **macrophages**. The resultant low-grade systemic inflammatory response alongside increased lipolysis contributes to insulin resistance and metabolic syndrome (discussed in Chapter 13). Obesity is a major risk factor for a number of chronic diseases, e.g. diabetes mellitus, **cardiovascular disease**, cancer and musculoskeletal disorders, especially **osteoarthritis**.

ACTIVITY 12.1: APPLY

Reflection

Considering the physiological changes that occur in someone who is overweight and has obesity, reflect on how society may treat or judge someone in these clinical states. Does this knowledge of the biological mechanisms involved change your thoughts and beliefs? How will you respond and how does this fit with being a person-centred practitioner?

DISORDERS OF THE UPPER GASTROINTESTINAL TRACT

Hiatal hernia

Hiatal hernia (also referred to as **hiatus hernia**) is a diaphragmatic protrusion (herniation) of the stomach (upper part) through the diaphragm into the thorax. There are four types of hiatal hernia: type I, type II, type III and type IV, discussed below (Figure 12.2):

Type II (True paraoesophageal)

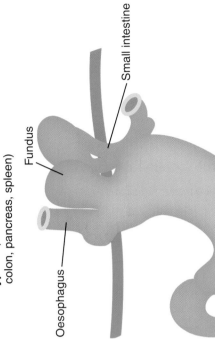

Fundus

Oesophagus

Gastroesophageal junction

Diaphragm

Pyloric sphincter

Greater curvature

Stomach

Lesser curvature

Type I (Sliding)

Gastroesophageal junction

Fundus

Oesophagus

Cardiac sphincter

Diaphragm

Pyloric sphincter

Greater curvature

Lesser curvature

Stomach

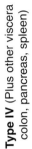

Type IV (Plus other viscera colon, pancreas, spleen)

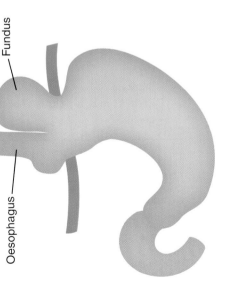

Small intestine

Fundus

Oesophagus

Illustrated by Shaun Mercier © SAGE Publications

Type III (Mixed)

Fundus

Oesophagus

Figure 12.2 Types of hiatal hernia

- *Type I* is known as a sliding hiatal hernia; the gastroesophageal junction (the point where the oesophagus and stomach join) moves above the diaphragm, the stomach remains in its usual alignment and the **fundus** remains below the gastroesophageal junction.
- *Type II* is a pure paraoesophageal hernia (PEH); the gastroesophageal junction remains in its usual anatomic position, however a portion of the fundus protrudes through the diaphragmatic hiatus beside the oesophagus.
- *Type III* is a mixed hiatal hernia and is a combination of type I and type II. Both the gastroesophageal junction and the fundus lie above the diaphragm.
- *Type IV* is a hiatal hernia that is characterised by the presence of another structure (other than the stomach), e.g. **omentum** (a fold of visceral peritoneal tissue that hangs from the stomach), small intestine or colon within the hernia sac.

Gastroesophageal reflux disease (GORD/GERD)

Gastroesophageal reflux disease develops when there is persistent reflux of stomach contents, i.e. acid, pepsin and bile salts, into the oesophagus, causing oesophagitis. The cause of GERD/GORD is unknown, however it is thought to be linked with abnormalities of the lower oesophageal sphincter (LOS) that allows the reflux of stomach contents to occur (Lee and McColl, 2013). It is also linked with oesophageal motility and prolonged oesophageal clearance, diminished saliva production, impaired mucosal resistance and delayed gastric emptying (Lee and McColl, 2013). Predisposing factors for the development of GORD are listed in Box 12.2. The severity of the oesophagitis associated with GORD depends on the composition of gastric contents and the length of time that the oesophageal mucosa is exposed to them. Injury to the **mucosa** occurs when there are frequent and prolonged episodes of reflux.

Box 12.2   Predisposing factors for development of GORD

- Hiatal hernia
- Obesity
- Pregnancy
- Smoking
- Certain foods, e.g. citrus, chocolate, caffeine, alcohol, fatty and fried foods, spicy foods, garlic, onions

---

Signs and symptoms

Signs and symptoms of GORD can be classified as either oesophageal or extraoesophageal (Table 12.4).

Table 12.4   Classifications of GORD

Oesophageal	Extraoesophageal
Heartburn	Sore throat, hoarseness
Chest pain	Frequent clearing of throat
Water brash	Loss of dental enamel
Regurgitation (food and liquid)	Cough
	Asthma
	Aspiration **pneumonia**

Gastroesophageal reflux disease in children

Gastroesophageal reflux is considered a normal physiological event in infants and children, however GORD occurs whenever the process causes symptoms severe enough to warrant medical intervention (Davies et al., 2015). An infant's stomach only has a small capacity; alongside this there is a regular spontaneous decrease in LOS pressure, both of which contribute to reflux. The LOS is weakened or relaxes when it shouldn't; this may be caused by being born prematurely, hiatal hernia, being overweight, exposure to second-hand smoke, or neurological conditions, e.g. **cerebral palsy** (Davies et al., 2015). It is usual for children to grow out of this by the age of 1 (Davies et al., 2015).

Signs and symptoms

There are a number of signs and symptoms that may indicate that an infant or child has GORD, and these include:

- Refusing to eat/feeding problems
- Not gaining weight
- Pain when swallowing
- Heartburn
- **Haematemesis** (vomiting of blood)
- Regurgitation associated with recurrent **otalgia** (ear pain – occurs through referral from vagus nerve in oesophagus to ear)
- **Dyspnoea**
- Laryngospasm
- Apnoea
- **Bradycardia**
- Dental caries (tooth decay)
- Halitosis (bad breath)
- In severe reflux, the child may tilt their head to one side and arch their back

APPLY

Lifestyle changes and drugs required with GORD

GORD may be successfully treated by making some lifestyle changes. These include:

- Weight loss (if necessary)
- Eat smaller meals
- Avoid high fat or spicy foods
- Wear loose-fitting clothing, especially around abdominal region
- Stay upright for 3 hours after eating
- Avoid reclining/slouching when sitting
- Sleep at a slight angle - raise head of bed by 15-20 cm

It may also be necessary to take drugs to treat GORD. These include:

- H_2 blockers, e.g. ranitidine
- PPIs, e.g. omeprazole
- Prokinetics, e.g. metoclopramide

Gastritis

The gastric mucosa is protected by a number of mechanisms, including: an epithelial surface that is impermeable, the secretion of hydrogen and bicarbonate ions and the production of gastric **mucus**. Together these form the gastric mucosal barrier and prevent autodigestion of the stomach wall by the hydrochloric acid it secretes. Gastritis is inflammation of the gastric mucosa and can be acute or chronic. There are numerous causative factors that can contribute to the development of either form.

Acute gastritis

Acute gastritis is most commonly associated with taking regular non-steroidal anti-inflammatory drugs or aspirin, increased alcohol intake or bacterial toxins (van der Post and Carneiro, 2017). It is usually transient and self-limiting in nature with the gastric mucosa completely regenerating within a few days following removal of the causative factor. Acute gastritis is characterised by an acute inflammatory response and may be accompanied by bleeding into the gastric mucosa.

Signs and symptoms

Signs and symptoms associated with acute gastritis may vary according to the causative factor:

* Aspirin- or NSAID-related – may be unaware of the condition, only symptom may be heartburn.
* Increased alcohol consumption – gastric distress, vomiting, in severe cases there may be haematemesis.
* Bacterial toxins – abrupt onset usually within 5 hours following exposure to the infective agent, vomiting and gastric distress.

Chronic gastritis

In chronic gastritis there are chronic inflammatory changes that lead to atrophy of the glandular gastric **epithelium**, but there is an absence of excessive visible erosions. There are three different types of chronic gastritis: *Helicobacter pylori* (*H. pylori*) gastritis, chronic autoimmune gastritis and **chemical gastropathy**.

Signs and symptoms

There are numerous signs and symptoms associated with chronic gastritis, including:

* Upper abdominal pain
* Indigestion
* Bloating
* Nausea/vomiting
* Belching
* Anorexia/loss of appetite
* Weight loss

GO DEEPER

Types of chronic gastritis

H. pylori gastritis

H. pylori gastritis is the most common cause of chronic gastritis and affects the antrum and body of the stomach. H. pylori bacteria cause chronic inflammation of the gastric mucosa by producing enzymes and toxins that disrupt the protection of the gastric mucosa from acid and produce a continuous inflammatory response with **infiltration** of **neutrophils** followed by T and B **lymphocytes**. Microbial and host factors both play a role in H. pylori infection, hence the reason why the clinical course will vary from person to person. Inflammation may only occur within the superficial gastric epithelium or it may spread deeper into the gastric glands, therefore there will be varying degrees of atrophy and **metaplasia** (the reversible transformation of one differentiated cell type to another).

Signs and symptoms

Acute infection may cause nausea and abdominal pain that can last several days. The person may then become asymptomatic although chronic inflammation will persist. Chronic infection may lead to the development of **peptic ulcer disease** and gastric atrophy. It is also linked to an increased risk of gastric **adenocarcinoma** and low-grade B-cell gastric lymphoma (Zucca et al., 2014).

Chronic autoimmune gastritis

Chronic autoimmune gastritis affects the body and fundus of the stomach. It is linked to other autoimmune conditions such as type 1 diabetes mellitus and Hashimoto thyroiditis (a form of hypothyroidism). Production of autoantibodies to the parietal cells and intrinsic factors, leading to faulty gastric acid secretion and vitamin B_{12} deficiency, will eventually lead to pernicious **anaemia**. There is increased risk of gastric adenocarcinoma due to metaplastic changes caused by atrophy of the fundic glands (oxyntic glands that secrete hydrochloric acid and intrinsic factors) and chief cells (peptic cells that release **pepsinogen** and chymosin).

Signs and symptoms

Chronic autoimmune gastritis is characterised by slow onset and **progression**; people affected by the condition may not be diagnosed for a number of years. Signs and symptoms are usually related to anaemia. Vitamin B_{12} deficiency may also lead to malabsorptive diarrhoea, atrophic glossitis and neuropathies in particular peripheral neuropathies, leading to **paraesthesia** and numbness. Cerebral neuropathies may be distinguished by mild personality changes and memory loss.

Chemical gastrophy

Chemical gastrophy refers to the injury caused to gastric mucosa from long-term reflux into the stomach of duodenal contents, pancreatic secretions and bile. It can be linked to the presence of a gastric ulcer or gall bladder disease. It is more commonly associated with those who have undergone surgical procedures for gastroduodenostomy or gastrojejunostomy.

Peptic ulcer disease

Gastroduodenal mucosa can withstand the digestive action of hydrochloric acid, pepsin and bile due to a number of mechanisms; this highly acidic environment aids the digestive process but also has the potential to damage the mucosa, resulting in ulceration. Peptic ulcer disease is a term used to describe

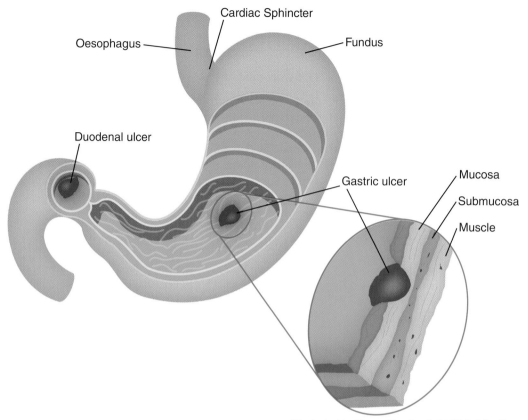

Illustrated by Shaun Mercier © SAGE Publications

Figure 12.3 Peptic ulcer disease

ulceration that occurs in the gastric or intestinal mucosal lining. Ulcers can be single or multiple, superficial or deep and acute or chronic.

Excessive acid secretions can lead to the destruction of the mucous membrane and decreased mucus production can leave the mucosal lining unprotected. All layers of the stomach or duodenum may be affected and the ulcer may penetrate only the mucosal layer or it could extend into the layers of smooth muscle (Figure 12.3). As healing occurs the muscularis layer is replaced with scar tissue. Whilst regeneration of the muscle layer occurs over the scar tissue, it may be imperfect, contributing to repeated episodes of ulceration; spontaneous **remission**s and exacerbations are common. Numerous risk factors have been identified as contributing to the development of peptic ulcer disease and these are summarised in Box 12.3.

Box 12.3   Risk factors for peptic ulcer disease

- *Helicobacter pylori* (*H. pylori*) infection of gastric and/or duodenal mucosal tissue
- Long-term use of non-steroidal anti-inflammatory drugs (NSAIDs) or aspirin
- Ageing
- Genetic factors that make people more susceptible include:
  - people with Type O blood – blood group **antigen**s correlate with peptic ulcer disease (Rubin, 2012)
  - people who do not secrete antigens in their saliva or gastric juices (Rubin, 2012)

- Excessive alcohol intake
- Smoking
- Obesity
- Long-term conditions, e.g. **rheumatoid arthritis**, diabetes, **emphysema**
- Psychological stress

Gastric ulcer

Gastric ulcers are those that occur in the stomach and affect both men and women equally, usually between the ages of 55 and 65. Most gastric ulcers develop in the antral region of the stomach (initial portion of the pylorus – near the bottom of the stomach) adjacent to the acid-secreting mucosa. The mucosal barrier increases its permeability to hydrogen ions, there may be a reduction in parietal cell mass and gastric secretion may be normal or less than normal. Gastric ulcers may occur as a consequence of chronic gastritis that may precipitate the formation of an ulcer by limiting the mucosa's ability to secrete a protective mucus layer. Other factors that may precipitate the development of gastric ulcers include:

- *H. pylori* infection: *H. pylori* secretes urease that converts blood urea to ammonia which weakens the blood mucosal barrier, secretes toxins that destroy epithelial cells and produces **platelet-activating factor**.
- NSAIDs (non-steroidal anti-inflammatory drugs which relieve pain, reduce inflammation and reduce fever): inhibit the enzyme cyclooxygenase and reduce the synthesis of prostaglandin (PGE_2) and prostacyclin (PGI_2) from arachidonic acid. The arachidonic acid is converted to lipoxygenase which leads to increased production of leukotriene (LTB_4), causing neutrophil adhesion to the **endothelium** of the small mucosal blood vessels. This leads to **ischaemia**, **hypoxia** and the release of **proteases** and **reactive oxygen species** from neutrophils.
- Decreased mucosal synthesis of **prostaglandins**.
- Duodenal reflux of bile and pancreatic enzymes that subsequently damages the mucosal membrane.

Once the mucosal barrier is broken, hydrogen ions diffuse into the mucosa and change the permeability and cellular structure. **Histamine** is released from the damaged mucosa, leading to increased secretion of acid and production of pepsinogen, increased blood flow and capillary permeability, leading to **oedema** and the loss of plasma proteins. Bleeding is due to the destruction of small blood vessels. The characteristics of gastric ulcers are similar to those of duodenal ulcers and are presented in Table 12.5.

Duodenal ulcer

Duodenal ulcers occur in the duodenum and are the most common type of peptic ulcer occurring between the ages of 20 and 50 years and are more common in males than females. They are associated with *H. pylori* infection and prolonged NSAID use. Increased acid and pepsinogen concentrations in the duodenum penetrate the mucosal barrier, resulting in the formation of an ulcer. Activation of T and B lymphocytes and infiltration of neutrophils happen in response to *H. pylori* infection. Gastric epithelium is destroyed due to the release of inflammatory cytokines. Inflammation and **apoptosis** of gastric epithelium are due to cytotoxin-associated gene A (*Cag A*) (an *H. pylori* virulence factor) producing **vacuolating toxin** (*VacA*).

Table 12.5 Characteristics of gastric and duodenal ulcers

Characteristic	Gastric ulcer	Duodenal ulcer
Pain	Epigastric	Epigastric
	Intermittent	Intermittent
	Immediately after eating	2–3 hours after eating
		Empty stomach
		Relieved by eating or antacids
Weight loss	Yes	No
Vomiting	Yes	No
Healing time	Slowly	Quickly
Remission and exacerbations	No - chronic	Yes

Stress ulcers

Stress ulcers are an acute form of peptic ulcer that occur alongside periods of physiological stress associated with major trauma or illness. Multiple sites of ulceration occur throughout the stomach and duodenum. Stress ulcers can be categorised as either ischaemic ulcers or Cushing ulcers:

- *Ischaemic ulcers* can develop following haemorrhage, multisystem trauma, severe burns, **heart failure** or sepsis and occur within hours. They result in shock, **anoxia**, sympathetic nervous system activation and in ischaemia, tissue acidosis and bile salts entering the stomach. They are usually found in the fundus of the stomach and proximal duodenum.
- *Cushing ulcers* are usually found in the stomach, duodenum and oesophagus and are associated with brain trauma or brain surgery. They occur due to hypersecretion of gastric acid and decreased mucosal blood flow caused by overstimulation of vagal nuclei by increased intracranial pressure, resulting in damage to the mucosal barrier and in erosion and ulceration.

APPLY

Treatment of peptic ulcer

- Antibiotic therapy - clarithromycin and amoxicillin or metronidazole if allergic to penicillin.
- Proton pump inhibitors inhibit gastric acid secretion by blocking the hydrogen-potassium adenosine triphosphatase enzyme system (the 'proton pump') of the gastric parietal cell, e.g. pantoprazole.
- H_2-receptor **antagonists** reduce gastric acid output as a result of histamine H_2-receptor blockade, e.g. ranitidine.

Recommended regimens for *H. pylori* eradication in adults

- **First-line treatment:** Offer people who test positive for *H. pylori* a 7-day, twice-daily course of treatment with:
  - a PPI and
  - amoxicillin and
  - either clarithromycin or metronidazole.

- **Second-line treatment:** Offer people who still have symptoms after first-line eradication treatment a 7-day, twice-daily course of treatment with:

  o a PPI **and**

  o amoxicillin **and**

  o either clarithromycin or metronidazole (whichever was not used first-line).

Source: National Institute for Health and Care Excellence (NICE), 2014

DISORDERS OF THE LOWER GASTROINTESTINAL TRACT

Malabsorption syndromes

Malabsorption syndromes refer to disorders that interfere with intestinal absorptive processes. They have been previously classified as maldigestion or malabsorption. Maldigestion infers a failure of the chemical processes associated with digestion that occur within the intestinal lumen. It is commonly caused by a reduction in digestive enzymes, inadequate secretion of bile salts or inadequate reabsorption of bile. Malabsorption refers to the inability of the intestinal mucosa to absorb digested nutrients. It is usually due to mucosal disruption as a consequence of gastric or intestinal resection, intestinal disorders or vascular disorders.

Failure to digest and absorb nutrients leads to a wide range of signs and symptoms (Table 12.6). A distinctive feature associated with malabsorption of nutrients is **steatorrhoea**, i.e. fatty, yellow-grey coloured foul-smelling stools. Diarrhoea, flatulence, bloating, abdominal pain/cramps and weight loss are also very common.

Table 12.6 Signs and symptoms of malabsorption syndromes

Nutrient	Site of absorption	Requirements	Signs and symptoms
Carbohydrates – starch, sucrose, lactose, maltose and fructose	Small intestine	**Amylase**, maltase, sucrase and lactase enzymes	Diarrhoea, flatulence, abdominal distension
Protein	Small intestine	Pancreatic enzymes	Weakness, oedema, loss of muscle mass
Fat	Jejunum	Pancreatic **lipase**, bile salts, lymphatic channels	Steatorrhoea, weight loss, deficiency of vitamins A, D, E and K (fat-soluble vitamins)
Vitamins A, B_9 (folic acid), B_{12}, D, E and K	Small intestine	Biles salts and intrinsic factor	Depends on vitamin lack: Dry eyes, night blindness, glossitis, neuropathies, **fractures**, bone pain, increased bruising/bleeding
Iron	Upper small intestine (duodenum and jejunum)	Hydrochloric acid	Iron deficiency anaemia, glossitis
Calcium	Duodenum	Vitamin D, parathyroid hormone	Fractures, bone pain, tetany

Pancreatic exocrine insufficiency

Pancreatic exocrine insufficiency refers to the inability to produce pancreatic enzymes, e.g. lipase, amylase, **procarboxypeptidase**, **trypsinogen** and **chymotrypsinogen**, that are essential for the digestion of carbohydrates, fats and proteins (macronutrients). Extensive damage or loss of pancreatic tissue may occur prior to a significant decrease in the levels of enzymes produced to cause maldigestion of nutrients. **Cystic fibrosis**, **chronic pancreatitis** and pancreatic cancer are the main causative factors associated with damage/loss of pancreatic tissue. Whilst maldigestion of all the macronutrients are affected by pancreatic insufficiency, it is the maldigestion of fat (decreased levels of pancreatic lipase) that is the key issue. Activation of pancreatic enzymes that may be present is inhibited by the acidic environment due to the absence of pancreatic bicarbonate (see Chapter 8 in Boore et al., 2016). Steatorrhoea, weight loss and fat-soluble vitamin deficiency are primary indicators due to pancreatic exocrine insufficiency.

Lactose intolerance

A genetic fault in the production of lactase leads to a deficiency of disaccharidase at the brush border. The breakdown of lactose into monosaccharides is prevented by lactase deficiency, thereby inhibiting the digestion and absorption of lactose across the intestinal wall; this results in lactose intolerance. Lactase deficiency may also be due to a number of diseases of the intestine, including **coeliac disease**, bacterial overgrowth and inflammation of the small intestine. Undigested lactose leads to the development of gases as it undergoes bacterial fermentation. This gives rise to excess intraluminal gas that can cause flatus, abdominal distension and **borborygmus** (a rumbling sound made by the movement of intestinal fluid/gas) (Deng et al., 2015). The osmotic gradient in the intestine increases due to the undigested lactose, causing irritation and osmotic diarrhoea. People who are lactose intolerant may complain of bloating, flatulence, crampy abdominal pain and diarrhoea if they consume products containing lactose as a result of these physiological processes.

Coeliac disease

Coeliac disease, a condition in which there is malabsorption in the small intestine with associated inflammation, is one of the most common genetic diseases worldwide. It is associated with the **major histocompatibility complex (MHC)** class II allele, human leucocyte antigen (HLA), HLA-DQ$_2$ and HLA-DQ$_8$ and causes an inappropriate T-cell-mediated response against **gliadin** (a protein that is a component of gluten) (Koning et al., 2015). There is an increase in **antibodies** to a range of antigens including transglutaminase, gliadin and endomysin. The immunological response produces an intense

ACTIVITY 12.2: APPLY

Living with coeliac disease

As a person-centred practitioner, it is important that you understand the lived experience of coeliac disease in order to understand the social reality of people in your care. Watch the following video to gain insight into the lived experience. If you are using the eBook just click on the play button. Alternatively go to **https://study.sagepub.com/essentialpatho/videos**

COELIAC DISEASE (4:42)

inflammatory response that has a toxic effect on the small intestine, resulting in villi atrophy and subsequent loss of absorptive surfaces and a reduction in enzyme production. Extensive **lesions** can impair the absorption of both macro and micro nutrients.

Signs and symptoms associated with coeliac disease vary with age. Younger children may have diarrhoea, abdominal distension and fail to thrive. In older children, signs and symptoms include short stature, constipation, dental caries and anaemia. In adults, the most common presenting feature is diarrhoea accompanied by abdominal pain. Iron deficiency anaemia and **osteoporosis** are also found in adults who have coeliac disease.

Irritable bowel syndrome (IBS)

Irritable bowel syndrome (IBS) is a gastrointestinal (GI) disorder affecting approximately 10–15% of the population worldwide (Lovell and Ford, 2012) and tends to affect young and middle-aged women primarily. It is associated with recurrent abdominal pain and altered bowel habits and can be either diarrhoea-prevalent or constipation-prevalent. Whilst the aetiology of IBS is unknown, evidence attempts to explain the various symptoms and presentations, particularly in relation to **dysbiosis** (microbial imbalance/maladaptation in the GIT), food intolerances, **epigenetics** (psychosocial factors), changes in GI motility and secretions (Catanzaro et al., 2014; Vaiopoulou et al., 2014).

--- **GO DEEPER** ---

Various presentations of irritable bowel syndrome (IBS)

1. Visceral *hypersensitivity/hyperalgesia* – increased sensitivity to visceral pain; may originate via the peripheral or central nervous system. It may be caused by dysregulation of the gut-brain axis (Mayer et al., 2014), affecting the function of serotonin-secreting cells of gut-brain pain modulation. Changes in metabolite production by gut microbiota and activation of gut immune system, increased visceral permeability and sensitivity and altered motility (Cross-Adame and Rao, 2014) are also contributory factors.
2. *Abnormal GI motility, permeability and secretion* – those with diarrhoea-prevalent IBS have decreased colonic transit time and increased permeability. Those with constipation-prevalent IBS experience increased colonic transit time and decreased permeability. It is thought to occur due to dysregulation of the gut-brain axis.
3. *Post-inflammatory* – diagnosed based on the presence of at least two of the following: fever, vomiting, diarrhoea and positive stool culture. Bacterial enteritis is commonly associated with symptoms and tends to be related to alterations in gut microbiota and immune activation in gut tissues, in particular innate immunity involving macrophages and innate lymphoid cell (Serkis et al., 2018).
4. *Dysbiosis* – alteration in gut microbiota changes sensory, motor and immune systems of the gut and interaction with higher brain centres. Serkis et al. (2018) found that intestinal microbiota from people with IBS-d (IBS with diarrhoea) and with comorbidity of anxiety have altered multiple immune and neural system pathways involved in the regulation of gut function.
5. *Food intolerances/allergies* – food antigens may initiate the mucosal immune system, alter intestinal microbiota or cause hypersensitivity reactions. Rajilić-Stojanović et al. (2015) reported that between 64% and 89% of IBS sufferers stated that their IBS symptoms were triggered by meals or specific foods.
6. *Epigenetic/psychosocial factors* – symptoms may be caused by emotional stress, or early life trauma, interacting with and affecting neuroendocrine, neuroimmune and pain modulatory responses (Foster et al., 2017). Thakur et al. (2017) found that emotional awareness and expression training significantly reduced IBS symptom severity.

Inflammatory bowel disease (IBD)

Inflammatory bowel disease (IBD) is a group of idiopathic chronic inflammatory disorders of the GIT that includes two major phenotypes: **Crohn's disease** and **ulcerative colitis** (UC). The two diseases have features in common, however they are characterised by different clinical features and a different course of the immune response (Kmeic et al., 2017) (Table 12.7). Crohn's disease can affect all of the GIT but most commonly affects the distal portion of the small intestine and proximal colon, whereas ulcerative colitis tends to be confined to the rectum and colon (Figure 12.4). Whilst the exact aetiology of IBD remains unknown, it is thought that the disease results from an excessive immune response directed against microbial or environmentally derived antigens which can be triggered by the disruption of the intestinal epithelial barrier integrity (Kmeic et al., 2017). A genetic predisposition to IBD has been suspected and genetic association studies have found 215 risk loci for the development of IBD (de Lange et al., 2017). Cellular events involved in the pathogenesis of Crohn's and UC involve the activation of macrophages, lymphocytes and polymorphonuclear cells with the release of inflammatory mediators. Environmental factors associated with IBD include stress, smoking and diet. Alongside the manifestations that occur due to the involvement of the GIT, there are also extraintestinal manifestations (EIM). EIM occur frequently in IBD and may significantly affect the quality of life of those with IBD (Vavricka et al., 2015); specific treatment may be required depending on the organ(s) affected. The joints, skin and eyes are most frequently affected although the liver, lungs and pancreas may also be involved. It is thought that EIM occurs due to diseased GI mucosa triggering an immune response at an extraintestinal site due to shared epitopes (part of an antigen molecule that an antibody attaches to) (Vavricka et al., 2015). Association of EIM in IBD with the major histocompatibility complex (MHC) loci have been demonstrated, e.g. in ulcerative colitis HLA-DR$_{103}$ has been identified and in Crohn's disease HLA-A$_2$, HLA-DR$_1$ and HLA-DQ$_{W5}$ have been identified. It has also emerged that genetic factors are found in 70% of parent–child pairs and 84% between siblings (Vavricka et al., 2015).

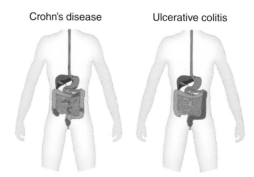

Crohn's disease   Ulcerative colitis

Illustrated by Shaun Mercier © SAGE Publications

Figure 12.4   Areas affected by inflammation in Crohn's disease and ulcerative colitis (indicated in red)

Table 12.7   Features of Crohn's disease and ulcerative colitis

Feature	Crohn's disease	Ulcerative colitis
Age of onset	10-30 years of age	10-40 years of age
Gender	Slightly more women than men affected	Men and women affected equally
Inflammation type	**Granulomatous**, cobblestone appearance	Ulcerative, exudative
Level of involvement	Submucosal (primarily) or **transmural**	Mucosal (primarily)

Feature	Crohn's disease	Ulcerative colitis
Extent of involvement	Skip lesions	Continuous
Area involved	Ileum, colon, right side more common May affect all of GIT	Rectum, colon left side more common
Diarrhoea	May or may not be present	Frequent; four or more times per day
Rectal bleeding	Infrequent	Frequent
Formation of fistulas	Frequent	Infrequent
Strictures	Frequent	Infrequent
Development of perianal abscesses	Frequent	Infrequent
Cancer development	Infrequent	Frequent
Exacerbations and remissions	Yes	Yes
Comorbidities	Extraintestinal manifestations (EIM)	Extraintestinal manifestations (EIM)
Smoking	Increases risk of development of disease and greater severity of disease	Less severe disease Nicotine withdrawal may cause exacerbation

ACTIVITY 12.3: APPLY

Living with inflammatory bowel disease

As a person-centred practitioner, it is important that you understand the lived experience of inflammatory bowel disease in order to understand the social reality of people in your care. Watch the following video to gain insight into the lived experience. If you are using the eBook just click on the play button. Alternatively go to **https://study.sagepub.com/essentialpatho/videos**

INFLAMMATORY BOWEL
DISEASE (4:05)

Crohn's disease

Crohn's disease is a recurrent granulomatous type of inflammatory response that can affect any part of the GIT from the mouth to the anus. It is slowly progressive and can be a life-limiting and disabling disease. In 40% of people lesions are restricted to the small intestine, in 30% the large bowel is affected only and in the remaining 30% both the large and small bowel are affected. Inflammation usually starts in the intestinal submucosa and spreads with irregular transmural involvement. The sharply demarcated granulomatous lesions are surrounded by normal-appearing mucosal tissue and referred to as skip lesions. The disease involves all layers of the bowel (transmural), however the submucosal layer is most affected. There are marked inflammatory and fibrotic changes of the submucosal layer that can cause ulceration. **Fissures** and crevices develop, surrounded by areas of mucosal oedema; the fissures are separated by thickened elevations or nodules which give the bowel a cobblestone appearance. Over time, the bowel wall becomes thickened and inflexible. Destruction of the wall leads to an impaired ability of the small intestine to process and absorb food. The inflammation also stimulates intestinal motility, decreasing the time available for digestion and absorption. The adjacent mesentery may become inflamed and regional lymph nodes and channels become enlarged. Over time, nutritional deficiencies may occur, caused by absorptive surfaces being disrupted and malabsorption.

Signs and symptoms

A person with Crohn's disease may have no specific symptoms for years and they vary according to the area of GIT involved. However, colicky pain in the right lower quadrant with intermittent diarrhoea are the principal symptoms; this is related to the inflammatory response and associated increase in intestinal mobility. Anorexia, weight loss, **malaise** and fatigue are also common as a result of malabsorption of nutrients. As the disease progresses, there is an increased risk of developing anaemia and fluid and electrolyte imbalances. Ulcers may penetrate the intestinal wall, causing abscesses, and fistulas may form as the ulcer erodes through the intestinal wall. Perianal fistulas that originate in the ileum are also common.

Ulcerative colitis

Ulcerative colitis (UC) is a non-specific inflammatory condition of the colon and rectum. The disease usually begins in the rectum (proctitis), and lesions form in the crypts of Lieberkühn (mucus-secreting **goblet cells** found in the base of the mucosal layer) and may spread proximally into the colon (pancolitis). The inflammatory process is confluent and continuous, affecting primarily the mucosal layer but may extend into the submucosal layer. The mucosa becomes hyperaemic and the inflammatory process leads to the formation of pinpoint haemorrhages that **suppurate** and become crypt abscesses that necrotise and develop into ulcers. The mucosal layer may develop **pseudopolyps** (tongue-like projections that resemble polyps) and thickening of the bowel wall may occur in response to repeated ulcerations.

Signs and symptoms

The disease presents as a relapsing disorder marked by attacks of diarrhoea with blood and mucus due to involvement of the mucosal layer. Diarrhoea may persist for days, weeks or months then subside only to recur after an asymptomatic interval of several months. Symptoms depend on the severity of the disease; it can be classified as mild, moderate, severe or fulminant:

Mild: With mild disease the person may have up to four stools per day with or without blood; no systemic signs of toxicity and normal erythrocyte sedimentation rate (ESR).

Moderate: In moderate disease they may experience greater than four stools per day with minimal signs of toxicity.

Severe: With severe disease they may experience more than six bloody stools per day, demonstrate signs of toxicity, demonstrated by fever, **tachycardia**, anaemia and elevated ESR.

Fulminant: In fulminant disease the person may have more than 10 stools per day, experience continuous bleeding, fever and other signs of toxicity, abdominal tenderness and distension. They may require blood transfusions.

There is a risk of developing toxic megacolon secondary to an extensive inflammatory response with involvement of neural and vascular components of the bowel. The person may also complain of mild abdominal cramping, particularly in the lower quadrant, anorexia, fatigue and weakness.

Dehydration, fluid and electrolyte imbalances, weight loss and anaemia may result from inflammation, fluid loss and bleeding. Development of anal fissures and perirectal abscesses may occur, and obstruction may be caused by oedema, strictures and fibrosis.

Diverticular disease

Diverticulae are herniations (protrusions) of mucosa and submucosa through muscle layers and occur primarily in the wall of the sigmoid colon. **Diverticulitis** refers to inflammation of the diverticula. The aetiology of diverticular disease is unknown, however predisposing factors include: ageing, physical inactivity, low residue diet, smoking and long-term use of aspirin or NSAIDs (Humes and Spiller, 2014).

Diverticulae can occur anywhere in the GIT, usually at weak points in the colon wall. They are usually multiple, ranging from one to several hundred. The diverticulae result from the unique structure and increased liminal pressures within the colon. The muscular layers of the colonic wall differ from that of the small intestine; there are three separate longitudinal bands of muscle (**teniae coli**) as opposed to a continuous layer. Contraction of the colon occurs due to bands of circular muscle. The lack of continuous longitudinal muscle combined with the contraction of circular muscle causes the intestine to bulge outwards into pouches (**haustra**). Diverticulae form between the longitudinal muscle bands of the haustra, and increased intraluminal pressure within the haustra creates enough force to develop the herniations. If pressure increases too much it may cause the diverticula to rupture, causing inflammation and diverticulitis. Complications associated with diverticulitis include abscess or fistula formation, obstruction, **perforation** and haemorrhage.

Signs and symptoms

Most people with diverticular disease remain asymptomatic, however cramping pain in the lower left quadrant is the most common complaint. Nausea, vomiting, diarrhoea or constipation, abdominal distension and flatulence may accompany the pain. Inflammation of the diverticula may cause fever and **leucocytosis**.

Intestinal obstruction

Intestinal obstructions refer to the lack of/impaired movement of chyme (intestinal contents) through the intestinal lumen. They can be classified according to where they occur, onset, the extent of obstruction and the effects on the intestinal wall (Table 12.8). Intestinal obstructions may be caused by a number of factors, including: hernia (inguinal or femoral), **tumours**, diverticular disease and IBD. Intestinal obstruction may be either mechanical or functional:

- *Mechanical* – blockage of the intestinal lumen by intrinsic lesions, i.e. occurring within the lumen, such as a foreign body, or by extrinsic lesions originating outside the lumen, such as a hernia or tumour
- *Functional* – paralysis of musculature usually caused by trauma, infection (peritonitis) or electrolyte imbalances.

Obstruction causes gas and fluid to gather in the lumen proximal to the obstruction, leading to intestinal distension. Water and electrolytes are unable to be absorbed due to distension, therefore the secretion of fluid and electrolytes into the lumen is increased. Intestinal distension leads to the loss of fluids and electrolytes due to profuse vomiting, and extracellular fluid and plasma volumes decrease, causing

Table 12.8 Classifications of intestinal obstructions

Site of obstruction	Small bowel obstruction – caused by **adhesions**, hernia, tumours, Crohn's disease
	Large bowel obstruction – caused by colon/rectal cancer, diverticular disease
Onset	Acute – sudden onset due to twisting or herniation
	Chronic – slow, protracted onset due to tumour growth or formation of strictures
Extent	Partial – incomplete obstruction of lumen
	Complete – complete obstruction of lumen
Effects on intestinal wall	Simple – obstruction of lumen does not lead to impairment of blood supply
	Strangulated – obstruction of lumen causes decreased blood supply
	Closed loop – obstruction occurs at the end of each segment of intestine

hypotension, tachycardia, dehydration and electrolyte imbalances. Due to excessive loss of hydrogen through vomiting and an inability to absorb, metabolic **alkalosis** initially develops. However, if the obstruction is not removed, bicarbonate ions may not be able to be absorbed and **metabolic acidosis** may occur. Metabolic acidosis may be worsened by hypokalaemia due to malabsorption and vomiting and also by ketosis caused by the decreased availability of carbohydrates and increased amounts of lactate due to poor circulation. Occlusion of arterial circulation may occur depending on pressure caused by distension, resulting in ischaemia, **necrosis** and perforation. Ischaemia and necrosis will lead to **denervation** and stop **peristalsis**. Rapid growth of intestinal bacteria occurs with some producing **endotoxins** that may translocate across the mucosa and into systemic circulation, causing septicaemia and peritonitis (Figure 12.5).

Signs and symptoms

Signs and symptoms will vary depending on the degree of obstruction and the duration. They include:

* Severe colicky abdominal pain (mechanical obstruction) or continuous pain (functional obstruction)
* Borborygmus
* Nausea and vomiting
* Abdominal distension and tenderness
* No bowel movements
* Fever
* Leucocytosis
* Hypotension, tachycardia, **diaphoresis**

Appendicitis

Appendicitis is inflammation with or without infection of the vermiform appendix. It is common amongst children between the ages of 10 and 11 years and occurs frequently in people between the ages of 20 and 30 years, however it can occur at any age. Appendicitis occurs due to intraluminal obstruction caused by **faecalith** (hard piece of stool), tumour, foreign body or twisting (torsion). Intraluminal pressure increases due to the build-up of fluid (drainage of appendix is inhibited) and continued mucosal secretion, leading to decreased mucosal blood flow, causing hypoxia, ischaemia and necrosis which result in increased permeability. Bacteria and toxins move through the wall and may cause the formation of abscesses and localised peritonitis. Increasing pressure due to further inflammation and oedema causes further necrosis, **thrombosis** of luminal vessels and **gangrene** which may lead to perforation. If perforation occurs, the contents will be emptied into the peritoneal cavity, causing generalised peritonitis.

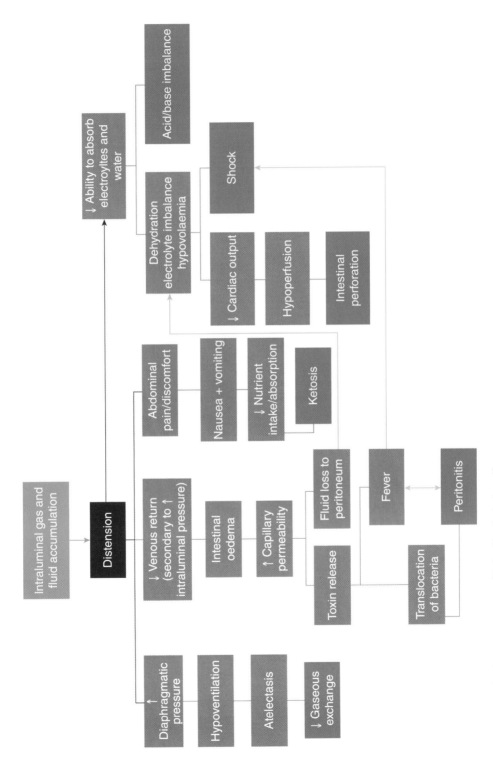

Figure 12.5 Consequences of intestinal obstruction

Signs and symptoms

Initially the person may complain of abdominal or periumbilical pain that occurs due to inflammation and stretching of the appendix. Pain increases in intensity and becomes localised in the lower right quadrant (extension of inflammation to surrounding tissues). Anorexia, nausea and vomiting accompany the pain; there may be a low-grade pyrexia and leucocytosis. In children, diarrhoea is commonly experienced.

Infectious enterocolitis

Enterocolitis refers to inflammation of both the small and large intestine. Infection of the GIT can be caused by a wide range of pathogens including viruses, e.g. Rotavirus, and bacteria, e.g. *Staphylococcus aureus, Escherichia coli* (*E. coli*), non-typhoid salmonella, campylobacter, *Clostridium difficile* (*C. diff.*) and *E. coli* O157:H7 (a specific **serotype** of *E. coli*) (Table 12.9). Bacterial infections tend to produce more severe effects than viral infections. A wide range of symptoms are caused by the infection and include diarrhoea, abdominal pain, fever, malaise, ulceration and haemorrhage (Table 12.9). Many pathogens are transmitted by faecally contaminated food and/or water. Some infections are seasonal or may occur as **epidemics**, e.g. Rotavirus. The infections are usually self-limiting although fluid and electrolyte replacement may be necessary if there is severe dehydration and loss of electrolytes.

Most viral infections affect the superficial epithelium of the small intestine, causing destruction of the cells and thereby limiting their absorptive function. Immature enterocytes repopulate the villi, and crypt secretory cells remain intact and lead to net secretion of water and electrolytes, leading to osmotic diarrhoea. Bacterial enterocolitis may be due to a number of causative factors: ingestion of contaminated food with preformed toxins, infection due to toxigenic organisms that multiply in the gut lumen and produce toxins, and infection by enteroinvasive organisms that multiply in the lumen and invade and destroy mucosal epithelial cells.

Table 12.9 Pathogens that cause enterocolitis

Pathogen	Incubation period	Pathogenesis	Signs and symptoms
Rotavirus	24-72 hours	Inflammation and loss of villi	Mild to moderate fever, vomiting, severe watery diarrhoea
Staphylococcus aureus	1-7 hours	Produces enterotoxins	Nausea, vomiting, abdominal cramps, below normal body temperature, hypotension, ± diarrhoea
Salmonella	6-72 hours	Inflammation and ulceration	Abdominal pain, sudden diarrhoea, fever, ± vomiting
Campylobacter	2-5 days	Tissue damage to jejunum, ileum and colon	Nausea, diarrhoea
C. difficile	Up to 7 days	Disruption of normal gut microbiota leads to overgrowth of spores	Lower abdominal cramps, severe watery diarrhoea
E. coli	10-12 hours	Releases enterotoxins, invades mucosa	Profuse watery diarrhoea ± blood and mucus, vomiting, abdominal cramps

Pathogen	Incubation period	Pathogenesis	Signs and symptoms
E. coli O157:H7	3-4 days	*Shigella*-like toxins attach to and destroy mucosal lining May access the circulatory system, damage the endothelium, initiate platelet activation	Bloody diarrhoea If access to circulation, it can cause haemolytic **uraemic syndrome** (**haemolytic anaemia, acute kidney injury** and **thrombocytopenia**) or thrombotic thrombocytopenic **purpura** (thrombocytopenia, acute kidney injury, fever and neurological changes)

APPLY

Clostridium difficile and antibiotic therapy

Clostridium difficile (*C. diff*) is a gram-positive spore-forming bacillus that forms part of the gut microbiome in some healthy people. However, virulent *C. diff* produces toxins that cause pseudomembranous colitis. Development of *C. diff* colitis requires disruption of the normal intestinal flora, overgrowth of bacilli, germination of spores and toxin production. Treatment with **broad spectrum antibiotics** can disrupt the normal protective flora of the colon, making the bowel susceptible to *C. diff.* colonisation and infection. Toxins produced bind to and damage the mucosa, causing inflammation, haemorrhage and necrosis. They also interfere with protein synthesis, increase permeability, attract inflammatory cells and promote intestinal peristalsis. The infection is usually acquired in hospital and tends to be more frequent, severe, resistant to treatment and to increase morbidity and mortality. New **strains** are more virulent with increased resistance to treatment.

First-line treatment involves the use of metronidazole, however if this is ineffective vancomycin may be used. Non-antibiotic therapy is being used in an attempt to break the cycle of recurrent infection, to restore the gut microbiota and protect gut mucosa. The use of probiotics when administered in adequate amounts may prevent potential *C. diff.* infection (Goldenberg et al., 2017); probiotics have the highest quality evidence among any cited prophylactic therapy (Goldenberg et al., 2017). It is also important that appropriate antibiotic use is facilitated, i.e. use the right antibiotic for the right pathogen; antibiotic stewardship aims to do just that. Baur et al. (2017) found that antibiotic stewardship programmes reduce the incidence of infections and colonisation with antibiotic-resistant bacteria and *C. diff* infection in hospital.

DISORDERS OF THE ACCESSORY ORGANS

As already identified, accessory organs of the digestive system include the salivary glands, gall bladder, liver and pancreas. We are going to discuss disorders that affect the gall bladder and pancreas; disorders of the liver are discussed in Chapter 13.

Disorders of the gall bladder

The function of the gall bladder is to store and concentrate bile. Bile contains bile salts, **cholesterol**, **bilirubin**, lecithin, fatty acids, water and electrolytes that are used to maintain the solubility of cholesterol. As food enters the intestine, the gall bladder contracts, causing the sphincter of the bile duct to relax and release bile into the duodenum. Pressure in the common bile duct is the regulatory factor controlling the passage of bile into the intestine. The gall bladder collects and stores bile; as it relaxes the pressure decreases, as the gall bladder contracts it empties bile; into the intestine. Common disorders affecting the gall bladder include: **cholelithiasis** (gallstones), **cholecystitis** (inflammation of the gall bladder) and **cholangitis** (inflammation of the common bile duct).

Cholelithiasis

Cholelithiasis (formation of gall stones) is caused by the solidification of substances found in bile, primarily cholesterol and bilirubin. There are three different types of gallstones: cholesterol (composed of approximately 70% cholesterol), pigmented (black and brown, containing less than 30% cholesterol) and mixed (Figure 12.6). Risk factors for the development of gallstones include: obesity, being female, rapid weight loss, gall bladder, pancreatic and ileal disease.

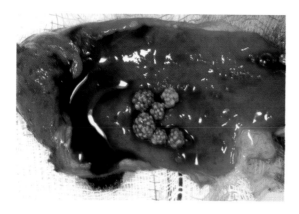

Figure 12.6a Cholesterol gallstones

Source: © Science Photo Library

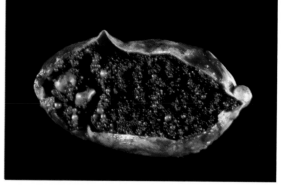

12.6b Pigmented gallstones

Three factors contribute to gallstone formation:

1. Abnormalities in the composition of bile salts, increased levels of cholesterol usually related to obesity, multiple pregnancies and the oral contraceptive pill all cause the liver to excrete more cholesterol into the bile. Increased levels of oestrogen in women taking the contraceptive pill reduce bile acid synthesis. Thickened gall bladder mucoprotein containing cholesterol crystals (gall bladder sludge) is thought to be a precursor to the development of gallstones. This sludge is thought to occur with rapid weight loss, starvation and pregnancy.

2. Stasis of bile leads to decreased levels of bile salts. Ileal disease or intestinal bypass can lead to malabsorption of bile salts and altering the solubility of cholesterol.

3. Inflammation of the gall bladder alters the absorptive characteristics of the mucosal layer, resulting in the excessive absorption of water and bile salts.

Signs and symptoms

Many people who have gallstones may be asymptomatic, and symptoms may only become apparent when the gallstones obstruct the flow of bile. However, clinical manifestations include:

* Epigastric and right hypochondrium pain with abrupt onset that may last for 2–8 hours and increases in intensity over this period of time
* Heartburn, epigastric discomfort
* Flatulence
* Food intolerance

Cholecystitis

Cholecystitis may be either acute or chronic, but regardless of what form, it is a diffuse inflammation of the gall bladder resulting from a gallstone becoming lodged in the cystic duct and causing obstruction of the gall bladder outlet.

Acute cholecystitis is widespread inflammation of the gall bladder. Calculous cholecystitis is the major cause of acute cholecystitis in the presence of gallstones accounting for approximately 85–90%. Acute calculous cholecystitis is caused by a gallstone becoming lodged in the cystic duct, causing an obstruction resulting in inflammation behind the obstruction. Due to obstruction of the cystic duct, the gall bladder epithelium releases mucosal phospholipase that disrupts the normal **glycoprotein** layer; subsequent destruction of mucosal epithelium occurs due to exposure to the concentrated bile salts. Acalculous cholecystitis (without gallstones) is associated with ischaemia resulting from sepsis, severe trauma or infection of the gall bladder. The cystic artery has no **collateral** circulation so a reduction in blood flow causes ischaemia that can quickly lead to gangrene and perforation of the gall bladder. Chronic cholecystitis is due to repeat episodes of acute cholecystitis or long-term irritation of the gall bladder from the presence of stones and is associated with varying degrees of inflammation.

Signs and symptoms

A person with acute cholecystitis may experience a sudden onset of persistent pain in the right upper quadrant or epigastric region. It may be accompanied by mild fever, anorexia, nausea and vomiting. The person may also have an elevated white blood cell count, mild elevation in AST, ALT, ALP (indicators of liver function) and bilirubin. Signs and symptoms usually subside within 24 hours but could persist for as long as 7–10 days if medical assistance is not sought. Signs and symptoms associated with chronic cholecystitis are not as clear but include food intolerances, in particular fatty foods, belching and abdominal discomfort. The person may experience colicky pain due to the presence of gallstones causing obstruction of biliary flow.

Choledocholithiasis and cholangitis

Choledocholithiasis occurs when there are stones in the common bile duct; these may originate in the gall bladder but formation may occur spontaneously within the common bile duct. Cholangitis refers to inflammation of the common bile duct. Signs and symptoms are similar to cholelithiasis and acute cholecystitis. The person will have a history of acute biliary colic and right upper abdominal pain accompanied by chills, fever and **jaundice**. Obstruction of the common bile duct leads to elevated serum bilirubin and bilirubinuria. The presence of stones in the common duct may also obstruct outflow of the pancreatic duct and cause secondary pancreatitis. Suppurative cholangitis is inflammation that is accompanied by pus in the common duct and represents a surgical or endoscopic emergency.

Disorders of the pancreas

The pancreas is a large gland that extends from the duodenum to the spleen and has both endocrine and exocrine functions. The exocrine functions include the production and secretion of **proteolytic enzymes** and amylase that are responsible for the digestion of fats, proteins, carbohydrates and nucleic acids. Pancreatic enzymes are produced in an inactive form and converted by other enzymes in the small intestine to their active form to prevent them from digesting pancreatic tissue. The **acinar cells** also secrete **trypsin** inhibitor, thereby preventing trypsin secretion and subsequent activation of other enzymes. The pancreas (epithelial cell) also releases large amounts of sodium bicarbonate that neutralises the acidic chyme in the small intestine, thus protecting the lining of the digestive tract. This chapter will discuss disorders of the exocrine function; disorders of endocrine function, namely diabetes mellitus, are discussed in Chapter 13.

Pancreatitis

Pancreatitis is inflammation of the pancreas and can either be acute or chronic; it affects men and women equally, usually occurring between the ages of 50 and 60. Risk factors for pancreatitis are presented in Box 12.4.

Box 12.4   Risk factors for pancreatitis

- Peptic ulcer disease
- Cholelithiasis
- Genetic factors, e.g. hereditary pancreatitis, cystic fibrosis
- Obesity
- Excessive alcohol intake
- Smoking
- Hyperlipidaemia
- Hypercalcaemia
- Smoking

Acute pancreatitis

Acute pancreatitis is reversible inflammation of the pancreas that occurs suddenly due to premature activation of pancreatic enzymes. It is caused by obstruction to the outflow of pancreatic digestive enzymes, usually the presence of gallstones. It may also result from direct injury to pancreatic tissue from long-term heavy alcohol consumption, viral infections or drugs. In pancreatitis due to obstructive disease there is a backup of pancreatic secretions and the activation and release of enzymes; activated trypsin leads to the activation of **chymotrypsin**, lipase and elastase within the pancreatic acinar cells, which subsequently causes autodigestion of pancreatic cells and tissues, resulting in a severe inflammatory response. Autodigestion of the pancreatic tissue leads to vascular changes, coagulative necrosis and fat necrosis; there is also the formation of pseudocysts. Further necrosis may occur from ischaemia caused by oedema within the pancreatic capsule. Local and systemic responses that occur with pancreatitis may be caused by independent activation of an inflammatory response within the acinar cells. Systemic effects are related to the release of pro-inflammatory cytokines (interleukin-6, **tumour necrosis factor**-alpha, platelet-activating factor) with the subsequent activation of leucocytes, damage to vessels walls, **vasodilation**, hypotension and shock. Pancreatitis due to excessive alcohol consumption is thought to occur due to the generation of toxic metabolites produced as the pancreatic acinar cells metabolise ethanol. These toxic metabolites damage the pancreatic acinar cells, causing the release of activated enzymes. Alcohol may cause a spasm of the sphincter of Oddi, resulting in obstruction; the obstruction causes the intrapancreatic release of activated enzymes that cause autodigestion and inflammation.

Complications associated with pancreatitis include cardiac failure, acute kidney injury, coagulopathies, intra-abdominal **hypertension**, **acute respiratory distress syndrome (ARDS)** and systemic inflammatory response syndrome (SIRS). Gastrointestinal bleeding and paralytic ileus may also occur; **translocation** of organisms of the gut microbiome into the bloodstream may cause peritonitis or sepsis. Activation of pancreatic stellate cells may result from recurrent inflammation, resulting in fibrosis, stricture and duct obstruction that can lead to the development of chronic pancreatitis.

Signs and symptoms

The clinical course of pancreatitis can range from mild with minimal organ dysfunction to severe and life-threatening; 20% of those with acute pancreatitis will be classified as severe with a mortality rate of 10–30%. Epigastric or mid-abdominal constant pain, ranging from mild discomfort to incapacitating, is the first symptom that someone will present with. Pain is caused by a number of factors, including: oedema that causes distension of the pancreatic capsule and ducts; irritation and inflammation of the peritoneum due to the release of chemicals; obstruction of the biliary tract; and inflammation of the nerves. Systemic signs are variable from person to person but may include: fever, hypotension, respiratory distress, **tachypnoea**, abdominal distension and tenderness. Nausea and vomiting may also occur due to paralytic ileus or peritonitis secondary to pancreatitis. Other findings include an increase in white blood cell count and leucocytosis, raised levels of inflammatory markers such as C-reactive protein, and hyperglycaemia due to the increased secretion of glucagon from damaged alpha cells in the islets of Langerhans.

Chronic pancreatitis

Chronic pancreatitis is the progressive and irreversible fibrotic destruction of the exocrine pancreas that over time leads to the destruction of the endocrine pancreas. The causes of chronic pancreatitis mirror those discussed in acute pancreatitis. The most common cause of chronic pancreatitis is long-term excessive alcohol intake, however genetic factors and smoking also increase the risk of developing it. Destruction of the islets of Langerhans and acinar cells occurs due to toxic metabolites and the long-term release of inflammatory cytokines. Over time, fibrous tissue replaces the pancreatic parenchyma and there is development of strictures, calcification, ductal obstruction and formation of pancreatic cysts. As mentioned previously, the disorder progresses to the extent that both exocrine and endocrine functions are impaired; at this point, signs of diabetes mellitus and malabsorption syndrome, e.g. weight loss, steatorrhoea, become apparent.

Signs and symptoms

Signs and symptoms associated with chronic pancreatitis are similar to those of acute pancreatitis but are less severe. The person will have persistent periods of pain in the epigastric and upper left quadrant that recur frequently and are exacerbated by excessive alcohol intake or overeating. The person may also experience flatulence, anorexia, constipation and vomiting.

CHAPTER SUMMARY

In this chapter you will have learned about disorders affecting the digestive system, nutrient supply and faecal elimination across the life span and how they impact not only physiologically but also how they influence health-related quality of life. These disorders can alter identity and significantly reduce independence and social integration. To be an effective person-centred practitioner, you need to be relational when considering these disorders; being compassionate and working with someone's belief system and values will enable you to care for them within the context of their culture and social structure.

KEY POINTS

- General GI disturbances include nausea, vomiting, constipation and diarrhoea.

- Anorexia is the lack of desire to eat associated with nausea, vomiting and abdominal pain and can be caused by stress, pain or as a side-effect of drugs.

- Malnutrition is the lack of nourishment from inadequate/inappropriate amounts of macronutrients and micronutrients.

- Obesity is a global epidemic; the development of obesity involves the interaction of central and peripheral pathways, the release of hormones and neurotransmitters.

- Gastritis is inflammation of the stomach mucosa and can be either acute or chronic. It is associated with long-term use of NSAID or aspirin, excessive alcohol intake and *H. pylori* infection.

- Peptic ulcers occur in either the stomach or duodenum and are caused by excessive acid secretion, *H. pylori* infection, or disruption of the mucosal barrier.

- Stress ulcers occur following severe illness, trauma or neurological injury/surgery.

- Malabsorption syndromes refer to disorders that interfere with intestinal absorptive processes.

- Intestinal obstruction refers to impaired movement of contents through the intestinal lumen and can be either mechanical (blockage within the lumen) or functional (paralysis of the musculature).

- Appendicitis is inflammation with or without infection of the vermiform appendix caused by intraluminal obstruction due to faecalith, tumour or foreign body.

- Diverticular disease has an unknown aetiology. Diverticula are herniations of the mucosa and submucosa and are primarily located in the sigmoid colon. Diverticulitis refers to inflammation of diverticula.

- **Infectious enterocolitis** refers to infection of the GIT and can be caused by numerous pathogens. It causes a wide range of symptoms, including: abdominal pain, diarrhoea, haemorrhage, perianal discomfort and ulceration.

- Irritable bowel syndrome is a complex multifaceted syndrome affecting 10–15% of the population worldwide. It can be either diarrhoea-prevalent or constipation-prevalent. It is thought to occur due to alterations in the gut–brain axis, dysbiosis, genetic predisposition, gut neuroendocrine cell function or epigenetic factors.

- Inflammatory bowel disease refers to two related inflammatory intestinal disorders: ulcerative colitis and Crohn's disease.

- Ulcerative colitis causes ulceration, abcess formation and necrosis of mucosa in the colon and rectum.

- Crohn's disease can affect any part of the GIT and involves all layers of the intestinal lumen. Main characteristics of the disease include skip lesions, fissures and granulomas.

- Disorders of the accessory organs include: gallstones, inflammation of the gall bladder and pancreatitis.

The content of this chapter will help you to understand the range of disordered functions of the GIT, and the number of different diseases that can occur. Revise the sections in turn then try to answer the questions below.

Answers are available online. If you are using the eBook just click on the answers icon below. Alternatively go to **https://study.sagepub.com/essentialpatho/answers**

REVISE

TEST YOUR KNOWLEDGE

1   Briefly explain the categories of primary constipation.

2   Explain the difference between osmotic and secretory diarrhoea.

3   Identify the hormones that are associated with the development of obesity.

4   Identify the various classifications of intestinal obstruction.

5   What signs and symptoms would you expect if someone presented with appendicitis?

6   What types of pathogens cause infectious enterocolitis? Provide examples.

7   Identify the predisposing factor for inflammatory bowel disease.

8   Differentiate between Crohn's disease and ulcerative colitis.

9   What are the three different types of gallstones?

10 Identify the risk factors associated with the development of pancreatitis.

- Further revision and learning opportunities are available online

- Test yourself away from the book with **Extra multiple choice questions**

- Learn and revise terminology with **Interactive flashcards**

If you are using the eBook access each resource by clicking on the respective icon. Alternatively go to **https://study.sagepub.com/essentialpatho/chapter12**

REVISE

ACE YOUR ASSESSMENT

CHAPTER 12 ANSWERS

EXTRA QUESTIONS

FLASHCARDS

REFERENCES

Babic, T. and Browning, K.N. (2014) The role of vagal neurocircuits in the regulation of nausea and vomiting. *European Journal of Pharmacology, 722*: 38–47.

Baur, D., Gladstone, B.P., Burket, F., Carrara, E., Foschi, F., Döbele, S. et al. (2017) Effect of antibiotic stewardship on the incidence of infection and colonization with antibiotic resistant bacteria and *Clostridium difficile* infection: a systematic review and meta-analysis. *The Lancet: Infectious Diseases, 17* (9): 990–1001.

Boore, J., Cook, N. and Shepherd, A. (2016) *Essentials of Anatomy and Physiology for Nursing Practice.* London: Sage.

Catanzaro, R., Occhipinti, S., Calabrese, F., Anazalone, M.G., Milazzo, M., Italia, A. et al. (2014) Irritable bowel syndrome: new findings in pathophysiological and therapeutic field. *Minerva Gastroenterologica Dietologica, 60* (2): 151–63.

Costilla, V.C. and Foxx-Orenstein, A.E. (2014) Constipation in adults: diagnosis and management. *Current Treatment Options in Gastroenterology, 12* (3): 310–324.

Cross-Adame, E. and Rao, S.S. (2014) Brain and gut interactions in irritable bowel syndrome: new paradigms and new understandings. *Current Gastroenterology Reports, 16* (4): 379.

Davies, I., Burman-Roy, S. and Murphy, S.M. (2015) Gastro-oesophageal reflux disease in children: NICE guidance. *BMJ: British Medical Journal (Online)*, published online 14 January. doi:10.1136/bmj.g7703.

de Lange, K.M., Moutsianas, L., Lee, J.C., Lamb, C.A., Luo, Y., Kennedy, N.A. et al.(2017) Genome-wide association study implicates immune activation of multiple integrin genes in inflammatory bowel disease. *Nature Genetics, 49*: 256–61.

Deng, Y., Misselwitz, B., Dai, N. and Fox, M. (2015) Lactose intolerance in adults: biological mechanism and dietary management. *Nutrients, 7* (9): 8020–35.

Dickson S.L., Egecioglu, E., Landgren, S., Skibicka, K.P., Engel, J.A. and Jerlhag, E. (2011) The role of the central ghrelin system in reward from food and chemical drugs. *Molecular and Cellular Endocrinology, 340*: 80–7.

Foster, J.A., Rinaman, L. and Cryan, J.F. (2017) Stress and the gut-brain axis: regulation by the microbiome. *Neurobiology of Stress, 7*: 124–36.

Goldenberg, J.Z., Yap, C., Lytvyn, L., Lo, C.K., Beardsley, J., Mertz, D. et al. (2017) Probiotics for the prevention of *Clostridium difficile* associated diarrhea in adults and children. *Cochrane Library* [online]. December 2017. doi:10.1002/14651858.CD006095.pub4.

Guérin, A., Mody, R., Fok, B., Lasch, K.L., Zhou, Z., Wu, E.Q. et al. (2014) Risk of developing colorectal cancer and benign colorectal neoplasm in patients with chronic constipation. *Alimentary Pharmacology & Therapeutics, 40* (1): 83–92.

Humes, D.J. and Spiller, R.C. (2014) Review article: the pathogenesis and management of acute colonic diverticulitis. *Alimentary Pharmacology and Therapeutics, 39* (4): 359–70.

Kmeic, Z., Cyman, M. and Slebioda, T.J. (2017) Cells of the innate and adaptive immunity and their interactions in inflammatory bowel disease. *Advances in Medical Sciences, 62* (1): 1–16.

Koning, F., Thomas, R., Rossjohn, J. and Toes, R.E. (2015) Coeliac disease and rheumatoid arthritis: similar mechanisms, different antigens. *Nature Reviews Rheumatology, 11* (8): 450.

Lacy, B.E., Levenick, J.M. and Crowell, M. (2012) Chronic constipation: new diagnostic and treatment approaches. *Therapeutic Advances in Gastroenterology, 5* (4): 233–47.

Lee, Y.Y. and McColl, K.E. (2013) Pathophysiology of gastroesophageal reflux disease. *Best Practice and Research: Clinical Gastroenterology, 27* (3): 339–51.

Lovell, R.M. and Ford, A.C. (2012) Global prevalence of and risk factors for irritable bowel syndrome: a meta-analysis. *Clinical Gastroenterology and Hepatology, 10*: 712–21.

Matthews, K.L., Capra, S.M. and Palmer, M.A. (2018) Throw caution to the wind: is refeeding syndrome really a cause of death in acute care? *European Journal of Clinical Nutrition, 72*: 93–8.

Mayer, E.A., Savidge, T. and Shulman, R.J. (2014) Brain–gut microbiome interactions and functional bowel disorders. *Gastroenterology*, *146* (6): 1500–12.

Mehanna, H., Nankivell, P.C., Moledina, J. and Travis, J. (2009) Refeeding syndrome: awareness, prevention and management. *Head and Neck Oncology*, *1*: 4.

Nasir, M., Zaman, B.S. and Kaleem, A. (2018) What a trainee surgeon should know about refeeding syndrome: a literature review. *Cureus*, *10* (3): e2388. Published online March 2018. doi:10.7759/cureus.2388.

NICE (2014) Gastro-oesophageal reflux disease and dyspepsia in adults: investigation and management. Clinical guideline [CG184]. National Institute for Health and Care Excellence. Available at: www.nice.org.uk/guidance/cg184 (accessed 10 December 2018).

NICE (2017) Nutrition support for adults: oral nutrition support, enteral tube feeding and parenteral nutrition. Clinical guideline [CG32]. National Institute for Health and Care Excellence. Available at: www.nice.org.uk/guidance/cg32 (accessed 10 December 2018).

Rajilić-Stojanović, M., Jonkers, D.M., Salonen, A., Hanevik, K., Raes, J., Jalanka, J. et al. (2015) Intestinal microbiota and diet in IBS: causes, consequences, or epiphenomena? *American Journal of Gastroenterology*, *110*: 278–87.

Rubin, R. (2012) The gastrointestinal tract. In R. Rubin and D.S. Strayer (eds), *Rubin's Pathophysiology: Clinicopathologic Foundations of Medicine*, 5th edn. Philadelphia, PA: Wolters Kluwer Health, Lippincott Williams and Wilkins.

Sáinz, N., Barrenetxe, J., Moreno-Aliaga, M.J. and Martínez, J.A. (2015) Leptin resistance and diet-induced obesity: central and peripheral actions of leptin. *Metabolism*, *64* (1): 35–46.

Scerif, M., Goldstone, A.P. and Korbonits, M. (2011) Ghrelin in obesity and endocrine diseases. *Molecular and Cellular Endocrinology*, *340*: 15–25.

Serkis, V., De Palma, G., Cocciolillo, S., Pigrau, M., Lu, J., Verdu, E. et al. (2018) A263 IBS-D microbiota induces gut-brain dysfunction by disrupting intestinal neural and immune pathways. *Journal of the Canadian Association of Gastroenterology*, *1* (Suppl 1): 458. First published online March 2018. doi.org/10.1093/jcag/gwy008.264.

Thakur, E.R., Holmes, H.J., Lockhart, N.A., Carty, J.N., Ziadni, M.S., Doherty, H.K. et al. (2017) Emotional awareness and expression training improves irritable bowel syndrome: a randomised controlled trial. *Neurogastroenterology & Motility*, *29* (12): e13143. First published online 22 June 2017. https://doi.org/10.1111/nmo.13143.

Vaiopoulou, A., Karamanolis, G., Psaltopoulou, T., Karatzias, G. and Gazouli, M. (2014) Molecular basis of the irritable bowel syndrome. *World Journal of Gastroenterology*, *20* (2): 376–83.

van der Post, C.R.S. and Carneiro, F. (2017) Acute gastritis. *Pathology of the Gastrointestinal Tract*. First published online 30 June 2017. doi:10.1007/978-3-319-40560-5_1607.

Vavricka, S.R., Schoepfer, A., Scharl, M., Lakatos, P.L., Navarini, A. and Rogler, G. (2015) Extraintestinal manifestations of inflammatory bowel disease. *Inflammatory Bowel Diseases*, *21* (8): 1982–92.

Vuckovic-Rebrina, S., Barada, L. and Smircic-Duvnjak, L. (2013) Diabetic autonomic neuropathy. *Diabetologia Croatica*, *42* (3): 73–9.

World Health Organisation (WHO) (2018) Health Topics: Obesity. [online]. Available at: www.who.int/topics/obesity/en/ (accessed 7 August 2018).

Zucca, E., Bertoni, F., Vannata, B. and Cavalli, F. (2014) Emerging role of infectious etiologies in the pathogenesis of marginal zone B-cell lymphomas. *Clinical Cancer Research*, *20* (20): 5207–16.

DISORDERS OF METABOLISM

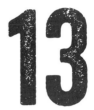

13

UNDERSTAND: CHAPTER VIDEOS

Watch the following videos to ease you into this chapter. If you are using the eBook just click on the play buttons. Alternatively go to **https://study.sagepub.com/essentialpatho/videos**

INSULIN AND GLUCAGON
(4:42)

THYROID GLAND HORMONES
(12:46)

CIRRHOSIS (5:35)

LEARNING OUTCOMES

When you have finished studying this chapter you will be able to:

1. State the main uses of energy in bodily function and outline the endocrine regulation and disturbances of metabolic rate.
2. Recognise some of the inherited disorders of carbohydrate metabolism.
3. Differentiate between the types of diabetes mellitus and recognise the complications that can occur.
4. Identify the main groups of disorders of lipid metabolism.
5. Outline some of the key disorders of amino acid metabolism.
6. Clarify the types of liver disorders and the metabolic disturbances that occur.

INTRODUCTION

This chapter will examine and discuss disorders of **metabolism**, the sum of **anabolism** and **catabolism**, i.e. the chemical reactions which occur in the body to maintain life. Nutrients taken into the body are used to create and store energy for bodily activities, and to form new structures. The two groups of chemical reactions are:

- *Anabolism*: the building up of large, more complex molecules from small ones, either for creating replacement structures in the body or for storing nutrients in larger molecules (e.g. glucose molecules combine to form **glycogen** which is stored until needed). Energy is needed for anabolism.
- *Catabolism*: the breakdown of ingested nutrients to provide energy for the chemical reactions of anabolism. The energy released is stored as **adenosine triphosphate (ATP)**.

REVISE: A&P RECAP

Anabolism and catabolism

Figure 9.5 in Chapter 9 of *Essentials of Anatomy and Physiology for Nursing Practice* (Boore et al., 2016) clarifies how anabolism and catabolism contribute to overall body function through energy management.

There are a number of chemical reactions involved in the metabolism of nutrients (carbohydrates, lipids and proteins) and energy management. Various disturbances can occur within these pathways, resulting in various metabolic disorders, some of which are discussed later in this chapter.

The major organ involved in nutrient metabolism and energy (and heat) production is the liver, so liver disorders have a significant influence on disorders of metabolism. In addition, hormones secreted from the thyroid gland regulate the level of cell metabolism; a raised level of secretion increases the metabolic rate while a decreased level results in reduced metabolism.

REVISE: A&P RECAP

Metabolic pathways

Figure 9.7 in Chapter 9 of *Essentials of Anatomy and Physiology for Nursing Practice* (Boore et al., 2016) outlines the major metabolic pathways and revision of these will be helpful in understanding some metabolic disorders.

PERSON-CENTRED CONTEXT: THE BODIE FAMILY

BODIE FAMILY
CASE NOTES

Disorders of metabolism are found in the Bodie family. Richard Jones was diagnosed with type 2 **diabetes mellitus** 5 years ago which means he must pay attention to his diet alongside maintaining a healthy cardiovascular system and weight. His body mass index (BMI) of 20.1 is within the healthy category and he eats a diet that has a low glycaemic index in order to help manage surges in blood sugar.

Maud has **hypothyroidism**, which can result in her feeling low in energy, impacting on her ability to engage in social activities and other energy-demanding activities.

IDENTIFICATION OF METABOLIC DISORDERS

These conditions fall into two main groups: genetically determined and **acquired** disorders. Individually, many of the genetically determined conditions are rare but overall not inconsiderable in number and many of the signs and symptoms may be associated with other conditions. Early identification, particularly with neonates, enables treatment to be started rapidly and, hopefully, the avoidance of complications and early death. Table 13.1 identifies the range of signs and symptoms that may occur and raise suspicion of such a **disease**.

ENERGY METABOLISM

A number of disorders are related to anabolism and catabolism in energy metabolism. This is a complex area involving some key concepts, including **metabolic syndrome**, central **obesity**, **insulin** resistance and thyroid function. We examine these in some detail below.

Table 13.1 Signs and symptoms of inherited metabolic disorders

Signs and symptoms	Causes
Growth delay	Decreased **anabolism** or increased **catabolism**; possibly reduced energy-generating substrates (e.g. **glycogen storage disease** - **GSD**) or inefficient energy or protein use (e.g. urea cycle defects)
Developmental delay	Chronic energy deficit in brain, decreased supply of carbohydrates that are non-energy substrates for the brain, or chronic amino acid deficit in the brain (e.g. tyrosine deficiency in **phenylketonuria**)
Neuromuscular symptoms	Acute energy deficit in brain **seizures** → muscle weakness, **hypotonia**, **myoclonus**, muscle pain, **stroke**, or **coma**, e.g., hypoglycaemic seizures in GSD, strokes in mitochondrial **oxidative phosphorylation** defects, muscle weakness in muscle forms of GSD, toxic compounds in brain
Congenital brain malformation	May be due to decreased availability of energy (e.g. decreased ATP output) or reduced precursors (e.g. **cholesterol**) during fetal development
Autonomic symptoms	Due to **hypoglycaemia** caused by increased glucose use or decreased glucose production (e.g. **vomiting**, sweating, pallor, **tachycardia** in GSD or fructose intolerance) or metabolic **acidosis** (e.g. vomiting and **Kussmaul respirations** in organic **acidaemias**)
Jaundice	After the neonatal period this is usually intrinsic hepatic disease, especially raised liver enzymes, but can be due to inherited disorders of metabolism (e.g. untreated galactosaemia, fructose intolerance, **tyrosinaemia**)
Unusual odours in body fluids	Odours due to specific compounds (e.g. sweaty feet in **isovaleric acidaemia**, smoky-sweet in **maple syrup urine disease**, mousy or musty in phenylketonuria, boiled cabbage in tyrosinaemia)
Change in urine colour	With exposure to air in some disorders (e.g. darkish brown in **alkaptonuria**, purplish brown in porphyria)
Organomegaly	Substrate accumulation within organ cells (e.g. **hepatomegaly** in hepatic forms of GSD and lysosomal storage diseases, cardiomegaly in GSD)
Eye changes	Cataracts in **galactokinase deficiency**/classic galactosemia; **ophthalmoplegia** and retinal degeneration in oxidative phosphorylation defects
Testing	Changed basic metabolic screening tests, including: glucose, **electrolytes**, complete blood count, liver function tests, ammonia levels, serum amino acid levels, urinalysis, urine organic acids, electrolyte measurements

Source: Adapted from Sanders, 2016

Metabolic syndrome

This is a complex of several pathophysiological conditions marked by:

* obesity
* cardiovascular changes
* significant insulin resistance.

Most individuals with metabolic syndrome have developed vascular and other complications before a diagnosis is made. Metabolic syndrome is becoming increasingly prevalent in adolescents and young adults, due to the increased incidence of childhood obesity. In addition, specific physiological parameters equate with the clinical criteria agreed internationally in the Consensus Statements initially developed in 2006 by the International Diabetes Federation: excess fat around the waist, **hypertension**, hyperglycaemia, abnormal cholesterol or **triglycerides** (Table 13.2) (IDF, 2017). Type 2 diabetes mellitus and **cardiovascular disease** (CVD) are two major health **epidemics** linked with metabolic syndrome. Obesity and insulin resistance are discussed in greater detail later in this chapter in the section on disorders of carbohydrate metabolism.

Table 13.2 The new International Diabetes Federation definition of metabolic syndrome

According to this definition, for a person to be defined as having the metabolic syndrome they must have:	
Central obesity (defined as waist circumference* within ethnicity-specific values) plus any two of the following four factors:	
Raised triglycerides	≥150 mg/dl (1.7 mmol/l) or specific treatment for this lipid abnormality
Reduced HDL cholesterol	<40 mg/dl (1.03 mmol/l) in males, <50 mg/dl (1.29 mmol/l) in females or specific treatment for this lipid abnormality
Raised blood pressure	Systolic BP ≥130 or diastolic BP ≥85 mmHg or treatment of previously diagnosed hypertension
Raised fasting plasma glucose (FPG)	(FPG) ≥100 mg/dl (5.6 mmol/l), or previously diagnosed type 2 diabetes If above 5.6 mmol/l or 100 mg/dl, an oral glucose tolerance test (OGTT) is strongly recommended but is not necessary to define presence of the syndrome

* If BMI is >30 kg/m^2, central obesity can be assumed and waist circumference does not need to be measured.

Source: IDF, 2017: 10

Thyroid hormones

The overall rate of metabolism of the body, and of all the cells comprising the body, is regulated by the thyroid hormones, and their secretion is controlled by TSH (thyroid-stimulating hormone). TSH is secreted from the anterior lobe of the pituitary gland and adjusted by negative feedback from thyroid hormone secretion to the pituitary gland. The metabolic rate is reflected in the activity of all the organs of the body. Both **hyperthyroidism** and hypothyroidism have been linked with disorders of carbohydrate metabolism, with the severity of the metabolic disease proportional to the hormone disorder. Impaired glucose tolerance in hyperthyroidism may be due to mainly hepatic insulin resistance, while it appears that insulin resistance of peripheral tissues is more common in hypothyroidism (Gierach et al., 2014).

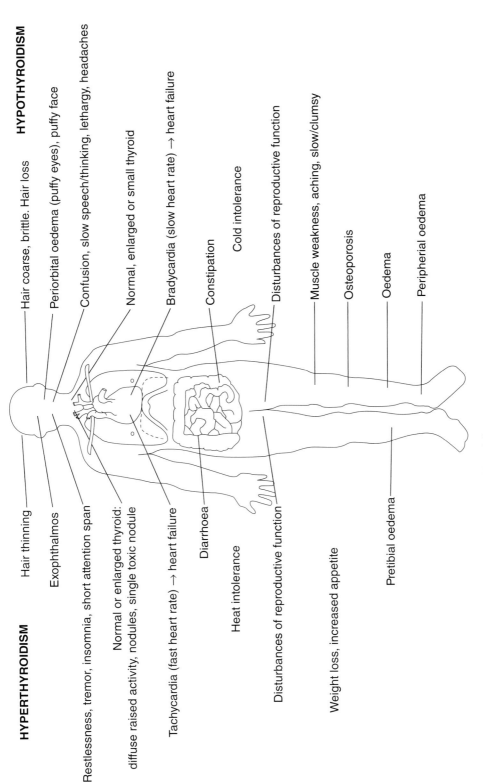

HYPERTHYROIDISM

Hair thinning

Exophthalmos

Restlessness, tremor, insomnia, short attention span

Normal or enlarged thyroid: diffuse raised activity, nodules, single toxic nodule

Tachycardia (fast heart rate) → heart failure

Diarrhoea

Heat intolerance

Disturbances of reproductive function

Weight loss, increased appetite

Pretibial oedema

HYPOTHYROIDISM

Hair coarse, brittle. Hair loss

Periorbital oedema (puffy eyes), puffy face

Confusion, slow speech/thinking, lethargy, headaches

Normal, enlarged or small thyroid

Bradycardia (slow heart rate) → heart failure

Constipation

Cold intolerance

Disturbances of reproductive function

Muscle weakness, aching, slow/clumsy

Osteoporosis

Oedema

Peripherial oedema

Figure 13.1 Disturbances in hyperthyroidism and hypothyroidism

Thyroid hormones are important in the regulation of lipid, cholesterol and glucose metabolism in the liver and, thus, in metabolic syndrome. They have important roles in controlling mitochondrial function, regulating metabolic genes, and balancing fatty acid formation (Sinha et al., 2014). In response to the supply of nutrients, hepatic **lipophagy** (the breakdown and elimination of lipids from cells) regulates intracellular lipid stores, levels of free lipids (e.g. fatty acids) and energy **homeostasis** (Liu and Czaja, 2013). Impairment of this function results in excessive fat being laid down in the cells.

The two main groups of disorders in this context are hypo- and hyperthyroidism with the clinical signs and symptoms indicated in Figure 13.1.

Hyperthyroidism/Thyrotoxicosis

Hyperthyroidism refers to a state of excess circulating thyroid hormones due to hyperfunction of the thyroid gland only, whereas **thyrotoxicosis** refers to a state of excess circulating thyroid hormones triggered by any cause, e.g. hyperfunction of thyroid gland or thyroid hormone overdose. Thyrotoxicosis may occur in the absence of hyperthyroidism, e.g. short-term thyrotoxicosis that occurs in destructive thyroiditis that causes the release of stored thyroid hormones (Carroll, 2014). Causes of thyrotoxicosis include giving birth (postpartum thyroiditis, common in women with type 1 diabetes mellitus), infection (subacute thyroiditis) and drug-induced, e.g. amiodarone (Carroll, 2014).

There are several causes of hyperthyroidism, including:

- Pituitary gland **tumour**, leading to raised TSH secretion stimulating thyroid hormone secretion.
- **Graves' disease**, which is the main cause of hyperthyroidism in the UK (80%) (McNicol and Foulis, 2014). It is an autoimmune condition in which the body's immune system is attacking its own tissues which stimulates growth of the thyroid gland and increased hormone secretion.
- Nodular thyroid disease, which tends to occur in response to the TSH increase at puberty, pregnancy, iodine deficiency, or infectious or genetic disorders.

High levels of thyroid hormones in the blood result in increased anabolism and metabolic rate with raised heat production leading to heat intolerance. In addition, the body's response to autonomic stimulation is increased.

APPLY

Hyperthyroidism

Signs and symptoms

Someone with hyperthyroidism will have a raised basal metabolic rate with: flushed skin, peripheral **vasodilation**, sweating to increase heat loss, increased cardiac activity, overactivity of the sympathetic nervous system, and sometimes a wide-eyed staring gaze.

Table 13.3 Systemic effects of hyperthyroidism

System	Effect
General	Weight reduction, irritability, heat intolerance, fatigue, poor sleep
Skin	Warm moist palms, urticarial, itching
Eye	Periorbital **oedema**, lid lag and retraction, exophthalmos, redness, loss of vision

System	Effect
Central nervous system	Worsening of mental ill-health, stupor, coma
Cardiovascular system	Tachycardia, cardiomegaly, heart failure, arrhythmias
Respiratory system	Dyspnoea
Bone	Decreased bone mineral density
Reproductive system	Gynaecomastia (breast development), amenorrhoea
Metabolic	**Hyperglycaemia, hypercalcaemia**
Gastrointestinal	Diarrhoea
Neuromuscular	Tremor, myopathy

Treatment

Treatment is to reduce secretion of thyroid hormones by:

- administering anti-thyroid drugs
- injecting radioactive iodine, which is absorbed by the thyroid gland and destroys some of the glandular tissue
- surgery to remove part of the gland
- administering **beta-blockers** to control raised sympathetic activity.

A **thyrotoxic crisis** or **thyroid storm** is an **acute** life-threatening hypermetabolic state caused by the excessive release of thyroid hormones in an individual with thyrotoxicosis, causing adrenergic hyperactivity (Idrose, 2015). The most common cause of thyroid storm is infection, although **diabetic ketoacidosis**, hypoglycaemia, hyperosmolar coma, **pulmonary embolism** and withdrawal of antithyroid medications may also contribute to its development (Idrose, 2015).

ACTIVITY 13.1: APPLY

Living with hyperthyroidism

Watch this video in order to hear how hyperthyroidism can affect a person. If you are using the eBook just click on the play button. Alternatively go to
https://study.sagepub.com/essentialpatho/videos

HYPERTHYROIDISM 1 (9:43)

Hypothyroidism

Hypothyroidism reflects a decrease in thyroid function and is one of the most common conditions seen in clinical practice (Drake, 2018). Thyroid hormones play a central role in the regulation of normal metabolism; therefore, reduced thyroid hormone levels that occur in hypothyroidism are associated with metabolic slowing (Drake, 2018). A wide range of signs and symptoms are associated with hypothyroidism, including bradycardia, fatigue, weight gain, cold intolerance, decreased exercise capacity, muscle weakness, constipation, depression and menstrual irregularities (Figure 13.1).

Hypothyroid disorders include:

- Pituitary gland dysfunction with diminished TSH and, thus, restricted secretion of thyroid hormones.
- Primary hypothyroidism with several causes. The commonest cause worldwide is iodine deficiency, although in first-world countries the addition of iodine to salt means that it is rare. Autoimmune changes cause inflammatory destruction of the glandular tissue.
- Congenital hypothyroidism is when a thyroid deficiency is present at birth. This needs immediate or rapid diagnosis and treatment as impaired mental development and stunted growth will occur without adequate treatment.
- Thyroid carcinoma is predominantly due to ionising radiation during childhood with the risk being related to the age of exposure and the dosage of radiation. The period between exposure and appearance of the **cancer** is at least 5–10 years (Iglesias et al., 2017).

Hypothyroidism is treated with hormone replacement therapy, often in the form of levothyroxine – a synthetic hormone.

Severe hypothyroidism can result in **myxoedema**, defined as: 'swelling of the skin and underlying tissues giving a waxy consistency, typical of patients with underactive thyroid glands' (Oxford Living Dictionary, 2017) and can include thickening of the tongue and mucous membranes of the larynx and pharynx, causing hoarse slurred speech (McCance and Huether, 2014).

Myxoedema coma, although rare, can cause life-threatening complications such as cardiogenic shock (Brahmandam et al., 2018). It occurs when a person has severe hypothyroidism and the neurological effects result in a reduced level of **consciousness**. This may happen because of an acute illness, infection, or use of sedative or narcotic drugs, and may occur in older people with vascular disease (McCance and Huether, 2014).

APPLY

MAUD BODIE
CASE NOTES

Hypothyroidism

Maud went to see her GP when she was 53 because she was getting headaches, feeling tired, and finding it difficult to walk any distance. She was also tending to feel cold and was wearing more clothes than usual. Her GP examined her, particularly looking for the signs and symptoms identified in Figure 13.1. Her pulse was a bit slow, her voice rather hoarse and, when asked, she said she was somewhat constipated.

Her GP thought that hypothyroidism was a strong possibility and took a blood sample for biochemical analysis (thyroid function test [TFT]). The results are compared with the reference range for normal of the particular laboratory used. Interestingly these reference ranges vary in different contexts, but the results documents always include the necessary information for interpretation of the individual's results. Maud's results confirmed the diagnosis of hypothyroidism:

- TSH (thyroid-stimulating hormone): high
- T_4 (thyroxine): low

She was commenced on levothyroxine daily to supplement her thyroxine level, has received regular check-ups since and has continued well.

Maud was started on levothyroxine but there are alternative treatments for hypothyroidism which are considered in the video below, which you should find interesting. If you are using the eBook just click on the play button. Alternatively go to

https://study.sagepub.com/essentialpatho/videos

HYPOTHYROIDISM 1 (2:02)

ACTIVITY 13.2: APPLY

Living with hypothyroidism

Watch this video in order to hear how hypothyroidism can affect a person. If you are using the eBook just click on the play button. Alternatively go to

https://study.sagepub.com/essentialpatho/videos

HYPOTHYROIDISM 2 (10:08)

DISORDERS OF CARBOHYDRATE METABOLISM

Inherited disorders of carbohydrate metabolism

These disorders include a number of different groups of conditions outlined in the Go Deeper box. The inheritance of most of these is **autosomal** recessive in nature, dependent on acquiring one gene for the disorder from each parent. A number of these conditions can be identified by post-natal screening and, with early diagnosis, some can be controlled and symptom development minimised by managing the individual's nutritional intake.

GO DEEPER

Table 13.4 Inherited disorders of carbohydrate metabolism

Fructose metabolism disorders	Fructose: a monosaccharide present in fruit and honey, a constituent of sucrose and sorbitol
Deficiency of fructose metabolising enzymes:	
Asymptomatic or hypoglycaemia	Ingestion of fructose → hypoglycaemia, **nausea** and vomiting, abdominal pain, sweating, tremors, confusion, lethargy, seizures, and coma. May → **cirrhosis**, mental deterioration, proximal **renal tubular acidosis** – loss of phosphate and glucose
Three **autosomal recessive** conditions:	
Fructose 1-phosphate aldolase (aldolase B) deficiency (acute)	
Fructokinase deficiency (benign)	Short-term treatment is oral or IV glucose for hypoglycaemia; long-term treatment is exclusion of dietary fructose, sucrose and sorbitol
Deficiency of fructose-1,6-biphosphatase (? fatal in infants)	

(Continued)

Table 13.4 (Continued)

Galactosaemia Deficiencies in enzymes that convert galactose to glucose Galactose: dairy products, fruits and vegetables Three autosomal recessive conditions: Galactose-1-phosphate uridyl transferase deficiency Galactokinase deficiency Galactose-1-phosphate uridyl transferase deficiency May vary in severity	Hepatic and renal dysfunction, cognitive deficits, cataracts, premature ovarian failure. Vomiting, hepatomegaly, poor growth, lethargy, diarrhoea, septicaemia, renal dysfunction, **metabolic acidosis** and oedema. **Haemolytic anaemia** may occur. Enzyme analysis of RBCs Without treatment, children remain short and develop cognitive, speech, gait and balance deficits, may have cataracts, **osteomalacia**, idiopathic **intracranial hypertension** Treatment elimination of galactose and lactose. Physical prognosis good, but cognitive and performance parameters are often subnormal
Glycogen storage diseases Enzyme deficiencies for glycogen synthesis or breakdown; in liver or muscles → hypoglycaemia or abnormal amounts or types of glycogen in tissues Autosomal recessive except for one which is **X-linked**	Age of onset, clinical manifestations and severity vary by type, but symptoms and signs are mainly those of hypoglycaemia and myopathy Diagnosis of glycogen storage diseases by history, examination, glycogen and intermediate metabolites in tissues. Diagnosis confirmed by decrease in enzyme activity in liver, muscle, skin **fibroblasts** depending on condition
Pyruvate metabolism disorders Normally acetyl CoA formed from pyruvate Deficiency results in elevation of pyruvate and thus lactic acid levels X-linked or autosomal recessive	Inability to metabolise pyruvate causes lactic acidosis and a variety of CNS abnormalities, e.g. cystic **lesions** of cerebral cortex, brain stem and basal ganglia; ataxia; psychomotor retardation Low-carbohydrate or ketogenic diet and dietary thiamine supplementation beneficial for some
Other carbohydrate metabolism disorders	Impaired **gluconeogenesis** results in symptoms and signs similar to hepatic forms of glycogen storage disease but without glycogen accumulation Deficiencies of glycolytic or pentose phosphate pathway enzymes → haemolytic anaemia

Acquired disorders of carbohydrate metabolism

The most significant acquired conditions in relation to the proportion of the population affected and the long-term influence on health status are diabetes mellitus type 1 and diabetes mellitus type 2. Diabetes mellitus (DM) is a **chronic**, life-long condition of glucose metabolism in which the body responds abnormally (insulin resistance) or does not produce enough insulin to control the blood glucose level.

The symptoms, which often take the person affected to their GP, include: thirst, **polyuria** (excessive amounts of urine passed), particularly nocturia, and fatigue. They may also include weight loss and muscle **atrophy**. **Glycosuria** is one of the earliest tests for diabetes followed by blood glucose levels, both of which indicate the current status of glucose metabolism. Glycated **haemoglobin** (HbA1c) is formed when haemoglobin combines with glucose in the blood and (because haemoglobin has a life span of approximately 4 months) it provides an overall picture of average blood glucose over the previous 2–3 months.

Monitoring the ongoing level of blood glucose facilitates control. The levels of blood glucose or glycated haemoglobin are compared with the standard levels shown on the results chart received from the biochemistry laboratory. It is important to recognise that different laboratories may use slightly different methods and, thus, have slightly different standards. In addition, most countries use SI units but the USA, Burma and Liberia do not; US Customary Units, developed from the original British units, are used instead. The Apply box below indicates SI levels recommended for individuals with different requirements.

APPLY

Blood glucose monitoring

The targets usually aimed for are as near to non-diabetic levels as possible:

  3.5-5.5 mmol/l before meals   less than 8 mmol/l 2 hours after meals

Type 1 DM (NICE, 2015, from Diabetes UK, 2017a)

Children with type 1 DM

> On waking and before meals   4-7 mmol/l
> After meals   5-9 mmol/l

Adults with type 1 DM

> On waking   5-7 mmol/l
> Before meals at other times   4-7 mmol/l
> 90 minutes after meals   5-9 mmol/l

Type 2 DM (Council of Healthcare Professionals, Diabetes UK, 2017a)

> Before meals   4-7 mmol/l
> 2 hours after meals   less than 8.5 mmol/l

Pregnant women with diabetes (NICE, 2015, from Diabetes UK, 2017a)

> Fasting below 5.3 mmol/l
> 1 hour after meals   below 7.8 mmol/l
> 2 hours after meals   below 6.5 mmol/l

Glycated haemoglobin levels (Diabetes UK, 2017a)

For most adults with diabetes the target is 48 mmol/mol (6.5%)

Levels in diagnosis:

> Normal below   42 mmol/mol
> Prediabetes   42-47 mmol/mol
> Diabetes   48 mmol/mol or over

Control of blood glucose

Blood glucose metabolism is controlled primarily by the hormonal secretions of the four types of cells in the Islets of Langerhans in the pancreas; see Revise box below.

————————————— **REVISE: A&P RECAP** —————————————

Control of blood glucose

Chapter 9 of *Essentials of Anatomy and Physiology for Nursing Practice* (Boore et al., 2016) gives details of the four different types of cell involved, the hormones secreted and the function of these hormones.

___

The balance between insulin and **glucagon** regulates the blood glucose level. Insulin is an anabolic hormone that promotes the synthesis of proteins, carbohydrates and nucleic acids, reduces blood glucose levels and facilitates entry into the cells of potassium (K^+), magnesium (Mg^{2+}) and phosphate (PO_4^{3-}). It is produced from a precursor (proinsulin) and stored as secretory granules in the Golgi body. Its secretion is calcium (Ca^{2+})-dependent, evoked primarily by raised blood glucose and amino acids, and regulated by chemical, hormonal (including gastrointestinal) and neural control. Its pulsed secretion occurs when beta cells are stimulated by the parasympathetic nervous system before eating. Insulin acts by binding to and activating the appropriate cell membrane receptors, causing glucose transporters to promote glucose uptake followed by diverse metabolic events through the body. Sensitivity of receptors is a key component in maintaining cellular function and insulin sensitivity if affected by: age, weight, abdominal fat and physical activity. Resistance of these receptors to insulin has been introduced above; exercise and weight loss are the most effective measures to increase sensitivity.

Glucagon promotes increased blood glucose; its release is stimulated by a fall in blood glucose, a rise in certain amino acids, sympathetic nervous stimulation and gut hormones, e.g. gastrin and cholecystokinin. It is inhibited by the factors which stimulate insulin release.

Diabetes mellitus

This is named from Greek (*diabetes* = 'going through') and Latin (*mellitus* = 'honey or sweet'). It was originally diagnosed by tasting for sweet urine.

It is a disorder of carbohydrate, protein and fat metabolism, resulting from a lack of insulin or a reduction in the biological effects of insulin. It can represent:

* an absolute or relative insulin deficiency which may be due to

  o impaired release of insulin
  o production of inactive insulin

* insulin resistance which may be due to

  o inadequate or defective insulin receptors or post-receptor regulation
  o insulin destroyed before it can carry out its action.

The classification of diabetes mellitus is shown in Table 13.5

Table 13.5 Classification of diabetes mellitus

Type 1 diabetes mellitus	Lack of insulin secretion→insulin dependent (see below)
Type 2 diabetes mellitus	Insulin resistance, often linked with obesity and managed by drug treatment (see below)
Gestational diabetes (GDM)	Develops during pregnancy, usually disappears afterwards 5%-10% develop type 2 later in life
Prediabetes	Blood glucose higher than normal but do not have diabetes. Can be: impaired glucose tolerance (IGT) or impaired fasting glucose (IFG)
Metabolic syndrome	Linked with insulin resistance (see earlier)

Source: NH3S England

Type 1 Diabetes mellitus (DM)

Type 1 DM is characterised by the destruction of pancreatic beta cells and can be subdivided into two categories: type 1A (immune-mediated diabetes) and type 1B (idiopathic diabetes). People with this condition are insulin-dependent as they produce no or very little insulin due to a loss of functioning beta cells in the Islets of Langerhans in the pancreas. Type 1 diabetes has a strong genetic component, evidenced by the fact that a close relative with the condition increases the risk for close relatives; substantial (>50) numbers of predisposing genes have been identified (de Beeck and Eizirik, 2016). These interact with environmental factors, including microbes, which trigger the autoimmune response when the body's immune system attacks its own beta cells and triggers **apoptosis**.

It appears that various microbes can both increase and decrease the risk of diabetes. Two hypotheses explain these findings:

- The hygiene hypothesis proposes that exposure to microbes as a child stimulates regulation of the immune system and limits autoimmune reactions.
- The triggering hypothesis suggests that specific microbes damage insulin-producing cells, with enteroviruses as the proposed main microbial risks. This relates to developing knowledge about the human **microbiome** and evidence that some microbes result in a reduced risk of diabetes (Kondrashova and Hyöty, 2014).

Type 1 diabetes mellitus occurs in about 1 in 250 of the UK population and usually develops in thin individuals relatively early in life: in children, adolescents or young adults (McNicol and Foulis, 2014). In young people, the symptoms of type 1 DM develop very quickly (days or weeks) but more slowly in adults. Those with this type of diabetes are prone to developing ketoacidotic coma.

Those affected with type 1 diabetes are dependent on balancing administered insulin with a healthy diet, regular exercise and careful monitoring of the condition. Careful management is necessary to minimise the risk of complications (NHS Choices, 2016a).

Type 1 DM may be subdivided into two categories: type 1A (immune-mediated diabetes) and type 1B (idiopathic diabetes).

Type 1A – immune-mediated DM

Type 1A is an autoimmune disorder that can develop due to a combination of a genetic predisposition and an environmental trigger such as an infection, e.g. mumps, rubella or cytomegalovirus. Abnormalities in immune cells and changes in beta cell antigens have been linked to deficient immune tolerance. Gene and environment interactions result in the formation of **autoantigens** expressed on beta cells (in the islets of Langerhans) and circulate in the bloodstream and lymphatics. Stimulation of **cell-mediated immunity** (T-cytotoxic cells and **macrophages**) and **humoral immunity** (autoantibodies) responses result in beta cell destruction and apoptosis. **Infiltration** of the islets by **lymphocytes** and macrophages lead to a release of inflammatory **cytokines**, the activation of **T-helper cells** and **cytotoxic T lymphocytes**, resulting in the death of beta cells. It is also mediated by the production of autoantibodies against islet cells, insulin, glutamic acid decarboxylase and other cytoplasmic proteins. This combination leads to autoimmune T-cell-mediated interaction with the beta cells, which slowly, progressively destroys them. With the destruction of these cells, insulin synthesis declines and hyperglycaemia develops. It is thought that 80–90% of beta cells must be destroyed for insulin synthesis to fall sufficiently to cause hyperglycaemia. Resultant **hypoinsulinaemia** leads to an increase in glucagon secretion, causing **glycogenolysis** and gluconeogenesis, with the function of both alpha and beta cells being abnormal and both contributing to hyperglycaemia (Figure 13.2).

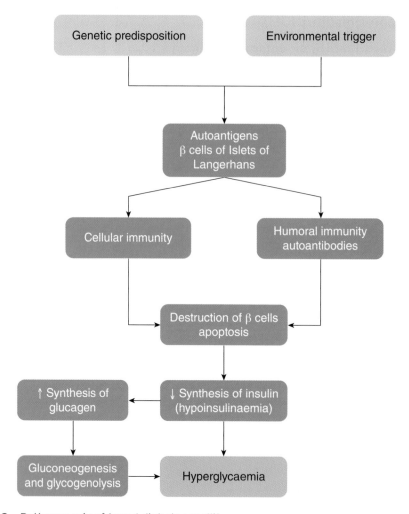

Figure 13.2 Pathogenesis of type 1 diabetes mellitus

GO DEEPER

Autoimmunity and type 1 diabetes mellitus

The **major histocompatibility complex (MHC)** codes for various elements of the immune system and is located on **chromosome** 6. It can be divided into three classes:

- Class I: on surface of virtually every cell, binds to CD8 receptors on cytotoxic T cells
- Class II: mainly on macrophages and B cells and present antigen to T-helper cells
- Class III: encode for other immune components such as complement or cytokines, e.g. **tumour necrosis factor-alpha**

The **human leucocyte antigen (HLA)** is the subset of MHC genes encoding for cell surface antigen-presenting antigens. HLA is classified into divisions: HLA-A, HLA-B and HLA-C belong to MHC class 1; HLA-D consists of six genes belonging to MHC class II.

Deviations in HLA genes increase the risk of developing autoimmune diseases, e.g. type 1 DM, **rheumatoid arthritis, coeliac disease** and **multiple sclerosis** (Hu et al., 2015). Numerous HLA genes increase the risk of type 1 DM; more than 90% of children with type 1 diabetes carry *HLA-DRB1, HLA -DQB1 (DR3-DQ2)* and/ or *DRB1-DQB1 (DR4-DQ8)*, and the highest risk *HLA-DR3-DQ2/DR4-DQ8* (Gillespie et al., 2014). *HLA-DRB1, HLA-DQA1* and *HLADQB1* have the largest allelic associations with type 1 DM (Hu et al., 2015).

It is proposed that two types of autoantibodies are produced, i.e. insulin autoantibodies and islet cell autoantibodies, leading to the destruction of islet beta cells. These may exist for years before hyperglycaemia occurs. In addition to MHC susceptibility genes for type 1, an insulin regulating and beta cell replication gene has been found on chromosome 11 (Porth, 2015).

Type 1B – idiopathic DM

Type 1B is used to describe those cases of beta cell destruction in which there is no evidence of **autoimmunity** present. It tends to be strongly inherited but affects only a small proportion of the population and people of African or Asian descent are more likely to fall into this category. It presents with varying degrees of insulin deficiency, with periods of absolute insulin deficiency leading to episodic ketoacidosis.

Signs and symptoms of type 1 DM

These result from the main physiological changes associated with hyperglycaemia, the raised level of blood glucose and altered fat metabolism. Hyperglycaemia results from decreased transport and uptake of glucose by cells. The raised amount of glucose in the blood filtered by the renal glomeruli is greater than can be reabsorbed from the filtrate back into the circulation. Glucose is a small osmotically active particle which carries water with it into the urinary filtrate, resulting in an increased volume of urine, polyuria, containing glucose (not normally present in urine), i.e. glycosuria. Table 13.6 shows the signs and symptoms resulting from these main alterations.

Table 13.6 Rationale for signs and symptoms of type 1 diabetes mellitus

Hyperglycaemia	Inadequate glucose available for metabolism
	Polyphagia: cellular starvation and depletion of cellular stores of carbohydrates, proteins and fats stimulate appetite
	Weight loss:
	• Loss of body fluids due to **osmotic diuresis**
	• Body tissue lost as lack of insulin forces body to use fat and protein stores for energy
	• Usually found in uncontrolled type 1; type 2 often have obesity
	Ketonuria
	• Increased metabolism of fats as energy → increased ketone bodies produced and excreted by kidney
	• People may have distinctive smell of acetone or 'pear drops' on their breath
	Fatigue: lowered plasma volume and lack of available glucose for energy needs
Glycosuria	Polyuria: **osmotic pressure** of glucose in urine carries excessive water → large volume of urine passed
	Polydipsia: high blood glucose → intracellular dehydration as water is pulled out of cells and excreted. Osmoreceptors detect change in osmolality of blood and stimulates excessive thirst. Large volume of fluid imbibed
Paraesthesia: temporary dysfunction of peripheral sensory nerves	
Skin infections: hyperglycaemia/glycosuria favour growth of yeast organisms	

Source: NHS England

APPLY

Treatment for type 1 DM

Insulins differ in their source (although most are now human or recombinant DNA, they used to be pork/beef), time of onset, peak effect and duration of action. Doses of insulin are highly individualised; the precise control of blood glucose levels, diet, amount of exercise, job etc. need to be taken into consideration when administering specific insulin doses.

Due to first pass metabolism insulin cannot be administered orally, therefore it is given by subcutaneous injection. There are various types of insulin available (Table 13.7).

Table 13.7 Treatment for type 1 diabetes mellitus

Action	Onset	Peak	Duration	Drug
Rapid	15-30 min	1 hour	3-4 hours	Insulin Aspart - NovoRapid
Short	30-60 min	2-4 hours	Up to 8 hours	Soluble Insulin - Humulin S, Actrapid
Intermediate	2-4 hours	6-7 hours	Up to 20 hours	Isophane Insulin - Humulin I, Insulatard
Long	1-3 hours	6-8 hours	20-24 hours	Insulin Detemir - Levemir Insulin Glargine - Lantus

Source: NHS England

As already noted, insulin regimes are highly individualised, however provided below are some examples of how an insulin regime may be prescribed:

- Multiple injection regimen: short-acting insulin or rapid-acting insulin analogue, before meals, with intermediate-acting or long-acting insulin, once or twice daily
- Short-acting insulin or rapid-acting insulin analogue mixed with intermediate-acting or long-acting insulin, once or twice daily (before meals)
- Intermediate-acting or long-acting insulin, once or twice daily, with or without short-acting insulin or rapid-acting insulin before meals

Type 2 diabetes mellitus

This type of diabetes occurs when an inadequate amount of insulin is produced or insulin resistance is present. Glucose then remains in the blood unused for energy. This type of diabetes occurs in about 1 in 25 of the population in the UK (McNicol and Foulis, 2014: 49) and is more common in those who are obese and over 40 years of age. Oral hypoglycaemic drugs, often different types in combination, are usually used in managing this condition. The key risk factors are indicated in Table 13.8.

This is a condition of hyperglycaemia related to insulin resistance and insulin deficiency. It is associated with:

- Genetic and acquired (environmental) factors
- Overconsumption of a diet rich in fats and **high glycaemic index carbohydrates** (foods with a relatively high ability to increase the level of glucose in the blood)
- Obesity
- Lack of exercise.

Table 13.8   Causes and risk factors in type 2 diabetes mellitus

	Risk factors	Presentation/ management
Age	Risk increases with age Caucasians over 40 South Asians Chinese African-Caribbean Black African — increased risk of developing the condition at a much earlier age In recent years younger people from all ethnic groups have been developing the condition. Also more common for young children (7 years) to develop type 2 diabetes due to childhood obesity (Singer and Lumeng, 2017)	Tend to gain weight and exercise less with age increasing risk Management: maintaining a healthy weight by eating a healthy, balanced diet and exercising regularly are ways of preventing and managing diabetes
Genetics	Major risk factor for type 2 diabetes Risk is increased if there is a close relative, e.g. parent, brother or sister, with the condition. The closer the relative, the greater the risk. A child with a parent with type 2 diabetes has about a one in three chance of also developing the condition	Early recognition of risk allows for early action to reduce risk factors and for introduction of treatment as soon as is necessary
Weight	Being overweight or obese increases risk UK, a body mass index (BMI) of: • 25+ in overweight range • 30+ in obese range • Asians with BMI of 23+ at increased risk • Asians with BMI of 27.5+ at high risk Central obesity increased risk Waist measurements also indicate raised risk level in the following: • Women with waist size 80 cm (31.5 inches)+ • Asian men with waist 89 cm (35 inches) + • White or black men with waist 94cm (37 inches) or more	Exercising regularly and reducing body weight by about 5% could reduce the risk of getting diabetes by more than 50% Read information and advice about losing weight
Other	Blood glucose level higher than normal, but not high enough to be diabetic, increases risk: known as prediabetes or impaired glucose tolerance Prediabetes can progress to type 2 diabetes if action not taken. Women with gestational diabetes during pregnancy have greater risk of diabetes in later life	Taking preventative steps, such as lifestyle changes including eating healthily, losing weight if overweight, and taking plenty of regular exercise can reduce risk

Source: Adapted from NHS Choices, 2016b

Genetic abnormalities alongside environmental factors result in the basic pathophysiologic mechanisms of type 2 DM, i.e. increased insulin resistance and decreased insulin secretion (Figure 13.3). Over 60 genes have been linked with the development of type 2 DM, genes that code for: beta cell mass, beta cell function, proinsulin and insulin molecular structures, insulin receptors, hepatic synthesis of glucose, glucagon synthesis and cellular responsiveness to insulin stimulation.

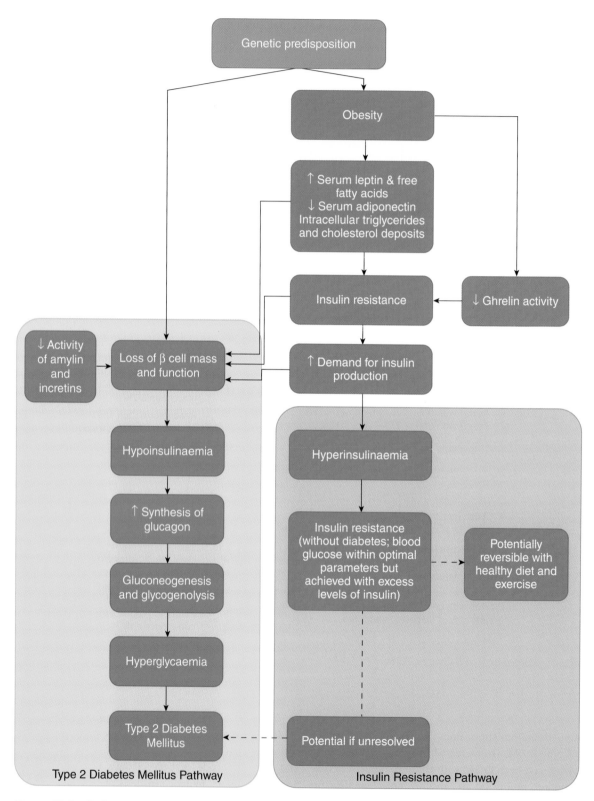

Figure 13.3 Pathogenesis of insulin resistance and type 2 diabetes

Insulin resistance and chronic hyperglycaemia are due to the contribution of many organs. Metabolic abnormalities involved include: insulin resistance, increased glucose production by the liver and deranged secretion of insulin by the pancreatic beta cells.

Obesity

Central (or abdominal) obesity is when excessive fat builds up around the stomach and abdomen, including within the peritoneal cavity, and may have a negative impact on health due to the correlation between central obesity, type 2 diabetes mellitus and cardiovascular disease. However, it is also associated with various other conditions including: **Alzheimer's disease**, asthma, **Cushing's syndrome**, and in **polycystic ovary syndrome**.

While obesity is an important contributory factor to insulin resistance and diabetes, it is important to note that not everyone who is obese will develop diabetes. Whilst all obese people have a degree of insulin resistance and compensatory **hyperinsulinaemia**, it is thought that only those with central obesity (a high waist [at the umbilicus] to hip [at the symphysis pubis] ratio) alongside a genetic defect will develop diabetes. It is not fully understood how obesity contributes to insulin resistance but a number of factors are believed to be involved and include:

- Increased **adipocytes** lead to increased levels of **adipokines** (cell-signalling proteins from adipose tissues), leading to increased serum levels of **leptin** and decreased levels of **adiponectin** (involved in controlling blood glucose). These changes are associated with **inflammation** and can decrease insulin sensitivity of the cells.
- Increased serum free fatty acids (FFAs) and intracellular triglycerides and cholesterol can interfere with intracellular insulin signalling and decrease the response of tissues to insulin. This may also alter the action of **incretins** (see below) and promote inflammation.
- Inflammatory cytokines from intra-abdominal adipocytes or adipocyte-associated mononuclear cells, lead to induced insulin resistance and are cytotoxic to beta cells.

Hyperinsulinaemia and decreased insulin receptor density are correlated to obesity. The clinical appearance of diabetes may be masked for many years due to compensatory hyperglycaemia. However, over time beta cell dysfunction will occur and lead to a deficiency in insulin and the development of diabetes.

Insulin resistance

Glucose metabolism is disrupted in insulin resistance. Normally insulin acts by linking with specific receptors on cell membranes, particularly of adipocytes (fat cells), **hepatocytes** (liver cells) and striated muscle cells to enable glucose to enter the cells. In insulin resistance these cells do not respond normally to the hormone and, thus, levels of glucose in the blood become raised. This reduced sensitivity occurs at one of three points: pre-receptor, receptor and post-receptor, and glucose is prevented from entering the cells and getting metabolised normally. Insulin resistance may present linked with a variety of disorders such as type 2 diabetes mellitus, **hypercholesterolaemia**, **hypertriglyceridaemia**, obesity and arterial hypertension. The effect of sub-clinical disorders is still being considered but the relationship between thyroid hormones and insulin resistance is significant.

It is thought that there are various mechanisms involved in irregularities in the insulin signalling pathway and subsequent development of insulin resistance. The mechanisms thought to be involved include:

- Changes to molecular structure of insulin
- Increased levels of insulin antagonists
- Downregulation of insulin receptors (reducing or suppressing response to a stimulus) (e.g. reduced response to insulin due to decreased receptors on cell surface)
- Changes to glucose transporter (GLUT) proteins

The genetic factors alongside environmental factors such as ageing, sedentary lifestyle and obesity, increase the propensity for development of insulin resistance. As insulin resistance develops, beta cell production of insulin increases to compensate and maintain the blood glucose level in the narrow range needed for normal bodily function. If insulin resistance persists or increases over time (usually years), beta cells will start to fail due to genetic defect, glucose and/or fat toxicity, or exhaustion. Eventually beta cells will fail and insulin secretion will decrease, resulting in elevated blood glucose levels leading to the development of diabetes.

GO DEEPER

Insulin deficiency

Insulin deficiency in type 2 DM is different from in type 1 DM as it is not mediated by the immune system. It may be due to:

- Beta cell exhaustion from hypersecretion of insulin
- Glucose and lipid toxicity to the beta cells
- Genetic factors

Probably a combination of these factors has differing importance for different people.

Toxicity to beta cells is a major factor in decreased insulin production. As glucose levels begin to rise slightly from beta cell exhaustion or other factors, damage to the beta cells results in decreased insulin production and a further increase in glucose levels (a vicious cycle is beginning).

Lipids, especially triglycerides, are also toxic to beta cells. Insulin deficiency, relative or absolute, activates **lipase** enzyme in fat cells. Incipient diabetes leads to the accumulation of intra-abdominal fat that can drain triglycerides directly into the portal system and thus into the pancreas of the person. These are toxic to beta cells, causing damage, loss of beta cells and loss of beta cell function.

It has been estimated that 50% of beta cell insulin production is lost by the time the diagnosis of type 2 DM is made.

Signs and symptoms of type 2 DM

The signs and symptoms associated with type 2 DM may be non-specific: the person may be overweight, hypertensive and hyperglycaemic. They exhibit some of the signs and symptoms associated with type 1 DM, specifically polyuria and **polydipsia**. However, it may be more common for the person to present with recurrent infections, fatigue, visual changes or complaints of paraesthesia.

APPLY

Treatment choices for type 2 DM

There is a wide range of drugs available to treat type 2 DM. These include:

Insulin sensitisers

Biguanides (metformin)

Action: Reduces glucose **absorption**. Reduces peripheral insulin resistance. Inhibits liver glucogenesis. Increases insulin sensitivity. Enhances effect of insulin in peripheral tissue (muscles) where it increases insulin-mediated glucose uptake.

Side-effects: Gastrointestinal upset.

Contraindications: Renal, liver and severe cardiovascular disease.

Thiazolidinediones (pioglitazone)

Action: Combine with a receptor inside the cell nucleus – peroxisome proliferator-activated receptor-gamma. They enhance the response of the tissues to insulin and so target insulin resistance. They aid insulin action by promoting glucose utilisation in the tissues. Decrease hepatic glucose production.

Side-effects: Weight gain, headache, fluid retention.

Secretagogues

Sulphonylureas (gliclizide, glibenclamide, tolbutamide)

Action: Stimulate the beta cells to secrete more insulin by binding to a receptor on the beta cell in the pancreas and allowing an influx of calcium into the cell. This stimulates the release of preformed insulin and results in a fall in plasma glucose concentrations.

Side-effects: Hypoglycaemia, weight gain, gastrointestinal disturbance, facial flushing.

Administration: Take 20–30 minutes before food. Education on relationship between diet, exercise and medication is necessary.

Interaction with other drugs: Warfarin can increase effect and increase risk of hypoglycaemia.

Prandial insulin releasers (repaglinide)

Action: Stimulates extra insulin release. Shorter acting – fewer hypoglycaemic episodes.

Administration: Take 15 minutes before food.

Side-effects: Gastrointestinal, nausea, skin rash.

Alpha-glucosidase inhibitor (acarbose)

Action: Delays carbohydrate absorption by inhibiting the enzyme alpha-glucosidase in the brush border of the intestine and so delays the splitting down of complex sugars to monosaccharides. This delays the absorption of glucose and rescues the post meal rise in blood glucose levels.

Side-effects: Gastrointestinal effects.

Newer drugs

Sitagliptin

Action: An inhibitor of the enzyme dipeptidylpeptidase-4 (DPP-4). It increases insulin secretion and lowers glucagon secretion.

Exenatide

Action: An incretin mimetic that increases insulin secretion and suppresses glucagon secretion and slows gastric emptying.

Administration: Given by subcutaneous injection twice daily.

Vildagliptin

Action: An oral DPP-4 inhibitor that inhibits the enzyme that breaks down incretins, thus allowing them to accumulate and having similar effect to exenatide. It prolongs the action of insulin and reduces the glucagon secretion.

GO DEEPER

Incretins and treatment of diabetes

These peptides are released from the gastrointestinal tract in response to food intake, increasing insulin secretion and decreasing glucose production by the liver. They have many positive effects on metabolism without causing hypoglycaemia.

GLP-1 glucagon-like peptide controls post-prandial glucose levels by:

- promoting glucose-dependent insulin secretion
- stimulating insulin **gene expression**
- inhibiting insulin synthesis and
- delaying gastric emptying.

It also reduces beta cell apoptosis and induces pancreatic **acinar cells** to differentiate into new beta cells, thus enhancing beta-cell mass and replenishing intracellular stores of insulin.

Incretin hormones and enhancers are now being used to treat diabetes mellitus, e.g. GLP-1 receptor **agonists** and dipeptidyl peptidase IV inhibitors (which block breakdown of incretins). They may also cause weight loss, improved B/P, serum lipids and myocardial function, thus decreasing the risk of associated complications.

ACTIVITY 13.3: APPLY

Lived experiences of diabetes

Living with diabetes can have an impact on the life of the person and it is important that nurses, as person-centred practitioners, can appreciate this in order to support people. Access the following resources in order to learn about that impact and reflect on how this may influence your practice:

Diabetes mellitus: www.diabetes.org.uk/diabetes-and-me

Living with diabetes: www.diabetes.org.uk/your-stories

Then watch the video for further insight into the lived experience of diabetes. If you are using the eBook just click on the play button. Alternatively go to

https://study.sagepub.com/essentialpatho/videos

DIABETES MELLITUS (4:02)

Complications of diabetes

People with diabetes are at risk of developing acute or **chronic** complications.

Acute complications

The acute complications involve loss of control of blood glucose levels and associated metabolic effects and there are three main complications, two associated with high and one with a fall in blood glucose.

DIABETIC KETOACIDOSIS (DKA) IN TYPE 1 DM

The metabolic changes are: hyperglycaemia, ketosis and metabolic acidosis. Ketoacidosis is due to insulin deficiency causing rapid breakdown of energy stores from muscle and fat, leading to increased amino acids entering the liver for conversion to glucose and fatty acids and subsequent conversion to **ketones**. Ketones lead to increased adrenaline (epinephrine). Metabolic acidosis is caused by ketoacids which are buffered by bicarbonate, leading to decreased levels in the serum and a fall in blood pH.

Hyperglycaemia leads to osmotic diuresis, dehydration and the critical loss of electrolytes. Hyperosmolality of extracellular fluids is due to hyperglycaemia, causing water and potassium shifts from intracellular to extracellular compartments. **Hypotension** and tachycardia are due to decreased fluid volume and compensatory mechanisms. Kussmaul respiration prevents a further decrease in pH by excreting extra carbon dioxide (acid).

HYPEROSMOLAR HYPERGLYCAEMIC NON-KETOTIC SYNDROME (HHNKS) IN TYPE 2 DM

HHNKS is characterised by hyperglycaemia, **hyperosmolarity**, dehydration and absence of ketones (limited insulin present prevents conversion of fats and proteins to ketones). Glycosuria causes dehydration; as plasma volume contracts **renal insufficiency** develops, leading to even higher blood glucose levels. Increased serum osmolarity pulls water out of body cells, resulting in dehydration, polyuria and polydipsia and may cause weakness. Neurological signs and symptoms such as **hemiparesis**, **aphasia**, seizures and coma can result from the effect on brain cells.

HYPOGLYCAEMIA

Hypoglycaemia or **insulin shock** is caused by insulin overdose, failure to eat or excessive or very high intensity exercise. It quickly affects the nervous system because fats or proteins are not the preferential energy source for **neurons**. It has a rapid onset and signs and symptoms are caused by altered cerebral function, i.e. headache, difficulty in problem solving, disturbed or altered behaviour, slurred speech, staggering gait, coma and seizures. Hypoglycaemia causes activation of the autonomic nervous system (parasympathetic then sympathetic activation) causing signs and symptoms that include: hunger, anxiety, tachycardia, sweating and cool clammy skin.

Chronic complications

Complications are commonly associated with hyperglycaemia, the accumulation of glycated end products and the activation of metabolic pathways that damage the tissues. These are classified as microvascular (damage to capillaries) or macrovascular (damage to larger vessels) (Maitra, 2015). Complications can be reduced with strict control of blood glucose levels.

MICROVASCULAR COMPLICATIONS

These are mainly due to a thickening of the basement membrane and a cross-linking of molecules, resulting from the raised blood glucose level. These changes can cause the blocking of smaller blood vessels (microvascular), resulting in **hypoxia** and ischaemia of the tissues. The major organs and systems affected are:

- Kidneys (nephropathy) – can lead to renal failure
- Eyes (**retinopathy**) – causing impaired vision and blindness. Commonest cause of blindness in working-age people. Annual screening is recommended for people over the age of 12 with diabetes
- Nervous system (neuropathy) – can affect central nervous system, sensorimotor nerves, autonomic nervous system. The most frequent pattern damages the sensation and movement of the legs.

MACROVASCULAR COMPLICATIONS

These cause damage to medium and larger blood vessels and the organs supplied. Common conditions include

- Atherosclerotic changes, causing
  - coronary artery disease
  - stroke
  - peripheral vascular disease
- Damage to the feet. This can become infected and loss of sensation may mean that diabetic foot ulcers are not noticed until serious damage has occurred. This can result in lower limb amputation (i.e. above the ankle), which has a six times higher incidence in diabetics than in non-diabetics (Ajibade et al., 2013) although the rate has diminished (Ahmad et al., 2016).

Managing diabetes

While type 1 and type 2 diabetes are different in some ways, the principles of management are very similar (NHS Choices, 2016a; NHS Choices, 2016b) and involve taking considerable care of one's health. Diabetes UK (2017b) provides useful guidance on living with diabetes. The aim is to minimise the development of complications of diabetes, or minimise the risk of the condition developing if at risk of type 2 diabetes. The following lifestyle factors are important, in conjunction with regular blood glucose monitoring:

- A healthy balanced diet
- Maintaining a healthy weight and losing weight if necessary
- Stopping smoking if undertaken
- Drinking alcohol only in moderation
- Undertaking regular exercise.

APPLY

Managing care

RICHARD JONES
CASE NOTES

Richard saw his GP about 5 years ago when he was feeling somewhat unwell, with reduced energy, complaining of polydipsia (excessive thirst) and polyuria (excessive urination). The GP arranged to have a fasting blood glucose test taken the next morning. The result came back showing a blood glucose above 7.0 mmol/L - an indication of diabetes mellitus.

Richard and his wife met with the dietitian for advice on the diet that he needed to take to lose a little weight and maintain a balanced nutritional intake. This also covered advice on diet for the children to reduce their risk of becoming obese and increasing their risk of diabetes. He was also referred to the Diabetic Nurse Specialist to learn how to monitor his blood glucose level, to understand the drugs he was prescribed, the importance of exercise and keeping his body weight under control, caring for his feet to prevent complications and how to contact her if he had any queries about his condition.

DISORDERS OF LIPID METABOLISM

There are two main groups of lipid disorders: disorders of **lipoproteins** and lipid-storage disorders.

REVISE: A&P RECAP

Lipids

Lipids are covered in Chapter 8 of *Essentials of Anatomy and Physiology for Nursing Practice* (Boore et al., 2016), which also includes some dietary advice on food stuffs that help to lower blood cholesterol levels.

Disorders of lipoproteins

Lipoproteins are large molecules which play a central role in the absorption of lipids, and in transporting cholesterol, triglycerides and fat-soluble vitamins through body fluids to and from peripheral tissues and the liver (Rader and Hobbs, 2015). These fall into four major classes, each group varying somewhat in density, size and protein. The density of the lipoprotein is determined by the quantity of lipid in the molecule:

- **Chylomicrons** are produced and easily absorbed from the small intestine, and converted to triglycerides in adipocytes.
- High-density lipoproteins (HDLs) pick up cholesterol in the blood and carry it to the liver for **excretion** in the bile.
- Low-density lipoproteins (LDLs) are largely formed of cholesterol which are transferred into cells and LDL is broken down to release the cholesterol.
- **Very low density lipoproteins** (**VLDLs**) transport most plasma triglyceride which is removed in the adipocytes and these VLDLs become LDLs.

The level of the different lipoproteins, particularly LDLs and HDLs, in the blood influences the risk of cardiovascular disease. LDL is known as 'bad' cholesterol as it contributes to the development of **atherosclerosis** as plaque builds up and narrows arteries. The risk of myocardial infarction, stroke and peripheral vascular disease is increased. HDL is known as 'good' cholesterol as it carries LDL cholesterol from the arteries and back to the liver from where it is eliminated from the body. Usually one-third to one-quarter of cholesterol is carried by HDL and this high level of HDL protects against stroke and heart disease (American Heart Association, 2017).

Pharmacological treatment is used to adjust the levels of the relevant lipoproteins and to reduce the incidence of heart disease. However, there can be side-effects to medications, leading a lot of people to use natural products that are proven to reduce cholesterol without the side-effects. These can be effective initially and may reduce or eliminate the need for medication if successful alongside a healthy diet.

Lipid-storage disorders

These are disorders involving lipids which may result in insufficient enzymes to break down the lipids appropriately, or the enzymes do not work properly and the fats cannot be used for energy (Mohamad, 2017). Lipids then build up in the body and may damage the tissues of the brain, peripheral nervous system, liver, spleen and bone marrow. These are autosomal **recessive inheritance** disorders except one (**Fabry disease**), which is X-linked recessive. Neonates are screened by taking a heel prick, and parents can have their carrier status identified. The Go Deeper box identifies some of these conditions and key characteristics. Those affecting infants are usually fatal while those in children and adults are variable in survival.

Lipids are a part of all cell membranes and disorders of their metabolism result in alterations of organs and tissues that modify specific functions. For example, neurodegeneration occurs with the accumulation of specific lipids in the central nervous system. Other presentations can also occur including enlargement of organs (**organomegaly**) and abnormalities of the skeleton. **Gene therapy** and bone marrow transplant may improve outcomes (Di Donato and Taroni, 2015).

GO DEEPER

Examples of lipid storage diseases

Table 13.9 summarises some examples of lipid storage diseases and their characteristics.

Table 13.9 Examples of lipid storage diseases

Disorder	Inheritance and affected populations	Characteristics of disorder
Gangliosidoses	Autosomal recessive Two distinct genetic causes	Accumulation of lipids known as gangliosides
Gaucher disease	Autosomal recessive Ashkenazi Jews Type 3 common in Norrbottnian region of Sweden (1 in 50,000)	Glucocerebroside deposited in cells of macrophage-monocyte system
Niemann-Pick disease types A and B	Autosomal recessive Ashkenazi Jews (type A) Rarely survive beyond 2 years	Sphingomyelinase deficiency Hepatosplenomegaly, pulmonary infections and central nervous system involvement in infancy
Niemann-Pick disease type C	Autosomal recessive High incidence in Nova Scotia Those of Hispanic descent in parts of the SW USA A Bedouin group in Israel	Neurodegenerative disease affects infants, children and adults Accumulation of lipids (fats) in the liver, brain and spleen
Tay-Sachs disease	Autosomal recessive Ashkenazi Jews Increased incidence in French Canadians (1 in 10,000) Cajuns from Louisiana, Old Order Amish in Pennsylvania	At 3-6 months of age loss of ability to turn over, sit, or crawl. Seizures, hearing loss, inability to move, death usually occurs in early childhood Milder - later childhood/adults
Fabry disease	X-linked recessive Late-onset form has increased incidence in Italy (1 in 4,600)	Deficiency of an enzyme alpha-galactosidase A. Affects skin, eyes, gastrointestinal system, kidney, heart, brain and nervous system
Fucosidosis	Autosomal recessive	Reduced/lost activity of alpha-L-fucosidase enzyme. Complex sugars in parts of body lead to death

Disorder	Inheritance and affected populations	Characteristics of disorder
Metachromatic leukodystrophy (MLD)	Autosomal recessive High incidence in Habbanite Jewish in Israel (1 in 75) Israeli and Christian Israeli Arabs (1 in 10,000) Western portion of Navajo nation in the United States (1 in 2,500)	Sulphatides in myelin-producing cells covering nerve cells cause progressive destruction of white matter in nervous system Deterioration of intellectual and motor skills, peripheral neuropathy, incontinence, seizures, paralysis, inability to speak, blindness and hearing loss. Loss of awareness
Krabbe disease	Autosomal recessive	Enzyme deficiency leads to lack of myelin and neurodegeneration
Farber disease	Autosomal recessive	Fatty material accumulates, leading to abnormalities of joints, liver, throat, tissues and central nervous system. Many signs/symptoms
Wolman disease	Autosomal recessive	Lysosomal acid lipase (LAL) deficiency, fats accumulate in tissues and organs, causing: abdominal distension, vomiting, enlargement of liver or spleen. Life-threatening

APPLY

Drug therapy for lipid disorders

There is a wide range of drug therapies available for the treatment of lipid disorders, and these include: HMG-CoA reductase inhibitors (**statins**), bile acid sequestrants, niacin, fibric acid agents and cholesterol absorption inhibitors.

Drugs used in dyslipidaemia include:

- atorvastatin
- simvastatin
- fluvastatin
- rosuvastatin
- colestyramine
- nicotinic acid
- fenofibrate
- gemifibrozil
- ezetimibe

Spotlight on statins

Statins are a group of drugs that are used in the treatment of lipid disorders. Statins can produce a reduction in LDL-cholesterol levels by 20-40%; they can also decrease triglyceride and VLDL levels

(Continued)

(Continued)

and increase the levels of HDL cholesterol (Adams et al., 2014). HMG-CoA reductase (3-hydroxy-3-methyglutaryl coenzyme A reductase) is an enzyme involved in the synthesis of cholesterol and serves as a primary regulatory site. This pathway is usually controlled by negative feedback, i.e. when there are high levels of LDL in the blood production of HMG-CoA reductase will be reduced, thereby turning off this pathway.

Statins act by inhibiting the production of HMG-CoA reductase; the resultant effect is a reduction in cholesterol synthesis. Due to the decrease in LDL production, the liver responds by increasing the number of LDL receptors on liver cells; this in turn helps to increase the removal of LDL from the blood, thereby leading to reduced blood levels of cholesterol and LDL.

The reduction in lipids is not permanent, therefore it is necessary that the person remains on the therapy long term. All statins are given orally; for some drugs with a short half-life they are usually administered at night as cholesterol synthesis is higher at this time (Adams et al., 2014).

DISORDERS OF AMINO ACID METABOLISM

REVISE: A&P RECAP

Amino acids

Fundamental information related to the amino acids is included in *Essentials of Anatomy and Physiology for Nursing Practice* (Boore et al., 2016). The structure of the amino acids is demonstrated in Figure 9.11. Table 8.3 lists the different groups of amino acids: essential, conditionally essential and non-essential. Formation of proteins is discussed in Chapter 2.

There are some hundreds of amino acids, of which only 20 are used in human cells coded for by the genetic code. Of these 20, nine are essential (one of these in infants) and must be present in the diet, another six are conditionally essential, meaning that their formation in the body can be inhibited by pathophysiological conditions, and the remaining five are formed within the body. Amino acids are used in the formation of proteins and **neurotransmitters**. There is a wide range of disorders of amino acid metabolism, some of which result in the build-up of specific amino acids in the bloodstream which can lead to serious neurological complications in the individual concerned. Neonates are screened for several of these shortly after birth, with the aim of minimising complications by dietary management from an early age. Phenylketonuria is one example; other examples of such disorders are shown in the Go Deeper box (Preece, 2017).

Phenylketonuria

Phenylalanine is an essential amino acid and is metabolised to tyrosine, a non-essential amino acid. However, in this disorder the enzyme required to convert phenylalanine to tyrosine is missing and, thus, phenylalanine accumulates in the blood. Tyrosine is not synthesised and thus becomes an essential amino acid for these children. In the UK, neonates are screened for this condition within a few days of birth and, if positive, treatment is commenced as soon as possible. Without such treatment, the children can develop significant intellectual disability (Preece, 2017).

APPLY

Heel prick test

When Danielle was born, she had a heel prick taken shortly after birth and the blood was tested to check whether she has the genetic disorder of phenylketonuria. This condition has serious effects on development if not treated adequately. A special diet, low in phenylalanine but containing tyrosine, is needed throughout childhood, with regular monitoring of phenylalanine levels. The diet can be relaxed in adolescence and adulthood, although many will continue with it for life.

Luckily, Danielle does not have this condition.

DANIELLE ZUMA
CASE NOTES

GO DEEPER

Amino acid disorders

Table 13.10 below summarises amino acid disorders.

Table 13.10 Amino acid disorders

Tyrosinaemia type 1	Normally synthesised from phenylalanine. Abnormal metabolism leads to defect of melanin formation, resulting in oculocutaneous albinism Person has fair skin, white/fair hair, reduced eye colour, risk of skin damage from sun Can cause: acute liver failure, renal tubule dysfunction, rickets and chronic liver failure Abdominal and neurological crises due to tyrosine metabolites	Nitisinone inhibits metabolic changes Diet with limited phenylalanine and tyrosin begins as soon as possible
Homocystinuria	Methionine metabolism disrupted. Methionine and homocysteine accumulate and systems disrupted Developmental delay and psychiatric disorders Dislocation of eye lenses, blood clots, osteoporosis and other bone abnormalities	Dietary treatment to keep amino acid levels normal
Maple syrup urine disease (Meisenberg and Simmons, 2017)	Three-branched amino acids (valine, leucine, isoleucine) metabolism disordered Sweet-smelling ear wax and urine, ketosis Baby lethargic, irritable, feels poorly Encephalopathy can develop if brain damaged	Diet managed to keep blood leucine within normal limits

Source: Preece, 2017

METABOLISM AND LIVER DISORDERS

The liver plays a major role in carrying out the metabolic functions necessary for life. Under normal conditions, the liver carries out large numbers of complex functions to keep the body working, including (NHS Choices, 2014):

- fighting infections and illness
- removing toxins (poisons) and drugs from the body
- regulating cholesterol levels
- helping blood clotting
- releasing bile

A range of acute or chronic liver disorders can threaten life; liver disease follows only heart, cancer, stroke and respiratory disease as a cause of death in England and Wales (British Liver Trust, 2017) and is still increasing. NHS Choices (2014) report that there are more than 100 types of liver disease, with some key groups shown in Table 13.11.

Table 13.11 Examples of liver disorders

Hepatitis	Inflammation (swelling) of the liver caused by various viral infections or poisons, autoimmunity or hereditary conditions Numerous types, see Table 13.12
Cirrhosis	Formation of fibrous tissue in liver, replacing dead liver cells. Death of liver cells can be caused by viral hepatitis, alcoholism or other liver-toxic chemicals
Haemochromatosis	Hereditary disease: usually in white northern Europeans, particularly Celtic, e.g. Ireland, Scotland and Wales, gradual build-up of iron in body, eventually leads to liver damage. Starts between 30 and 60 years Common symptoms: fatigue, weight loss, weakness, joint pain, (men) erectile dysfunction, (women) irregular or absent periods; can damage body parts, e.g. liver, joints, pancreas and heart
Budd-Chiari syndrome	Obstruction of the hepatic vein
Gilbert's syndrome	A genetic disorder of bilirubin metabolism, found in about 5% of the population
Glycogen storage disease type II	Build-up of glycogen causes progressive muscle weakness (myopathy) throughout the body and affects various body tissues, particularly in the heart, skeletal muscles, liver and nervous system
Primary biliary cirrhosis	Rare, long-term liver disease damages bile ducts, causes build-up of bile in liver, eventually leading to cirrhosis
Cholangitis	No symptoms in early stages: later fatigue, itchy skin, dry eyes and mouth, pain or discomfort in upper right abdomen

Source: NHS Choices, 2014

Acute liver disease

Acute liver disease can be described as having an acute onset with coagulopathy but with no previous evidence of liver disease. It may occur for a number of reasons including:

- Viral infection: viral hepatitis (Table 13.12); cytomegalovirus, herpes viruses 1, 2 and 6, Epstein–Barr **virus**
- Drug-induced: e.g. paracetamol

- Toxins: e.g. *Amanita phalloides* (death cap mushroom, organic solvents)
- Acute fatty liver of pregnancy
- Vascular conditions: e.g. Budd–Chiari syndrome, heat stroke
- Other causes: e.g. Wilson's disease, autoimmune hepatitis, liver tumour

Enhanced understanding and new approaches to treatment have greatly improved outcomes of interventions used.

Regardless of the cause of acute liver failure, the presentation is similar and includes:

> prolonged prothrombin time, decline in mental function, peripheral vasodilation, indications of systemic inflammatory response syndrome (inflammatory state of the whole body due to immune system response to inflammation - often related to sepsis), and eventually multi-organ failure (Bernal et al. 2015).

Hepatotoxicity

Hepatotoxicity refers to damage of the liver that is chemically induced, e.g. by drugs. Willet et al. (2004) also found that herbal or dietary supplements might induce hepatotoxicity. Drug-induced liver injury (DILI) is a common diagnosis in people with acute liver injury where the aetiology is unknown (Björnsson, 2016). There are a number of mechanisms responsible for either inducing hepatic injury or worsening the damage process. Many chemicals can cause damage to the **mitochondria**; its subsequent dysfunction leads to the release of excessive amounts of oxidants that, in turn, injure hepatic cells (Valente et al., 2016). Activation of some enzymes in the cytochrome P-450 system such as CYP2E1 also lead to **oxidative stress**. Injury to hepatocytes and bile duct cells leads to accumulation of bile acid inside the liver, thus causing further liver, damage. Non-parenchymal cells such as Kupffer cells, fat-storing stellate cells and leucocytes (i.e. neutrophil and monocyte) may also play a role in the mechanism.

APPLY

Drugs most commonly known to cause hepatotoxicity

There is a wide range of drugs that can cause hepatotoxicity, and these include: antiarrhythmic, non-steroidal anti-inflammatory drugs (NSAIDs), antimicrobials, immunosuppressants, antiepileptics and anticoagulants. In a recent study, azathioprine and infliximab were noted as being the highest risk for causing hepatotoxicity (Björnsson, 2016).

Drugs:

- allopurinol (treatment for gout)
- amiodarone, quinidine (antiarrhythmic)
- amoxicillin-clavulanate; erythromycin, flucloxacillin (antimicrobial)
- atorvastatin, simvastatin (statin)
- azithioprine, 6-mercaptopurine, infliximab (immunosuppressant)
- carbamazepine, valproate (antiepileptic)
- chlorpromazine (antipsychotic)
- contraceptives
- diclofenac, ibuprofen (NSAID)
- isoniazid rifampicin (antituberculosis)
- ketoconazole (antifungal)

APPLY

Paracetamol overdose and hepatotoxicity

Paracetamol overdose is the commonest cause of acute liver failure in the UK with about 75.4% of these patients having taken an intentional (rather than unintentional) overdose. Those taking an unintentional overdose had an increased mortality rate, were older, have acute and chronic alcohol abuse, and a staggered pattern of overdose (Craig et al., 2011).

Paracetamol is normally metabolised to NAPQI (N-acetyl-p-benzoquinoneimine), is conjugated with glutathione and excreted. However, if an overdose is taken, there is more NAPQI than can be conjugated and the unmetabolised molecule accumulates in the liver, reacts with cell membranes, resulting in damage to hepatocytes and causes centrilobular **necrosis** which may progress to liver failure (Kumar et al., 2015).

Acetylcysteine is the usual antidote administered according to the UK's Commission of Human Medicines 2012 guidance (Bateman et al., 2014). This has some adverse effects including rash, urticaria, vomiting and anaphylaxis (rarely fatal) (Buckley and Eddleston, 2007). Further research is needed to determine the most effective management for this condition. Yoon et al. (2016) believe that research regarding treatment needs to focus on the underlying molecular signalling pathways as opposed to antidotal knowledge at the molecular level.

Hepatitis

Hepatitis is an important type of liver disorder and there are numerous different types of hepatitis outlined in Table 13.12. Some conditions will resolve without lasting problems, but others can be long lasting and may result in cirrhosis or liver cancer. Acute hepatitis may have no specific characteristics but signs and symptoms can include: nausea and vomiting, fatigue, feeling unwell, loss of appetite, pyrexia (38°C/100.4°F), muscle and joint pain, abdominal pain, jaundice, dark-coloured urine and pale faeces, and **pruritus** (itchy skin). As the condition develops, jaundice, oedema of legs, ankles and feet, mental confusion and blood in faeces or vomit can occur.

Table 13.12 Types of hepatitis

Hepatitis A	Hepatitis A virus spreads through faeces of infected person, thereby infecting food/drink. Unpleasant, not usually serious. Rarely causes liver failure. Vaccine available
Hepatitis B	Hepatitis B virus, double-stranded DNA, spreads in blood of infected person. Uncommon in UK, most are infected where infection more common, e.g. Southeast Asia and sub-Saharan Africa. Can spread from infected pregnant women to their babies, or child-to-child contact; rarely, by unprotected sex and injecting drugs. Most adults recover within a few months. Children may develop long-term infection – chronic hepatitis B can lead to cirrhosis and liver cancer. Affects 350 million people worldwide
	Vaccination for high-risk groups, e.g. health care workers, drug injectors, practising homosexuals, children of mothers with hepatitis B, travellers to where more common
	UK 2017, hepatitis B vaccine part of routine **immunisation** programme
Hepatitis C	Hepatitis C virus, single-strand RNA virus (most common cause of chronic viral hepatitis), usually spreads through blood-to-blood contact with infected person, e.g. through sharing needles for drugs. Poor health care practices and unsafe medical injections are main method of spread outside UK. Often no or flu-like symptoms. Around 25% will become virus-free. In others, it stays in the body for many years as chronic hepatitis C and can cause cirrhosis and liver failure. Antiviral medications are effective, but no vaccine available

Hepatitis D	Hepatitis D virus, only affects those already infected with hepatitis B; it needs hepatitis B virus to survive in the body
	Hepatitis D usually spreads through blood-to-blood or sexual contact. Uncommon in UK, but more widespread in other parts of Europe, Middle East, Africa and South America. Long-term infection with hepatitis D and B can increase risk of serious problems, such as cirrhosis and liver cancer
	No vaccine for hepatitis D, but the hepatitis B vaccine can help protection
Hepatitis E	Hepatitis E virus. Now commonest cause of acute hepatitis in UK. Mainly due to eating raw/undercooked pork meat or offal, wild boar meat, venison and shellfish. Generally mild and short-term infection needing no treatment, but may be serious in some, e.g. those with a weakened immune system
	No vaccine available. Reduce risk by good food and water hygiene
Alcoholic hepatitis	Excessive alcohol over many years. Common in UK and usually does not cause symptoms, although sudden jaundice and liver failure sometimes occur. Stopping alcohol may allow liver recovery; continued excessive alcohol can lead to cirrhosis, liver failure or liver cancer. Recommended intake of no more than 14 units of alcohol a week
Autoimmune hepatitis	A rare cause of long-term hepatitis – immune system attacks and damages the liver, so that it stops working properly. Cause unclear
	Medications used suppress the immune system and reduce inflammation

Source: NHS Choices, 2016c

Chronic liver disease

Liver disease develops over time where there is repeated damage to the cells of the liver. This can be due to viral infections, including hepatitis (Table 13.12); chronic viral hepatitis is a most common cause of chronic hepatitis, cirrhosis and hepatocellular cancer. Chronic liver disease is a condition where damage to the liver tissue develops over a period of 6 months or more and results in fibrosis and cirrhosis. Sometimes an acute episode occurs on top of this (**acute on chronic** liver disease) (Asrani et al., 2015). Two other major categories are alcohol-related liver disease and non-alcoholic fatty liver disease (NAFLD).

Alcohol-related liver disease

A liver damaged due to years of excessive alcohol intake can result in cirrhosis (scarring of the liver). Stages of severity are:

* *Reversible alcoholic fatty liver (steatosis)*: Increased lipogenesis and cholesterol result in increased fat deposition in the liver due to synthesis and decreased fatty acid oxidation. It is the mildest form of alcoholic liver disease and may be reversible on the cessation of alcohol consumption.
* *Alcoholic steatohepatitis*: This is due to increased fat storage, inflammation and degeneration and the death of hepatocytes. **Neutrophils** and lymphocytes infiltrate the liver. This is reversible if the person stops drinking permanently. If severe, it is serious and life-threatening.
* *Alcoholic cirrhosis*: Alcohol metabolism causes toxic effects on the liver, leading to immunological alterations, the release of inflammatory mediators, oxidative stress from lipid peroxidation, and **malnutrition**. The damage may be caused by acetaldehyde or other metabolites. Acetaldehyde activates hepatic stellate cells and impedes the mitochondrial electron transport system (oxidative metabolism and generation of ATP); hydrogen ions are shunted into lipid synthesis and ketogenesis. Kupffer cell activation attracts neutrophils, promoting inflammation, **endotoxins** accumulate from the translocation of gut bacteria and **cell-mediated immunity** is suppressed. Acetaldehyde

promotes **collagen** synthesis and fibrogenesis. Fibrosis and scarring cause alteration in the structure of the liver and can lead to the obstruction of biliary and vascular channels. The amount of alcohol required depends on size, age, sex and ethnicity but it is thought that the high end range is 80 g/day for 10–12 years.

Symptoms with severe damage are: nausea, weight loss, loss of appetite, jaundice, swelling in ankles and abdomen, confusion or drowsiness, vomiting blood or passing blood in faeces.

Non-alcoholic fatty liver disease (NAFLD)

This pattern of disease is related to obesity, hypercholesterolaemia, metabolic syndrome, type 2 diabetes mellitus, and is due to the infiltration of hepatocytes with fat (triglycerides). NAFLD may develop to NASH (see below) with hepatocellular injury, inflammation and fibrosis.

There is a build-up of fat within liver cells, usually in overweight or obese people. There are four main stages:

* *Simple fatty liver (steatosis)*: harmless build-up of fat in liver cells
* *Non-alcoholic steatohepatitis (NASH)*: a more serious form of NAFLD; liver inflamed
* *Fibrosis*: inflammation causes scar tissue around liver and near blood vessels; liver still functions normally
* *Cirrhosis*: most severe stage; after years of inflammation, liver shrinks, is scarred and lumpy; permanent damage can lead to liver failure and liver cancer.

Symptoms may include: dull or aching pain over the lower right side of the ribs, fatigue, unexplained weight loss, or weakness. If cirrhosis develops, more severe symptoms occur such as jaundice and yellowing of whites of the eyes, itchy skin, and swelling of legs, ankles, feet or abdomen.

Cirrhosis

Cirrhosis is the end point consequence of chronic liver disease and is an irreversible, inflammatory, fibrotic liver disease in which hepatocytes are destroyed faster than they can be regenerated. Liver tissue changes from fatty liver, becomes scarred and destroyed through inflammation and fibrosis, to irreversible cirrhosis when the regeneration of liver tissue is no longer possible.

Structural injury to the liver results from injury and fibrosis, through the infiltration of leucocytes, release of inflammatory mediators and activation of hepatic stellate cells and myofibroblasts. Liver tissue is replaced by fibrotic scar tissue as well as regenerative nodules, leading to progressive loss of liver function. Formation of macro- and micro-nodules affects the liver structure and its blood supply. These structural changes impede blood flow through the liver, causing **portal hypertension** (high pressure in the hepatic portal vein). To compensate for this increased pressure, **collateral** vessels form to divert blood from the high pressure hepatic portal vein. This leads to decreased life expectancy and quality of life.

Symptoms are:

* Tenderness in right upper quadrant of the abdomen, with fluid accumulating in the abdomen (**ascites**) leading to abdominal distension
* Peripheral fluid accumulation which leads to peripheral oedema
* Jaundice (yellow discolouration of the skin and whites of the eyes)
* Pruritus (diffuse itching of the skin)
* **Anorexia** (loss of appetite), malnutrition and fatigue
* Bruising and bleeding tendencies

Management of individuals with cirrhosis is primarily supportive, including the use of diuretics, vitamin K, blood products, antibiotics and appropriate nutritional care.

Complications

- *Portal hypertension*: blood normally carried from the intestines and spleen through the hepatic portal vein flows more slowly and the pressure increases.
- *Ascites*: accumulation of fluid in the peritoneal cavity. Cirrhosis damages the liver's ability to function in the metabolism of all food products. There is a decrease in the formation of plasma proteins, which will decrease colloid osmotic pressure. Due to the changes in the architecture of the liver, there is obstruction to blood flow, with a resultant increase in portal hypertension. Fluid leaks into the peritoneal cavity and there is a decreased blood volume. The decreased blood volume will increase the reabsorption of sodium and water. The increased reabsorption of sodium and water and the increased portal hypertension will increase **hydrostatic pressure**. The increase in hydrostatic pressure, with a concomitant decrease in colloid osmotic pressure, can increase the leakage of fluid into the abdominal cavity. Ascites may become infected with bacteria normally present in the intestine; this is known as **spontaneous bacterial peritonitis (SBP).**
- *Oesophageal varices*: collateral blood flow through vessels in the stomach and oesophagus. These blood vessels become enlarged and are more likely to burst.
- *Hepatic encephalopathy*: the liver has a very important function related to the metabolism of proteins. Protein metabolism produces ammonia, which is then converted into urea for excretion by a normally functioning liver. Ammonium normally diffuses into hepatic portal circulation and is converted to urea, however in cirrhosis, blood bypasses the liver which prevents the conversion of ammonia to urea; ammonia moves into general circulation and into cerebral circulation, affecting cerebral functioning. An increased level of ammonia is one of the factors responsible for the development of hepatic encephalopathy. It refers to the totality of central nervous system (CNS) manifestations of liver failure, characterised by neural disturbances, e.g. neglect of personal appearance, unresponsiveness, forgetfulness, trouble concentrating or changes in sleep pattern, coma and **convulsions.**
- *Splenomegaly*: enlargment of the spleen due to portal hypertension and the inability of blood cells to be released, leading to **thrombocytopenia.**
- *Anaemia*: increased haemolysis of RBC's and impaired formation.
- *Bruising and bleeding*: due to decreased production of coagulation factors. As Factors V, VII, IX and X, prothrombin and fibrinogen are not synthesised by the liver, there is an increased risk of bleeding. **Malabsorption** of vitamin K contributes further to a lack of production of coagulation factors.

ACTIVITY 13.4: APPLY

Personal stories – cirrhosis

Watch this video to hear a selection of personal stories of people living with cirrhosis. Reflect on these stories and consider how you would apply this understanding and insight to your practice. If you are using the eBook just click on the play button. Alternatively go to

https://study.sagepub.com/essentialpatho/videos

CIRRHOSIS (2:35)

CHAPTER SUMMARY

This chapter has examined some of the disorders of metabolism which occur. Many of these, such as cystic fibrosis, are inherited and need early identification so that the appropriate dietary intervention can be provided. In some instances, this can enable the individual concerned to develop normally and have a near normal life span. The range of disorders is wide.

KEY POINTS

- Knowledge of the signs and symptoms of inherited metabolic disorders enables early identification of such disorders and appropriate interventions.

- Metabolic syndrome plays an important role in the development of disorders such as cardiovascular disease, stroke and diabetes which are increasing **morbidity** and mortality rates in the UK and other developed countries.

- There are numerous genetic disorders affecting the metabolism of different nutrients, carbohydrates, lipids and amino acids. While individually these are rare, in total they affect a substantial number of individuals. Most are transmitted by autosomal recessive inheritance.

- Diabetes mellitus types 1 and 2 are the commonest acquired disorders of carbohydrate metabolism (although with a genetic component to their development). These are largely due to lifestyle factors with increasing rates in the population. The complications of these conditions adversely affect the health and independence of those with these disorders.

- The liver plays a vital role in metabolism and there are a number of different liver disorders. Paracetamol (acetaminophen – US) overdose is one of the commonest causes of acute liver failure in the UK.

REVISE

TEST YOUR KNOWLEDGE

There are numerous issues related to metabolism of the human body which can go wrong and result in physiological disorders and you will come across a number of people with these. To provide high-quality care you need to understand the physiological disturbances and be able to use your understanding of the PCN Framework to provide the care needed by the person affected and their family. Check your understanding by answering the questions below.

Answers are available online. If you are using the eBook just click on the answers icon below. Alternatively go to **https://study.sagepub.com/essentialpatho/answers**

1   Explain the main groups of metabolic reactions and discuss the range of physiological disturbances that can occur when someone has a disorder of metabolism.

2   What do you understand by 'metabolic syndrome' and what is its significance for a number of conditions?

3   Discuss the main disorders of the thyroid gland and their effect on physiological functioning.

4   Analyse the changes in glucose metabolism that occur in diabetes mellitus (DM). Differentiate between DM type 1 and DM type 2.

5 Discuss the causes of and implications for care of the complications of diabetes mellitus.

6 Discuss the implications for health of acute and chronic liver disorders.

- Further revision and learning opportunities are available online

- Test yourself away from the book with **Extra multiple choice questions**

- Learn and revise terminology with **Interactive flashcards**

If you are using the eBook access each resource by clicking on the respective icon. Alternatively go to **https://study.sagepub.com/essentialpatho/chapter13**

REVISE

ACE YOUR ASSESSMENT

CHAPTER 13 ANSWERS

EXTRA QUESTIONS

FLASHCARDS

REFERENCES

Adams, S.P., Sekhon, S.S. and Wright, J.M. (2014) Rosuvastatin for lowering lipids. *Cochrane Database of Systematic Reviews Issue 11*. DOI: 10.1002/14651858.CD010254.pub2 (accessed 6 July 2018).

Ahmad, N., Thomas G.N., Gill, P. and Torella, F. (2016) The prevalence of major lower limb amputation in the diabetic and non-diabetic population of England, 2003–2013. *Diabetes & Vascular Disease Research, 13* (5): 348–53.

Ajibade, A., Akinniyi, O. and Okoye, C. (2013) Indications and complications of major limb amputations in Kano, Nigeria. *Ghana Medical Journal. 47* (4): 185–8.

American Heart Association (2017) HDL (good), LDL (bad) cholesterol and triglycerides. Dallas: American Heart Association. Available at: www.heart.org/HEARTORG/Conditions/Cholesterol/HDLLDLTriglycerides/HDL-Good-LDL-Bad-Cholesterol-and-Triglycerides_UCM_305561_Article.jsp#.WcfmsbJ97IU (accessed 24 September 2017).

Asrani, S.K., Simonetto, D.A. and Kamath, P.S. (2015) Acute-on-chronic liver failure. *Clinical Gastroenterology and Hepatology, 13* (12): 2128–39.

Bateman, D.N., Carroll, R., Pettie, J., Yamamoto, T., Elamin, M.E.M.O., Peart, L., etc. (2014) Effect of the UK's revised paracetamol poisoning management guidelines on admissions, adverse reaction and costs of treatment. *British Journal of Clinical Pharmacology, 78* (3): 610–18.

Bernal, W., Lee, W.M., Wendon, J., Larsen, F.S. and Williams, R. (2015) Acute liver failure: a curable disease by 2024? *Journal of Hepatology, 62*: S112–S120.

Björnsson, E.S. (2016) Hepatotoxicity by drugs: the most common implicated agents. *International Journal of Molecular Sciences, 17* (2): 224.

Boore, J., Cook, N. and Shepherd, A. (2016) *Essentials of Anatomy and Physiology for Nursing Practice*. London: Sage.

Brahmandam, S., Price, J.D. and Nunley, D.R. (2018) Myxedema coma causing cardiogenic shock treated with a percutaneous cardiac assist device (a novel approach in management of cardiogenic shock in myxedema coma). *American Journal of Respiratory and Critical Care Medicine*. Available at: www.atsjournals.org/doi/pdf/10.1164/ajrccm-conference.2018.197.1_MeetingAbstracts.A3472 (accessed 10 October 2018).

British Liver Trust (2017) *Facts about Liver Disease*. Bournemouth: British Liver Trust. Available at: www. britishlivertrust.org.uk/about-us/media-centre/facts-about-liver-disease/ (accessed 25 August 2017).

Buckley, N. and Eddleston, M. (2007) Paracetamol (acetaminophen) poisoning. *BMJ Clinical Evidence*, *2007*: 2101. Available at: www.ncbi.nlm.nih.gov/pmc/articles/PMC2943815/ (accessed 6 September 2017).

Carroll, P.V. (2014) Hyperthyroidism, thyrotoxicosis and thyroiditis: causes, investigations and management. *Journal of ENT Masterclass. Year Book 2014*, 120–6. Available at: www.entmasterclass. com/journals/ENT_Journal_Vol7_2014.pdf#page=123 (accessed 10 October 2918).

Craig, D.G.N., Bates, C.M., Davidson, J.S., Martin, K.G., Hayes, P.C. and Simpson, K.J. (2011) Overdose pattern and outcome in paracetamol-induced acute severe hepatotoxicity. *British Journal of Clinical Pharmacology*, *70* (2): 273–82.

de Beeck, A.O. and Eizirik, D.L (2016) Viral infections in type 1 diabetes mellitus – why the β cells? *Nature Reviews Endocrinology*, *12* (5): 263–73.

Diabetes UK (2017a) Diabetes and checking your blood sugars. [online]. Available at: www.diabetes.org. uk/guide-to-diabetes/managing-your-diabetes/testing (accessed 7 December 2017).

Diabetes UK (2017b) Diabetes UK – Know diabetes. Fight diabetes. [online]. Available at: www.diabetes. org.uk/home (accessed 10 December 2017).

Di Donato, S. and Taroni, F. (2015) Disorders of lipid metabolism. In R. Rosenberg and J. Pascual (eds), *Rosenberg's Molecular and Genetic Basis of Neurological and Psychiatric Disease*, 5th edn. London: Elsevier Academic Press. pp. 559–76.

Drake, M.T. (2018) Hypothyroidism in clinical practice. *Mayo Clinical Proceedings*, *93* (9): 1169–72.

Gierach, M., Gierach, J. and Junik, R. (2014) Insulin resistance and thyroid disorders. *Endokrynologia Polska*, *65* (1): 70–6.

Gillespie, K.M., Aitken, R.J., Wilson, I., Williams, A.J.K. and Bingley, P.J. (2014) Early onset of diabetes in the proband is the major determinant of risk in HLA DR3-DQ2/DR4-DQ8 siblings. *Diabetes*, *63*: 1041–7.

Hu, X., Deutsch, A.J., Lenz, T.L., Onengut-Gumuscu, S., Han, B., Chen, W-M. et al. (2015) Additive and interaction effects at three amino acid positions in HLA-DQ and HLA-DR molecules drive type 1 diabetes risk. *Nature Genetics*, *47* (8): 898–905.

IDF (2017) *The IDF Consensus Worldwide Definition of the Metabolic Syndrome*. Brussels: International Diabetes Federation. Available at: www.idf.org/e-library/consensus-statements/60-idfconsensus-worldwide-definitionof-the-metabolic-syndrome.html online (accessed 6 December 2017).

Idrose, A.M. (2015) Acute and emergency care for thyrotoxicosis and thyroid storm. *Acute Medicine and Surgery*, *2* (3): 147–57.

Iglesias, M.L., Schmidt, A., Ghuzlan, A.A., Lacroix, L., Vathaire, F., Chevillard, S. et al. (2017). Radiation exposure and thyroid cancer: a review. *Archives of Endocrinology and Metabolism*, *61* (2): 180–7.

Kondrashova, A. and Hyöty, H. (2014) Role of viruses and other microbes in the pathogenesis of type 1 diabetes. *International Reviews of Immunology*, *33* (4): 284–95.

Kumar, V., Abbas, A.K. and Aster, J.C. (2015) *Robbins and Cotran Pathologic Basis of Disease*. Philadelphia: Elsevier Saunders.

Liu, K. and Czaja, M.J. (2013) Regulation of lipid stores and metabolism by lipophagy. *Cell Death and Differentiation*, *20*: 3–11.

Maitra, A. (2015) The endocrine system. In Kumar, V., Abbas, A.K. and Aster, J.C. (eds), *Robbins and Cotran Pathologic Basis of Disease*. Philadelphia, PA: Elsevier Saunders.

McCance, K.L. and Huether, S.E. (2014) *Pathophysiology: The Biologic Basis for Disease in Adults and Children*, 7th edn. St Louis, MO: Elsevier Mosby.

McNicol, A.M. and Foulis, A. (2014) Endocrine system. In C.S. Herrington (ed.), *Muir's Textbook of Pathology*, 15th edn. London: CRC Press/Taylor and Francis.

Meisenberg, G. and Simmons, W.H. (2017) *Principles of Medical Biochemistry* 4th ed. Philadelphia: Elsevier

Mohamad, T.N. (2017) Lipid storage disorders. Medscape, emedicine. Available at: http://emedicine.medscape.com/article/945966-overview (accessed 23 September 2017)

NHS Choices (2014) Liver disease. [online]. Available at: www.nhs.uk/conditions/liver-disease/Pages/Introduction.aspx (accessed 31 August 2017).

NHS Choices (2016a) Type 1 diabetes. [online]. Available at: www.nhs.uk/Conditions/Diabetes-type1/Pages/Introduction.aspx (accessed 17 September 2017).

NHS Choices (2016b) Type 2 diabetes. [online]. Available at: www.nhs.uk/conditions/Diabetes-type2/Pages/Introduction.aspx?url=Pages/what-is-it.aspx (accessed 17 September 2017).

NHS Choices (2016c) Hepatitis. [online]. Available at: www.nhs.uk/Conditions/Hepatitis/Pages/Introduction.aspx (accessed 1 September 2017).

NICE (2015) Type 2 diabetes in adults: management. NICE guidance [NG28] (Updated 2017). National Institute for Health and Care Excellence. Available at: www.nice.org.uk/guidance/ng28 (accessed 8 December 2017).

Oxford Living Dictionary (2017) Myxoedema. Available at: https://en.oxforddictionaries.com/definition/myxoedema (accessed 14 December 2018).

Porth, C.M. (2015) *Essentials of Pathophysiology*, 4th edn. Philadelphi, PA: Wolters Kluwer.

Preece, M.A. (2017) Inherited metabolic disorders and newborn screening. In N. Ahmed (ed.), *Clinical Biochemistry*, 2nd edn. Oxford: Oxford University Press.

Rader, D.J. and Hobbs, H.H. (2015) Disorders of lipoprotein metabolism. In D. Kasper et al. (eds), *Harrison's Principles of Internal Medicine*, 19th edn. New York: McGraw-Hill Education.

Sanders, L.M. (2016) Introduction to inherited disorders of metabolism. *MSD Manual Professional Version*. Available at: www.msdmanuals.com/professional/pediatrics/inherited-disorders-of-metabolism/introduction-to-inherited-disorders-of-metabolism (accessed 18 August 2017).

Singer, K. and Lumeng, C.N. (2017) The initiation of metabolic inflammation in childhood obesity. *Journal of Clinical Investigation, 127* (1): 65–73.

Sinha, R.A., Singh, B.K. and Yen, P.M (2014) Thyroid hormone regulation of hepatic lipid and carbohydrate metabolism (Review). *Trends in Endocrinology and Metabolism, 25* (10): 538–45. Available at: www.ncbi.nlm.nih.gov/pubmed/25127738 (accessed 9 September 2017).

Valente, M.J., Araújo, A.M., de Lourdes Bastos, M., Fernandes, E., Carvalho, F., Guedeside de Pinho, P. et al. (2016) Editor's highlight: characterization of hepatotoxicity mechanisms triggered by designer cathinone drugs (β-keto amphetamines). *Toxicological Sciences, 153* (1): 89–102.

Willet, K.L., Roth, R.A. and Walker L. (2004) Workshop overview: hepatotoxicity assessment for botanical dietary supplements. *Toxicological Sciences, 79* (1): 4–9.

Yoon, E., Babar, A., Choudhray, M., Kutner, M. and Pyrsopoulos, N. (2016) Acetaminophen-induced hepatotoxicity: a comprehensive update. *Journal of Clinical and Translational Hepatology, 4* (2): 131–42.

DISORDERS OF OXYGENATION AND CARBON DIOXIDE ELIMINATION

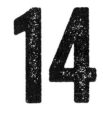

14

UNDERSTAND: CHAPTER VIDEOS

Watch the following videos to ease you into this chapter. If you are using the eBook just click on the play buttons. Alternatively go to **https://study.sagepub.com/essentialpatho/videos**

CHRONIC OBSTRUCTIVE PULMONARY DISEASE (5:02) ASTHMA (10:29) PNEUMOTHORAX (10:52) CYSTIC FIBROSIS (2:49) CYSTIC FIBROSIS A–Z (6:36)

LEARNING OUTCOMES

When you have finished studying this chapter you will be able to:

1. Identify terms associated with disorders of the respiratory system.
2. Describe the pathophysiology of upper and lower respiratory tract infections.
3. Explain what happens when there is damage to the pleura.
4. Explain the pathophysiological changes that occur in pulmonary disorders.
5. Explain the pathophysiology of asthma and chronic obstructive pulmonary disease.
6. Describe the changes that occur with cystic fibrosis.
7. Identify the changes that occur when there are interruptions to the pulmonary circulation.
8. Explain the changes that occur in the respiratory system during acute lung disorders.

INTRODUCTION

In this chapter, you will consider disorders of pulmonary function; various types of **disease** can disrupt the normal processes associated with gaseous exchange. Pulmonary disease may be classified as infectious or non-infectious, acute or chronic, obstructive or restrictive. We look at these various diseases and the impact that they have on the person. Additionally, you will also consider the emotional/psychological and social implications of such pathophysiological changes, a central element of person-centred nursing.

Every cell in the body requires a constant supply of oxygen to undertake their metabolic function. In doing so, they produce carbon dioxide (a waste product) that must be removed. The respiratory system is therefore vital to how we function physically and is essential in maintaining **homeostasis**.

BODIE FAMILY
CASE NOTES

PERSON-CENTRED CONTEXT: THE BODIE FAMILY

As a person-centred nurse, it is imperative that you understand that disorders of the respiratory system can have a significant impact on health-related quality of life; many conditions are long-term, progressive and can be life-limiting. The mature members of the family may start to notice changes in their respiratory systems. For example, Maud (age 77) and George (age 84) will have structural changes and may have reduced lung capacity that could impact on their activity levels as they may become short of breath more readily. They may also be more susceptible to respiratory tract infections such as **pneumonia** or bronchitis due to the decrease in the number of alveolar **macrophage**s; thus they receive the flu vaccine each year.

Derek Jones has asthma and needs to monitor his condition closely as exacerbations of his condition may occur; also due to his condition he needs to be careful that he does not develop chest infections. Danielle, as the youngest member of the family, may be susceptible to many respiratory tract infections as she does not yet have a fully developed immune system.

REVISE: A&P RECAP

Before reading this chapter, you may want to revise Chapter 10 in *Essentials of Anatomy and Physiology for Nursing Practice* (Boore et al., 2016). These videos may also help with revision. If you are using the eBook just click on the play button. Alternatively go to
https://study.sagepub.com/essentialpatho/videos

CONTROL OF
RESPIRATION (7:48)

RESPIRATORY SYSTEM (15:47)

The principal function of the respiratory system is to ensure that the body extracts enough oxygen (O_2) from the atmosphere and that excess carbon dioxide (CO_2) is expelled (Boore et al., 2016). The process by which this happens consists of three distinct phases: pulmonary **ventilation**, external respiration and internal respiration (Boore et al., 2016). If for whatever reason these processes are interrupted, pulmonary function may become dysfunctional. There are a number of terms associated with pulmonary dysfunction presented in Table 14.1; it is essential that you understand these terms as they will be referred to frequently as we move through the rest of the chapter.

Table 14.1 Terms associated with pulmonary dysfunction

Term	Definition
Dyspnoea	Difficulty in breathing
Hyperventilation	Ventilation in excess of what is needed for normal elimination of CO_2
Hypoventilation	Decreased ventilation, unable to eliminate adequate amounts of CO_2
Hyperpnoea	Increase in rate and depth of breathing (normal during exercise)
Tachypnoea	Increased respiratory rate
Bradypnoea	Decreased respiratory rate
Orthopnoea	Difficulty in breathing when lying flat
Hypoxia	Reduction in tissue oxygenation
Hypoxaemia	Decreased levels of oxygen in the blood
Hypercapnia	Increased levels of carbon dioxide content of the blood
Acidosis (can be either respiratory or metabolic)	Clinical condition as a result of a low blood pH (<7.35)
Alkalosis (can be either respiratory or metabolic)	Clinical condition as a result of a high blood pH (>7.45)
Atelectasis	Lack of gas exchange within alveoli, due to alveolar collapse or fluid **consolidation**
Cyanosis	Bluish discolouration of skin and/or mucous membrane due to increased levels of deoxygenated blood in the small vessels
Ventilation	The amount of air that enters the alveoli
Perfusion	The amount of blood perfusing the capillaries around the alveoli. Also refers to the delivery of blood to capillary bed in systemic circulation
Ventilation/Perfusion (V/Q) mismatch	Abnormal ventilation/perfusion ratio, e.g. when areas of the lungs are better perfused by blood than they are ventilated (e.g. lack of alveoli), or better ventilated than perfused with blood (e.g. lack of blood supply to a well-ventilated lung with sufficient alveoli)
Cough	Protective reflex that helps clear the airways
Acute cough	Resolves within 2-3 weeks of onset of illness or with treatment
Chronic cough	Persistent, does not resolve with treatment
Haemoptysis	Coughing up of blood or bloody secretions
Minute volume	Volume of air/gas inhaled (inhaled minute volume) or exhaled (exhaled minute volume) from a person's lungs in one minute.

Let's have a look at a few of these terms in more detail and how/why they occur.

HYPOVENTILATION AND HYPERVENTILATION

Hypoventilation refers to inadequate **alveolar ventilation** compared to the metabolic demands of the body. It occurs when the minute volume is reduced and is caused by changes in the mechanics of breathing or due to changes in the neurological control of breathing. Hypoventilation results in the accumulation of CO_2 (rate of production exceeds rate of excretion), leading to hypercapnia that may result in respiratory acidosis and affect the normal functioning of many tissues throughout the body.

Hyperventilation refers to increased alveolar ventilation that exceeds the metabolic demands of the body. It occurs when the excretion rate of CO_2 exceeds that which is produced by cellular **metabolism**, leading to hypocapnia that may result in respiratory alkalosis that can also affect the normal functioning of body tissues.

HYPOXIA AND HYPOXAEMIA

Hypoxia refers to a reduction in tissue oxygenation and can result from pulmonary alterations, or other abnormalities that are not related to pulmonary function, e.g. decreased **cardiac output**. **Hypoxaemia** refers to a reduction of oxygen in arterial blood and is caused by pulmonary dysfunction and may lead to hypoxia. There are four types of hypoxia:

1. **Ischaemic hypoxia** – when blood supply to the tissue is inadequate
2. **Anaemic hypoxia** – when blood is unable to carry enough oxygen to the tissues
3. **Hypoxic hypoxia** – when inadequate amounts of oxygen enter the lungs
4. **Histotoxic hypoxia** – when cells are unable to effectively use the oxygen reaching them.

Hypoxaemia may result from a number of factors. Hypoventilation, caused by neurological or muscular disorders restricting chest expansion, can lead to retention of CO_2 and a decrease in O_2. Ventilation/perfusion mismatch; either low V/Q, i.e. inadequate ventilation of well perfused areas of the lungs causing shunting (e.g. atelectasis, asthma, **pulmonary oedema** or pneumonia) or high V/Q, i.e. poor perfusion of lung areas that are well ventilated (e.g. pulmonary **embolus**). Signs and symptoms of hypoxaemia include cyanosis, altered mental state and confusion, **tachycardia** and decreased urinary output (Table 14.2).

HYPERCAPNIA

Hypercapnia refers to an increase in the CO_2 content of arterial blood and is usually caused by disorders that lead to hypoventilation or V/Q mismatching. Increased CO_2 production may result from increased metabolic activity, e.g. exercise, a rise in body temperature, disorders of respiratory muscle function or disorders of neural control of respiration. Hypercapnia can have profound effects on the body and its ability to function normally (Table 14.2).

Table 14.2 Effects of hypoxia and hypercapnia on the body

Hypoxia	Hypercapnia
Energy production reduced – anaerobic metabolism produces less ATP	Respiratory system – chemoreceptors stimulated – increased respiratory rate
pH – Increased lactic acid production ($\downarrow$ pH)	Cardiovascular system – vasodilation of blood vessels, tachycardia, **diaphoresis**
Cell – oedema due to $\uparrow$ Na$^+$ and $\downarrow$ H$_2$O inside cell, $\uparrow$ membrane permeability, $\downarrow$ mitochondrial activity	Nervous system – vasodilation of cerebral vessels – headache, disorientation, coma
Central nervous system – restlessness, agitation, uncoordinated movements, impaired judgement, delirium, coma	
Cardiovascular system – tachycardia, peripheral vasoconstriction (cool moist skin), increased BP. Later leads to **bradycardia** and hypotension	
GI system – reduced gut function – **constipation, anorexia**. Reduced liver function – reduced plasma protein production	
Muscles – reduced function – fatigue	
Pulmonary circulation – **pulmonary hypertension** (vessels constrict in response to hypoxia), **pulmonary oedema**	
Cyanosis – excessive concentration of deoxygenated **haemoglobin** (5g/100 ml blood)	

PHASES IN RESPIRATORY DISEASE

Respiratory disease can be categorised into three phases: respiratory impairment, respiratory insufficiency and **respiratory failure**.

- Phase I: Respiratory impairment
  - Normal healthy adult has a very large functional reserve
  - Although having respiratory impairment, they will have no symptoms
  - Reduced respiratory function only identified through respiratory function tests

- Phase II: Respiratory insufficiency
  - Person becomes aware of respiratory discomfort during exertion
  - Exercise tolerance becomes progressively impaired
  - Blood gases remain within normal limits

- Phase III: Respiratory failure
  - Person loses the ability to maintain normal arterial blood gases at rest
  - PO_2 is low at rest
  - PCO_2 is raised at rest

In your practice as a nurse, you will be caring for people across this range of phases and so it is important to consider the physiological impact and what phase of respiratory disease this person is in. This will influence how much care they may require as a result of the impact on their independence and it may also require you to consider if they and their family need end of life care.

INFECTIONS OF THE RESPIRATORY TRACT

Respiratory tract infections (RTIs) refer to an infectious disease that can affect any part of the respiratory tract; they tend to be discussed in terms of upper respiratory tract infections (URTIs), i.e. infection of nose, oropharynx or larynx, or lower respiratory tract infections (LRTIs), i.e. lower airways and lungs. Diao et al. (2018) state that RTIs comprise as many as 34 kinds of infections. Whilst any **pathogen** can cause infection of the respiratory tract, **viruses** are the most frequent cause. RTIs are the most common diseases in humans; Hull et al. (2013) found that adults usually experience one to three episodes of URTIs per year. Signs and symptoms of RTIs depend on the structure infected, the severity of the infection and the person's age and health status. They are usually relatively limited, consisting mainly of sore throat, fever, cough, productive cough, rhinorrhoea with or without pus, shortness of breath, headache and/or general discomfort, earache and/or tinnitus (Diao et al., 2018).

Upper respiratory tract infections

The upper respiratory tract consists of the nasal cavity, sinuses, pharynx and larynx. The upper respiratory tract is continuously exposed to potential pathogens which are usually dealt with by the mucociliary escalator and coughing. Despite these defence mechanisms, infections are fairly common and include the common cold, **influenza**, **rhinitis**, **sinusitis** and **otitis media**.

Common cold

The common cold is the most frequent cause of upper respiratory tract infection and is usually caused by one of a number of viruses, including rhinovirus, coronavirus, **adenovirus**, parainfluenza, influenza and respiratory syncytial types, which together have around 200 **serotypes** (Hemilä and Chalker, 2017). Due to the large number of causative agents, it would be impossible for a person to develop immunity to all, hence they can occur frequently throughout the year. The common cold is spread by respiratory droplets that can be directly inhaled or **acquired** through contamination of objects by infected secretions. It is highly contagious, especially during the first three days following onset of signs and symptoms; incubation may last up to five days. Signs and symptoms include nasal congestion, **rhinorrhoea**, sneezing, increased secretions and watery eyes. As the nose is congested, mouth breathing may be common and there may be a change in the person's voice. The person may also complain of a sore throat, headache, mild fever and general **malaise**.

Influenza

Influenza is a viral infection that can affect both the upper and lower respiratory tract. Influenza is caused by viruses that belong to the Orthomyxoviridae family; there are three different groups of influenza virus that cause disease in humans: type A (most prevalent), type B and type C. Regardless of the type, they mutate constantly, meaning that initiating an effective immune response for a long time is prevented. Influenza type A and type B can cause seasonal epidemics (World Health Organisation [WHO], 2018a) (see Go Deeper box). Influenza C is responsible for causing mild URTIs in adults and children. Influenza may cause three types of infection: uncomplicated URTI, viral pneumonia (discussed later) and respiratory viral infection that is then followed by a **bacterial** infection. Once a virus establishes an URTI, it then targets and destroys mucus secreting cells, ciliated **epithelium** and other epithelial cells, thereby leaving large spaces between the underlying basal cells, allowing extracellular fluid to escape, i.e. rhinorrhoea. If the infection spreads to the lower respiratory tract, it can cause diffuse shedding of bronchial and alveolar cells.

Signs and symptoms of flu are usually similar to those of other viral infections. Onset is abrupt with fever, chills, malaise, **myalgia**, headache, rhinorrhoea, non-productive cough and a sore throat.

GO DEEPER

Influenza subtypes/lineages

- *Influenza A* viruses can be categorised into subtypes based on two **glycoproteins**: haemagglutinin (H) that allows the virus to anchor to the epithelium of the respiratory tract and neuraminidase (N) that facilitates digestion of host secretions and release of viral particles from host cells (Labella and Merel, 2013). There are 16 variants of haemagglutinin (H1– H16) and nine variants of neuraminidase (N1-N9). For example, in the winter of 2017/2018 the main **strains** circulating were Influenza A(H3N2) and A(H1N1).
- *Influenza B* viruses are not classified into subtypes but can be broken down into lineages, e.g. B-Victoria lineage, B-Yamagata lineage.
- *Influenza C* virus does not present public health importance as it is detected less frequently and usually only causes mild infections (WHO, 2018a).

Epidemics (type A and type B) and pandemics (only caused by type A) result from the ability of viruses to mutate and develop new subtypes against which the population has no protection. Worldwide, these annual epidemics are estimated to result in about 3-5 million cases of severe illness, and about 290,000 to 650,000 deaths (WHO, 2018a).

In winter 2017/2018, influenza A H3N2 caused widespread disease as it is a particularly virulent strain of influenza type A, mutating at a faster rate and being more dominant. This particular strain spreads with much more severity, is harder to vaccinate against and increases health complications.

Rhinitis

Rhinitis refers to **inflammation** of the nasal passages. B cells produce immunoglobulin (Ig) IgE against **allergens**. IgE binds to **mast cells** and causes degranulation with the release of **histamine**, **proteases**, **prostaglandins**, cysteinyl leukotrienes and **cytokines**. These inflammatory mediators cause the acute symptoms including sneezing, itch, rhinorrhoea and nasal congestion. Allergens presented to T cells cause the release of **interleukins** (IL), IL-4 and IL-13, that further stimulate B cells to release IL-5, IL-9 and granulocyte macrophage colony-stimulating factor. This results in a switch from a T-**helper cell** 1 (T_h1) response to a T_h2 response to activate **eosinophils**, **basophils**, **neutrophils** and T **lymphocytes**, leading to nasal obstruction, hyper-reactivity and **anosmia**.

Sinusitis

Sinusitis refers to inflammation/infection of the paranasal sinuses, caused mainly by *Streptococcus pneumoniae* and *Haemophilius influenzae*; occasionally it may be caused by a fungal infection. The infection leads to obstruction and prevents drainage of the paranasal sinuses into the nasal cavity. Pressure builds up inside the sinus cavity due to the accumulation of exudate, causing severe facial pain that can be confused with toothache (due to blockage of the maxillary sinus) or headache (blockage of the ethmoid sinus).

Otitis media

Otitis media, whilst technically not an infection of the respiratory tract, refers to infection of the middle ear seeded from an upper respiratory tract infection through the eustachian tube. *Streptococcus pneumoniae* and *Haemophilius influenzae* are the most common bacteria that cause otitis media. Infection causes inflammation of the middle ear **mucosa** and inflammatory exudate in the middle ear space. It usually presents with **otalgia** (ear pain) and hearing disturbances. If it does not resolve it can lead to tympanic membrane **perforation** and discharge.

Croup

Croup is a condition that affects the airways of babies and young children aged between 3 months and 3 years (NICE, 2017c). It is usually caused by viruses, and the parainfluenza virus accounts for 75% of cases (Johnson, 2014) with the remaining 25% caused by **adenoviruses**, respiratory syntical virus and influenza types A and B (Zoorob et al., 2011). Whilst the disease is well defined in children, it remains an uncommon cause of respiratory distress in adults (Patel et al,. 2018). However, it is believed that adult croup syndrome takes a more severe course than in children and may require definitive airway management and intensive care monitoring (Patel et al., 2018). Croup is characterised by abrupt onset although it is usually preceded by upper respiratory tract infections. Symptoms are most often worse at night and can fluctuate rapidly depending on whether the child is calm or agitated (Bjornson and Johnson, 2013). As the larynx and subglottic area become inflamed, oedema and exudate can cause obstruction, leading to the characteristic barking cough, hoarse voice, inspiratory stridor and respiratory distress. Symptoms are usually short-lived, with about 60% of children having resolution of the barking cough within 48 hours; less than 2% of children have symptoms persisting for more than 5 nights (Bjornson and Johnson, 2013).

LOWER RESPIRATORY TRACT INFECTIONS

Pneumonia

Pneumonia refers to infection of the pulmonary parenchyma, i.e. bronchioles and alveoli. It may develop as an acute primary infection or may occur as a secondary infection due to another respiratory or systemic condition. In the majority of cases, organisms enter the lungs by inhalation, aspiration or **translocation** of resident bacteria that spread along the mucosa. Pneumonia can be classified in a number of ways based on the pathogen (typical or atypical) or the area of infection (lobar pneumonia or bronchopneumonia). Pneumonia may also be classified according to the setting in which they occur and referred to as community-acquired pneumonia (CAP), hospital-acquired pneumonia (HAP), health care-associated pneumonia (HCAP) or ventilator-associated pneumonia (VAP) (Table 14.3).

Table 14.3 Classification of pneumonia

Pathogen	Typical - bacterial
	Atypical - variety of organisms including: *Mycoplasma pneumoniae*, viruses and **fungi**
Area of infection	Lobar pneumonia - confluent consolidation involving one or more lung lobes. Most often due to *Streptococcus pneumoniae* (the pneumococcus)
	Bronchopneumonia - widespread small patches usually affecting both lungs, especially lower lobes. Causative organisms more varied including: *Streptococcus pneumoniae*, *Haemophilus influenza*, *Staphylococcus*, anaerobes, coliforms
Setting	Community-acquired - describes infection caused by organisms (bacterial or viral) found in the community, begins outside the hospital or develops within 48 hours after admission to hospital
	Health care-associated - occurs in someone who has had a recent hospitalisation or resides in a care home, receiving chronic dialysis or home infusion therapy
	Hospital-acquired - nosocomial infection, LRTI not present on admission or develops 48 hours or more following admission
	Ventilator-associated - nosocomial infection that occurs in a person requiring mechanical ventilation 48 hours or more following intubation. May occur in 9-27% of ventilated patients (Kalanuria et al., 2014)

The areas of lung below the bronchi are usually sterile despite the entry of pathogens into the airways by inhalation or aspiration of nasopharyngeal secretions. A number of defence mechanisms exist to protect the lower respiratory tract and prevent infections; these include: cough reflex, **mucociliary escalator**, alveolar macrophages, **immunoglobulins** (Ig) (IgA and IgG) and **cell-mediated** and **humoral immunity**. Loss of one or more of these defence mechanisms predisposes the lower respiratory tract to colonisation and subsequent infection. Those that are critically ill or have a long-term condition are more susceptible to pneumonia as their epithelial cells are much more receptive to binding pathogens that cause pneumonia. Colonisation of the tracheobronchial tree is also enhanced in those that smoke, have diabetes or **chronic bronchitis**.

If a pathogen gains entry to the lower respiratory tract, especially the alveolar region, local host defences (**antibodies**, complement and cytokines) prepare the bacteria for ingestion by alveolar macrophages. Macrophages present the **antigens** to the adaptive immune system, thereby activating both cell-mediated and humoral immunity with the release of T and B cells. Macrophages also release inflammatory cytokines, e.g. **tumour necrosis factor**-alpha, interleukin (IL)-1, while mast cells and **fibroblasts** release **chemokines** and chemotactic signals that result in neutrophil recruitment from the lungs into the alveoli. Intense cytokine-mediated inflammation ensues, resulting in the destruction of bronchial mucous membranes and alveolocapillary membranes which leads to vascular **engorgement**, oedema and the production of **fibrinopurulent** exudate which infiltrates the **acini** and terminal bronchioles. Dyspnoea, V/Q mismatching and hypoxaemia result. Consolidation of lung tissue may occur if certain bacteria release toxins that further damage the lung tissue.

Typical pneumonia (acute bacterial)

Typical pneumonia is caused by bacteria, with the most common causative agent being *Streptococcus pneumoniae* (the pneumococcus). This type of pneumonia is often referred to as pneumococcal pneumonia and is a frequent cause of lobar pneumonia. Bronchopneumonia may be caused by one or more species of microorganism; infection usually begins in the bronchial mucosa and spreads to adjacent alveoli. **Legionnaires' disease** is a type of pneumonia caused by *Legionella pneumophila* (gram-negative bacteria), which thrive in warm, moist environments, e.g. air conditioning units, spas. The infection can cause severe congestion and consolidation and necrosis of lung tissue that potentially may have fatal consequences. Signs and symptoms associated with typical pneumonia include: sudden onset with pyrexia and chills, fatigue, dyspnoea, tachypnoea, tachycardia, productive cough and pleuritic pain.

Atypical pneumonia

Atypical pneumonia, or primary atypical pneumonia, can be caused by either viral or mycoplasmic pathogens and is associated with a patchy involvement of the lung that is predominantly confined to the alveolar septum or **interstitium** (support tissue). The term atypical refers to the lack of consolidation, absence of alveolar exudate, production of moderate amounts of white sputum and a slightly elevated white blood cell count. The most common causative agents of atypical pneumonia are *Chlamydia pneumoniae, Mycoplasma pneumoniae* and *Legionella pueumophila* (Arnold et al., 2016) and it is common in older children and young adults. Viruses responsible for causing atypical pneumonia include influenza types A and B, respiratory syncytial virus, adenovirus, rhinovirus, rubella and varicella viruses (Gu et al., 2017). Pathogens responsible for atypical pneumonia cause initial destruction of ciliated epithelium of the distal airway cellular material and impair respiratory defences. In doing so they predispose the respiratory tract to secondary bacterial infections. Signs and symptoms associated with atypical pneumonia are usually vague but can include a non-productive cough (absence of exudate in alveoli), mild fever, malaise, myalgia, headache, hoarseness and a sore throat.

Tuberculosis

Tuberculosis (TB) is an infection caused by *Mycobacterium tuberculosis* (MTB) (an acid-fast bacilli), usually affecting the lungs but it may invade other body systems, e.g. skin (cutaneous TB), kidneys

(Fogel, 2015). It is highly contagious and spread is airborne by means of droplet nuclei that are harboured in the respiratory secretions of persons with active tuberculosis (Zuma et al., 2013). TB is the ninth leading cause of death worldwide and it is the leading cause of death from a single infectious agent (WHO, 2017). Cruz-Knight and Blake-Gumbs (2013) state that approximately one-third of the world's population is latently infected with MTB. Whilst the incidence of TB is dropping globally at a rate of approximately 2% annually, the burden remains high with over 6 million new cases being diagnosed annually (WHO, 2017). Drug-resistant TB remains a threat; of the new cases reported in 2016, 600,000 were resistant to rifampicin (the most effective first-line drug) and, alarmingly, 490,000 of these cases were multidrug resistant (MDR-TB) (WHO, 2017).

As previously stated, MTB is spread from person-to-person via airborne droplets. Salgame et al. (2015) identify that a specific, complex interplay between host and pathogen with the environment determines the outcome of MTB infection, resulting in one of three possible outcomes: cure, latency or active disease. The virulence of the strain, intensity of exposure, size of bacterial inoculum and host factors (e.g. age, comorbidities) can contribute to the possible outcomes (Salgame et al., 2015). The majority of people mount an effective response with successful inhibition of the growth of MTB and the bacteria becomes dormant and inactive, i.e. latent (Thillai et al., 2014). Immunocompetent latent individuals infected with MTB do not present symptoms and do not transmit the disease to others (Fogel, 2015). Risk groups and factors for the development of the disease are presented in Box 14.1.

Box 14.1 Risk groups and factors for the development of tuberculosis

- Young adults – male > female
- People living in developing countries
- Poverty (higher level = higher risk)
- Health care workers who are exposed to disease on a frequent basis
- Those with compromised/weakened immune systems
- Cancer
- Human immunodeficiency virus (HIV)
- Smoking
- Host deficiency in IL-2-promoting T-helper 1 response (de Martino et al., 2014)
- Foreign-born individuals living in impoverished areas
- Undernutrition

Sources: Fogel, 2015; WHO, 2017

Once inhaled, MTB droplets pass down the bronchial tree and deposit in peripheral alveoli and cause non-specific pneumonitis (localised inflammation). Some MTB may migrate through the lymphatic system and lodge in the lymph nodes where they encounter lymphocytes and initiate an immune response. Activation of alveolar macrophages leads to bacilli being engulfed by **phagocytes**. Macrophages initiate a cell-mediated immune response and the infection is contained. Whilst the bacilli are phagocytosed and contained, they resist lysosomal killing and continue to multiply inside the alveolar macrophage. Macrophages degrade the bacilli and present the antigens to helper CD4+ T lymphocytes. The sensitised T cells further stimulate the macrophages to increase the concentration of **lytic enzymes,** increasing the ability to destroy the bacilli. However, they also damage the lung tissue. In the immunocompetent person, this cell-mediated immune response leads to the development of a **granulomatous lesion** known as a **Ghon focus**. The Ghon focus contains tubercle bacilli, modified macrophages and other immune cells.

Infected tissue inside the Ghon focus dies and undergoes necrosis that subsequently produces a cheese-like material of dead cells known as caseous necrosis. Tubercle bacilli (free or inside macrophages) drain along lymph channels to the tracheobronchial lymph nodes of the affected lung and stimulate the formation of caseous **granulomas**. The primary lung lesion and lymph node granulomas are collectively known as the **Ghon complex** (Figure 14.1). As the Ghon complex heals it undergoes shrinkage, fibrous scarring and calcification. Tuberculosis may remain dormant for life; however, reactivation and progressive disease may occur when the immune system is compromised or impaired.

Signs and symptoms are not always initially apparent but may include: mild fever, cough with **purulent** sputum, fatigue and night sweats. As the disease progresses, dyspnoea, wheezing, **haemoptysis**, chest pain, weight loss and anorexia may become apparent.

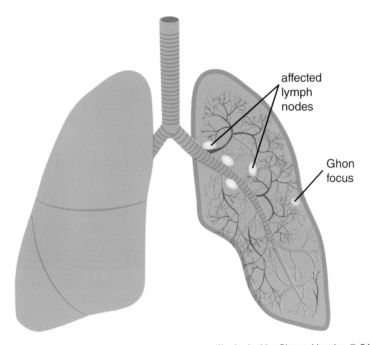

affected lymph nodes

Ghon focus

Illustrated by Shaun Mercier © SAGE Publications

Figure 14.1 Ghon complex

Primary TB

Primary TB develops in previously unexposed, unsensitised people (Zuma et al., 2013). Most people with primary TB are asymptomatic and go on to develop latent TB whereby the cell-mediated response (T lymphocytes and macrophages) limits the spread as the organisms are surrounded by granulomas. In approximately 5% of people newly infected with MTB there will be an inadequate response that leads to progressive primary tuberculosis with the destruction of lung tissue and spread to multiple sites within the lung (Zuma et al., 2013). Most commonly affected are young children with immature immune systems, those with HIV infection or other **immunodeficiency** disorders, or those receiving immunosuppressive therapy.

Secondary TB

Secondary TB refers to the reinfection or reactivation of the disease in a person with some immunity. The tubercle ruptures and re-establishes an active infection, and bacteria can spread through the lungs via the bronchioles. The disease tends initially to remain localised, often in apices of the lung. It tends to recur when there are impaired body defence mechanisms.

BRONCHIOLITIS

Bronchiolitis is the most common lower respiratory tract infection in the first year of life, affecting one in five children with 2–3% of these requiring hospitalisation (Ricci et al., 2015). It is caused by a range of viruses, including the respiratory syncytial virus, parainfluenza virus and adenoviruses (Meissner, 2016). However, **mycoplasmas** may also cause the disease. Children usually present with a **coryzal illness** (head cold, inflammation of nasal cavities) that progresses over 3–5 days to a troublesome cough, dyspnoea, tachypnoea, wheeze, crackles and difficulty feeding (Ricci et al., 2015). It is associated with an increased risk of chronic respiratory conditions such as asthma. However, it is unknown if it actually causes these conditions (NICE, 2017b).

The infection produces an inflammation and necrosis of the small bronchi and bronchioles accompanied by oedema, increased secretions and reflex **bronchospasm** that lead to obstruction (partial or complete). Partial obstruction of the lungs may cause hyperinflation and air trapping or alveolar collapse. In complete obstruction, air becomes trapped distal to the obstruction and may cause atelectasis or non-aeration, hypoxaemia and in severe cases hypercapnia.

DISORDERS OF THE PLEURA

The pleura is a thin double-layered serous membrane that surrounds the lungs consisting of the parietal pleura (attached to the inside of the thoracic cavity) and the visceral pleura (attached to the surface of the lungs). Between the two layers is the pleural cavity, filled with pleural fluid that allows the layers to move freely over each other, preventing friction when breathing (Boore et al., 2016). The pleura and pleural fluid create a pressure gradient that assists with lung inflation. Anything that interferes with the pleura can have a negative impact on the ability to breathe properly and maintain effective gaseous exchange. The two disorders we are going to discuss in this chapter are **pneumothorax** and **pleural effusion**.

Pneumothorax

A pneumothorax refers to the presence of air in the pleural cavity caused by rupture of either the parietal or visceral pleura. Separation of the parietal and visceral pleural disrupts the negative pressure and changes the balance between elastic recoil forces of the lung and chest wall. A pneumothorax can cause either partial or complete collapse of the affected lung, which recoils towards the hilum (Figure 14.2). There are various types of pneumothorax: open/traumatic, closed/**spontaneous** and **tension**.

- *Spontaneous*: occurs when an air-filled bleb or blister on the surface of the lung ruptures (Weldon and Williams, 2012). Blebs are usually situated at the apices of the lungs. Following rupture of the bleb, atmospheric air from the airways enters the pleural cavity and changes the pressure gradient. Alveolar pressure is greater than pleural pressure so air flows from the alveoli to the pleural space; air takes up space, thereby restricting lung expansion and causing the lung to collapse. Spontaneous pneumothoraces can be further subdivided into primary and secondary (Weldon and Williams, 2012).

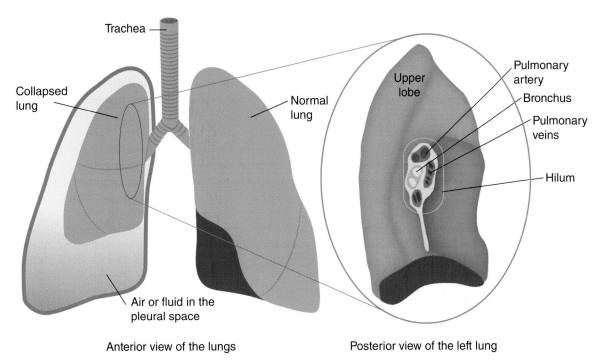

Anterior view of the lungs   Posterior view of the left lung

Illustrated by Shaun Mercier © SAGE Publications

Figure 14.2 Pneumothorax

- ○ Primary spontaneous – spontaneous rupture of blebs that occur unexpectedly in healthy individuals (predominantly males) between the ages of 20 and 40 years. Tall, thin people are at higher risk as it is suggested that pleural pressure from top to bottom of the lung is greater and thus may contribute to the development of blebs (Weldon and Williams, 2012). Smoking is also a contributory factor as it is thought to cause inflammation of the small airways.
- ○ Secondary spontaneous – occurs as a complication associated with underlying lung disease and tends to be more serious. Various types of lung disease may be associated with secondary spontaneous pneumothorax, including asthma, tuberculosis, cystic fibrosis and sarcoidosis.

- *Traumatic*: may be caused by either penetrating or non-penetrating chest injuries. The most common cause is fractured or dislocated ribs that subsequently puncture the pleura.
- *Tension*: occurs when intrapleural pressure exceeds atmospheric pressure (Walden and Williams, 2012). Air enters the pleural cavity on inhalation but cannot leave on exhalation, resulting in a rapid increase in pressure within the chest, making it a life-threatening condition. Due to the increased pressure, compression of the unaffected lung and mediastinal shift to the opposite side occurs, leading to compression of the vena cava. This reduces venous return to the heart and results in reduced cardiac output.

Signs and symptoms associated with a pneumothorax include **dyspnoea**, cough and chest pain. **Atelectasis** also manifests and there will be reduced air entry and breath sounds on the affected lung(s). There may also be unequal, asymmetrical chest rise and fall and mediastinal shift depending on the severity of pneumothorax; this may cause tracheal deviation. Over time, **hypoxia** results and initiates a sympathetic nervous system response, leading to tachycardia, pallor and anxiety; decreased venous return will lead to hypotension.

Pleural effusion

Pleural effusion refers to an abnormal collection of fluid in the pleural cavity (Saguil et al., 2014). Whilst a small amount of fluid is usually present to allow for lubrication of the pleural membrane, a pleural effusion occurs when there are large amounts of fluid in the pleural cavity. This excess fluid firstly increases the pressure within the pleural cavity and then causes separation of the pleural membranes. This prevents cohesion during inspiration, thereby preventing expansion of the lung, leading to atelectasis. Atelectasis on the affected side and shift of the mediastinal contents towards the unaffected lung limit expansion and gaseous exchange. Venous return in the inferior vena cava and cardiac filling become impaired due to increased pressure in the mediastinum when the pleural effusion is large. There are a number of types of pleural effusions that are characterised by the presence of substances in them: **hydrothorax** (serous fluid, transudative or exudative), **empyema** (pus), **chylothorax** (chyle) and **haemothorax** (blood) (Weldon and Williams, 2012):

- *Hydrothorax*: refers to the collection of serous fluid in the pleural cavity caused by increased **hydrostatic pressure** or decreased **osmotic pressure** in blood vessels, leading to a shift of fluid out of blood vessels into the potential space in the pleural cavity. May occur secondary to cardiac failure, liver or kidney disease.
- *Empyema*: refers to infection in the pleural cavity, resulting in pus (purulent fluid containing glucose, proteins, leukocytes and debris from dead cells and tissue) accumulation. It usually occurs as a result of infection, usually pneumonia.
- *Chylothorax*: refers to the presence of lymphatic fluid in the pleural space secondary to leakage from the thoracic duct or one of its main tributaries due to trauma, **malignant infiltration** that prevents the transport of chyle from thoracic duct to central circulation or inflammation.
- *Haemothorax*: refers to the presence of blood in the pleural cavity due to chest trauma, tumours, aortic **aneurysm** rupture or chest **surgery**.

Signs and symptoms associated with pleural effusion will vary according to the cause (Weldon and Williams, 2012). However, as previously noted, lung expansion on the affected side will be decreased proportionally to the amount of fluid collected in the pleural cavity. Dyspnoea is the most common symptom associated with it; the person may also complain of chest discomfort/pleural pain. There will also be decreased breath sounds on auscultation and dullness on percussion. If the person has an empyema, they may also present with fever, tachycardia and cough.

PULMONARY DISORDERS

Atelectasis

The term atelectasis is derived from the Greek words *ateles* and *ektasis*, which mean incomplete expansion or collapse resulting in reduced or absent gas exchange. Atelectasis may affect all or part of a lung. There are three different types of atelectasis: compression atelectasis, **absorption** atelectasis and surfactant impairment (Table 14.4). It may be present at birth (primary atelectasis) or develop later in life (acquired atelectasis).

Signs and symptoms associated with atelectasis include dyspnoea, **tachypnoea**, cyanosis, signs of hypoxaemia (e.g. altered **consciousness** levels), tachycardia, reduced chest expansion and absence of breath sounds on the affected side.

Obstructive lung disorders

This is a group of disorders caused by an obstruction or limitation to airflow characterised by a reduction in expiratory airflow and respiratory symptoms. The main disorders of obstructive lung disease are **asthma**, chronic bronchitis and **emphysema**.

Table 14.4   Different types of atelectasis

Type	Cause
Compression atelectasis	External pressure exerted by tumour, fluid or air in pleural space, or by abdominal distension, causing alveolar collapse
Absorption atelectasis	Removal of air from obstructed/hypoventilated alveoli, inhalation of: **anaesthetic agents, concentrated** O_2
Surfactant impairment	Decreased production or inactivation of surfactant due to premature birth, **acute respiratory distress syndrome (ARDS),** anaesthetics, mechanical ventilation

Bronchial asthma

Bronchial asthma is a chronic inflammatory disease and the most prevalent chronic respiratory disease. The World Health Organisation (WHO, 2018a) states that between 100 million and 150 million people worldwide suffer from asthma and this number continues to grow. Asthma is linked to genetic and environmental factors and it is classified as atopic/allergic (triggered by allergic **sensitisation**) or non-atopic/non-allergic. The Global Initiative for Asthma defines asthma as a disease characterised by chronic airway inflammation with a history of wheeze, shortness of breath, chest tightness and cough (GINA, 2018). This can be due to inflammation, oedema and mucus production (Papi et al., 2018).

Asthma is associated with the release of inflammatory mediators from mast cells in the airways and this leads to a response clinically manifested as expiratory wheeze, experience of chest tightness, dyspnoea, tachypnoea and cough. In atopic (allergic) asthma the inflammatory response is triggered by allergens and is often associated with other allergic conditions such as **eczema**, rhinitis or food allergy and a positive family history of the disease (Papi et al., 2018). Non-atopic (non-allergic) asthma occurs in people with no history of allergy and often develops in middle age. In both types, bronchospasm is triggered by exposure to a stimulant such as viral respiratory infection, smoke, exercise and cold air.

Living with asthma

As a person-centred practitioner, it is important to understand the lived experience of asthma in order that you can support people in their illness. Watch the following video to help you gain some insight into that lived experience and reflect on how it may help you in your practice. If you are using the eBook just click on the play button. Alternatively go to

https://study.sagepub.com/essentialpatho/videos

ASTHMA (3:38)

Allergic (atopic) asthma

The allergic (atopic) form of asthma is associated with exposure to a stimulant, usually an allergen, that induces a type 1 **hypersensitivity** response (see Chapter 7). The mechanisms of response can be described in two distinct phases: the early phase and the late or delayed phase. During the early phase response following antigen exposure to the bronchial mucosa, dendritic cells activate T-helper-2 cells to produce interleukins (ILs) IL-5, IL-4, IL-13.

IL-5 activates eosinophils and IL-4 and IL-13 stimulate B lymphocytes to produce immunoglobulin E (IgE) (Russell and Brightling, 2017). IL-13 also stimulates mucus production and eosinophil recruitment to the lung mucosa. IgE antibodies attach to the receptors on the mast cell surface, causing them to degranulate their contents. The inflammatory mediators histamine, **bradykinins**, interleukins, tumour necrosis factor, prostaglandins and **leukotrienes** are released, causing vasodilation and altered capillary permeability and resulting in mucosal oedema and smooth muscle contraction with subsequent bronchospasm and mucous secretion (Figure 14.3), narrowing the airways and obstructing airflow. Eosinophil products cause damage directly to the lung epithelial tissue and may also cause **bronchoconstriction** through the release of leukotrienes (Diver et al., 2018).

The late phase response occurs 4–8 hours after the early phase and involves the recruitment of more eosinophils, neutrophils and lymphocytes to the lung tissue, which increases and sustains the inflammatory response. Recurrent episodes of inflammation lead to injury to the epithelium and the formation of scar tissue (Kudo et al., 2013). Ciliated epithelial cells are damaged and mucous accumulates in the lumen of the airways. Long-term airway damage leads to airway remodelling that results in goblet cell **hyperplasia**, epithelial damage and cilia dysfunction with increased smooth muscle mass and increased vascularity. This leads to a thickening of the airway wall and narrowing of the airway lumen (Brightling et al., 2012). This, along with an increased production of mucus, can lead to smaller airways becoming completely blocked (Russell and Brightling, 2017).

Non-allergic (non-atopic) asthma

Asthma can be triggered by non-allergic stimulants, for example exercise, drug-induced or respiratory infection. Exercise can induce bronchoconstriction and is thought to be due to heat loss, **dehydration** and increased **osmolarity** of the respiratory mucosa, triggering bronchospasm (Smoliga et al., 2016). Drug-induced asthma is mainly associated with aspirin ingestion and can lead to bronchospasm, rhinorrhoea (when the nasal cavity is filled with large amounts of mucus), rash and itching. It is thought to involve abnormal pathways in prostaglandin metabolism and release of leukotrienes, causing bronchoconstriction (Rajan et al., 2015). Respiratory tract infection (RTI), particularly viral infection, causes epithelial damage and stimulates IgE antibodies against the virus (Wos et al., 2008). It has been suggested that there is an increased risk for asthma development associated with recurrent RTIs in childhood (Del Giacco et al., 2017). RTIs also increase hyper-responsiveness of the airways to other triggers. Airway hyper-responsiveness is a feature of asthma where airway smooth muscle is hypercontractile, resulting in airway narrowing. This can result from direct or indirect stimuli; the degree of hyper-responsiveness is determined by the number of mast cells affected (Diver et al., 2018).

Bronchoconstriction, inflammation and secretions lead to airway obstruction. Constriction of the smooth muscle in the walls of the airways narrows the lumen and increases resistance to airflow, particularly on expiration (Figure 14.4). Normally during expiration, the elastic recoil of the lungs decreases the diameter of the airways but air can still flow out. Where there is high airway resistance the airways collapse just before expiration, trapping air in the alveoli and causing hyperinflation; this leads to non-uniform ventilation. Alveolar gas pressure increases and perfusion decreases, leading to ventilation–perfusion (V/Q) mismatching. Hypoxaemia results. However, due to hyperventilation, CO_2 levels initially remain normal or may fall with associated respiratory alkalosis. Continued hyperinflation reduces the effectiveness of the respiratory muscles, leading to hypoventilation and reduced tidal volumes that subsequently result in systemic hypoxaemia, hypercapnia and respiratory acidosis.

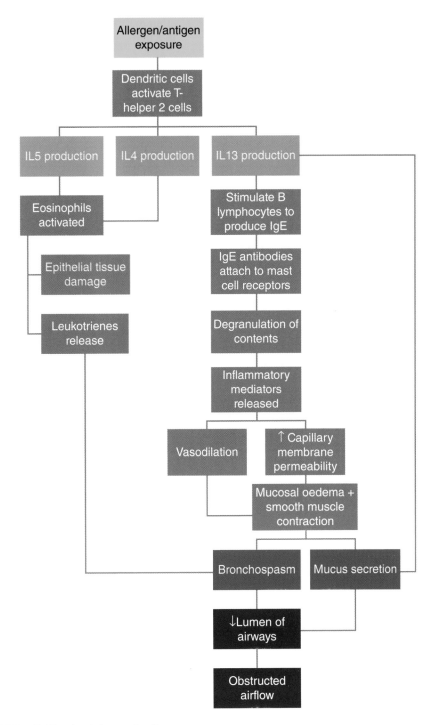

Figure 14.3 Pathophysiology of asthma

Healthy bronchial tube

Inflammed bronchial tube in a person with asthma

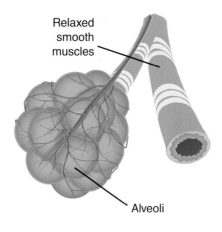
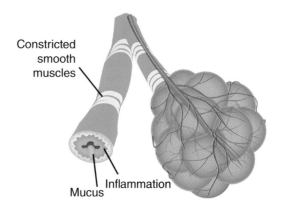

Relaxed smooth muscles

Alveoli

Constricted smooth muscles

Mucus Inflammation

Illustrated by Shaun Mercier © SAGE Publications

Figure 14.4 Normal bronchial tube and the bronchial tube in asthma

APPLY

Asthma

Signs and symptoms

A person with asthma is often asymptomatic in between attacks and the severity of an attack will determine the physical effects. A mild attack shows signs of expiratory wheezing, dyspnoea, tachypnoea and the person may complain of chest tightness and fatigue. A more severe attack is associated with dyspnoea, use of the sternocleidomastoid and scalene accessory muscles, and inspiratory as well as expiratory wheeze. Oxygen saturations may fall below 90% and arterial blood gases indicate hypoxaemia and later hypercapnia.

Status asthmaticus occurs where bronchospasm has not responded to bronchodilators and or anti-inflammatory drugs. Hypoxaemia worsens, and hypercapnia leads to respiratory acidosis. The person may appear cyanotic and there may be very little airflow and ventilation, requiring emergency medical intervention and mechanical ventilation.

Diagnosis

Diagnosis is based on history, including family history of asthma or allergens, and history of recurrent episodes of cough and wheezing or shortness of breath. Pulmonary function tests are an important part of diagnosis and management, using spirometry. A forced expiratory volume test measures the amount of air that can be forcibly expired in one second (FEV_1) and peak expiratory flow rate (PEFR), measured in litres per second, is the fastest rate air can flow out on expiration. These tests provide an indication of expiration ability and airway obstruction. Forced vital capacity (FVC) is the amount of air exhaled forcefully and quickly after inhaling as much as you can. A FEV_1/FVC ratio of less than 70% is a positive test for obstructive airway disease.

Source: NICE, 2017a

Treatment

Self-management and education play a key role in the approach to asthma management. Avoidance of known triggers and risk factors should reduce the frequency and risk of asthmatic attacks. Pharmacological therapy needs to be monitored and adjusted to find the minimum effective dose for the individual. A short-acting inhaled beta-2 agonist is used to relax bronchial smooth muscle and is used in people with low risk for exacerbations and who have symptoms less than twice per month (GINA, 2018). A regular low-dose inhaled **corticosteroid** to reduce inflammation and improve symptom control is used in combination with the short-acting beta-2 agonist. A long-acting beta-2 agonist can be used where symptoms are not well controlled (GINA, 2018).

Severe or uncontrolled asthma is where there is poor symptom control and frequent severe exacerbations (Chung et al., 2014). IgE monoclonal antibodies have been used to treat moderate to severe allergic asthma (Olin and Wechsler, 2014). Omalizumab was the first monoclonal antibody used for severe asthma and it works by binding to IgE to prevent it from attaching to the receptor on the surface of the mast cell, basophils and dendritic cells (Diver et al., 2018).

APPLY

Asthma and long-term treatment

DEREK JONES
CASE NOTES

Referring back to the Bodie family, Derek Jones has had mild persistent asthma since childhood. Among children, asthma prevalence is higher in boys than girls and atopic asthma is common in adults with childhood onset asthma (Del Giacco et al., 2017). Derek is taking a beta-2 agonist and a low dose corticosteroid inhaler. This is considered standard treatment and should be effective in symptom control and reducing risk of exacerbations.

Chronic obstructive pulmonary disease (COPD)

Chronic obstructive pulmonary disease (COPD) refers to a group of respiratory disorders that are characterised by persistent respiratory symptoms and airflow limitation due to abnormalities caused by exposure to noxious particles or gases (GOLD, 2016). It is a progressive disease and is associated with risk factors, in particular tobacco smoking, and exposure to respiratory irritants such as dust, chemicals and environmental pollution (Kim and Criner, 2013). COPD is the fourth leading cause of death in the world, accounting for 6% of all deaths globally. It is a major cause of **morbidity** and mortality and is in most cases a preventable disease (GBD [2015 Chronic Respiratory Disease Collaborators], 2017). There are two types of obstructive airway disease associated with COPD: emphysema, and chronic bronchitis. Whilst the two conditions have many similarities, they also display distinct differences. Table 14.5 identifies the characteristics of emphysema and chronic bronchitis.

Table 14.5 Characteristics of emphysema and chronic bronchitis

Feature	Emphysema	Chronic bronchitis
Health history	Generally healthy, but smoker	Recurrent chest infections Exacerbation of symptoms by irritants and cold air, smoker
Cough/sputum	Minor	Significant/copious, purulent
Physical examination and general appearance	Cachetic, history of weight loss and protein calorie **malnutrition**	Tendency towards **obesity**, cyanotic, polycythaemia, oedematous, distended neck veins
Dyspnoea	Slowly progressive	Variable, often late in illness
Breath sounds	Quiet or diminished	Scattered wheezing, ronchi, rales
Chest appearance	Increase in anteroposterior diameter, barrel chest, prominent accessory muscles of respiration, limited diaphragmatic excursion	Slight to marked increase in anteroposterior diameter, **pulmonary hypertension**
ABGs	Near normal, $\downarrow PaO_2$, normal or $\downarrow PaCO_2$, hypercapnia (late stages)	$\downarrow PaO_2$, $\uparrow PaCO_2$
Chest X-ray	Hyperinflation, flat diaphragm, widened intercostal margins	Congested lung fields, cardiac enlargement

Chronic bronchitis

The Global Initiative for Chronic Obstructive Lung Disease defines chronic bronchitis as a persistent cough and sputum production for at least 3 months per year for two consecutive years (GOLD, 2016). Exposure to respiratory irritants such as tobacco smoke or acute and chronic respiratory infections causes airway inflammation and the overproduction of mucus by **goblet cells** and hypersecretion from increased degranulation by neutrophil-mediated elastase (Kim and Criner, 2013). There is difficulty in clearing mucus due to poor ciliary function and ineffective cough. This causes narrowing of the lumen of the airway and obstruction to airflow. Initially, the larger airways are affected but with disease **progression** all airways are involved.

Inflammatory mechanisms responsible for mucus overproduction are attributed to Th1 cells (T-helper cells type 1) and specifically the subset Th17 cells (Kim and Criner, 2013). Interleukin 6 (IL-6) and interleukin 17 (IL-17) induce the production of proteins called mucins by lung epithelial cells which contribute to thick mucus production and the formation of mucus plugs, blocking the airway lumen. Impaired **mucociliary clearance** due to dysfunction and loss of cilia leads to the consolidation of mucus in the lungs.

Inflammatory infiltration of neutrophils, lymphocytes and macrophages in the bronchial wall leads to oedema of the bronchial mucosa and eventually fibrosis. These changes extend to the alveoli and further contribute to airway obstruction. Bacterial and viral infections are common and lead to exacerbations of COPD and amplification of alveolar injury (Tuder and Petrache, 2012). The narrowed airways increase resistance to airflow and cause obstruction, resulting in ventilation–perfusion mismatch with hypoxaemia and hypercapnia. Pulmonary blood vessels constrict in response to hypoxaemia, leading to pulmonary hypertension (Portillo et al., 2015) which can eventually lead to right-sided **heart failure**.

The classic signs of chronic bronchitis are a productive cough and prolonged expiration. Dyspnoea occurs late in the disease progression and cyanosis is often present as a result of hypoxaemia. The person usually has a history of smoking.

Emphysema

Emphysema is an obstructive airway disease characterised by destructive changes of the alveolar walls and irreversible enlargement of the alveolar sacs with loss of surface area for gas exchange (Tuder and Petrache, 2012) (Figure 14.5). The main characteristic of emphysema is the destruction of lung tissue rather than mucus production and inflammation as in chronic bronchitis. Abnormal, permanent enlargement of gas-exchange airways accompanied by destruction of alveolar walls without obvious fibrosis of the small airways contributes to airflow obstruction.

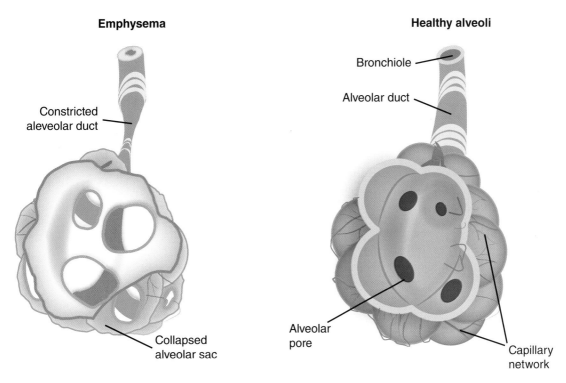

Illustrated by Shaun Mercier © SAGE Publications

Figure 14.5   Structural alveolar changes in emphysema

The distribution of damage to terminal respiratory units (acini) within the respiratory lobule and the extent of alveolar wall damage are used as a basis for the classification of emphysema. **Centriacinar** and **panacinar** emphysema are the most common forms of emphysema:

*   *Centriacinar emphysema*: refers to the central or proximal parts of the acini and is associated with smokers. It is often seen in COPD.
*   *Panacinar emphysema*: involves the acini at the terminal alveoli and is associated with alpha(α)-1-antitrypsin deficiency, an **autosomal recessive** inherited disorder. This enzyme inhibits the action of **proteolytic enzymes** released by neutrophils during inflammation. Absence of alpha-1-antitrypsin increases the risk of developing emphysema (Baraldo et al., 2015), particularly if the person smokes, as proteolytic enzymes are not inhibited and contribute to the damage of acini.

Prolonged exposure to a respiratory irritant such as tobacco smoke stimulates the inflammatory response and infiltration of inflammatory cells such as neutrophils and inflammatory mediators (i.e. leukotrienes, IL-8 and tumour necrosis factor [TNF]) in the lung tissue (Goldklang and Stockley, 2016). Proteases (enzymes that break down proteins) are released and there is inadequate production of protective antiproteases to counteract the action of the proteases, resulting in the breakdown of **elastin** and destruction of alveolar walls.

The destruction of alveoli results in large air spaces known as **bullae**; these are not effective in gaseous exchange, leading to ventilation–perfusion mismatch and hypoxia. The loss of the elastic recoil makes expiration difficult and leads to air-trapping in the alveoli (Gelb et al., 2015). This causes hyperexpansion of the chest and increases the work of breathing. Destruction of pulmonary capillaries leads to pulmonary hypertension and **cor pulmonale** (enlargement of the right side of the heart secondary to lungs or pulmonary blood vessel disease) with right-sided heart failure.

People with emphysema have a history of increasing dyspnoea, particularly on exertion. Use of accessory muscles is evident and expiration is prolonged through pursed lips in an effort to exhale as much air as possible before the alveoli and small airways collapse. They may or may not have a cough and a wheeze. Hyperinflation of the lungs produces an increase in the anteroposterior dimensions of the chest, resulting in a barrel-shaped chest typical of a person with emphysema which further contributes to dyspnoea and activity limitation (Langer et al., 2014). The person with emphysema will often have a history of smoking.

Bronchiectasis

Bronchiectasis is characterised by the permanent dilation of the bronchi caused by destruction of the bronchial wall and elastic supporting tissue. There may be a genetic predisposition, or it may occur in conjunction with another respiratory disease such as cystic fibrosis and tuberculosis and a compromised host defence to infection (King, 2018). Bronchiectasis is associated with recurrent infection of the lower respiratory tract, which leads to a persistent inflammatory response and permanent dilation of the medium-sized bronchi and bronchioles (Chen et al., 2018). Chronic inflammation causes destruction of the central bronchial wall with collapse of the peripheral bronchi and bronchioles. Loss of ciliated columnar epithelium and production of copious secretions lead to obstruction of airflow (Pasteur et al., 2010). The microorganisms that cause infection in bronchiectasis are present in the **microbiome** of the upper respiratory tract and include *Streptococcus pneumoniae*, *Haemophilus influenzae* and *Pseudomonas aeruginosa* (King, 2018).

A chronic productive cough with copious foul-smelling sputum is characteristic of bronchiectasis as a result of these pathophysiological changes. The person may have a fever, dyspnoea, wheezing and haemoptysis. Systemic manifestations include night sweats, **anaemia** and weight loss (due to the increased work of breathing and associated energy expenditure). In severe cases, clubbing may be present in the fingertips. Clubbing is enlargement of the distal segment of the digit (fingers or toes). It is thought that **vascular endothelial growth factor (VEGF)** (a platelet-derived factor) is an important component in its development (Rajagopalan and Schwartz, 2018). Hypoxia stimulates the release of VEGF that induces vascular hyperplasia, oedema and **proliferation** of fibroblasts/**osteoblasts** at a peripheral level in the nail (Rajagopalan and Schwartz, 2018). Large **megakaryocyte** fragments enter the systemic circulation and affect distal sites, releasing growth factors including VEGF. Platelets in the vasculature of the fingertips release platelet-derived growth factor that subsequently stimulates growth, increased vascular permeability and monocyte and neutrophil **chemotaxis**, leading to the proliferation of vascular smooth muscle cells and fibroblasts (Figure 14.6). It is associated with disorders such as bronchiectasis and **cystic fibrosis** and the severity of clubbing reflects the severity of the respiratory disease.

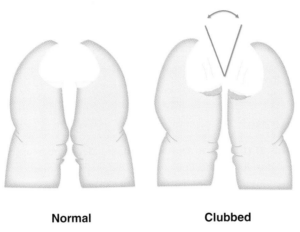

Normal   **Clubbed**

Illustrated by Shaun Mercier © SAGE Publications

Figure 14.6 Finger clubbing

Cystic Fibrosis (CF)

Cystic fibrosis is an inherited autosomal recessive disorder of the exocrine glands and is a major cause of severe respiratory disease in children and young adults. It affects 70,000 people worldwide and improved survival has led to increasing numbers reaching adulthood, with average survival to 40 years (Elborn et al., 2016).

Cystic fibrosis is a genetic disorder arising from a **mutation** on the cystic fibrosis transmembrane conductance regulator (*CFTCR*) gene on **chromosome** 7, resulting in a defective CFTCR protein (Stolz et al., 2015). This protein normally functions as a chloride channel in the epithelial cells lining the airways, the bile duct, the pancreas and the vas deferens. The defective protein means that chloride transport is impaired and both secretion and reabsorption can be affected. In the lung, the transport of chloride into the airway lumen is impaired which leads to increased absorption of sodium and water into the circulation, resulting in the secretion of thick tenacious mucus and dehydration of the mucociliary layer with a subsequent reduction in ciliary mobility and an ineffective clearing of mucus. The build-up of mucus obstructs the airways and provides a medium for recurrent pulmonary infection. Neutrophils release tissue-damaging proteases and oxidants that induce airway cells to destroy immunoglobulin G (IgG) and produce interleukin 8 (IL-8), which attracts more neutrophils and stimulates mucus secretion. Airway obstruction from mucus plugs and chronic inflammation and infection results in respiratory signs and symptoms.

Respiratory symptoms of CF include a persistent cough and the production of thick sputum and recurrent respiratory infections. Dyspnoea, tachypnoea and wheeze may be present. Over time, structural changes in the bronchial wall lead to bronchiectasis, and later signs of barrel chest and digital clubbing may be present. Chronic recurrent infection is common and microorganisms such as *Staphylococcus aureus* and *Haemophilus influenzae* are common in younger children (King, 2018). *Pseudomonas aeruginosa* colonises the lungs and leads to a decline in lung function (Harun et al., 2016).

Other manifestations of CF result from the impaired chloride transport in the sweat glands and the exocrine glands of the pancreas. In the sweat glands, the reabsorption of chloride and the subsequent reabsorption of sodium into the ducts of the glands fail, leading to a high concentration of sodium chloride in the sweat of the person with CF. The pancreatic and biliary ducts are affected by impaired sodium, chloride and potassium resorption, resulting in thick mucus production which blocks the pancreatic ducts. This in turn blocks the flow of digestive enzymes, leading to **malabsorption** of proteins, fats, carbohydrates and vitamins. Degenerative and fibrotic changes occur in the pancreas and gastrointestinal tract and diabetes can develop from the destruction of beta cells in the pancreas.

Diagnosis is based on clinical signs and diagnostic tests. Newborn screening includes a sweat chloride test to detect sodium and chloride levels in the sweat in excess of 60 mEq/l and blood tests for **immunoreactive trypsinogen** (IRT) (Farrell et al., 2017). IRT is a pancreatic enzyme precursor and it is elevated in infants and children with CF. Genetic testing for mutations in the *CFTR* gene can also be carried out (Farrell et al., 2017).

Interstitial lung disease

Interstitial lung disease (ILD) refers to a group of diffuse parenchymal lung disorders associated with substantial morbidity and mortality (Antoniou et al., 2014). They exert their effects on the **collagen** and elastic **connective tissue** found in the interstitium of the alveolar walls (Behr, 2012). ILD may occur in isolation or it may coexist alongside systemic disease (Behr, 2012); diminished lung compliance resulting in 'stiff' lungs that are difficult to inflate is the definitive hallmark of the condition. Increased work of breathing ensues as greater pressures need to be generated to inflate the lungs. Impaired gas exchange and hypoxaemia result due to damage of the alveolar epithelium and interstitial vasculature. As the disease progresses, respiratory failure may develop and may be associated with pulmonary hypertension or cor pulmonale.

ILD is initiated by some form of injury to the alveolar epithelium that causes an inflammatory response involving both the alveoli and the interstitium. Persistent injury leads to an accumulation of inflammatory and immune cells that cause damage to the lung tissue and development of fibrous scar tissue. Further development of fibrosis occurs as alveolar macrophages secrete a range of fibrogenic factors (e.g. fibroblast growth factor, platelet-derived growth factor) that attract fibroblasts and encourage their multiplication. Destruction of type I alveolar cells alongside an increase in type II alveolar cells chemotactically attracts further macrophages, cytokines and growth factors that further contribute to fibrotic changes.

Two of the most common ILDs are **idiopathic pulmonary fibrosis** (IPF) and sarcoidosis, therefore we will discuss both these disorders as they are frequently encountered in the people we care for.

Idiopathic pulmonary fibrosis

Idiopathic pulmonary fibrosis (IPF) is the most common disorder diagnosed among people with ILD; Antoniou et al. (2014) report that it is the most lethal disorder amongst ILDs. IPF is a chronic, progressive ILD of unknown aetiology that is difficult to diagnose and usually requires collaborative expertise to do so (NICE, 2017d). NICE (2017d) identifies clinical features that should be considered so that an early diagnosis can be made (Box 14.2). Two-thirds of those affected are people over the age of 60 years at the time of presentation. It affects men more than women. Risk factors for the disease include smoking and some occupations (e.g. farming, hairdressing, stone cutting and metal cutting) (Behr, 2012).

Box 14.2   Clinical features of IPF

- Age over 45 years
- Persistent breathlessness on exertion
- Persistent cough
- Bilateral inspiratory crackles when listening to the chest
- Clubbing of the fingers
- Normal spirometry or impaired spirometry, usually with a restrictive pattern but sometimes with an obstructive pattern

---

People presenting with IPF experience symptoms of breathlessness/dyspnoea initially on exertion and a cough (productive or non-productive); over time they will develop decreased lung function, cyanosis and cor pulmonale and have a reduced quality of life and ultimately death.

The rate of disease progression can vary greatly from person to person; the median survival time of someone with IPF is approximately 3 years from time of diagnosis, however 20% of people may live for more than 5 years (NICE, 2017d). Meyer (2014) acknowledges that ILD with extensive fibrosis is difficult to treat but appropriate therapies, including immunosuppressive anti-inflammatory therapies, oxygen therapy and pulmonary rehabilitation, can have a positive impact on quality of life and symptom palliation.

ACTIVITY 14.2: APPLY

Living with pulmonary fibrosis

As a person-centred practitioner, it is important to understand the lived experience of pulmonary fibrosis in order that you can support people in their illness. Watch the following video to help you gain some insight into that lived experience and reflect on how it may help you in your practice. If you are using the eBook just click on the play button. Alternatively go to
https://study.sagepub.com/essentialpatho/videos

INTERSTITIAL PULMONARY
FIBROSIS (1:53)

Sarcoidosis

Sarcoidosis is a systemic granulomatous disease process that may impact on any organ (in particular the lung) and can mimic other disease processes, especially malignancy or infection, making it difficult to diagnose (Parker et al., 2016). The disease usually affects people younger than 40 years but can occur in older people, affecting more females than males. The aetiology of sarcoidosis remains unclear. However, it is thought it may be linked to defective **human leucocyte antigen (HLA)** genes located in the **major histocompatibility complex (MHC)** (Baughman et al., 2011). The pathogenesis of sarcoidosis seems to involve the interplay of antigen, HLA class II molecules and T-cell receptors, with specific combinations of these three facets required for sarcoidosis to develop (Baughman et al., 2011). Sarcoidosis most likely requires exposure to one or more exogenous antigens. Infectious agents have long been suspected as possible causes of sarcoidosis; although it is unclear at present what these are specifically, it is thought that mycobacteria or *Propionibacterium acnes* may contribute to the disease (Baughman et al., 2011). Baughman et al. (2011) believe that the triggering antigen may vary depending on ethnicity, geographic location and individual genetic background.

The immune response is focused on the alveoli and is characterised by chronic inflammation, starting with polarisation of T lymphocytes to a Th1 phenotype, followed by cellular recruitment, especially macrophages and lymphocytes, that multiply and differentiate with the subsequent formation of the sarcoid granulomas (Baughman et al., 2011). The sarcoid granulomas do not show evidence of necrosis, however Chen et al. (2010) demonstrated that granulomas in sarcoidosis are characterised by extensive deposition of **serum amyloid**, a protein capable of starting an immune response and triggering cytokine release.

Signs and symptoms are variable, progression of the disease is unpredictable and any organ can be affected although mostly lungs, eyes and skin are involved. People may present with respiratory symptoms such as dyspnoea, non-productive cough and chest pain. They may also complain of fever, diaphoresis, anorexia, weight loss, fatigue and myalgia. The presence of skin plaques and **papules** is noted when there is skin involvement; involvement of the eyes leads to inflammation of the middle layer of the eye, i.e. **uveitis**. The person may experience periods of progressive chronicity, activity interspersed with periods of **remission**.

DISORDERS OF PULMONARY CIRCULATION

Disruption to blood flow through the lungs can be caused by the occlusion of blood vessels, increased pulmonary vascular resistance and destruction of the vascular bed that can lead to ventilation/perfusion mismatching. The effects of disrupted blood flow can range from mildly dysfunctional to severe and life-threatening. Two major problems associated with disruption in pulmonary blood flow are **pulmonary embolism** and pulmonary hypertension, both of which will be discussed.

Pulmonary embolism

Pulmonary embolism (PE) occurs when a blood-borne substance lodges in a branch of the pulmonary artery, occluding pulmonary vasculature (Figure 14.7). PE can originate from numerous sources, including **deep vein thrombosis** (DVT) (commonly in the lower extremities), tumours, fat (e.g. from a **fracture**), amniotic fluid, foreign bodies, air and **sepsis** (NICE, 2018). The most common source of PE is DVT; thrombus formation in the venous system occurs as a result of venous stasis, trauma (endothelial injury) and hypercoagulability. Collectively, these factors are known as Virchow's triad (Merli et al., 2018). Risk factors for the development of PE are presented in Table 14.6.

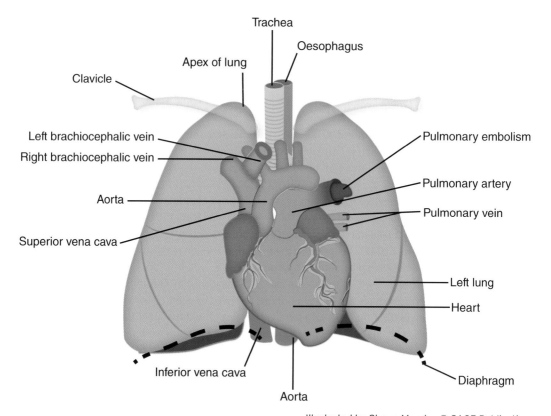

Illustrated by Shaun Mercier © SAGE Publications

Figure 14.7 Pulmonary embolism

Table 14.6 Risk factors for the development of pulmonary embolism

Stasis of blood flow	Prolonged immobilisation
	Long aeroplane or other journeys
	Diagnosis of DVT
	Varicose veins
Endothelial injury	Surgery within last 2 months
	Fractures
	Hypertension
	Contact with substances that promote coagulation: e.g. implants, medical devices, cell membranes (platelets, monocytes in chronic inflammation)
Hypercoagulability	Advancing age
	Obesity
	Malignancy
	Genetic factors: factor V Leiden, prothrombin gene mutations, inherited coagulation disorders
	Hormones: pregnancy, use of oral contraceptive pill, hormone replacement therapy

In PE, the lung tissue is ventilated but not perfused, causing a V/Q mismatch that creates intrapulmonary dead space, resulting in impaired gas exchange and loss of alveolar surfactant. Over a period of several hours the alveoli collapse, resulting in worsening hypoxaemia. There is a reduction in blood flow to a cross-sectional area of the pulmonary bed that leads to the elevation of pulmonary arterial pressure and decreased cardiac output. The affected area of the lung is no longer perfused and may infarct, although this only happens on rare occasions as oxygen continues to be supplied by bronchial circulation and the airways (Merli et al., 2018).

Signs and symptoms of PE depend on the size and location of the obstruction. If the embolus is small and lodged in peripheries of the pulmonary artery, it may go unnoticed and be clinically silent, particularly in the elderly or acutely ill. If the embolus is moderate in size, the person may complain of chest pain, dyspnoea and a sense of apprehension. In some cases, they may present with haemoptysis or syncope. Persons with a large embolus usually present with a sudden collapse or crushing substernal chest pain; they may be cyanotic, tachycardic, hypotensive and diaphoretic; they may also have distension of the jugular vein. PEs are potentially life-threatening if they completely occlude the pulmonary vasculature as this can lead to right ventricular failure, cardiac arrest and ultimately death.

Pulmonary hypertension

Pulmonary hypertension is defined as an increase in mean pulmonary arterial pressure (PAPm) greater than 25 mmHg at rest as assessed by right heart catheterisation (Galiè et al., 2016). It is a relatively common complication of chronic obstructive pulmonary disease and diffuse pulmonary lung disease (including ILD) that may have serious implications for the function of the right ventricle (Tseng et al., 2018). Pulmonary hypertension causes profound functional limitations and results in a poor quality of life (Babu et al., 2016). It can be categorised into five groups (Galiè et al., 2016):

1. Pulmonary arterial hypertension
2. Pulmonary hypertension due to left heart disease

3. Pulmonary hypertension due to lung disease with or without hypoxia
4. Chronic thromboembolic pulmonary hypertension
5. Pulmonary hypertension with unclear and/or multifactorial mechanisms.

ACTIVITY 14.3: GO DEEPER

Classification of pulmonary hypertension

To find out more about the five groups of pulmonary hypertension, read the 2015 ESC/ERS Guidelines for the diagnosis and treatment of pulmonary hypertension. The article is openly available online but if you are using the eBook just click on the icon to access it.

ARTICLE: PULMONARY
HYPERTENSION

The pathophysiology of pulmonary hypertension focuses on endothelial dysfunction and the interplay between the overproduction of powerful vasoconstrictors (e.g. thromboxane, endothelin) and the underproduction of the vasodilators (e.g. prostacyclin and **nitric oxide**). Remodelling (fibrosis and thickening) of the vessel walls occurs due to the release of growth vascular factors and subsequent narrowing of the lumen and abnormal vasoconstriction (Gao and Raj, 2017). Resistance to pulmonary blood flow ensues, thereby increasing pressure within the pulmonary arteries and right ventricle; there is a reduction in lung volumes and gas exchange is impaired. Right ventricular workload is increased as pressure and resistance continue to rise, resulting in right ventricular **hypertrophy** followed by right-sided heart failure.

Signs and symptoms of pulmonary hypertension are non-specific and are mainly related to the progression of right-sided heart failure (Galiè et al., 2016). Initially symptoms are induced by exertion and include dyspnoea, shortness of breath, fatigue, weakness, **angina** and syncope. On occasion, the person may present with a dry cough and exercise-induced **nausea** and **vomiting** (Galiè et al., 2016). As the disease progresses and reaches advanced stages, symptoms begin to occur at rest, with increased right ventricle dysfunction, abdominal distension and ankle oedema more likely to develop.

ACUTE RESPIRATORY DISORDERS

Acute respiratory disorders refer to disruptions in gaseous exchange that are life-threatening with a high morbidity and mortality rate. Acute respiratory disorders include **acute lung injury (ALI)**, acute respiratory distress syndrome (ARDS) and acute respiratory failure.

Acute lung injury and acute respiratory distress syndrome

Acute lung injury (ALI) and acute respiratory distress syndrome (ARDS) are manifestations of an inflammatory response of the lung to an insult either directly or indirectly (Ragaller and Richter, 2010). ALI and ARDS are characterised by severe hypoxaemia, hypercapnia, diffuse infiltrate on chest X-ray and substantial reduction in lung compliance. ALI can be defined as an acute lung disease with bilateral pulmonary infiltrate consistent with oedema and with no evidence of left atrial hypertension (Ragaller and Richter, 2010).

ARDS can be defined as an acute inflammatory lung injury associated with increased pulmonary vascular permeability, increased lung weight and loss of aerated tissue (Bellani et al., 2016). The conditions are differentiated by the difference in the extent of hypoxaemia determined by the ratio of partial pressure of oxygen in arterial blood (PaO_2) to the fraction of inspired oxygen (FiO_2) (Saguil and Fargo, 2012). ALI and ARDS can be caused by a variety of insults, including aspiration of gastric contents, trauma, sepsis, **acute pancreatitis**, **disseminated intravascular coagulation** and reactions to drugs/toxins.

The pathophysiology of ALI and ARDS is unclear although both local and systemic inflammatory responses occur. Mattihay et al. (2012) suggest that dysregulation of the inflammatory response, the accumulation of neutrophils, uncontrolled activation of coagulation pathways and altered permeability of the endothelium and disruption of endothelial barriers play a role in their development. Activation and migration of neutrophils across the alveolar epithelial surfaces result in the release of cytokines, proteases and **reactive oxygen species** that cause increased permeability and damage to alveolar type I and type II cells. Increased permeability allows the movement of fluid, plasma protein and blood cells from the vascular compartment to move into the interstitium and alveoli of the lung. Pulmonary oedema, hyaline membrane formation and the loss of alveolar surfactant decrease lung compliance, increasing intrapulmonary shunting of blood (V/Q mismatching), impairing gas exchange and resulting in hypoxaemia. At the bedside, ALI and ARDS culminate in life-threatening hypoxia, hypercapnia, acidosis and pulmonary hypertension, and require a fast and goal-oriented therapy without further lung damage (Ragaller and Richter, 2010).

Acute respiratory failure

Respiratory failure refers to the failure of the respiratory system to oxygenate the body or to eliminate carbon dioxide from the body. It may be due to acute disorders or trauma or can develop as a result of the course of a chronic disease. Respiratory failure is divided into two types: hypoxaemic respiratory failure (type I) and hypercapnic/hypoxaemic respiratory failure (type II) (Saguil and Fargo, 2012).

- *Type I (hypoxaemic)*: characterised by low O_2 and normal or low PCO_2, often due to a dysfunction of gaseous exchange. Two major factors contribute to a decrease in oxygen level: V/Q mismatching and impaired diffusion. V/Q mismatching occurs when areas of the lungs are perfused but not ventilated, or ventilated but not perfused. This could be due to hypoventilation or decreased cardiac output. Impaired diffusion refers to the disruption in gaseous exchange between the alveoli and pulmonary circulation due to permeability of the alveolar surface or an increase in the distance for diffusion.
- *Type II (hypercapnic)*: characterised by low O_2 with high PCO_2, often caused by a dysfunction of alveolar ventilation. Type II respiratory failure is usually caused by conditions that occur outside of the respiratory system, including depression of the central nervous system (drug/alcohol induced, brain injury); conditions that affect nerve supply to the respiratory system (**Guillain-Barré syndrome**, spinal cord injury); disorders of the respiratory muscles (muscular dystrophy); or thoracic cage disorders (**scoliosis**).

Signs and symptoms of acute respiratory failure are associated with hypoxaemia or hypercapnia and the clinical manifestations that occur because of this.

CHAPTER SUMMARY

In this chapter you will have learned about disorders of the respiratory system across the life span and how they impact not only physiologically but also how they influence health-related quality of life. To be an effective person-centred practitioner, you need to be relational when considering these disorders; being compassionate and working with someone's belief system and values will enable you to care for them within the context of their culture and social structure.

- Hypoventilation refers to inadequate alveolar ventilation compared to the metabolic demands of the body. It occurs when the minute volume is reduced and is caused by changes in the mechanics of breathing or due to changes in the neurological control of breathing.

- Hyperventilation refers to increased alveolar ventilation that exceeds the metabolic demands of the body. It occurs when the excretion rate of CO_2 exceeds that which is produced by cellular metabolism.

- Hypoxia refers to a reduction in tissue oxygenation and can result from pulmonary alterations, or other abnormalities that are not related to pulmonary function, e.g. decreased cardiac output. Hypoxaemia refers to a reduction of oxygen in arterial blood and is caused by pulmonary dysfunction and may lead to hypoxia.

- Hypercapnia refers to an increase in CO_2 content of arterial blood and is usually caused by disorders that lead to hypoventilation or V/Q mismatching.

- Respiratory disease can be categorised into three phases: respiratory impairment, respiratory insufficiency and respiratory failure.

- Respiratory tract infections (RTIs) refer to infectious diseases that can affect any part of the respiratory tract; they tend to be discussed in terms of upper respiratory tract infections (URTIs), i.e. infection of nose, oropharynx or larynx, or lower respiratory tract infections (LRTIs), i.e. lower airways and lungs.

- Infections of the upper respiratory tract include: the common cold, influenza, rhinitis, sinusitis and otitis media. Infections of the lower respiratory tract include: bronchiolitis, pneumonia and tuberculosis.

- Pneumonia refers to infection of the pulmonary parenchyma, i.e. bronchioles and alveoli. It occurs when the normal defence mechanisms are bypassed and a pathogen gains access to the lower respiratory tract, causing an extensive inflammatory response. Pneumonias can be classified in a number of ways based on the pathogen (typical or atypical) or the area of infection (lobar pneumonia or bronchopneumonia). Pneumonias may also be classified according to the setting in which they occur and referred to as community-acquired pneumonia (CAP), hospital-acquired pneumonia (HAP), health care-associated pneumonia (HCAP) or ventilator-associated pneumonia (VAP).

- Tuberculosis (TB) is an infection caused by *Mycobacterium tuberculosis* (MTB) (an acid-fast bacilli), usually affecting the lungs but it may invade other body systems. It is highly contagious and the spread is airborne by means of droplet nuclei that are harboured in the respiratory secretions of persons with active tuberculosis. It is the ninth leading cause of death worldwide and is the leading cause of death from a single infectious agent.

- A pneumothorax refers to the presence of air in the pleural cavity caused by rupture of either the parietal or visceral pleura. A pneumothorax can cause either partial or complete collapse of the affected lung.

- Pleural effusion refers to an abnormal collection of fluid in the pleural cavity. Types of pleural effusions are characterised by the presence of substances in them: hydrothorax (serous fluid, transudative or exudative), empyema (pus), chylothorax (chyle) and haemothorax (blood).

- Obstructive lung disorders are a group of diseases caused by obstruction or limitation to airflow. The main disorders of obstructive lung disease are asthma, chronic bronchitis and emphysema.

- Chronic obstructive pulmonary disease (COPD) is an umbrella term for a group of disorders that cause airway obstruction, particularly chronic bronchitis and emphysema. Tobacco smoke is a primary risk factor for COPD.

- Bronchiectasis is characterised by the permanent dilation of the bronchi caused by destruction of the bronchial wall and elastic supporting tissue.

- Cystic fibrosis is an autosomal recessive disorder of defective chloride transport, resulting in thick mucus production in the airways and the glandular ducts.

- Interstitial lung disease (ILD) refers to a group of diffuse parenchymal lung disorders that exert their effects on the collagen and elastic connective tissue found in the interstitium of the alveolar walls. Two of the most common ILD are idiopathic pulmonary fibrosis and sarcoidosis.

- Pulmonary embolism (PE) occurs when a blood-borne substance lodges in a branch of the pulmonary artery occluding pulmonary vasculature.

- Pulmonary hypertension is defined as an increase in mean pulmonary arterial pressure (PAPm) greater than 25 mmHg at rest as assessed by right heart catheterisation.

- Acute lung injury (ALI) and acute respiratory distress syndrome (ARDS) are manifestations of an inflammatory response of the lung to an insult either directly or indirectly. They are characterised by severe hypoxaemia, hypercapnia, diffuse infiltrate on chest X-ray and substantial reduction in lung compliance.

- Respiratory failure refers to the failure of the respiratory system to oxygenate the body or to eliminate carbon dioxide from the body. It can be divided into two types: hypoxaemic respiratory failure (type I) and hypercapnic/hypoxaemic respiratory failure (type II).

REVISE

TEST YOUR KNOWLEDGE

In this chapter you will have learned about a variety of disorders of oxygenation and carbon dioxide elimination; these can be complex and in order to check your understanding, the following questions will help you confirm your knowledge and application.

Answers are available online. If you are using the eBook just click on the answers icon below. Alternatively go to **https://study.sagepub.com/essentialpatho/answers**

1 Identify and briefly explain the different types of hypoxia.

2 Identify and briefly explain the defence mechanisms of the respiratory tract function.

3 Briefly discuss the pathophysiology of pneumonia, indicating the different types.

4 Identify the risk groups and factors for developing tuberculosis.

5   What are the signs and symptoms of tuberculosis?

6   Briefly explain what a pleural effusion is and identify the different types.

7   What are the different types of atelectasis?

8   Explain the inflammatory response in atopic asthma.

9   Describe the physiological mechanism of 'air trapping'.

10   Explain the inflammatory mechanisms responsible for mucous overproduction in chronic bronchitis.

11   Describe the types of emphysema.

12   Explain the physiological mechanisms that lead to thick mucus secretions in cystic fibrosis.

13   Identify the sources that can cause pulmonary embolism.

14   Differentiate between Type I and Type II respiratory failure.

REVISE

———

ACE YOUR ASSESSMENT

- Further revision and learning opportunities are available online
- Test yourself away from the book with **Extra multiple choice questions**
- Learn and revise terminology with **Interactive flashcards**

If you are using the eBook access each resource by clicking on the respective icon. Alternatively go to **https://study.sagepub.com/essentialpatho/chapter14**

CHAPTER 14 ANSWERS

EXTRA QUESTIONS

FLASHCARDS

REFERENCES

Antoniou, K.A., Margaritopoulous, G.A., Tomasetti, S., Bonella, F., Costabel, U. and Poletti, V. (2014) Interstitial lung disease. *European Respiratory Review*, *23* (131): 40–54.

Arnold, F.W., Summersgill, J.T. and Ramirez, J.A. (2016) Role of atypical pathogens in the etiology of community-acquired pneumonia. *Seminars in Respiratory and Critical Care Medicine*, *37* (6): 819–28.

Babu, A.S., Padmakumar, R., Maiya, A.G., Mohapatra, A.K. and Kamath, R.L. (2016) Effects of exercise training on exercise capacity in pulmonary arterial hypertension: a systematic review of clinical trials. *Heart, Lung and Circulation, 25* (4): 333–41.

Baraldo, S., Turato, G., Lunardi, F., Bazzan, E., Schiavon, M., Ferrarotti, I. et al. (2015) Immune activation in α1-antitrypsin-deficiency emphysema: beyond the protease–antiprotease paradigm. *American Journal of Respiratory and Critical Care Medicine, 191* (4): 402–9.

Baughman, R.P., Culver, D.A. and Judson, M.A. (2011) A concise review of pulmonary sarcoidosis. *American Journal of Respiratory and Critical Care Medicine, 183* (5): 573–81.

Behr, K. (2012) Approach to diagnosis of interstitial lung disease. *Clinics in Chest Medicine, 33* (1): 1–10.

Bellani, G., Laffey, J.G., Pham, T., Fan, E., Brochard, L., Esteban, A. et al. (2016) Epidemiology, patterns of care, and mortality for patients with acute respiratory distress syndrome in intensive care units in 50 countries. *JAMA, 316* (8): 788–800.

Bjornson, C.L. and Johnson, D.W. (2013) Croup in children. *CMAJ: Canadian Medical Association Journal, 185* (15): 1317–23.

Boore, J., Cook, N. and Shepherd, A. (2016) *Essentials of Anatomy and Physiology for Nursing Practice.* London: Sage.

Brightling, C.E., Gupta, S., Gonem, S. and Siddigui, S. (2012) Lung damage and airway remodeling in severe asthma. *Clinical and Experimental Allergy, 42* (5): 638–49.

Chen, E.S., Song, Z., Willett, M.H., Heine, S., Yung, R.C., Liu, M.C., Groshon, S.D. et al. (2010) Serum amyloid A regulates granulomatous inflammation in sarcoidosis through Toll-like receptor-2. *American Journal of Respiatory and Critical Care Medicine, 181*: 360–73.

Chen, Z.G., Li, Y.Y., Wang, Z.N., Li, M., Lim, H.F. et al (2018) Aberrant epithelial remodeling with impairment of cilic architecture in non-cystic fibrosis bronchiectasis. *Journal of Thoracic Disease, 10* (3): 1753–64.

Chung, K.F., Wenzel, S.E., Brozek, J.L., Li, M., Lim, H.F., Zhou Y.Q. et al. (2014) International ERS/ATS guidelines on definition, evaluation and treatment of severe asthma. *European Respiratory Journal, 43*: 343–73.

Cruz-Knight, W. and Blake-Gumbs, L. (2013) Tuberculosis: an overview. *Primary Care, 40* (3): 743–56.

De Martino, M., Galli, L. and Chiappini, E. (2014) Reflections of the immunology of tuberculosis: will we ever unravel the skein? *BMC: Infectious Diseases, 14* (Suppl 1) [online] doi: 10.1186/1471-2334-14-S1-S1].

Del Giacco, S.R., Bakirtas, A., Be, L.E., Custovic, A., Diamant, Z., Hamelmann, E. et al. (2017) Allergy in severe asthma. *Allergy,: 72*: 207–20.

Diao, M., Shen, X., Cheng, J., Chai, J., Feng, R., Zhang, P. et al. (2018) How patients' experiences of respiratory tract infections affect healthcare-seeking and antibiotic use: insights from a cross-sectional survey in rural Anhui, China. *BMJ Open, 8* (2) [online] doi: 10.1136/bmjopen-2017-019492.

Diver, S., Russell, R.J. and Brightling, C.E. (2018) New and emerging drug treatments for asthma. *Clinical and Experimental Allergy, 48* (3): 241–52.

Elborn, J.S., Bell, S.C., Madge, S.L., Burgel, P.R., Castellani, C., Conway, S. et al. (2016) Report of the European Respiratory Society/European Cystic Fibrosis Society task force on the care of adults with cystic fibrosis. *European Respiratory Journal, 47* (2): 420–8.

Farrell, P.M., White, T.B., Ren, C.L., Hempstead, S.E., Accurso, F., Derichs, N. et al. (2017) Diagnosis of cystic fibrosis: consensus guidelines from the cystic fibrosis foundation. *Journal of Paediatrics, 181* (Suppl): S4–S15.

Fogel, N. (2015) Tuberculosis: a disease without boundaries. *Tuberculosis, 95* (5): 527–31.

Galiè, N., Humbert, M., Vachiery, J-L., Gibbs, S., Lang, I., Torbicki, A. et al. (2016) 2015 ESC/ERS guidelines for the diagnosis and treatment of pulmonary hypertension: the Joint Task Force for the Diagnosis and Treatment of Pulmonary Hypertension of the European Society of Cardiology (ESC) and the European Respiratory Society (ERS). Endorsed by the Association for European Paediatric and Congenital Cardiology (AEPC), International Society for Heart and Lung Transplantation (ISHLT). *European Heart Journal, 37* (1): 67–119.

Gao, Y. and Raj, J.U. (2017) Pathophysiology of pulmonary hypertension. *Colloquium Series on Integrated Systems Physiology: From Molecule to Function, 9* (6): i–104. doi.org/10.4199/ C00158ED1V01Y201710ISP078. Available at: www.morganclaypool.com/doi/10.4199/ C00158ED1V01Y201710ISP078 (accessed 10 August 2018).

GBD (2015 Chronic Respiratory Disease Collaborators) (2017) Global, regional, and national deaths, prevalence, disability-adjusted life years, and years lived with disability for chronic obstructive pulmonary disease and asthma, 1990–2015: a systematic analysis for the Global Burden of Disease Study 2015. *The Lancet Respiratory Medicine, 5* (9): 691–706.

Gelb, A.F., Yamamoto, A., Verbeken, E.K. and Nadal, J.A. (2015) Unravelling the pathophysiology of the asthma-COPD overlap syndrome. *Chest, 148* (2): 313–20.

GINA (2018) GINA 2018 Report, Global Strategy for Asthma Management and Prevention. Global Initiative for Asthma. [online]. Available at: https://ginasthma.org/2018-gina-report-global-strategy-for-asthma-management-and-prevention/ (accessed 6 August 2018).

GOLD (2016) Global Strategy for the Diagnosis, Management and Prevention of COPD. Global Initiative for Chronic Obstructive Lung Disease. [online]. Available at: https://goldcopd.org/ (accessed 8 August 2018).

Goldklang, M. and Stockley, R. (2016) Pathophysiology of emphysema and implications. *Chronic Obstructive Pulmonary Diseases, 3* (1): 454–8.

Gu, K., van Caeseele, P., Dust, K. and Ho, J. (2017) Atypical pneumonia due to human bocavirus in an immunocompromised patient. *CMAJ: Canadian Medical Association Journal, 189* (19): E697–E699.

Harun, S.N., Wainwright, K. and Henning, S. (2016) A systematic review of studies examining the rate of lung function decline in patients with cystic fibrosis. *Paediatric Respiratory Reviews, 20*: 55–66.

Hemilä, H. and Chalker, E. (2017) Zinc for preventing and treating the common cold. *Cochrane Database of Systematic Reviews, 9.* [online]. Available at: www.cochranelibrary.com/cdsr/ doi/10.1002/14651858.CD012808/ (accessed 6 August 2018).

Hull, J.D., Barton, I.P., Torgersen, J. and McNeil, C.M. (2013) A survey of the experiences and impact of acute upper respiratory tract infections on people in six countries in the 2011/2012 common cold and flu season. *Open Journal of Respiratory Disease, 3*: 175–87.

Johnson, D.W. (2014) Croup. *BMJ: Clinical Evidence*, published online 29 September 2014. Available at: www.ncbi.nlm.nih.gov/pubmed/25263284 (accessed 6 August 2018).

Kalanuria, A.A., Zai, W. and Mirski, M. (2014) Ventilator-associated pneumonia in the ICU. *Critical Care, 18*: 208.

Kim, V. and Criner, J.G. (2013) Chronic bronchitis and chronic obstructive pulmonary disease. *American Journal of Respiratory and Critical Care Medicine, 187* (3): 228–37.

King, P.T. (2018) The role of the immune response in the pathogenesis of bronchiectasis. *BioMed Research International, 2018* (6802637): 1–12. [online]. Available at: www.hindawi.com/journals/ bmri/2018/6802637/ (accessed 10 August 2018).

Kudo, M., Ishigatsubo, Y. and Aoki, I. (2013) Pathology of asthma. *Frontiers in Microbiology, 4* (263): 1–16.

Labella, A.M. and Merel, S.E. (2013) Influenza. *Medical Clinics of North America, 97* (4): 621–45.

Langer, D., Ciavaglia, C.E., Neder, J.A., Webb, K.A. and O'Donnell, D.E. (2014) Lung hyperinflation in chronic obstructive pulmonary disease: mechanisms, clinical implications and treatment. *Expert Review of Respiratory Medicine, 8* (6): 731–49.

Mattihay, M.A., Ware, L.B. and Zimmerman, G.A. (2012) The acute respiratory distress syndrome. *Journal of Clinical Investigation, 122* (8): 2731–40.

Meissner, H.C. (2016) Viral bronchiolitis in children. *New England Journal of Medicine, 374* (1): 62–72.

Merli, G., Eraso, L.H., Galanis, T. and Ouma, G. (2018) Pulmonary embolism. *BMJ Best Practice*. Available at: https://bestpractice.bmj.com/topics/en-gb/116#referencePop1 (accessed 10 August 2018).

Meyer, K.C. (2014) Diagnosis and management of interstitial lung disease. *Translational Respiratory Medicine, 2*: 4. doi: 10.1186/2213-0802-2-4.

NICE (2017a) Asthma: diagnosis, monitoring and chronic asthma management. NICE guideline [NG80]. National Institute for Health and Care Excellence. Available at: www.nice.org.uk/guidance/ng80 (accessed 9 August 2018).

NICE (2017b) Bronchiolitis in children: diagnosis and management. NICE guideline [NG9]. National Institute of Health and Care Excellence. Available at: www.nice.org.uk/guidance/ng9 date (accessed 8 August 2018).

NICE (2017c) Croup. Clinical Knowledge Summaries. National Institute of Health and Care Excellence. Available at: https://cks.nice.org.uk/croup (accessed 6 August 2018).

NICE (2017d) Idiopathic pulmonary fibrosis in adults: diagnosis and management. Clinical guidance [CG163]. National Institute of Health and Care Excellence. Available at: www.nice.org.uk/guidance/cg163 (accessed 8 August 2018).

NICE (2018) Venous thromboembolism in over 16s. Reducing the risk of hospital-acquired deep vein thrombosis or pulmonary embolism. NICE guideline [NG89] Volume 1: Methods, evidence and recommendations. National Institute for Health and Care Excellence. Available at: www.nice.org.uk/guidance/ng89/evidence/full-guideline-volume-1-pdf-4787002765 (accessed 9 August 2018).

Olin, J.T. and Wechsler, M.E. (2014) Asthma: pathogenesis and novel drugs for treatment. *British Medical Journal, 349*: g5517. Available at: https://doi.org/10.1136/bmj.g5517 (accessed 6 August 2018).

Papi, A., Brightling, C.E., Pedersen, S.E. and Reddel, H.K. (2018) Asthma. *The Lancet, 391*: 783–800.

Parker, C., Allen, K. and Browning, S. (2016) Can a leopard change its spots? Metastatic breast cancer or sarcoidosis. *American Journal of Respiratory and Critical Care Medicine, 193*: A5051. Available at: www.atsjournals.org/doi/pdf/10.1164/ajrccm-conference.2016.193.1_MeetingAbstracts.A5051 (accessed 8 August 2018).

Pasteur, M.C., Bilton, D. and Hill, A.T. (2010) British Thoracic Guideline for non-CF bronchiectasis. *Thorax, 65*: 11–58.

Patel, P.P., Jacob, C., Thind, G.S., Loehrke, M. and Stryker, H. (2018) Croup in adults: all bite and no bark? *American Journal of Respiratory and Critical Care Medicine, 197*: A6748. Available at: www.atsjournals.org/doi/abs/10.1164/ajrccm-conference.2018.197.1_MeetingAbstracts.A6748 (accessed 7 August 2018).

Portillo, K., Torralba, Y., Blanco, I., Burgos, F., Rodriguez-Roisin, R., Rios, J. et al. (2015) Pulmonary haemodynamic profile in chronic obstructive pulmonary disease. *International Journal of Chronic Obstructive Pulmonary Disease, 10*: 1313–20.

Ragaller, M. and Richter, T. (2010) Acute lung injury and acute respiratory distress syndrome. *Journal of Emergencies, Trauma and Shock, 3* (1): 43–51.

Rajagopalan, M. and Schwartz, R.A. (2018) Assessment of clubbing. *BMJ Best Practice*. Available at: https://bestpractice.bmj.com/topics/en-gb/623#referencePop2 (accessed 16 August 2018).

Rajan, J.P., Wineinger, N.E., Stevenson, D.D. and White, A.A. (2015) Prevalence of aspirin-exacerbated respiratory disease among asthmatic patients: a meta-analysis of the literature. *Journal of Allergy and Clinical Immunology, 135* (3): 676–81.

Ricci, V., Delgado, V., Murphy, S.M. and Cunningham, S. (2015) Bronchiolitis in children: summary of NICE Guidance. *BMJ, 350*: h2305.

Russell, R.J. and Brightling, C. (2017) Pathogenesis of asthma: implications for precision medicine. *Clinical Science (London), 131*: 1723–35.

Saguil, A. and Fargo, M. (2012) Acute respiratory distress syndrome: diagnosis and management. *American Family Physician*, *84* (4): 352–8.

Saguil, A., Wyrick, K. and Hallgren, J. (2014) Diagnostic approach to pleural effusion. *American Family Physician*, *90* (2): 99–104.

Salgame, P., Geadas, C., Collins, L., Jones-López, E. and Ellner, J.J. (2015) Latent tuberculosis infection: revisiting and revising concepts. *Tuberculosis*, *95* (4): 373–84.

Smoliga, J.M., Weiss, P. and Rundell, K.W. (2016) Exercise induced bronchoconstriction in adults: evidence based diagnosis and management. *British Medical Journal*, *352*: h6951.

Stolz, D.A., Meyerhols, M.J. and Welsh, M.J. (2015) Origins of cystic fibrosis lung disease. *New England Journal of Medicine*, *372* (4): 351–62.

Thillai, M., Pollock, K., Pareek, M. and Lalvani, A. (2014) Interferon-gamma release assays for tuberculosis: current and future application. *Expert Review of Respiratory Medicine*, *8* (1): 67–78.

Tseng, S., Stanziola, A.A., Sultan, S., Henry, K., Saggar, R. and Saggar, R. (2018) Pulmonary hypertension related to chronic obstructive pulmonary disease and diffuse parenchymal lung disease: a focus of right ventricle (dys)function. *Heart Failure Clinics*, *14* (3): 403–11.

Tuder, R.M. and Petrache, I. (2012) Pathogenesis of chronic obstructive pulmonary disease. *Journal of Clinical Investigation*, *122* (8): 2749–55.

Weldon, E. and Williams, J. (2012) Pleural disease in the emergency room. *Emergency Medicinal Clinics of North America*, *30*: 475–99.

World Health Organisation (WHO) (2017) Global Tuberculosis Report 2017. Geneva: WHO. Available at: http://apps.who.int/medicinedocs/en/m/abstract/Js23360en (accessed 8 August 2018).

World Health Organisation (WHO) (2018a) Bronchial asthma. Factsheet No. 206. [online]. Available at: www.who.int/mediacentre/factsheets/fs206/en/ (accessed 16 August 2018).

World Health Organisation (WHO) (2018b) Influenza (seasonal). Factsheet. [online]. Available at: www.who.int/en/news-room/fact-sheets/detail/influenza-(seasonal) (accessed 7 August 2018).

Wos, M., Sanak, M., Soja, J., Olechnowicz, H., Busse, W.W. and Szczeklik, A. (2008) The presence of rhinovirus in lower airways of patients with bronchial asthma. *American Journal of Respiratory and Critical Care Medicine*, *177* (10): 1082–9.

Zoorob, T., Sidani, M. and Murray, J. (2011) Croup. *American Family Physician*, *83* (9): 1067–73.

Zuma, A., Raviglione, H., Hafner, R. and van Reyn, C.F. (2013) Tuberculosis. *New England Journal of Medicine*, *368* (8): 745–55.

DISORDERS OF THE CARDIOVASCULAR SYSTEM

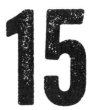
15

UNDERSTAND: CHAPTER VIDEOS

Watch the following videos to ease you into this chapter. If you are using the eBook just click on the play buttons. Alternatively go to **https://study.sagepub.com/essentialpatho/videos**

HYPERTENSION (5:10)

CORONARY ARTERY DISEASE (13:31)

LEARNING OUTCOMES

When you have finished studying this chapter you will be able to:

1. Describe the pathophysiology and classifications of hypertension.
2. Recognise how heart failure occurs and the impact it has systemically and on gaseous exchange.
3. Discuss the causes of oedema.
4. Describe the causes of arrhythmogenesis (initiating cardiac arrhythmias) and the characteristics of major cardiac arrhythmias.
5. Outline the major congenital heart conditions and their structural elements.

INTRODUCTION

The heart lies at the centre of the circulatory system, providing blood to the lungs for gaseous exchange and to the whole body through the circulatory system. It is therefore a key organ for the delivery of nutrients to tissues and the delivery of waste products to various sites for their elimination. **Cardiovascular disease** therefore represents a major risk to survival and the maintenance of **homeostasis**. Cardiovascular **diseases** are major causes of death and **morbidity** globally and understanding their origins and impact is central to a nurse being able to engage in preventative health strategies, understand the principles underpinning holistic care and be aware of the wider impact of conditions on the person and their family.

In this chapter we will reflect on **coronary artery disease** and then consider **hypertension**; the latter is a common characteristic in many cardiovascular diseases and so it is important to understand it first. We will then focus on the major cardiovascular diseases and also consider those that occur at the beginning of life.

It is important to read Chapter 8 in this book before progressing through this chapter. This is because many of the factors that affect blood supply to the tissues will lead to disorders of the cardiovascular system and so these two chapters interrelate closely.

PERSON-CENTRED CONTEXT: THE BODIE FAMILY

BODIE FAMILY
CASE NOTES

The heart is at the centre of life; it is central to homeostasis and the ability of the body to meet metabolic demands; this means it needs to be functioning effectively and efficiently if we are to have energy for daily activities, including working, engaging in hobbies, being independent and being able to experience joy and fear. Cardiovascular health is therefore central to our health-related quality of life, not just in terms of physical functioning but also in terms of our social roles, independence and our ability to gain joy out of life.

Consider Maud Bodie, who was diagnosed with **heart failure** 3 years ago (right ventricular failure). This means she will have a reduced pumping of blood to the lungs and a reduced ability to manage the volume of blood coming into the right side of the heart, causing a backlog in the systemic circulation. This can give her oedema in her peripheries but will also lead to her having less energy to engage with her great-grandchild. She also had a heart attack (**myocardial infarction**) and so we know there is coronary artery disease present. This means she needs to eat well, exercise and adopt lifestyle changes that promote cardiovascular health. She is also **overweight** and so should be working to lose some weight to achieve optimal health.

Her husband, George, also has a history of raised blood **cholesterol**, which indicates a risk of developing **atherosclerosis**. He also needs to ensure he makes lifestyle choices that maximise his cardiovascular health.

Richard Jones has diabetes and this can also place him at risk of cardiovascular disease; managing his blood sugar levels through diet and lifestyle is therefore a very important preventative strategy.

--- **REVISE: A&P RECAP** ---

Cardiovascular system: structure and functions

We recommend that you revise the structure and functions of the cardiovascular system by reading Chapter 12 in *Essentials of Anatomy and Physiology for Nursing Practice* (Boore et al., 2016). This will help you to better understand the content of this chapter.

CORONARY ARTERY DISEASE

Coronary artery disease (CAD) (also referred to as ischaemic heart disease/cardiovascular disease/**coronary heart disease**) dominates as a leading cause of death worldwide. CAD is responsible for 1 in every 5 deaths; the morbidity, mortality and socioeconomic impact of CAD on society is significant and it is the focus of many issues on health care agendas worldwide. While Chapter 8 focused on disorders of the blood supply, this chapter will take a more focused look at diseases of the heart itself, recognising the interplay of an impaired blood supply with these conditions.

HYPERTENSION

We are going to start this chapter by focusing on hypertension as it is often a precursor to disorders of the cardiovascular system. First, we need to think back to what controls blood pressure. Remember that blood pressure is the force exerted on the arterial walls by the blood circulating through them. It is therefore expressed in the formula:

Blood Pressure = Cardiac Output × Peripheral Resistance

If you recall **cardiac output**, it is the volume of blood pumped out of the heart in a minute and so is represented by the following formula:

Cardiac Output = Heart Rate × Stroke Volume

It is also important to remember how blood pressure is regulated within the body. You will recall that there are short-acting and long-acting control systems, largely through the nervous and endocrine systems respectively:

* *Neurological*: The cardiovascular centre in the medulla detects falls and rises in blood pressure through **baroreceptors**. The sympathetic nervous system responds to an increase in blood pressure and the parasympathetic nervous system to decreased blood pressure (Figure 15.1).
* *Endocrine*: The renin–angiotensin aldosterone system (RAAS) (Figure 15.2) is the primary hormonal system that regulates blood pressure. Other hormones, such as **catecholamines** (e.g. adrenaline/epinephrine and noradrenaline/norepinephrine), also influence blood pressure as they are vasoactive substances that cause **vasoconstriction** through the contraction of smooth muscle in arterioles, raising blood pressure, and also by stimulating the heart to beat fast. Both will increase cardiac output.

Other factors, such as being warm or cold, can influence blood pressure, as can the presence of any other substances that are vasoactive, e.g. carbon dioxide.

Now that we have refreshed our knowledge on what controls blood pressure, we can consider hypertension itself. Hypertension, persistently elevated blood pressure, is one of the most common health problems experienced by adults and is the leading risk factor for cardiovascular disease. Approximately one-third of adults (men and women) have hypertension, with the condition being more prevalent as people get older (Nadella and Howell, 2015).

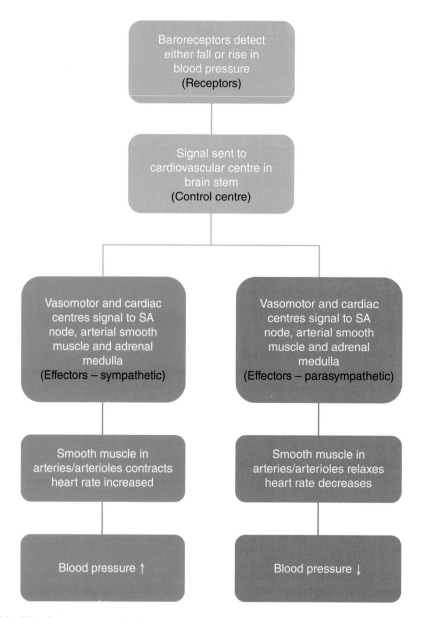

Figure 15.1 Blood pressure control

Classification

There are three main classifications of hypertension:

- *Primary hypertension*: This is when blood pressure is elevated without evidence of another disease causing it. In essence, the set point for blood pressure control is elevated and therefore homeostatic mechanisms work to that set point. The exact causes of primary hypertension are therefore unclear but thought to be multifactorial, including a potential genetic predisposition and a complex interrelationship between the renal system, a hyperactive sympathetic nervous system and a hypersensitive RAAS (Nadella and Howell, 2015). There is significant evidence of increased noradrenaline outflow in primary hypertension with a selective increase in sympathetic outflow to the heart and the

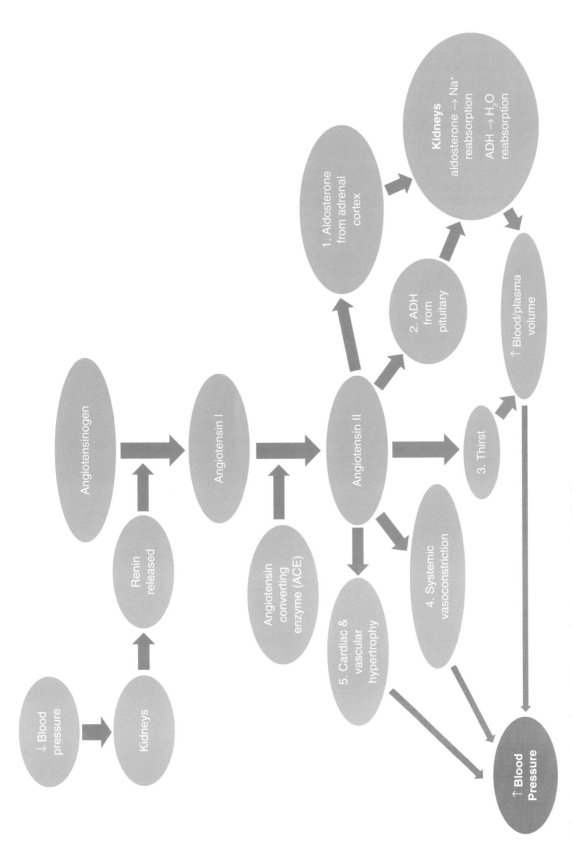

Figure 15.2 The renin–angiotensin aldosterone system (RAAS)

kidney (Hering et al., 2017). The trigger for this is thought to be through the RAAS. Additionally, an imbalance between vasodilators and vasoconstrictors occurs in primary hypertension that results in changes in vascular **endothelium**. The endothelium has a role in controlling vascular tone and blood pressure through locally releasing **nitric oxide** and endothelin (peptides that are major regulators of vascular tone and blood pressure). This endothelial activation and damage can alter vascular tone and reactivity, and also alter coagulation and **fibrinolytic** pathways. This form of hypertension is referred to as essential or **idiopathic hypertension**.

- *Secondary hypertension*: This form of hypertension is when another disorder causes blood pressure to rise; about 5% of people with hypertension have this form (Nadella and Howell, 2015). This can be seen in renal disease, responses to medication, altered hormonal regulation and physiological factors such as coarctation of the aorta (**congenital** narrowing of the aorta).
- *Malignant hypertension (hypertensive crisis)*: This form of hypertension occurs rapidly to extreme levels (systolic >180 mmHg) and can lead to organ damage. This severe hypertension occurs in association with bilateral retinal haemorrhages and/or exudates (± **papilloedema**) (Shantsila et al., 2010). It therefore has serious implications and can be difficult to control.

In addition to these classifications of hypertension, the National Institute for Health and Care Excellence (NICE) (2011) has classified the stages of hypertension (Table 15.1).

Table 15.1 NICE (2011) definitions of hypertension

Stage 1	Stage 2	Severe
• Clinical blood pressure of 140/90 mmHg or higher • Subsequent ambulatory blood pressure monitoring (ABPM) daytime average or home blood pressure monitoring (HBPM). Average blood pressure is 135/85 mmHg or higher	• Clinical blood pressure of 160/100 mmHg or higher • Subsequent ABPM daytime average or HBPM average blood pressure is 150/95 mmHg or higher	• Clinical systolic blood pressure is 180 mmHg or diastolic blood pressure is 110 mmHg or higher

Source: NHS Reproduced under the terms of the NICE UK Open Content License

In 2013, the European Society of Hypertension (ESH) and the European Society of Cardiology (ESC) Task Force (Mancia et al., 2013) further classified blood pressure for the cut-off values used to facilitate decisions about treatment (Table 15.2).

Table 15.2 Classifications of blood pressure and cut-off values

	Optimal	Normal	High normal	Grade 1 hypertension	Grade 2 hypertension	Grade 3 hypertension	Isolated systolic hypertension
Systolic (mmHg)	<120	120-129	130-139	140-159	160-179	≥180	≥140
Diastolic (mmHg)	<80	80-84	85-89	90-99	100-109	≥110	<90

APPLY

Diagnosis of hypertension

The accurate diagnosis of hypertension needs to follow particular criteria (NICE, 2011). This normally involves ABPM with at least two measurements taken per hour during the person's usual waking hours. The average of at least 14 measurements is used to determine if hypertension can be diagnosed.

For HBPM, two consecutive blood pressure measurements are taken, at least 1 minute apart and with the person seated. Blood pressure is recorded twice daily, ideally for seven days but for a minimum of four.

For full details on the NICE (2011) guidelines go to www.nice.org.uk and search for 'Hypertension in adults: diagnosis and management'. If you are using the eBook you can access this by clicking the icon.

It is important to remember that automated devices may not measure blood pressure accurately if the heart rate is irregular. In this situation, blood pressure should be measured manually using a stethoscope and sphygmomanometer. Additionally, an electronic device requires that it is regularly maintained and recalibrated, and readings are validated.

ARTICLE: HYPERTENSION
DIAGNOSIS

APPLY

Treatment of hypertension

With hypertension so prevalent in society, it is important that we know how to treat it holistically. From the point of investigation and assessment, the person will need education and ongoing support to help them understand the process and what is happening. Remember, this could be frightening for that person and their family, particularly if they have experience of cardiovascular disease in the family and may therefore have seen the negative impact it can have on everyday life. Support and compassion are therefore essential.

Risk management is important from the outset. This requires screening for effects on systems of the body (renal, cardiac, nervous) to determine the potential for hypertensive-related complications.

Lifestyle changes may be required to promote optimal cardiovascular health such as a healthy diet, increased exercise, modification of alcohol and caffeine intake and smoking cessation. Support groups and other local initiatives may be available to help that person and their family to adapt.

NICE (2011) advocates that pharmacological treatment should be considered as follows:

Stage 1 Hypertension

- Antihypertensive drug treatment for people aged under 80 years with stage 1 hypertension with one or more of the following conditions – organ damage, established cardiovascular or renal disease, diabetes, and a 10-year cardiovascular risk of 20% or greater.
- Those under 40 with stage 1 hypertension who do not have these conditions should have specialist evaluation for a secondary cause.

Stage 2 Hypertension

- People with stage 2 hypertension of any age should be offered antihypertensive drug treatment.

The specifics of how to manage medication therapy can be found at www.nice.org.uk. Search for 'Hypertension in adults: diagnosis and management' and then click on section 1.6. If you are using the eBook you can access the guidelines directly by clicking the icon to the right.

ARTICLE: HYPERTENSION
TREATMENT

It is important to remember that hypertension is the most important risk factor for cardiovascular disease worldwide. Combined, they can accelerate the development of coronary atherosclerosis (Chapter 8) and the range of conditions this can lead to.

ACTIVITY 15.1: APPLY

Living with hypertension

Watch this video and listen to Carol's story in order to understand her family history of hypertension and how it has impacted upon her and her health. If you are using the eBook just click on the play button. Alternatively go to **https://study.sagepub.com/essentialpatho/videos**

LIVING WITH HYPERTENSION (2:23)

HEART FAILURE

Heart failure (also known as **congestive heart failure**) is the failure of the heart to effectively pump blood around the body, so that its ability to respond to increased demands for cardiac output is impaired (Rogers and Bush, 2015). Coronary artery disease and hypertension are leading causes of heart failure and the prognosis for the condition is poor; over one-third of people with the diagnosis die within a year. The ageing population has seen the incidence of hospital admissions with this condition rise and it is anticipated to rise further as society ages.

Table 15.3 Right- and left-sided heart failure

Left-sided heart failure	Right-sided heart failure
Occurs when the left ventricle cannot pump out enough blood	Occurs when the right ventricle cannot pump out enough blood
Blood gets backed up behind the pump in the pulmonary circulation	Blood gets backed up in the systemic circulation
Pulmonary oedema occurs as hydrostatic pressure increases in the pulmonary circulation	Systemic oedema can occur as a result of increased hydrostatic pressure in the venous circulation, preventing fluid returning from the tissues to the venous end of capillaries
In addition, this back-up means the right ventricle is pumping against increased pressure and may lead to right-sided heart failure over time	
Decreased cardiac output leads to reduced tissue perfusion and an inability to respond to any increased physical demands (e.g. increased activity)	
Pulmonary oedema can lead to impaired gaseous exchange – this can exacerbate the condition as increased respiration is needed to compensate, creating an additional physical demand for the failing heart to respond to	

Heart failure occurs as a result of systolic and/or **diastolic dysfunction** that leads to a drop in cardiac output. It occurs as a result of myocardial oxygen demand surpassing supply and can occur as a result of impeded or occluded coronary circulation. With oxygen supply lower than demand, **hypoxia** occurs, resulting in cell injury or death and leading to a **myocardium** that can no longer beat with its usual strength and efficiency. In response, cardiac **myocyte**s expand and stretch to compensate, becoming hypertrophied and less effective. When these changes are progressive and large scale, the heart appears enlarged as a result of **hypertrophy**. As myocytes are less effective in this state, the ability of the heart to pump efficiently is impaired.

Hypertension and diabetes mellitus can lead to impaired coronary circulation; hypertension increases the pressure on the endothelial walls of the coronary circulation that can result in atherosclerosis (Chapter 8). Additionally, diabetes mellitus can lead to microvascular damage due to raised blood sugar and its impact on the walls of blood vessels, also described in Chapter 8.

When heart failure occurs, there can be impaired **perfusion** of the tissues in front of the pump (i.e. to the lungs or the rest of the body) and there may also be congestion behind the pump. This congestion can occur in the pulmonary circulation or systemically (or both), depending on which side of the heart is affected. In heart failure, cardiac output decreases and this can result in a backup of blood in the circulation behind the affected side of the heart (Table 15.3) (Figure 15.3).

Failure in compensation

When cardiac output drops, the body will deploy a variety of systemic mechanisms to attempt to compensate. The sympathetic nervous system is stimulated to release adrenaline and noradrenaline which increase peripheral vascular resistance, heart rate and contractility (Rogers and Bush, 2015). In turn, a drop in cardiac output will trigger the RAAS which will deploy a variety of mechanisms to increase blood pressure (Figure 15.2). One measure is the release of aldosterone which increases sodium reabsorption, pulling with it water and thereby increasing the blood volume. These factors, while attempting to compensate, presume that the heart is working well. However, the increased volume and pressure inside the cardiovascular system create the conditions for the heart to have to work harder, pumping against higher resistance and with increased volume overloading it.

Systolic and diastolic dysfunction

Systolic dysfunction is when the heart is thin and dilated, leading to a myocardium that is incapable of maintaining adequate cardiac output (Rogers and Bush, 2015) (Figure 15.4). It is usually caused by **myocardial infarction**, is the common form of heart failure and **ejection fraction** is less than 40%. This is commonly referred to as heart failure with reduced ejection fraction.

Diastolic dysfunction occurs when the myocardium loses elasticity and therefore has reduced filling (as it cannot stretch as much) (Figure 15.4). There is decreased compliance and contraction as a result, leading to hypertrophy in an attempt to compensate for the increased workload. **Stroke volume** is decreased and therefore so is cardiac output. However, ejection fraction remains greater than 50% (heart failure with preserved ejection fraction).

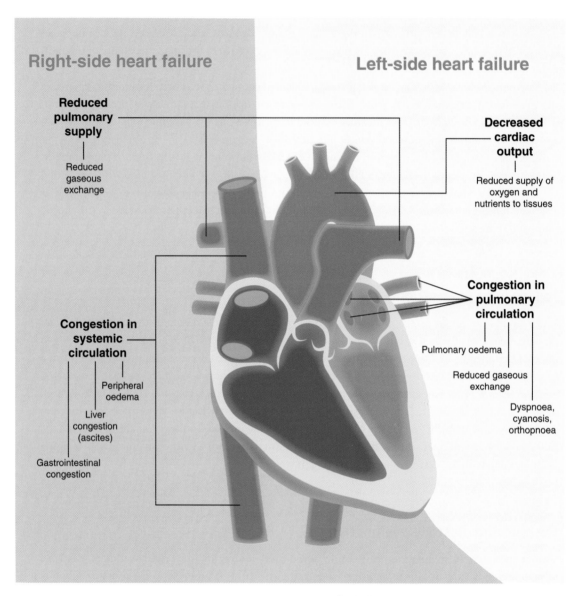

Right-side heart failure

Left-side heart failure

Reduced pulmonary supply

Reduced gaseous exchange

Decreased cardiac output

Reduced supply of oxygen and nutrients to tissues

Congestion in systemic circulation

Peripheral oedema

Liver congestion (ascites)

Gastrointestinal congestion

Congestion in pulmonary circulation

Pulmonary oedema

Reduced gaseous exchange

Dyspnoea, cyanosis, orthopnoea

Illustrated by Shaun Mercier © SAGE Publications

Figure 15.3 Right- and left-sided heart failure

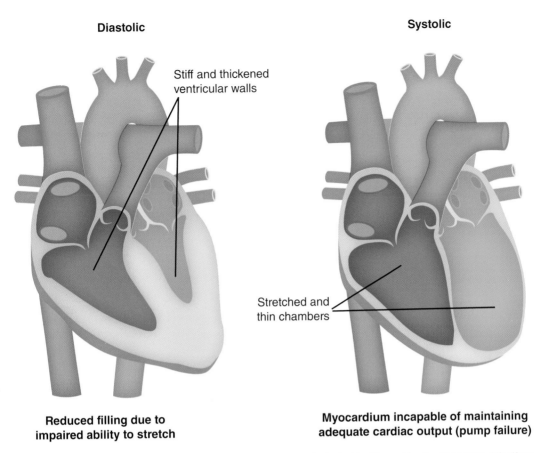

Diastolic

Stiff and thickened
ventricular walls

Systolic

Stretched and
thin chambers

**Reduced filling due to
impaired ability to stretch**

**Myocardium incapable of maintaining
adequate cardiac output (pump failure)**

Illustrated by Shaun Mercier © SAGE Publications

Figure 15.4 Systolic and diastolic dysfunction in heart failure

APPLY

Symptoms of heart failure

There are a variety of signs and symptoms of heart failure that you will observe and it is important to understand why they occur.

- *Dyspnoea*: Laboured breathing occurs as a result of pulmonary congestion, causing increased pulmonary capillary pressure, forcing fluid into the alveoli and resulting in pulmonary oedema. This decreases gaseous exchange and requires the person to increase their work of breathing (e.g. respiratory rate) to compensate.
- *Orthopnoea*: This is dyspnoea that occurs when a person lies back: the resulting shift in fluid increases the work of the left ventricle with which it cannot cope. This results in increased pulmonary capillary pressure, forcing fluid into the alveoli. The affects are similar to dyspnoea but only occur when the person lies back and is relieved when they sit up.
- *Cough*: This may be present in response to clearing any fluid accumulating in the alveoli.

(Continued)

(Continued)

- *Oedema*: As described in Table 15.3, this can result from increased hydrostatic pressure in the venous end of the capillaries in right-sided heart failure.
- *Weight gain*: This may occur due to reduced activity tolerance without a reduction in calorific intake.
- *Fatigue*: As the heart is unable to meet the increased activity demand (and increasingly baseline activity), the person will experience fatigue.
- *Chest pain*: Heart failure is associated with coronary artery disease, resulting in an inefficient supply of oxygen to the myocardium. This will cause chest pain, particularly if cardiac demands are increased (e.g. through activity).
- *Jugular venous distension*: The jugular veins in the neck may become distended due to a back-up of blood in the superior vena cava in right-sided heart failure.

APPLY

Assessment

The following investigations are usually undertaken in the person with suspected/actual heart failure:

- *Chest auscultation*: The assessor can listen for lung sounds (coarse/fine crackles, basal crepes) that could indicate pulmonary oedema.
- *Pulse*: Rhythm may be irregular and rate faster in an attempt to meet systemic requirements.
- *Urinalysis*: To check renal function – heart failure signs and symptoms can be similar to those of renal disease.
- *Chest X-ray*: To look for cardiac hypertrophy and pulmonary disorders.
- *BNP and NT-proBNP*: **B-type natriuretic peptide (BNP)** and **N-terminal pro b-type natriuretic peptide (NT-proBNP)** are produced and released when the heart is stretched and working hard to pump blood. Elevated levels can support a diagnosis of heart failure.
- *ECG*: As people with heart failure often have some damage to the myocardium, the conduction system can be affected. A 12-lead electrocardiogram (ECG) enables examination of this.
- *Echocardiogram*: To test ejection fraction and determine if there is systolic or diastolic dysfunction.

Heart failure, although a chronic condition, can occur acutely or chronically. There is no cure as the myocardium has been irreversibly damaged by some disease process. The focus of care is upon improving health-related quality of life as much as possible for as long as possible.

OEDEMA

Oedema is the observable accumulation of excess interstitial fluid secondary to an imbalance between capillary filtration and lymph drainage (Atkin, 2014). It is an indicator of ill-health that should be investigated. Oedema is classified as chronic once it is present for 3 months or more and, left untreated, will lead to lymphatic changes that result in lymphovenous oedema; both lymphatic and venous drainage are affected. This chronic form can lead to a reduced perfusion of tissues that then compromises tissue viability.

--- **REVISE: A&P RECAP** ---

Movement of fluid and nutrients between fluid compartments

Review Figure 12.15 in Chapter 12 of *Essentials of Anatomy & Physiology for Nursing Pratice* (Boore et al., 2016). The illustration shows the movement of fluid and nutrients between fluid compartments and will be useful for refreshing your knowledge.

Causes of oedema can be summarised as follows:

- *Venous hypertension*: As explained in the section on heart failure, systemic and pulmonary oedema can occur as a result of an increase in hydrostatic pressure in the venous circulation in systemic and pulmonary circulations respectively. This impacts upon capillary filtration by preventing the effective return of fluid back into capillaries.
- *Lymphatic insufficiency*: If the lymphatic circulation is chronically overloaded by excess capillary filtrate, then lymphatic vessels will eventually fail. This will cause **lymphoedema**. Another cause is when lymph vessels are surgically removed (e.g. as part of **surgery** for breast cancer) and lymphatic drainage is no longer available or is insufficient.
- *Malnutrition*: **Malnutrition** can cause a reduction in the amount of plasma protein in the systemic circulation, most notably albumin. Plasma proteins provide **osmotic pressure** that holds fluid in the plasma and draws it from the interstitial fluid. If this osmotic pressure in the circulation drops, then fluid is lost to the interstitial space and may not be picked up by the lymphatic system. This can lead to oedema formation.
- *Inflammatory response*: An inflammatory response (**inflammation**) will cause localised oedema as a result of increased vascular permeability. This can be seen at a systemic level in **sepsis** and in thermal injuries (burns) (Chapter 10).

ARRHYTHMIAS

Arrhythmias are disorders of the cardiac conduction cycle. They can be atrial (or **supraventricular**) or ventricular in origin. Those that are atrial in origin occur in the atrial wall, sino-atrial node (SA node), atrioventricular node (AV node) or in the junctional tissues. Ventricular arrhythmias originate in the ventricular muscle or conduction system and are generally life-threatening, requiring urgent treatment.

Arrhythmogenesis

So, what causes these disturbances in the cardiac cycle? While **arrhythmogenesis** is not fully understood, largely, causes can be isolated to a disruption of ion distribution (e.g. a low serum potassium) and/or conduction abnormalities. However, other substances can be **arrhythmogenic**, such as drugs that may impact on the action potential in the cardiac cycle. Table 15.4 indicates the causes in summary form (Khan, 2006).

Table 15.4 Causes of arrhythmogenesis →

Category	Trigger	Mechanism of action	Causes
Ionic	Increase in positive ions	Triggers release of calcium; excess free calcium results in cellular contraction	• Ionic imbalance • Myocardial infarction (free radicals and excess calcium in re-perfused tissues) • Loss of energy (removal of calcium involves active transport) • Decrease in pH (impairs calcium regulation as hydrogen, sodium and calcium are co-regulated) • Heart failure (sodium-calcium exchange process is impaired)
Conduction	Myocardial re-entry	Occurs when myocardium depolarises or repolarises later than surrounding myocardium	Localised **ischaemia**, fibrosis and loss of cell-to-cell conduction
	Purkinje myocardial junction re-entry	A Purkinje fibre divides into two branches joining with a single muscle fibre; one branch conducts normally, the other experiences conduction block due to disease (e.g. ischaemia). The **depolarisation** wave travels down healthy conduction fibre. But, diseased branch may repolarise and trigger further depolarisation	Branched Purkinje fibre that connects with a single muscle fibre
	AV node re-entry **tachycardia**	Abnormal conduction down one of two distinct conduction tracts in AV node. Depolarising wave goes along antegrade path (slow conduction fibre) and then up **retrograde** conduction path (fast fibre) (slow/fast). Each conduction event goes around the circuit and it depolarises ventricles and atria, resulting in tachycardia through increased ventricular firing rate	In diseased states the AV conduction fibres act not only as antegrade conduction pathways but also become retrograde conduction pathways
	Atrioventricular reciprocating tachycardia	Normally antegrade pathway is formed by AV node but a second abnormal accessory pathway enables retrograde conduction for depolarisation wave back to atria. In this case, both the atria and ventricular rates are increased	Accessory pathway (bundle of Kent, James bypass and Mahaim fibres)

In this chapter we are going to focus on some of the main forms of arrhythmias that you will encounter in practice.

Atrial disturbances

Atrial fibrillation (AF)

Atrial fibrillation (AF) is the most common sustained cardiac arrhythmia, with an increasing prevalence; 1–2% of the global population is affected and this is set to double with an ageing society in the next 50 years (Berry et al., 2015). It is primarily a disorder with uncoordinated atrial activation that results in a deterioration of atrial function. Irregular atrial discharge is thought to occur through one of three conductive processes (Iwasaki et al., 2011):

- Local **ectopic** rapidly discharging driver that gives rise to an irregular atrial response
- Single localised reentry circuit
- Multiple functional reentry circuits

Andrade et al. (2014) highlight that ion channel dysfunction, calcium regulation abnormalities, structural remodelling and autonomic dysregulation are the primary causes of these irregular processes. Therefore, the following conditions are linked with AF:

- **Ischaemic heart disease**
- Thyroid dysfunction (leading to calcium dysregulation)
- Heart valve dysfunction
- Hypertension
- Heart failure
- Infections (impact on ion channel function)
- **Electrolyte** imbalance (ion channel and calcium dysregulation)

As the atria are depolarising irregularly (giving rise to fibrillation waves on ECG), there is a variable response at the AV node that causes an irregular ventricular rate with a normal QRS complex (the dysfunction is only at the atrial level). There are four sub-classifications of AF (Table 15.5) (Berry et al., 2015). A fifth category is sometimes referred to, that of lone/idiopathic AF which occurs in those under the age of 60 with no clinical symptoms or identifiable structural heart disease.

Table 15.5 Sub-classifications of atrial fibrillation (AF)

Sub type	Description
Paroxysmal AF	This recurrent form lasts for longer than 30 seconds and ends spontaneously within 7 days
Persistent AF	This form lasts longer than 7 days (sinus rhythm may be restored through pharmacological or electrical cardioversion)
Long-standing persistent AF	This form lasts for ≥1 year
Permanent AF	This form is longstanding and a return to normal sinus rhythm is no longer an option

Over time, the irregularity of the conduction cycle in AF can lead to thrombus formation in the atria. The risk here is that this can then release emboli and lead to a pulmonary or cerebral **embolus**; AF is therefore a risk factor for stroke and **pulmonary embolism**. Table 15.6 outlines the differences between sinus rhythm and atrial fibrillation and how these are represented on ECG, while Figure 15.5 illustrates the electrical pathways.

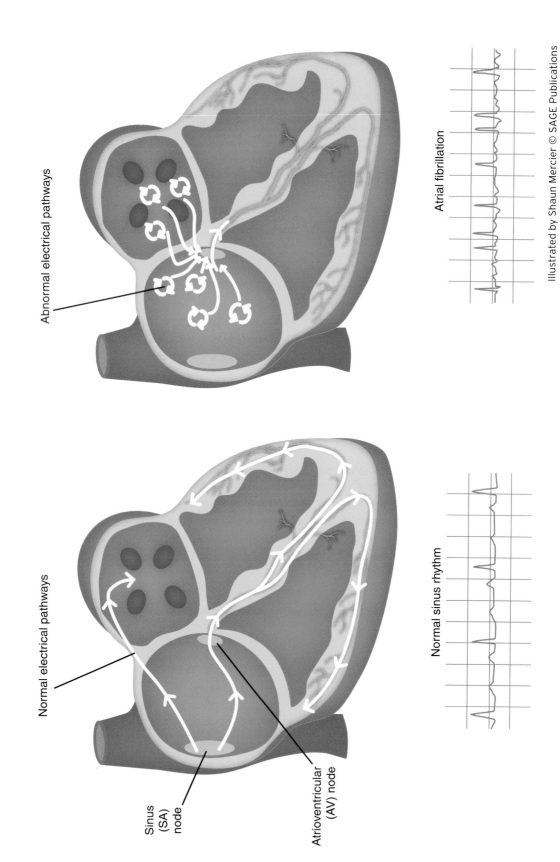

Figure 15.5 Electrical pathways in atrial fibrillation

Table 15.6 Sinus rhythm versus atrial fibrillation

Sinus rhythm	Atrial fibrillation
Regular rhythm	Irregular rhythm
Normal impulse formation and conduction	Atrial impulses are faster than those generated in SA node
Normal PR interval	These impulses take multiple, chaotic, random pathways through the atria. They lead to no clear, definable P waves on ECG (therefore PR interval cannot be measured)
QRS complex normal	
	QRS usually normal

APPLY

Management of AF

The first thing to remember is that any condition of the heart can be very frightening to a person and their family. They need to be treated with compassion and provided with support throughout as often the physiological care becomes the priority.

NICE (2014) identifies how AF should be managed. The UK guidelines advocate the following:

Acute AF:

- Achieve rate and rhythm control (pharmacological or electrical cardioversion under certain criteria)
- Consider anticoagulation therapy.

Chronic AF:

- Consider drug treatment for long-term rhythm control
- Consider approaches to prevent stroke, including anticoagulation.

Read the full guidelines in context here: www.nice.org.uk/guidance/cg180

Atrial flutter

Atrial flutter is different to fibrillation in that there is an organised atrial rhythm with a rate of typically 250–350 beats per minute. The most common form (typical type 1) is located in the right atrium and occurs as a result of a large reentry anticlockwise circuit around the anterior tricuspid annulus (Eftekhari and Darlison, 2014). This reentry circuit gives rise to the classic sawtooth pattern of atrial activity on ECG (Figure 15.6). Atrial flutter is not a stable rhythm and may progress to fibrillation as the rate of atrial contraction is unsustainable at such a fast rate.

Narrow complex tachycardia

Narrow complex tachycardias are a type of arrhythmia, commonly referred to as paroxysmal supraventricular tachycardias, that originate in the atria. The three most common of these are atrioventricular nodal reentrant tachycardia (AVNRT), atrioventricular reciprocating tachycardia (AVRT) and atrial tachycardia (AT). We will briefly examine each of these (Colucci et al., 2010):

- *AVNRT*: This is the most common form and is normally not associated with a structural heart disease. It is an AV node reentry tachycardia which is when a reentrant circuit forms within or just next to the AV node. This will then increase the heart rate by resulting in more conduction cycles being created.
- *AVRT*: This is the second most common form and occurs as a result of reentry mechanisms secondary to accessory pathways (antegrade or retrograde conduction through the AV node).
- *AT*: This is the third most common form and usually occurs as a result of a single atrial focus with a definitive localised origin. Multifocal AT can also occur in people with heart failure or **chronic obstructive pulmonary disease**.

Until the rhythm is slowed down (pharmacologically or electrically), it is not possible to determine the nature of the full cardiac cycle on ECG.

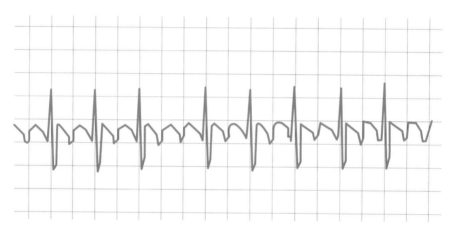

Figure 15.6   Atrial flutter

VENTRICULAR DISORDERS

Ventricular tachycardia (VT) and ventricular fibrillation (VF)

These arrhythmias originate in the ventricles and are often secondary to myocardial disturbances whereby multiple factors, such as myocardial ischemia and its associated electrolyte dysregulation, **necrosis**, reperfusion, healing and scar formation, can lead to ventricular dysfunction (John et al., 2012; Podrid et al., 2018).

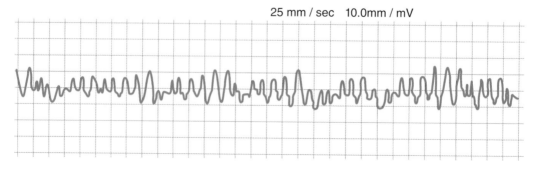

25 mm / sec   10.0mm / mV

Figure 15.7   Ventricular fibrillation

In VF, the hypoxic myocardium can result in myocardial cells that are hyperirritable. These can function as pacemakers, becoming arrhythmogenic. However, the ventricles now become stimulated by more than one source, leading to multiple action potentials that cause the ventricles to fibrillate; this fibrillation (quivering) does not produce a contraction that produces cardiac output and so technically this is a cardiac arrest (cardiac output has arrested). In order to restore a functional cardiac cycle, the abnormal electrical activity (Figure 15.7) must be cleared in the hope that the regular pathways of conduction can resume. This is achieved through defibrillation, the outcome of which is more successful the sooner it occurs.

In VT (the monomorphic form where the increased rate occurs from one single point of reentry) the impulse is generated from increased automaticity at a single point in either the left or the right ventricle, or due to a reentry circuit within the ventricle. Scarring of the heart muscle from a previous myocardial infarction is a common cause; the scar cannot conduct electrical activity but a potential circuit around the scar exists that gives rise to a reentry point that leads to tachycardia. This is similar to the reentry process seen in atrial flutter. As a result, the rate is fast but organised due to a single reentry point (Figure 15.8).

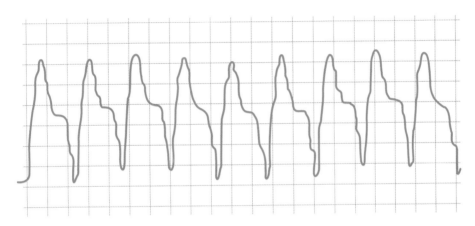

Figure 15.8 Ventricular tachycardia

Sinus arrhythmias

Sinus arrhythmias occur as a result of disordered sympathetic stimulation and other homeostatic alterations in temperature, oxygen availability and metabolic changes:

- **Sinus bradycardia**: In this arrhythmia, the PQRST complex is normal but the ventricular rate is slow (less than 60 beats per minute in an adult) (Figure 15.9). It can occur from parasympathetic regulation of the vagus nerve that slows conduction.

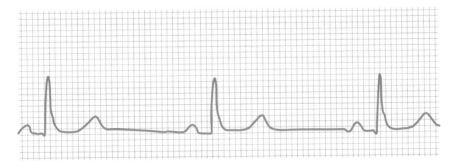

Figure 15.9 Sinus bradycardia

APPLY

Bradycardia in healthy people

While the normal pulse rate is between 60 and 100, athletes and people who exercise regularly can have a pulse rate that is normally as low as 50 beats per minute. The heart's pumping ability is enhanced by exercise so that fewer heart contractions are needed.

- **Sinus tachycardia**: In this arrhythmia, the PQRST complex is normal but the ventricular rate is fast (greater than 100 beats per minute in an adult) (Figure 15.10). It is usually as a result of sympathetic stimulation.

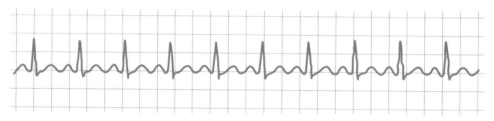

Figure 15.10   Sinus tachycardia

Sudden arrhythmic death syndrome (SADS) and sudden cardiac death

While having a variety of names, **sudden arrhythmic death syndrome (SADS)** refers to the sudden, untimely death of a young, apparently fit and healthy person. When that death is thought to be as a direct result of cardiac disease, it is referred to as a **sudden cardiac death**. In SADS the origins are thought to be arrhythmogenic and often have no identifiable cause at all. SADS occurs in 50–100 per 100,000 every year in Europe and North America. Coronary artery disease and **acute myocardial infarction** are common causes in older adults, whereas disorders with genetic origins are more prevalent in those aged 40 and under (Semsarian et al., 2015). Of these sudden deaths, half are attributable to ventricular tachycardia or ventricular fibrillation (John et al., 2012). Multiple single gene **mutations** have been isolated that cause these potentially fatal arrhythmias by ionic dysregulation or through pathophysiological processes that lead to the development of **cardiomyopathy**. Unfortunately, victims of SADS are largely asymptomatic. These causes can be isolated down to the following (John et al., 2012; Link et al., 2014):

1. *Abnormalities of repolarisation and the QT interval.* In these cases, there is prolonged repolarisation that extends the QT interval, leading to syncope or cardiac arrest as a result of a polymorphic VT. A rare cause is short QT syndrome which can also lead to a polymorphic VT.
2. *Catecholaminergic polymorphic VT.* Catecholaminergic polymorphic VT is also characterised by syncope or cardiac arrest and is related to emotional state/upset and physical exertion. This is as a result of calcium dysregulation in the presence of catecholamine release.
3. *Inherited* **cardiomyopathies**. A genetically inherited condition, **hypertrophic cardiomyopathy** has been isolated as the most common genetic cardiac disorder that results in sudden death before 35 years of age. In cardiomyopathy, the ventricles stretch and become less effective. There can be a development of scar tissue which can lead to VT, particularly polymorphic VT, and VF (see pathophysiological causes under VT and VF above).

These conditions are profound. Young lives are taken suddenly and the impact on family, friends and community groups is extensive. Genetic screening and other fitness screening practices have emerged since SADS has become more prominent, with further work necessary to continue to maximise preventative impact in this area.

CARDIOMYOPATHIES

Cardiomyopathies are a group of cardiac disorders that affect the myocardium. They can be primary or secondary (Table 15.7) (Figure 15.11).

Table 15.7 Primary and secondary cardiomyopathies

Primary (unknown origin)	Secondary (secondary to another disorder)
Dilated	Myocardial infarction
Hypertrophic	Hypertension
Restrictive	Valve disease
Peripartum	Congenital heart defect
	Coronary artery disease
	Toxins/medications

CONGENITAL ABNORMALITIES

A number of congenital cardiac abnormalities exist that can lead to dysfunction in the body. Some are more common than others and in this chapter we will deal with some of the more prevalent conditions.

Aortic stenosis

Aortic stenosis is the narrowing of the aorta that restricts the blood flow leaving the left ventricle. It can be congenital, occurring in the first 8 weeks of pregnancy, or **acquired**. Acquired forms are secondary to endothelial damage due to mechanical stress, inflammation, fibrosis and calcification (Joseph et al., 2017). This calcification leads to a stiffened aortic valve and a pressure gradient across the valve. This can gradually worsen over time and lead to left ventricular pressure overload, left ventricular hypertrophy and eventually left ventricular failure (heart failure) (Joseph et al., 2017).

Dilated Cardiomyopathy

- This type of cardiomyopathy can be inherited (autosomal dominant or recessive, or X-linked) and associated with infection, toxins, immunological disorders and metabolic disorders. The heart becomes dilated, which results in the walls of the myocardium thinning with a consequent impaired ability to pump, which gives rise to symptoms of heart failure. The ventricles are primarily affect. Scarring and atrophy of the myocytes occurs and as the disorder progresses, mural thrombi (thrombi in the walls of the myocardium) and arrhythmias can develop alongside heart failure

Hypertrophic Cardiomyopathy

- In this form, hypertrophic changes of the myocardium occur, including of the ventricular septum which becomes somewhat obstructive. There are genetic links with the disorder (autosomal dominant) and the condition is seen in younger adults. The exact cause is unknown but the myofibrils are found to be disorganised which leads to the myocardium being ineffective in contracting and can lead to arrhythmias.

Restrictive

- This is an uncommon form in Western society in which the ventricular walls become rigid and inflexible, leading to restricted ventricular filling. The cause is linked with amyloidosis whereby amyloid proteins infiltrate the myocardium, generating amyloid fibrils. Heart failure can develop in advanced stages of the disease.

Peripartum Cardiomyopathy

- This form of cardiomyopathy develops in the last month of pregnancy up to five months after delivery. The cause is unknown and the prognosis worrying as around half of the people affected will not survive. Myocarditis is linked with the disorder which results in left ventricular dysfunction.

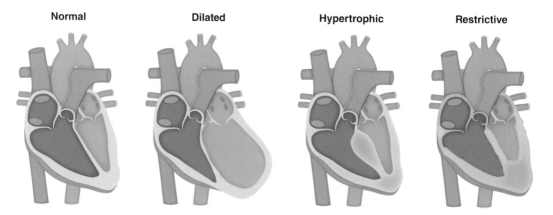

Normal   Dilated   Hypertrophic   Restrictive

Illustrated by Shaun Mercier © SAGE Publications

Figure 15.11 Pathophysiology of primary cardiomyopathies

Atrial septal defect

These defects are the third most common form of congenital heart abnormalities and have no identifiable causes. They involve the shunting of blood between the systemic and the pulmonary circulations via one of three primary mechanisms. The two most common forms are:

- *Patent foramen ovale*: In almost all babies born, the **foramen ovale** is patent (open). The pressure in the left ventricle is usually greater than the right and this helps the foramen ovale to progressively seal over. In some cases, this does not occur and can lead to a shunt of blood from the right atrium to the left.
- *Secundum atrial septal defect*: Such defects usually occur as a result of an enlarged foramen ovale, inadequate growth of the **septum secundum** (a tissue growth that descends from the upper wall of the right atrium and which, after birth, closes the foramen ovale by fusing with **the septum primum**), or excessive **absorption** of the septum primum (the septum primum is the tissue growth down in the single atrium of the developing heart in the human embryo, which will result in the single atrium being divided into two atria) (Geva et al., 2014). Some 10–20% of people with this form of **atrial septal defect** have mitral valve prolapse. There are some autosomal dominant genetic links identified with this form of defect (Geva et al., 2014).

Other forms exist though all lead to the same shunting effect at atrial level but may include the pulmonary veins, superior vena cava or coronary sinus.

Coarctation of the aorta

Coarctation of the aorta (CoA) is a localised narrowing of the aortic lumen secondary to medial wall thickening and infolding aortic wall tissue. It represents 5–8% of all congenital heart abnormalities, is more common in males and occurs in 4 out of every 1,000 births (Dijkema et al., 2017). There are three known potential causes of CoA:

- Atypical embryogenetic development
- Reduced intrauterine aortic blood flow, leading to aortic underdevelopment
- Anomalous patent ductus arteriosus (see below) tissue in the aorta that narrows the lumen at the isthmus (the final section of the aortic arch, the connection between the ascending and descending aorta) and which regresses postnatally

CoA results in left ventricular dysfunction secondary to a sudden increase in afterload that occurs after the closure of the **ductus arteriosus**. There is hypertension in the upper body as a result.

Atrioventricular septal defect

Atrioventricular septal defect (AVSD) is one of the most common congenital heart diseases. The condition is associated with chromosomal abnormalities such as Down syndrome and complex syndromes such as cardiosplenic syndrome (Gómez and Martinez, 2018). AVSD is a spectrum of defects where there is incomplete development of the atrioventricular septum alongside atrioventricular (AV) valve abnormalities (Kharbanda et al., 2018). AVSD is characterised by abnormal fusion of the superior and inferior endocardial cushions in the atrial and ventricular septum. Additionally, the AV node and **AV bundle**, or **bundle of His**, are displaced inferiorly. These structural abnormalities make it possible for blood to be shunted to and from both sides of the heart and for arrhythmias to occur. Essentially, there is a common atrioventricular junction where a normal heart has separate right and left atrioventricular junctions. In a partial AVSD, the defect is in the atrial septum; in complete AVSD there is a large ventricular involvement. Figure 15.12 illustrates the three types of shunting that can occur.

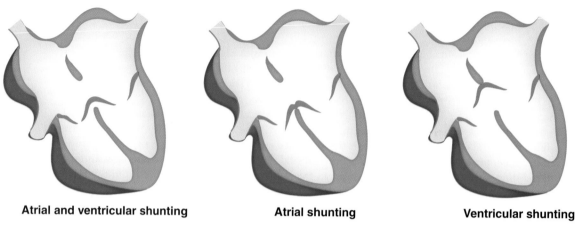

Atrial and ventricular shunting   **Atrial shunting**   **Ventricular shunting**

Illustrated by Shaun Mercier © SAGE Publications

Figure 15.12   Types of shunting in AVSD

Double-inlet ventricle

Double-inlet ventricle is where more than half of both atria are joined to one dominant ventricle through either two separate atrioventricular (AV) valves or a common AV valve (Martin and Poirier, 2018) (Figure 15.13). You can see in the image that there is one dominant and functional ventricle and one minor and, for all practical purposes, dysfunctional ventricle. As a result of both atria filling primarily one ventricle (the size of each ventricle and how much each atria fill are variable), there is a mixing of oxygenated and deoxygenated blood. The condition normally occurs early in pregnancy and the cause is largely unknown.

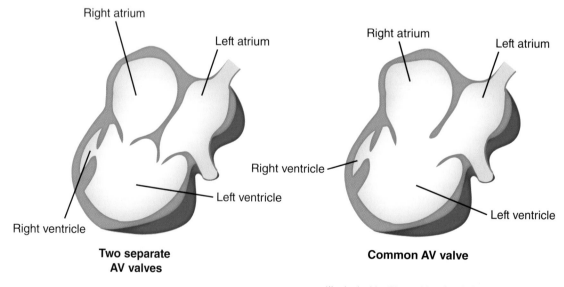

**Two separate
AV valves**   **Common AV valve**

Illustrated by Shaun Mercier © SAGE Publications

Figure 15.13   Double-inlet ventricle (separate and common AV valves)

Hypoplastic left heart syndrome

This syndrome is characterised by the left-sided heart structures being underdevelope, therefore resulting in a left ventricle that is unable to pump with enough force to meet the needs of the systemic circulation (Mussa and Barron, 2017) (Figure 15.14). As a result, life is unsustainable in most cases unless there is surgical intervention; such interventions uses the preserved function of the right ventricle to meet the needs of the body. No causative gene has been isolated for the condition but it is linked with Turner syndrome, Edwards syndrome and Patau syndrome.

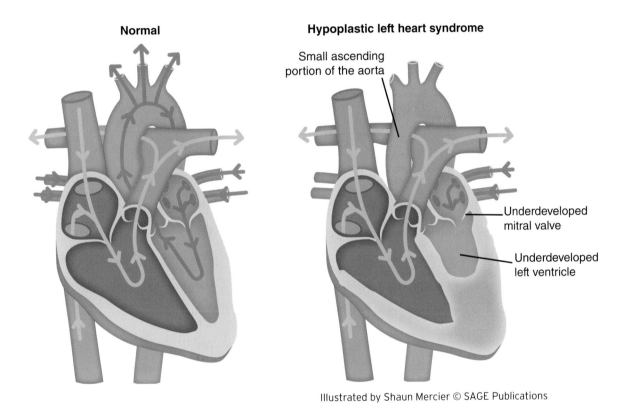

Illustrated by Shaun Mercier © SAGE Publications

Figure 15.14 Hypoplastic left heart syndrome

Ventricular septal defect

Ventricular septal defects (VSDs) are characterised by openings in the ventricular septum and commonly occur alongside other cardiac abnormalities. They are the most common congenital cardiac anomaly and the cause is largely unknown although there is an increased incidence in Down syndrome (Uebing and Kaemmerer, 2018). With a passage existing between the two ventricles, blood can shunt from one side to the other; the degree of this depends on the size of the defect and the degree of pulmonary vascular resistance (Figure 15.15). Normally, the shunting occurs from the left ventricle to the right as a result of the left ventricle being larger and pumping with more force. In cases where this shunting is significant, there is increased pulmonary blood flow and subsequent pulmonary venous return to the left side of the heart; as a consequence, there can be left atrial ventricular overload and associated hypertrophy over time (Uebing and Kaemmerer, 2018). These defects can be surgically repaired with good success rates. Minor VSDs can close themselves over time in neonates.

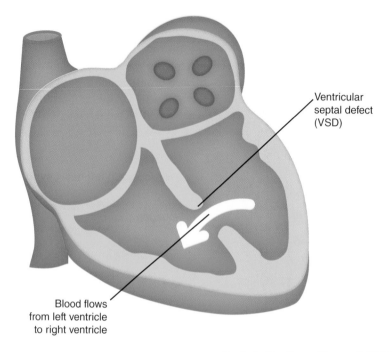

Ventricular
septal defect
(VSD)

Blood flows
from left ventricle
to right ventricle

Figure 15.15 Shunting in ventricular septal defect

Pulmonary artery

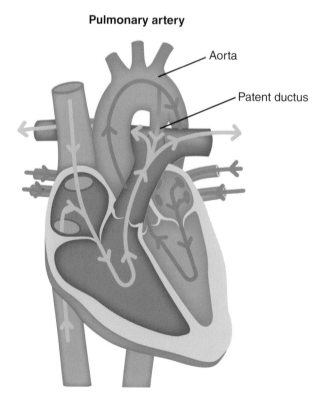

Aorta

Patent ductus

Figure 15.16 Patent ductus arteriosus

Patent ductus arteriosus (PDA)

PDA is when the fetal ductus arteriosus fails to close after birth (Figure 15.16). The ductus arteriosus is a vessel that connects the main pulmonary artery to the aorta in order for blood to bypass the lungs; fetal gaseous exchange occurs in the placenta in utero and so blood does not need to go to the lungs for such gaseous exchange. However, after birth, the ductus arteriosus closes within approximately 48 hours; PDA describes the situation when this does not occur. The presence of the duct allows for the shunting of blood, usually from left to right, and depending on the degree of shunting, can result in left ventricular distension (Clyman, 2018). The increase can raise pulmonary venous pressure and result in pulmonary congestion and subsequently pulmonary oedema and/or respiratory distress syndrome. The increased pressure on the left ventricle can lead to hypertrophy over time and heart failure if severe and uncorrected.

Pulmonary stenosis

Pulmonary stenosis occurs when there is a narrowing at one or more points between the right ventricle and the pulmonary artery. This condition is the most common form of right-sided obstruction in the heart. There is fusion of the valve leaflets, resulting in a conical-shaped pulmonary valve with a narrow opening at its apex (Chaix and Dore, 2018). With a narrowing of the passageway that takes all blood from the right ventricle leading out to the lungs (Figure 15.17), there is an increase in right ventricular pressure as the same volume of blood is being forced through a smaller space. This can lead to right ventricular hypertrophy over time. The condition is associated with a variety of genetic and **chromosome** disorders (e.g. Costello syndrome).

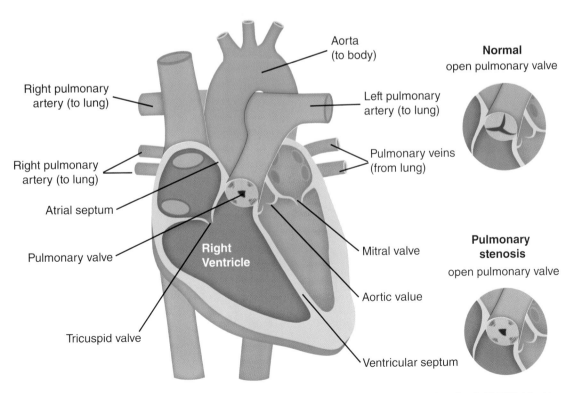

Illustrated by Shaun Mercier © SAGE Publications

Figure 15.17   Pulmonary stenosis

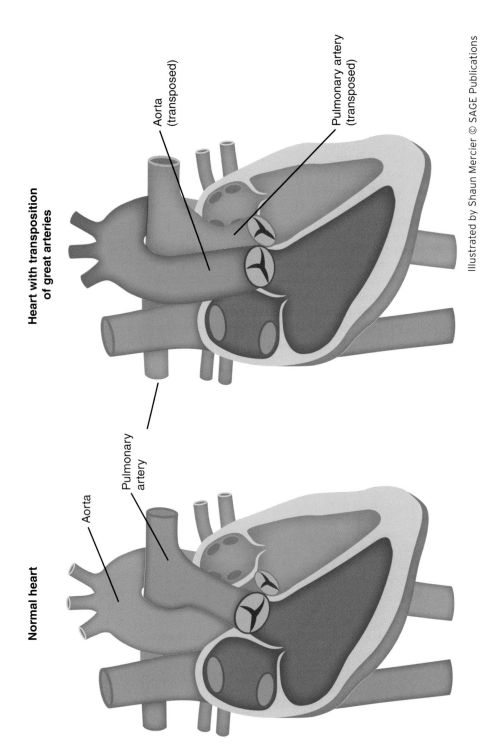

Normal heart

Aorta

Pulmonary artery

Heart with transposition of great arteries

Aorta (transposed)

Pulmonary artery (transposed)

Illustrated by Shaun Mercier © SAGE Publications

Figure 15.18 Transposition of the great arteries

Transposition of the great arteries

Transposition of the great arteries (TGA) is characterised by the aorta arising from the right ventricle and the pulmonary artery from the left ventricle, i.e. the opposite to the normal location of these vessels (Figure 15.18). Approximately half of the people with this condition have other cardiac abnormalities, such as VSD and CoA (Hornung and O'Donnell, 2018). The misalignment of these vessels is problematic; oxygenated pulmonary venous blood does not end up in the systemic circulation and systemic venous blood does not get oxygenated (Sheikh et al., 2012). Unless a VSD or PDA exists, or other similar connections that will allow some correction, the infant will not survive. Surgical intervention is necessary to correct the vasculature.

CHAPTER SUMMARY

In this chapter you will have learned about how cardiovascular disease can occur across the life span, at fetal development and throughout life, influenced in part by lifestyle and partly by genetics. The consequence of cardiovascular disease is profound in that it impacts not only on physiological homeostasis, but also upon our identity – our ability to parent, to fulfil our social roles, to be independent and to have the energy and ability to engage in activities that are central to health-related quality of life. Person-centred practice is not only about understanding and responding to the physiological issues, which are highly important, but is also about relating to the impact on the person and their family in a wider context.

KEY POINTS

- Cardiovascular disease is a leading cause of mortality and morbidity globally.

- Understanding the causes of preventable cardiovascular disease is central to engaging in strategies at individual, group and strategic levels (e.g. government, global approaches) to reduce the risk of cardiovascular disease.

- A variety of cardiovascular disorders originate during fetal development, some with unknown causes and others with strong genetic links.

- Genetic influences are well documented in a number of cardiovascular disorders; screening practices have the potential to improve outcomes in this area.

- Understanding the pathophysiology of cardiovascular disorders is central to effective nursing practice; signs and symptoms are evident in people affected and the effective practitioner must be able to recognise these, understand what their presentation indicates and act promptly to ensure care is effective and timely, in collaboration with other members of the multiprofessional team.

REVISE

TEST YOUR KNOWLEDGE

This chapter has addressed many complex issues with regards to disorders of the cardiovascular system. These are prevalent in society and so it is important that, as a person-centred practitioner, you understand these disorders so that you can support those in your care. Use the following revision questions to test your understanding.

Answers are available online. If you are using the eBook just click on the answers icon below. Alternatively go to **https://study.sagepub.com/essentialpatho/answers**

1   What is hypertension and how common is it?

2   What are the three classifications of hypertension?

3   How does NICE categorise the stages of hypertension?

4   What is heart failure?

5   What are the main causes of heart failure?

6   What are the defining characteristics of heart failure?

7   How do right- and left-sided heart failure individually impact on circulation?

8   What is oedema?

9   What are the main causes of oedema?

10   What are arrhythmias?

11   Where do arrhythmias originate?

12   What is atrial fibrillation and how does it appear on an ECG?

13   What is SADS and sudden cardiac death and what are the primary causes in older adults and younger people?

14   What are the three primary categories of causes of SADS?

15   What are cardiomyopathies?

16   What is aortic stenosis and what is its eventual result (if untreated)?

17   What is atrioventricular septal defect?

- Further revision and learning opportunities are available online

- Test yourself away from the book with **Extra multiple choice questions**

- Learn and revise terminology with **Interactive flashcards**

REVISE

ACE YOUR
ASSESSMENT

If you are using the eBook access each resource by clicking on the respective icon. Alternatively go to **https://study.sagepub.com/essentialpatho/chapter15**

CHAPTER 15 ANSWERS   EXTRA QUESTIONS   FLASHCARDS

REFERENCES

Andrade, J., Khairy, P., Dobrev, D. and Nattel, S. (2014) The clinical profile and pathophysiology of atrial fibrillation: relationships among clinical features, epidemiology, and mechanisms. *Circulation Research, 114* (9): 1453–68.

Atkin, L. (2014) Lower-limb oedema: assessment, treatment and challenges. *British Journal of Community Nursing, 19* (Suppl 10): S22–S28.

Berry, E., Padgett, H. and Holton, C. (2015) Atrial fibrillation guidelines for management: what's new? *British Journal of Cardiac Nursing, 10* (9): 426–35.

Boore, J., Cook, N. and Shepherd, A. (2016) *Essentials of Anatomy and Physiology for Nursing Practice.* London: Sage.

Chaix, M. and Dore, A. (2018) Pulmonary stenosis. In M. Gatzoulis, G. Webb. and P. Daubeney (eds), *Diagnosis and Management of Adult Congenital Heart Disease*, 3rd edn. Philadelphia, PA: Elsevier Saunders. pp. 460–4.

Clyman, R.I. (2018) Patent ductus arteriosus, its treatments, and the risks of pulmonary morbidity. *Seminars in Perinatology, 42* (4): 235–42.

Colucci, R.A., Silver, M.J. and Shubrook, J. (2010) Common types of supraventricular tachycardia: diagnosis and management. *American Family Physician, 82* (8): 942–52.

Dijkema, E.J., Leiner, T. and Grotenhuis, H.B. (2017) Diagnosis, imaging and clinical management of aortic coarctation. *Heart, 103* (15): 1148–55.

Eftekhari, H. and Darlison, L. (2014) Treatment for atrial flutter in a patient with heart failure and mesothelioma: a case study. *British Journal of Cardiac Nursing, 9* (12): 599–602.

Geva, T., Martins, J.D. and Wald, R.M. (2014) Atrial septal defects. *The Lancet, 383* (9932): 1921–32.

Gómez, O. and Martinez, J.M. (2018) Atrioventricular septal defect. In *Obstetric Imaging: Fetal Diagnosis and Care*, 2nd edn. Philadelphia, PA: Elsevier Saunders. pp. 360–4.

Hering, D., Trzebski, A. and Narkiewicz, K. (2017) Recent advances in the pathophysiology of arterial hypertension: potential implications for clinical practice. *Polish Archives of Internal Medicine, 127* (3): 195–204.

Hornung, T. and O'Donnell, C. (2018) Transposition of the great arteries. In M. Gatzoulis, G. Webb and P. Daubeney (eds), *Diagnosis and Management of Adult Congenital Heart Disease*, 3rd edn. Philadelphia, PA: Elsevier Saunders. pp. 513–27.

Iwasaki, Y.K., Nishida, K., Kato, T. and Nattel, S. (2011) Atrial fibrillation pathophysiology: implications for management. *Circulation, 124* (20): 2264–74.

John, R.M., Tedrow, U.B., Koplan, B.A., Albert, C.M., Epstein, L.M., Sweeney, M.O. et al. (2012) Ventricular arrhythmias and sudden cardiac death. *The Lancet, 380* (9852): 1520–9.

Joseph, J., Naqvi, S.Y., Giri, J. and Goldberg, S. (2017) Aortic stenosis: pathophysiology, diagnosis, and therapy. *American Journal of Medicine, 130* (3): 253–63.

Khan, E. (2006) The pathological origins of arrhythmias. *British Journal of Cardiac Nursing, 1* (9): 408–17.

Kharbanda, R.K., Blom, N.A., Hazekamp, M.G., Yildiz, P., Mulder, B.J., Wolterbeek, R. et al. (2018) Incidence and risk factors of post-operative arrhythmias and sudden cardiac death after atrioventricular septal defect (AVSD) correction: up to 47 years of follow-up. *International Journal of Cardiology, 252*: 88–93.

Link, M.S., Laidlaw, D., Polonsky, B., Zareba, W., McNitt, S., Gear, K. et al. (2014) Ventricular arrhythmias in the North American multidisciplinary study of ARVC: predictors, characteristics, and treatment. *Journal of the American College of Cardiology, 64* (2): 119–25.

Mancia, G., Fagard, R., Narkiewicz, K., Redán, J., Zanchetti, A., Böhm, M. et al. (2013) 2013 practice guidelines for the management of arterial hypertension of the European Society of Hypertension (ESH) and the European Society of Cardiology (ESC): ESH/ESC Task Force for the Management of Arterial Hypertension. *Journal of Hypertension, 31* (10): 1925–38.

Martin, E. and Poirier, N. (2018) Double-inlet ventricle. In M. Gatzoulis, G. Webb and P. Daubeney (eds), *Diagnosis and Management of Adult Congenital Heart Disease*, 3rd edn. Philadelphia, PA: Elsevier Saunders. pp. 564–9.

Mussa, S. and Barron, D.J. (2017) Hypoplastic left heart syndrome. *Paediatrics and Child Health, 27* (2): 75–82.

Nadella, V. and Howell, S.J. (2015) Hypertension: pathophysiology and perioperative implications. *British Journal of Anaesthesia (BJA) Education, 15* (6): 275–9.

NICE (2011) Hypertension in adults: diagnosis and management. Clinical guideline [CG127]. National Institute for Health and Care Excellence. [online]. Available at: www.nice.org.uk/guidance/cg127 (accessed 17 December 2018).

NICE (2014) Atrial fibrillation: management. Clinical guideline [CG180]. National Institute for Health and Care Excellence. [online]. Available at: www.nice.org.uk/guidance/cg180 (accessed 17 December 2018).

Podrid, P.J., Knight, B.P. and Downey, B.C. (2018) Pathogenesis of ventricular tachycardia and ventricular fibrillation during acute myocardial infarction. UpToDate. [online]. Available at: www. uptodate.com/contents/pathogenesis-of-ventricular-tachycardia-and-ventricular-fibrillation-during-acute-myocardial-infarction (accessed 10 July 2018).

Rogers, C. and Bush, N. (2015) Heart failure: pathophysiology, diagnosis, medical treatment guidelines, and nursing management. *Nursing Clinics of North America, 50* (4): 787–99.

Semsarian, C., Ingles, J. and Wilde, A.A. (2015) Sudden cardiac death in the young: the molecular autopsy and a practical approach to surviving relatives. *European Heart Journal, 36* (21): 1290–6.

Shantsila, A., Shantsila, E. and Lip, G. (2010) Malignant hypertension: a rare problem or is it underdiagnosed? *Current Vascular Pharmacology, 8* (6): 775–9.

Sheikh, N., Hussain, M.Z., Islam, M.T. and Bhuiyan, M.M.R. (2012) Transposition of the great arteries. *University Heart Journal, 8* (1): 46–51.

Uebing, A. and Kaemmerer, H. (2018) Ventricular septal defect. In M. Gatzoulis, G. Webb and P. Daubeney (eds), *Diagnosis and Management of Adult Congenital Heart Disease*, 3rd edn. Philadelphia, PA: Elsevier Saunders. pp. 316–25.

SECTION 4

DISORDERS OF CONTROL AND COORDINATION

This section considers the disorders of those components dealing with the control and coordination of bodily function, neurological and endocrine control; in addition, reproductive systems are considered. These can affect any function of the body and all sections have serious interpersonal implications to take into account in person-centred nursing.

Chapter 16: Disorders of Neurological Control. This lengthy chapter examines the structural and physiological changes which lead to the range of different disorders, including: disturbed motor function; the epilepsies; synaptic dysfunction; brain hypoxia; raised intracranial pressure; meningitis and encephalitis. The principles of management are examined within the context of person-centredness with the person and their family needing care.

Chapter 17: Disorders of Endocrine Regulation. The causes and effects of the major disorders of endocrine function and implications for the individual concerned are considered. It is therefore particularly important that those caring for these individuals have a thorough understanding to support PCP.

Chapter 18: Disorders of the Female Reproductive System. This examines causes and effects of disorders of the female reproductive system and nurturing. In addition, issues concerned with the causes and management of infertility are considered. The emotional/psychological and social relationship with the pathophysiological changes are particularly important.

Chapter 19: Disorders of the Male Reproductive System. This chapter examines causes and effects of disorders of the male reproductive system, including of the prostate gland. The emotional/psychological and social implications of the pathophysiological changes are also addressed and are central to person-centred nursing.

DISORDERS OF NEUROLOGICAL CONTROL

16

LEARNING OUTCOMES

When you have finished studying this chapter you will be able to:

1. Discuss how trauma alters the physiology of the nervous system.
2. Describe the pathophysiological processes involved in degenerative conditions of the nervous system.
3. Explain the genetic influences in relation to disorders of the nervous system.
4. Identify the microbial contribution/influence to disorders of the nervous system.
5. Apply the pathophysiology of neurological disorders to practice and treatment.
6. Describe the impact of altered physiology of the nervous system on the person and their family.

INTRODUCTION

In this chapter, you will examine the structural and physiological changes which lead to the range of different neurological disorders. These disorders can be secondary to trauma, infection and/or a degenerative process. Others are **congenital** or their causes not fully understood. Considering the key role of the nervous system in defining who we are as people, these disorders will be considered from a person-centred perspective.

The role of the nervous system in maintaining **homeostasis** is vast; the nervous system is complex, not fully understood and has extensive connections with all other systems in the body, being a key regulator of activity. It is also the system that creates our identities and processes our experiences, thoughts and feelings throughout life. As a result, any neurological disorder, regardless of origin, has the potential to devastate a person's life and their ability to maintain homeostasis. Neurological disorders, including cerebrovascular **disease**, represented 7.1% of the total global burden of disease in 2010 in terms of **disability-adjusted life years** across all causes and ages (Chin and Vora, 2014), an increase from 6.3% in 2005 (World Health Organisation [WHO], 2005). With the predicted rise in the incidence of dementia (Prince et al., 2013), this global burden is set to increase. Within this context, the likelihood of a nurse caring for a person with a neurological disorder is high, necessitating sufficient understanding to provide informed person-centred care.

There are a considerable number of conditions within the neurological disorders and they are organised under key headings in this chapter as follows:

- Traumatic injuries
- Seizure disorders
- Inflammatory and infectious disorders
- Neurodegenerative disorders
- Headache
- Peripheral nerve disorders
- Congenital disorders

REVISE: A&P RECAP

The nervous system

We recommend you revise Chapters 5 and 6 in *Essentials of Anatomy and Physiology for Nursing Practice* (Boore et al., 2016) in order that you have refreshed your baseline knowledge on the structure, organisation and functions of the nervous system before working through this chapter.

While **stroke** is considered a neurological disorder, it is also considered a vascular disorder that leads to neurological impairment. In this regard, stroke is considered in Chapter 8 rather than in this chapter; it is important to remember that the result of brain injury from stroke will be similar to that of brain injury addressed in this chapter.

PERSON-CENTRED CONTEXT: THE BODIE FAMILY

BODIE FAMILY
CASE NOTES

The members of the Bodie family can influence their risk of developing a neurological disorder; a meta-analysis by Xu et al. (2015) identified that diet, specific medications (e.g. antihypertensives), biochemical exposure (**hyperhomocysteinaemia** resulting from deficiencies of vitamins B_6, B_9 and B_{12}), psychological conditions (**depression**), pre-existing disease and lifestyle are all modifiable risk factors that have the potential to reduce the risk of **Alzheimer's disease**. Indeed, quercetin, a component in coffee, has been identified as a neuroprotective in Alzheimer's disease and **Parkinson's disease** (Lee et al., 2016); those members of the Bodie family who consume coffee may actually be protecting themselves from neuro-degenerative conditions. In the United Kingdom, Danielle Zuma can have her risk of **meningitis** reduced by being vaccinated for meningococcal group B bacteria. Traumatic injuries to the brain and spinal cord require everyone in the family to maximise their own safety, although these injuries can occur as a result of the actions of others. George Bodie may already have indications of a neurological disorder; he has no conscious awareness of being thirsty, which may suggest a hypothalamic **lesion**.

TRAUMATIC INJURY TO THE NERVOUS SYSTEM

We are going to start with traumatic injuries to the brain and spinal cord; they are potentially devastating and can result in significant disability. These injuries can be some of the most traumatic life events for the injured person and their family, and so nurses working with people affected need to have the knowledge and skills to provide effective care and support.

APPLY

Classification of severity of brain injury

The severity of a head injury is determined using the Glasgow **Coma** Scale (GCS) (Teasdale and Jennet, 1974) as in Figure 16.1.

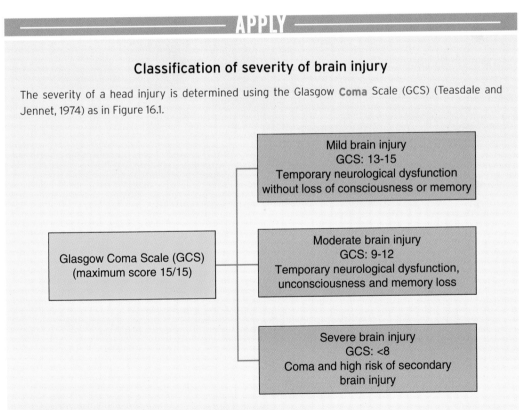

Figure 16.1   Classification of brain injury severity

To learn about the 2014 relaunch of the GCS, go to www.glasgowcomascale.org/

Within Europe, falls and traumatic brain injuries represent the leading causes of brain trauma, with peak incidence in older adults reported as being 262 per 100,000 for people admitted to hospital with traumatic brain injuries (Peeters et al., 2015) compared with 824 per 100,000 in the US (Centers for Disease Control and Prevention, 2014). Variations in incidence can be as a result of how cases are recorded, particularly with many not being recorded unless injury has required hospital admission. For traumatic spinal cord injury, the global figure ranges from 3.6 to 195.4 per million; again, recording and classification of incidence account for some of the variability in incidence (Jazayeri et al., 2015).

When we refer to trauma, there are two classifications of injury:

- **Primary injury**: referring to damage that occurs at the time of trauma, i.e. the physical effect of mechanical forces on the brain or spinal cord. This includes the microscopic damage of blood vessels, neurons and **neuroglia**.
- **Secondary injury**: referring to further damage occurring at cellular level as a result of the primary injury. This can occur over hours or days after the primary injury and includes **ischaemia**, hypoxia, infection and raised intracranial pressure. These changes are biomolecular and physiological (Greve and Zink, 2009).

Primary brain injury

We can do little about the primary injury other than reparative physical work, such as attending to **fractures** or managing a haemorrhage, thus the focus is largely on trying to prevent secondary brain injury, thus minimising the impact of the primary injury. Table 16.1 identifies a number of primary brain injuries and their pathophysiology.

Table 16.1 Primary brain injuries and their pathophysiology

Type of injury	Pathophysiology
Subdural haematoma (Figure 16.2)	A collection of blood below the dura above arachnoid membranes of the brain; resulting from rupture of a bridging cortical vein emptying into dural venous sinuses; arterial involvement is possible but less common. Torsional or shearing forces cause them and the haematoma forms along curvature of the brain. Trauma or coagulation problems are largely the cause of subdural haematomas; acceleration-deceleration of the brain is the primary cause although severe force is needed in older people to cause the venous bleed (Edlmann et al., 2017)
	Classified as:
	Acute - less than three days old
	Sub-acute - 3-7 days old
	Chronic - older than a week.
	The density of presentation on CT scan aids classification (e.g. acute subdural haematomas appear hyperdense (white) compared with the brain). Brain atrophy with advancing age may help to compensate for the haematoma as atrophy provides more space in the skull which the haematoma can fill. Otherwise, the haematoma may need surgical evacuation, usually the case if the person becomes neurologically unstable with signs of raised intracranial pressure when cerebral blood flow is largely compromised. With time, subdural haematomas tend to get bigger either through osmosis drawing fluid into the haematoma or through a change in mass as the haematoma begins to disintegrate. This explains deterioration in some people a week or so after the initial injury. Fluid accumulation is due to angiogenic stimuli forming weak blood vessels within the haematoma membrane wall. Inflammatory cells within the haematoma and its membrane trigger an inflammatory response, causing fluid accumulation (Edlmann et al., 2017)

Type of injury	Pathophysiology
Extradural (epidural) haematoma (Figure 16.2)	A collection of blood between the skull and the dura mater when a force has resulted in periosteal dura mater-bone cleavage. The effect is similar to a subdural haematoma. Approximately 60% are arterial in origin, due to direct cranial trauma, resulting in meningeal arterial rupture (Yilmazlar et al., 2005). The remainder result from venous dural sinus tears, rupture of emissary veins or rupture of venous collections of blood in the dura mater. Some occur from rupture of arachnoid granulations (Yilmazlar et al., 2005). As the dura is tightly connected to the skull, suture lines tend to stop the haemorrhage extending (Huisman and Tschirch, 2009). Unlike subdural haematomas, most extradural haematomas have a characteristic biconvex shape
Traumatic subarachnoid haemorrhage	Of all forms of primary brain injury, traumatic subarachnoid haemorrhage is considered a leading cause of mortality, morbidity and disability among primary brain injury (Modi et al., 2016). Rotational, stretching and tearing forces cause arteries to rupture with haemorrhage in the subarachnoid space, usually due to trauma. Leucocytes invade the CSF and phagocytose the erythrocytes present. The blood in the subarachnoid space can impair reabsorption of CSF, causing hydrocephalus to develop. As red blood cells are broken down, the byproducts can cause vasospasm of cerebral arteries, reducing their lumen by up to 50% and potentially exacerbating any existing brain injury; vasospasm can occur within 12 hours and up to 30 days after the initial haemorrhage (Modi et al., 2016). The blood is often thinly dispersed and the haemorrhage itself largely requires no intervention; usually vasospasm, hydrocephalus and prevention of secondary brain injury are the foci of care
Diffuse axonal injury (DAI)	DAI has become a recognised factor across the spectrum of traumatic brain injuries. It is when there is neuronal axonal damage from a variety of mechanisms; mechanical breaking/shearage of the axonal cytoskeleton, transport disruption along the axon, inflammation of the neuronal axon, or through secondary pathophysiological changes (Johnson et al., 2013). These axonal changes can be immediate but also can result in axonal degeneration over many years; this process is linked with the development of neurodegenerative conditions such as Alzheimer's disease (Johnson et al., 2013). All forms of axonal damage interrupt transport along its length, leading to neuronal dysfunction; while action potentials may not be able to travel down the axon, progressive inflammation can also result in axons disconnecting, also impairing synaptic transmission. Depending on the extent of DAI throughout the brain and spinal cord, a little to extensive neurological impairment can occur. Traumatic forces that result in head rotational acceleration/deceleration and the propagation of force through the brain are the primary cause of DAI (Siedler et al., 2014). The result is the presence of lesions in the white matter in multiple locations throughout the brain
Intracerebral haemorrhage/haematoma (ICH) (Figure 16.2)	ICH is a subset of stroke in which a rupture occurs in a cerebral blood vessel (typically arteries/arterioles), largely as a result of chronic hypertension damaging the vessel wall integrity over time (Schlunk and Greenberg, 2015). The weakened vessel walls develop aneurysms; thin walled micro balloons in the wall. Hypertensive pressure can result in rupture of these aneurysms, resulting in haemorrhage and haematoma formation in the cerebral parenchyma which can extend into the subarachnoid space. Other than hypertension, the other known cause of ICH is cerebral amyloid angiopathy (CAA) when proteins called amyloids are deposited on the walls of cerebral arteries, progressively weakening the wall (Schlunk and Greenberg, 2015). Once haemorrhage starts, it largely forms a haematoma rapidly (within 10 minutes). Haemorrhage may continue after the acute bleed depending on a variety of factors affecting the pressure at the site of haemorrhage. Secondary expansion of the haematoma may occur although the pathophysiology remains unclear; it may result from other nearby weakened vessels rupturing or be secondary to osmotic processes occurring in subdural haematomas. Nevertheless, expansion of the primary haematoma may occur, resulting in neurological deterioration

(Continued)

Table 16.1　(Continued)

Type of injury	Pathophysiology
Cerebral contusions	These are bruising to cerebral parenchyma, largely due to blunt trauma to the head, causing micro-haemorrhages either: *Gliding*: usually occurring alongside a DAI resulting from rotational forces *Surface*: usually occurring from direct forces from a skull fracture, **coup** (under the area of impact), or **contrecoup** (opposite side of the impact) injury. They can also occur from compressive forces as the brain herniates due to raised intracranial pressure Those with **contusions** may be asymptomatic or may develop signs of neurological compromise depending on the extent and depth of damage and surrounding **cerebral oedema**
Cerebral lacerations	Lacerations are tears to the brain tissue and are largely as a result of a high impact injury. They are often accompanied by another form of primary brain injury as the same forces that cause a laceration can cause haematomas and contusions
Concussion	This occurs when the brain is exposed to rapid acceleration, deceleration and rotational forces that stretch and distort neural structures, causing transient neurological dysfunction (Seifert and Shipman, 2015). This is caused by a cascade of physiological occurrences that disrupt axonal and membrane function but do not necessarily result in neuronal or glial death. They can impair cerebral blood flow and synaptic function. Repeated concussions are associated with neurodegenerative processes in the same way as DAI

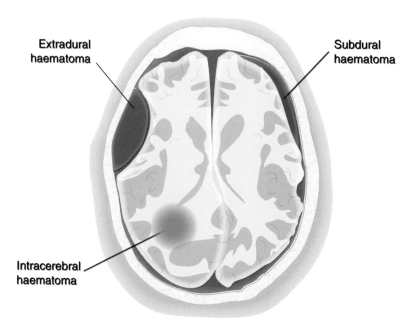

Extradural
haematoma

Subdural
haematoma

Intracerebral
haematoma

Illustrated by Shaun Mercier © SAGE Publications

Figure 16.2　Focal primary brain injuries

SECONDARY BRAIN INJURY

Cellular effect of secondary brain injury

In relation to secondary brain injury, we must consider what occurs at cellular level first; then examine the overall net effect. A primary brain injury has the potential to increase pressure in the brain and/or disrupt cerebral **autoregulation**. A rise in pressure is undesirable as it will compress the structures of the brain, most notably the vascular structures, reducing the nutrient and oxygen-rich blood supply to the cells of the brain and impairing the removal of waste products such as carbon dioxide. Once disruption of delivery and removal of nutrients and waste products occur, this leads to a series of undesirable events at cellular level. Figure 16.3 shows the lack of oxygen supply to the **neurons** and neuroglia, leading to a failure of **aerobic metabolism** (**metabolism** of glucose in the presence of oxygen), resulting in anaerobic glycolysis.

Anaerobic glycolysis is only a short-term solution to providing energy for the cell as it only produces two **ATP** molecules per glucose molecule (5% of the energy potential from aerobic metabolism of glucose). **Lactate** is also produced (by reducing pyruvate) but the failure in circulation at the site means the lactate cannot be removed and taken to the liver (where it can be converted back to glucose). This lactate production results in cellular **acidosis** and eventually a failure of ATP production. The **sodium–potassium pump**, central to neurons carrying action potentials, will therefore also fail. Cellular failure then results in potassium leaking out of the cell and sodium moving into the cell. The sodium brings water with it, increasing the intracellular fluid volume. Further fluid is drawn into the intercellular fluid, resulting in cerebral oedema. This further raises the intracranial pressure and makes the supply of nutrients (including oxygen) even more difficult, often extending the problem wider in the central nervous system. Damage to the neuronal membrane also causes an efflux of potassium into the extracellular fluid with **glutamate** also being released (Seifert and Shipman, 2015). This glutamate binds to ionic channels, causing **depolarisation** and an influx of calcium ions, depressing neuronal function and triggering the sodium–potassium pump (where intact). High mitochondrial calcium resulting from this influx can trigger **apoptosis** (Greve and Zink, 2009). Local levels of glucose are metabolised in this process, being used up through aerobic glycolysis.

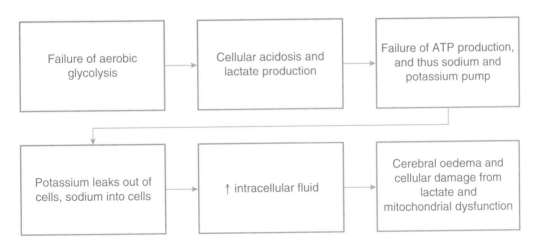

Figure 16.3 Cellular effect of secondary brain injury

This mechanism of secondary injury can be caused by (Martini et al., 2013):

* Impaired autoregulation of cerebral blood flow
* Hypotension
* Hypoxaemia

- Raised intracranial pressure (ICP) (**intracranial hypertension**)
- Increased cerebral metabolic demands (as a result of injury)

Understanding this cascade of effects at cellular level is central to your practice as a nurse. It emphasises the importance of preventing this form of secondary brain injury. If the intracranial pressure is kept within normal limits and the supply of oxygen and nutrients to the neurons and neuroglia is maintained, then we can prevent this occurrence. There are two key measurements used in practice to monitor how well the brain is being perfused: **cerebral perfusion pressure** and brain tissue oxygenation.

ACTIVITY 16.1: APPLY

Living with a brain injury

The impact of a traumatic brain injury can often be invisible; the injury is not always physically visible and so people can assume there are no issues. However, even a mild brain injury can result in significant changes to someone's life; personality, **cognition** and daily living are affected. Listen to Anna's story to gain some insight into the lived experience of a brain injury. If you are using the eBook just click on the play button. Alternatively go to

https://study.sagepub.com/essentialpatho/videos

BRAIN INJURY (2:55)

Cerebral perfusion pressure (CPP)

CPP is the net pressure gradient that causes cerebral blood to perfuse the tissues of the brain. Essentially it is the difference between the mean arterial blood pressure (MAP) and the intracranial pressure (ICP), giving us this formula:

CPP = MAP - ICP

Allen et al. (2014) highlight the need for CPP targets to be age-specific, recommending that lower limits for CPP should be 50–60 mmHg for adults, >50 mmHg for 6 to 17 year olds and >40 mmHg in those under 6 years of age. Other evidence suggests that:

- CPP >70 mmHg is associated with reduced mortality (Griesdale et al., 2015).
- CPP should be maintained between 50 and 70 mmHg to promote optimal **perfusion** while avoiding complications of high CPP (Prabhakar et al., 2014).

However, Kirkman and Smith (2014) highlight that the evidence to support using CPP as a guide for treatment is weak and still an emerging science.

Brain tissue oxygenation (pBtO$_2$)

Martini et al. (2013) highlight that even when ICP is normal and CPP within optimal parameters, ischaemic secondary brain injury can still occur. The measurement of **brain tissue oxygenation** was introduced for this reason, directly testing free, dissolved oxygen. This enables the identification of low cerebral tissue oxygenation and guides practitioners to seek the cause and address it; ongoing monitoring allows them to determine the effect of interventions on cerebral oxygenation (Lin et al., 2015):

- Homeostatic $PbtO_2$ is ≥20 mmHg.
- $PbtO_2$ values <20 mmHg are an indication for treatment.
- $PbtO_2$ values <10 mmHg represent severe cerebral ischemia.

Ideally, $PbtO_2$ should be maintained between 20 and 25 mmHg (Wilensky et al., 2005). While there is controversy over $PbtO_2$-informed therapy, it has better outcomes than CPP informed therapies (Lin et al., 2015).

Effect of primary and secondary brain injury on the nervous system

Now that we understand what happens at cellular level in secondary brain injury, we must think of the impact of that cellular change on the nervous system. The same applies to primary brain injury. Table 16.2 indicates how injury to particular lobes of the brain manifests, helping to determine which part of the brain is affected on presentation and anticipate the effects an injury may have on a person.

Table 16.2 Lobal effects of brain injury

FRONTAL LOBE	BRAIN STEM
Paralysis	Decreased vital capacity
Difficulty in sequencing (inability to plan a sequence of complex movements needed to complete multi-stepped tasks)	Dysphagia (difficulty swallowing)
	Difficulty with balance and movement
Loss of spontaneity in interacting with others	Vertigo (dizziness and nausea)
Loss of flexibility in thinking	Insomnia, sleep apnoea (sleeping difficulties)
Perseveration (persistence of a single thought)	
Difficulty attending (inability to focus on task)	
Emotionally labile (mood changes)	

PARIETAL LOBE	TEMPORAL LOBE
Inability to attend to more than one object at a time	Prosopagnosia (difficulty in recognising faces)
Anomia (inability to name an object)	Wernicke's aphasia (difficulty in understanding spoken words)
Agraphia (inability to locate the words for writing)	
Alexia (reading difficulties)	Disturbance with selective attention to what we see and hear
Difficulty drawing	Difficulty with identification of and verbalisation about objects
Difficulty in distinguishing left from right	
Dyscalculia (difficulty with mathematics)	Short-term memory loss
Apraxia (lack of awareness of certain body parts and/or surrounding space)	Interference with long-term memory
	Increased or decreased interest in sexual behaviour
Inability to focus visual attention	Inability to categorise objects
Difficulties with hand-eye coordination	Persistent talking (right lobe damage)
	Increased aggressive behaviour

(Continued)

Table 16.2 (Continued)

OCCIPITAL LOBE	CEREBELLUM
Visual field deficits	Asynergia (loss of coordination of motor movements)
Difficulty locating objects	
Colour agnosia (difficulty identifying colour)	Dysmetria (inability to judge distance and when to stop)
Production of hallucinations	
Visual illusions	Adiadochokinesia (inability to perform rapid alternating movements)
Inability to recognise words (word blindness)	Intention tremor
Difficulty recognising drawn objects	Abnormal/ataxic gait (staggering wide-based walking)
Movement agnosia (inability to recognise movement of an object)	Tendency to fall
Difficulty reading and writing	Hypotonia (weak muscles)
	Dysphonia (slurred speech)
	Nystagmus (abnormal eye movements)
	Loss of ability to coordinate fine movements

The next consideration is how both primary and secondary brain injury can increase intracranial pressure (ICP). ICP is the pressure inside the skull and indicates the pressure of the CSF in the ventricular system; traditionally ICP was measured from the ventricles using a catheter whereas now a sensor on the parenchyma of the brain is used.

Intracranial hypertension (raised intracranial pressure)

The brain and spinal cord are both encased within bone; the skull encases the brain and the spinal vertebrae encase the spinal cord. Thus, there is limited space for inflammation or **oedema** to occur before the pressure inside the skull and spine rises.

Within this limited space, we need to know what occupies the cranial and spinal cavities, which is:

* Blood (10%)
* CSF (10%)
* Brain tissue (80%)

Any increase in any one of these requires a proportional decrease in one or both of the other two; often this compensation is temporary and cannot be sustained in the long term. For example, oedema and inflammation will increase brain tissue volume and the brain will displace CSF and/or reduce cerebral blood flow to balance this; otherwise, intracranial pressure will rise. Figure 16.4 illustrates how the brain can tolerate an increase in volume without much impact in ICP initially. However, once a certain point is reached, the brain must compensate but can only manage a small volume. A critical point is then reached when the brain has no further ability to compensate and ICP rises rapidly; this may be to a point of no return. In the compensation phase, CSF is normally first displaced down towards the spinal cord as the brain will not want to reduce its oxygen supply by reducing cerebral blood flow. Factors inside and outside of the brain can result in raised ICP (Table 16.3).

Table 16.3 Intracerebral and extracerebral causes of raised ICP

Intracerebral causes	Extracerebral causes
Cerebral oedema	Movement
Hydrocephalus	Breathing/held breath
Tumours (space-occupying lesions)	Hepatic encephalopathy
Intracranial haemorrhage (including haematoma)	Obstructed cranial venous outflow
Vasodilation (including caused by low pCO_2)	
Abscess formation	
Intracranial hypertension	
Seizure activity	

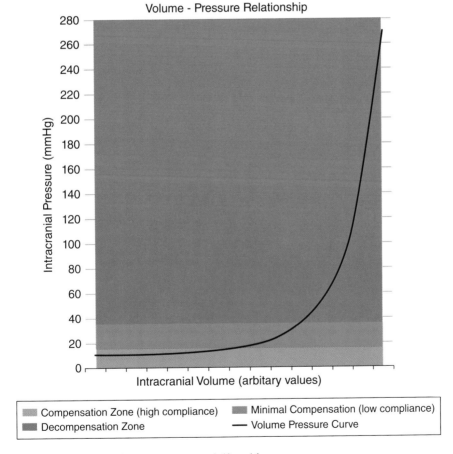

Figure 16.4 Intracranial volume-pressure relationship

When ICP reaches the point of irreversible decompensation, the brain will begin to herniate, forcing the brain to displace into any available space. This is referred to as **'coning'** and usually results in death.

GO DEEPER

Primary types of cerebral herniation

There are four primary forms of herniation (Figure 16.5):

- *Subfalcine/cingulate*: the brain herniates from below the falx cerebri across the midline, from one side to the other.
- *Transtentorial*: a descending or ascending form of herniation. In ascending transtentorial herniation, the cerebellum/posterior fossa contents are forced upwards. In descending transtentorial herniation, also known as uncal herniation, the temporal lobe descends into the anterior opening of the tentorium cerebelli. It also includes the symmetrical herniation of the thalamic region down through the opening of the tentorium cerebelli.
- *Tonsillar*: the cerebellar tonsils are displaced down through the foramen magnum, compressing the medulla.
- *External/transcalvarial*: the brain is forced through a skull defect, for example a burr hole, skull fracture or craniectomy site.

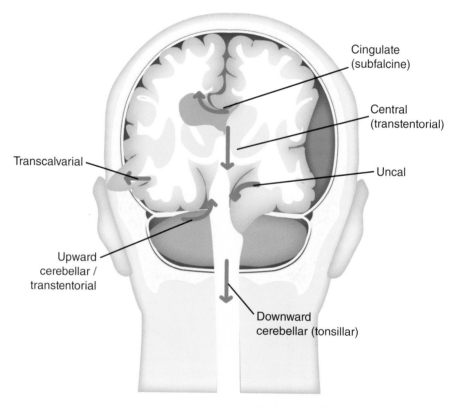

Illustrated by Shaun Mercier © SAGE Publications

Figure 16.5 Types of cerebral herniation

Cerebral oedema

Cerebral oedema is an increased accumulation of water in the intracellular and interstitial fluids within the brain. This can be localised or generalised and can contribute to increasing intracranial pressure. There are three main types of cerebral oedema:

- *Cytotoxic*: caused by intracellular swelling secondary to direct cell injury that results in failure of the sodium–potassium pump. It is common in people with severe cerebral injuries such as traumatic brain injury, DAI or hypoxic–ischaemic injury. It can also occur from water intoxication and this form is readily reversible.
- *Vasogenic*: occurs with increased permeability of capillary **endothelial cells**, permitting fluid to escape into the extracellular space. In this form, neurons are not primarily injured and this form of oedema often occurs with tumours, intracranial haematomas, cerebral **infarction**, cerebral abscesses and central nervous system infections.
- *Interstitial*: characterised by increased fluid in the periventricular white matter. Increased CSF **hydrostatic pressure**, as occurs with hydrocephalus, forces fluid across the **ependymal tissue** (lining the CSF-filled ventricles in the brain and the central canal of the spinal cord) into the periventricular white matter. Reducing CSF hydrostatic pressure allows homeostasis to be restored.

Hydrocephalus

Hydrocephalus is enlargement of the CSF-containing cavities, the ventricles, within the brain due to impairment of flow or **absorption** of the CSF. This increase in CSF volume increases intracranial volume and thus intracranial pressure (Figure 16.6). There are two main types of hydrocephalus:

- *Communicating/Non-obstructive*: In this form, there is a lack of absorption of CSF rather than impairment of its circulation. This may be due to subarachnoid blood preventing reabsorption of CSF or may be secondary to inflammation of the **meninges** or overproduction of CSF (Thompson, 2017); the latter is quite rare.
- *Non-communicating/Obstructive*: This form of hydrocephalus is caused by a blockage of the flow of CSF from its point of production through the ventricular system and eventually to the **arachnoid villi** where it is reabsorbed for return to the venous circulation. Common causes include tumours, congenital defects, intraventricular haemorrhage and cysts (Thompson, 2017). **Aqueduct stenosis** is a common congenital cause due to narrowing of the channel between the third and fourth ventricles. Idiopathic normal pressure hydrocephalus (iNPH) falls into this category. In this form, there is an increase in CSF volume over time without a significant rise in ICP. The exact cause is unknown but it is linked to altered cerebral blood and CSF flow, metabolic changes and degenerative changes similar to that seen in Alzheimer's disease (Nassar and Lippa, 2016); these are potentially reversible with treatment.

Cerebral ischaemia and infarction

When ICP is raised, and when there is damage to cerebral circulation, cerebral blood flow, perfusion and oxygenation can be reduced and result in cerebral ischaemia. This results in a temporarily reversible state of oxygen lack that results in neuronal dysfunction. The area of cells with ischaemia is called the **penumbra**; these cells are barely surviving but can be saved at this point. However, once cellular secondary brain injury sets in, as described earlier, cells will eventually die and ischaemia becomes an infarction. Unless homeostasis is restored to the cells surrounding the infarction, the area of infarction can extend.

Post-traumatic epilepsy (PTE)

Post-traumatic epilepsy (PTE), the most common cause of new-onset **epilepsy** in young adults, is a recurrent **seizure** disorder occurring due to traumatic brain injury. The pathophysiology of its development occurs in three stages; first, there is an injury which leads to the second stage – **epileptogenesis**. Finally, recurrent unprovoked seizures result from this epileptogenesis (Lamar et al., 2014). Essentially, molecular

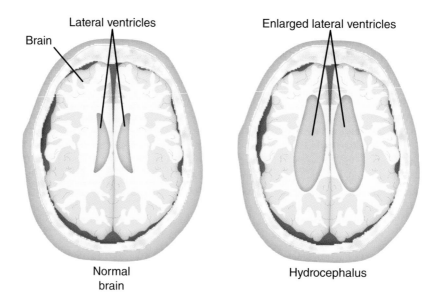

Illustrated by Shaun Mercier © SAGE Publications

Figure 16.6   Hydrocephalus

and neural cellular alterations that occur from brain injury increase neural excitability. The inflammatory response that occurs after injury is thought to generate epileptogenesis as a result of neuronal cell loss and **neuroplasticity** where new neural connections are created that enhance excitation, reduce inhibition and promote **hypersynchronisation** (Lamar et al., 2014). Changes in the neocortex and **hippocampus** in particular are identified as vulnerable to creating an imbalance between excitatory and inhibitory neurotransmission with the potential for spontaneous seizures (Hunt et al., 2013). As neuroplasticity occurs over a long period of time, excitability potential increases over time and so PTE may not manifest until years after injury.

REVISE: A&P RECAP

Neurotransmitters and synapses

Read about neurotransmitters and chemical synapses in Chapter 5 of *Essentials of Anatomy and Physiology for Nursing Practice* (Boore et al., 2016) in order to refresh your knowledge.

Disorders of consciousness

REVISE: A&P RECAP

Physiology of consciousness

Before reading this section on disorders of consciousness, it is advisable to refresh your memory on the physiology of consciousness in Chapter 5 of *Essentials of Anatomy and Physiology for Nursing Practice* (Boore et al., 2016).

When we think of disorders of **consciousness** (DOCs), it is usually coma that comes to mind. However, DOCs are more complex than this and represent chronic disorders where there is a disruption in the neural pathways within and between the frontoparietal and insular lobes and subcortical structures (Di Perri et al., 2014). Any factor that disrupts the **reticular formation**, reticular activating system, **thalamus, hypothalamus** and pre-frontal cortex has the potential to cause a disorder of consciousness as they all contribute to regulation of consciousness, including the sleep–wake cycle, environmental perception and emotional responses. Consciousness has two components: awareness and wakefulness. Awareness is largely aligned with the frontal and parietal lobes and wakefulness with brain stem function. Wakefulness largely precedes external awareness although internal awareness can exist in sleep states (Di Perri et al., 2014). Consciousness is thought to occur as stimuli ascend into a neural network in the dorsal pons and midbrain called the **reticular activating system (RAS)** from which they are projected to the thalamus and then bifurcate out to both cerebral cortices. Any disruption to this complex network can result in a DOC.

There are many components to DOCs; we will focus on coma, **vegetative state (VS)** and **minimally conscious state (MCS)**. There is debate about retention and preservation of arousal and awareness in all three states. New technology is emerging that can demonstrate the presence of these processes which cannot be measured by observation alone, and has resulted in a particular type of DOC being re-diagnosed. The primary causes of DOCs are (Royal College of Physicians, 2015):

- Trauma
- Intracranial haemorrhage, including intracerebral and **subarachnoid haemorrhage**
- Hypoxia
- Infection/inflammation
- Metabolic causes, including toxins

Coma

Coma is a state of unconsciousness where the person cannot be aroused and there is no detectable behavioural awareness. This state persists for at least 6 hours to be confirmed as a coma and the distinguishing characteristics are (Royal College of Physicians, 2015):

- The person cannot be awakened
- No response to pain, light or sound
- Absence of a sleep–wake cycle
- No voluntary movements or actions

Any impairment of the RAS–thalamic–cortex axis responsible for arousal and awareness can result in coma. However, both arousability and awareness must be absent and therefore impairment is extensive across this network.

Vegetative state

Vegetative state (VS) is also known as **unresponsive wakefulness syndrome (UWS)**. The person appears awake but displays no behavioural signs of awareness, although it may be present to some degree (Di Perri et al., 2014); paralysis or aphasia may result in misdiagnosis of VS. In VS, there is a sleep–wake cycle and there may be reflexive and spontaneous behaviours but not in response to stimuli (Royal College of Physicians, 2015). It is thought to be due to extensive diffuse axonal injury and damage to the thalamus, leading to loss of the thalamocortical connections in normal consciousness. In addition, there is significant, widespread disruption to the network in the frontoparietal cortex controlling awareness.

Minimally conscious state (MCS)

People in MCS have a shifting awareness of others and their environment, sometimes responding to some stimuli. In other words, responses are inconsistent but reproducible and indicate that the person is interacting with their environment to some degree (Royal College of Physicians, 2015). In recent years, MCS has been subdivided into MCS+ (plus) and MCS– (minus); if some language is understood, the person is categorised as MCS+; if not, but the criteria for MCS in general are met, they are categorised as MCS–. Emergence from MCS is defined as the return of reliable communication or functional use of objects. A complex network of neural connections in the frontoparietal cortex of the brain that responds to a variety of sensory inputs is primarily thought to control awareness. In MCS, there is partial damage to this network. Connections between this network and the thalamus are intact, at least partially.

APPLY

Prolonged disorders of consciousness

Caring for a person with a prolonged disorder of consciousness is complex as many ethical issues arise around treatments, long-term care and resuscitation, to name a few. The Royal College of Physicians has extensive guidelines around these factors, including on supporting families through what is an extremely challenging time. To read these go online and search for RCP + prolonged disorders of consciousness. If you are using the eBook just click on the icon.

ARTICLE: PROLONGED
DISORDERS OF
CONSCIOUSNESS

It is important to distinguish **locked in syndrome** from DOCs as a person in locked in syndrome has lost voluntary control of movement, usually from some form of brain stem damage/disorder, but they retain arousability and awareness, that is, they remain conscious (Royal College of Physicians, 2015). Additionally, brain stem death is not considered a DOC as it is not compatible with life; cardiac and respiratory function are not sustainable in brain stem death beyond a time and only through artificial means. In DOCs, cardiac and respiratory function remain spontaneous.

Spinal cord injury

Acute spinal cord injury is pathophysiologically similar to traumatic brain injury. Primary injury results from a mechanical force that leads to direct damage to the spinal column or underlying spinal cord. Vertebral fractures or **dislocations** are a common cause of injury to the cord alongside displaced bone and disc fragments; direct damage can occur to the axons and membranes of the spinal cord (Hagen, 2015). Haemorrhage may occur, exacerbating physical injury as the spinal cord is confined within a tight, narrow space with little space for additional volume. This increase in volume results in compression of the cord.

The vertebrae are vulnerable to injury at three main points (Figure 16.7); the C7/T1 junction, T12/L1 junction and at the level of T7. The C7/T1 and T12/L1 junctions are borders between the rigid thoracic spine and flexible cervical and lumbar spines, creating weak points. T7 is the apex of the largest primary curve in the spinal column, resulting in a buckling point for compressive forces. The spinal cord beneath these three points is vulnerable to injury.

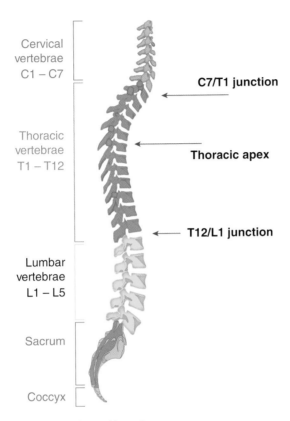

Figure 16.7 Vulnerable injury points on the spine

Cord injuries at the sixth thoracic vertebra can disrupt the descending sympathetic division of the autonomic nervous system in the sympathetic trunk (T1 to L2). Supraspinal sympathetic control is lost, resulting in reduced inhibition of the parasympathetic nervous system and increased sympathetic activity below the injury level (Hagen, 2015). This can result in cardiovascular, thermoregulatory and respiratory instabilities as well as losses of motor and sensory function; the latter is dependent on the level of injury and whether it is complete or incomplete. People with injuries below T6 will have intact autonomic regulation of the cardiovascular and respiratory system. Table 16.4 highlights likely impairments dependent on the level of spinal injury and spinal nerves affected.

Classification of spinal cord injury

Two primary classifications are used in people with spinal cord injury:

- **Tetraplegia**: Results from injury to the cervical spinal cord with associated loss of motor and/or sensory function in all four extremities.
- **Paraplegia**: Results from injury to the thoracic, lumbar, or sacral regions of the spinal cord, including the **cauda equina** and **conus medullaris**, resulting in loss of function of the lower body.

Table 16.4 Levels of injuries and associated impairments

High-cervical nerves (C1–C4)	Low-cervical nerves (C5–C8)	Thoracic nerves	Lumbar and sacral nerves

C1–C4
- Most serious injury
- Paralysis in arms, hands, trunk and legs
- May be unable to breathe independently
- Absent or weak cough
- Loss or impaired control of bowel and/or bladder
- May have tetraplegia/quadriplegia

C5
- May be able to breathe independently and speak normally
- Can raise arms and bend elbows
- Some or total paralysis of wrists, hands, thorax and legs
- Impaired ventilation

C6
- Impaired wrist extension
- Paralysis in hands, thorax and legs
- Able to bend wrists back
- Possible impaired ventilation
- Impaired voluntary control of bowel and/or bladder

C7
- May have preserved elbow and finger function
- Impaired control of bowel and/or bladder

C8
- May have impaired hand movement
- May have preserved ability to grasp and release objects
- Impaired control of bowel and/or bladder

T1–T5
- Impaired innervation to muscles of upper chest, mid-back and abdomen
- Arm and hand function preserved
- Thorax and lower limbs impaired (paraplegia)

T6–T12
- Impaired innervation to muscles of thorax (abdominal and back)
- Paraplegia normally present
- Functional upper body movement
- Mild to no impairment of truncal control
- Effective cough (if abdominal muscles not impaired)
- Impaired voluntary control of bowel and/or bladder

L1–L5
- Impaired innervation to muscles of hips and legs
- Impaired control of bowel and/or bladder
- Ability to walk depends on level of injury

S1–S5
- Impaired innervation to muscles of hips and legs
- Impaired control of bowel and/or bladder
- Probably able to walk

Illustrated by Shaun Mercier © SAGE Publications

Note: The images in this refer to vertebrae and the text below to the spinal nerves. For example, there are seven cervical vertebrae and eight pairs of cervical nerves.

Spinal injury can also be classified as being complete or incomplete:

- **Complete:**
    - ○ when no sensory or motor function is present below the level of injury
    - ○ when there is no **sacral sparing** (movement or sensation is not preserved in the sacrum)
    - ○ reflexes may be present.

- **Incomplete:**
    - ○ when some sensation is preserved (below the level of injury)
    - ○ when position sense is preserved
    - ○ when there is sacral sparing
    - ○ when there is voluntary movement of the lower limbs.

Incomplete injuries can result in one of a number of **syndromes**. The most common of these are identified in Table 16.5.

Neurogenic shock

Neurogenic shock is a triad of hypotension, **bradycardia** and hypothermia. It occurs more commonly in injuries above T6 and due to disruption to the sympathetic outflow from T1 to L2 and to unopposed vagal tone, causing a decrease in vascular resistance with vascular dilation. Neurogenic shock can persist for up to five weeks after injury (Hagen, 2015).

Spinal shock

Spinal shock is transient physiological (rather than anatomical) reflex depression of cord function below the level of injury with associated loss of all sensorimotor functions. There is an initial increase in blood pressure due to the release of **catecholamines**, followed by hypotension. **Flaccid paralysis** is usually present, including of the bowel and bladder. Sustained **priapism** can occur. Symptoms can last from hours to days until reflex arcs below the level of injury begin to function again.

Autonomic dysreflexia

Autonomic dysreflexia is a syndrome of massive imbalanced reflex sympathetic discharge occurring in people with spinal cord injury above the splanchnic sympathetic outflow (T5–T6). It occurs after the phase of spinal shock in which reflexes return and is provoked by stimuli below the level of injury (e.g. distended bladder or bowel) (Hagen, 2015). In this syndrome, large sympathetic outflow causes the release of various **neurotransmitters** (norepinephrine, **dopamine**-b-hydroxylase, dopamine). As a result, the person tends to present with **diaphoresis** above the level of injury and **piloerection** and pallor below this level. Extreme hypertension may present alongside bradycardia because of **vasoconstriction** below the level of injury and a corresponding vagal reflex slowing of the heart rate. Above the level of injury, vasodilation causes high colour and diaphoresis.

Table 16.5 Incomplete spinal injury syndromes

Syndrome	Description	Area of spinal cord affected
Anterior cord syndrome	Damage to the anterior two-thirds of the cord or the anterior spinal artery (which supplies this area of the spinal cord). The result is loss of motor function, pain and temperature sensation below area of injury/damage. As the posterior columns are preserved, proprioception, vibration, deep pressure and touch sensations are preserved This form of cord syndrome has the worst prognosis. Prognosis is more positive if recovery of function/sensation is apparent and progressive within first 24 hours. If no sacral response to sharp sensation or temperature present after first 24 hours, prognosis is pessimistic. Only 10–15% of patients demonstrate functional recovery	Posterior column, Corticospinal tract, Lateral spinothalamic tract, Anterior spinothalamic tract
Central cord syndrome	This acute cervical spinal cord injury presents with the person with disproportionately greater motor impairment in arms than legs, accompanying bladder dysfunction. The degree of sensory loss below the level of injury is variable. The presentation is due to anteroposterior compressive forces distributing pressure and damage onto the central spinal cord (pincer effect); this is where corticospinal tracts innervating arms are located (those controlling legs are more lateral). This is why arms are affected more than legs	Posterior column, Corticospinal tract, Lateral spinothalamic tract, Anterior spinothalamic tract
Brown–Séquard syndrome (lateral cord syndrome)	This is often secondary to a penetrating trauma or unilateral facet fracture/dislocation. Damage occurs to one side of the cord, resulting in ipsilateral muscle paralysis (corticospinal tract injury), ipsilateral loss of vibration and position sensation (posterior column injury). This is because motor fibres of the corticospinal tracts and the ascending dorsal column carrying a sensation of vibration and position decussate high in the spinal cord and medulla. Ascending pathways carrying pain and temperature sensation cross over at the level they enter the cord before ascending in the spinothalamic tract; therefore, pain and temperature sensations are lost contralaterally	**Same side as lesion:** Upper motor neuron weakness Loss of position & vibration; Posterior (dorsal) columns, Lateral corticospinal tract, Spinothalamic tract; **Side opposite lesion:** Loss of pain & temperature sensation

Syndrome	Description	Area of spinal cord affected
Posterior cord syndrome	This form of cord injury is less common and involves injury to the posterior third of the spinal cord or the posterior spinal artery. Usually one side is affected if the posterior spinal artery is involved as there are two of these arteries (the other is usually still intact). Motor function and sense of pain and temperature are preserved but light touch, vibration and proprioception are lost. People with this syndrome can walk but have poor coordination	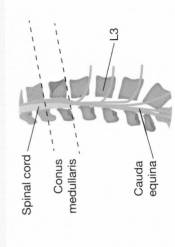 Posterior spinal artery · Anterior →
Cauda equina syndrome	Although technically not a spinal cord injury (the cauda equina is a bundle of nerve roots), this syndrome causes compression to the lumbar, sacral and coccygeal nerve roots extending from the conus medullaris, affecting innervation of legs, feet and pelvic organs. The person will present with weak or flaccid legs with some sensation preserved. They may have bladder and bowel dysfunction, depending on the severity	Point of compression · L3 · Spinal cord · Conus medullaris · Cauda Equina
Conus medullaris syndrome	Occurs from trauma to the spine, but also as a result of spinal cord infection, vertebral abnormality, spinal **stenosis** or a tumour. These injure the conus medullaris. Onset is normally sudden and symptoms can include **radicular pain** (pain that radiates into the lower extremity directly along the course of a spinal nerve root), bowel and bladder dysfunction, loss of sensation and lower limb weakness relative to the lumbar and sacral nerve pathways affected	L3 · Spinal cord · Conus medullaris · Cauda equina

Illustrated by Shaun Mercier © SAGE Publications

Neurogenic bowel and bladder

Spinal cord injury can result in bladder and bowel dysfunction as a result of impaired neuronal control of parts of the body that coordinate their function. Damage to the central spinal cord can result in dysfunction in the pontine and sacral micturition centres. Secondly, disruption to the parasympathetic supply to the **detrusor** muscle and sympathetic supply to the bladder neck can occur in addition to disruption to **somatic** innervation of the external urethral **sphincter**. Cortical control can remain unless there is associated head injury affecting the reticular formation (Benevento and Sipski, 2002). There are two broad classifications of **neurogenic bladder**:

- *Injury above S1 level*: In these injuries, parasympathetic and somatic pathways are preserved. These injuries occur between the pons and sacral spinal cord and will result in an overactive bladder as a result of an upper motor neuron lesion and detrusor overactivity. The person often will experience urge incontinence as both the bladder and external sphincter become spastic at the same time (detrusor–sphincter dyssynergia). Injury at the level of S2–S4 can impair detrusor contractility and pudendal nerve conduction, the latter of which innervates the distal sphincter.
- *Injury below S1 level*: Injuries that involve the sacral spinal cord or cauda equina result in a lower motor neuron lesion that results in detrusor areflexia. The bladder may be prevented from emptying and the person may not sense when the bladder is full, causing urinary retention that may be harmful.

Neurogenic bowel is a result of colon dysfunction secondary to impaired nervous control. There are two broad classifications:

- *Lower motor neuron (LMN) bowel syndrome or areflexic bowel*: This occurs when inhibition of parasympathetic pathways in the conus medullaris, cauda equina, or pelvic nerve occurs, causing spinal cord-mediated **peristalsis** to cease; segmental colonic peristalsis continues as it originates from the **myenteric plexus** (Benevento and Sipski, 2002). Reduced **chyme** propulsion can result in **constipation**. **Denervation** of the external anal sphincter and loss of tone to the levator ani muscles can lead to faecal incontinence.
- *Upper motor neuron (UMN) bowel syndrome or hyperreflexic bowel*: This syndrome is caused by a spinal lesion above the conus medullaris. Voluntary control of the external anal sphincter is lost, inhibiting relaxation (Benevento and Sipski, 2002). However, chyme propulsion is preserved and the result is faecal retention and constipation.

Spasticity

Spasticity is disordered sensorimotor control of the muscles of the body secondary to a UMN lesion, resulting in an intermittent or sustained involuntary activation of those muscles. In essence, spasticity occurs when an imbalance exists between the inhibitory and excitatory signals from the CNS (Keenan, 2009). This leads to **hypertonia** in the muscles during active or passive movement. Any form of trauma to the CNS can cause this, including traumatic brain injury, **multiple sclerosis** and stroke. The three primary lesion sites are:

- Brain stem
- Cerebral cortex (in primary, secondary and supplementary motor area)
- Spinal cord (pyramidal tract)

These neurological changes alter muscle properties and cause stiffness, fibrosis and atrophy; such changes may occur because of chaotic neuronal reorganisation following the initial trauma. There is increased excitation of spinal motor neurons and a reduced stimulus threshold when the frontal motor cortex and its connections are damaged. This overactivity results in spasticity. Similar results occur with damage in the motor and premotor cortex or the supramedullary corticospinal projections. Interestingly, damage to the motor cortex or corticospinal lesions at the level of the medulla do not result in spasticity. Damage from a spinal injury can cause spasticity below the level of injury.

Spasticity primarily affects the antigravity muscle groups and its effect varies with the speed of movement; resistance increases as the speed of stretch increases. In spasticity, the resistance occurs in the first few degrees of joint movement; it increases as movement continues and then releases suddenly. Box 16.1 identifies how spasticity affects the limbs of the body.

Box 16.1 Effects of spasticity in the limbs

Spasticity tends to occur with other disordered forms of movement:

- **Clonus**: involuntary rhythmic contractions triggered by stretch of the muscle.
- **Spasms**: sudden involuntary movements that often involve multiple muscle groups and joints. They can occur in response to somatic or visceral stimuli or spontaneously.
- **Spastic dystonia**: **tonic** muscle overactivity in the absence of any stimulus. It occurs when motor units are unable to stop firing after voluntary or reflex movement. This often leads to contractures.
- Spastic co-contraction: results from a lack of reciprocal inhibition of motor neuron activity, leading to inappropriate initiation of antagonistic muscles during voluntary activity.
- Increased tendon reflexes: these occur because of hyperexcitability of the stretch reflex.

APPLY

Benefits of mild spasticity

Not all spasticity needs to be treated. For example, the hypertonia present in spasticity may help with positioning a person. Spasticity can also reduce oedema and increase venous return. It can enhance the strength of a cough and therefore improve respiratory functioning through improved pulmonary clearance. Spasticity is usually only treated when it results in pain, or inhibits health-related quality of life or functional ability.

SEIZURE DISORDERS

Seizure disorders refer to any abnormality generating an electrochemical differential across cell membranes and depolarisation, i.e. an abnormality in an action potential, creating uncontrolled neuronal activity. This can result from variations in cell membrane permeability, the dispersal of ions across the neuronal cell membrane or an imbalance of neurotransmitters. The alteration in neuronal excitability can result in the transitory disturbance of electrical activity, affecting movement, sensation, emotions, behaviour or consciousness. A seizure manifests when many neurons in one or more brain regions generate synchronised, repetitive action potentials with the usual refractory period, resulting in prolonged neuronal membrane depolarisation (Henry, 2012). Generalised epileptic seizures involve the deep subcortical structures of the brain whereas partial seizures involve cortical areas. A seizure may be a one-off event or a disorder, largely epilepsy. Regardless, seizures are an indication of some form of CNS dysfunction.

Excitation of the neuron can occur as a result of sodium and calcium moving into the cells or as a result of excess glutamate or aspartate (both of which are neurotransmitters). A seizure can also be caused by too little **GABA (gamma-aminobutyric acid)**, although excess GABA in the developing brain in children can also trigger a seizure (Stafstrom and Carmant, 2015).

GO DEEPER

Epilepsy and genetics

In recent years, it has become evident that epilepsy can result from monogenic and polygenic **mutations** (Stafstrom and Carmant, 2015). A number of studies are investigating this complex issue with multiple gene defects causing altered neuronal cellular excitability.

Seizures versus epilepsy and convulsions

There is a clear difference between a seizure and epilepsy. A seizure is a single episode of electrical neuronal dysfunction in the brain, resulting in an acute, temporary change in neurological functioning. A seizure is therefore not epilepsy as it may be a one-off event triggered by a number of factors (e.g. metabolic disturbance, drug intoxication). Epilepsy is a seizure disorder characterised by recurrent seizures occurring unprovoked by any systemic or acute neurological event. It is important to consider the epileptogensis of the event, i.e. the underlying physiology resulting in hyperexcitability of the neuronal network. In addition, we must clarify that a **convulsion** is a motor manifestation of a seizure; seizure activity is not always accompanied by an outward, obvious physical presentation.

Epilepsy

Epilepsy is a distinct, chronic seizure disorder characterised by an imbalance between excitatory and inhibitory neurotransmitter activity in cerebral neuronal ions; this can be in a localised area of the cerebral cortex, resulting in focal seizures, or widespread across the cerebral cortex, resulting in generalised seizures. The imbalance can be attributed to either:

* Low levels of inhibitory neurotransmitters such as GABA
* High levels of excitatory transmitters such as glutamate

However, it may result from ionic disturbance or dysfunction of neuronal calcium channels. Epilepsy may also occur from injury, infection or the development of abnormal neuronal connections following brain injury (post-traumatic epilepsy) or during brain development. There is an abnormal response by the hyper-excitable cerebral cortex to a thalamic signal. The primary subcortical trigger results in abnormal cerebrocortical innervation.

There are two broad categories of epilepsy:

* **Idiopathic (primary) epilepsy**: There is no apparent cause.
* **Symptomatic (secondary) epilepsy**: There is a known cause, which may include head trauma, stroke, meningitis or brain tumour. Genetic causes can also be involved.

Figure 16.8 highlights the causes of epilepsy. The gaps between seizures can be anything from minutes to hours, days to months or even years, depending on the extent of the disorder and how well it is managed.

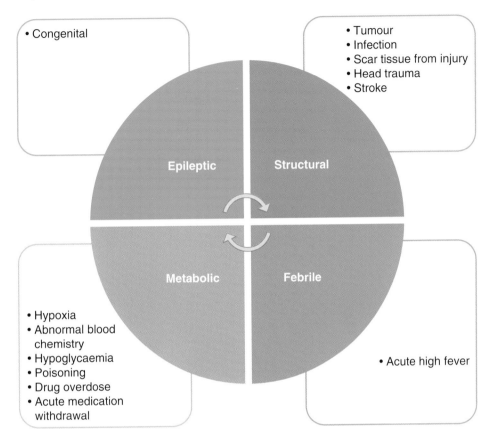

Figure 16.8 Causes of epilepsy

Types of seizures

Seizures are categorised as having an onset that is either focal, generalised or unknown (Table 16.6).

Table 16.6 Classification of seizures

Focal onset	Generalised onset	Unknown onset
These are 80% of adult epilepsies with three sub-categories (Berg et al., 2010)	These involve both cerebral hemispheres from the start	Includes motor seizures (tonic-clonic, epileptic spasms) and non-motor seizures (behaviour arrest)
Focal aware seizures	Non-motor	
No impairment of consciousness or awareness	Absence seizures	
	• Common in childhood	Seizures that cannot be classified also fall into this category
• Observable motor or autonomic components (*motor*)	• Brief diminished consciousness with reduced awareness or ability to respond to stimuli	
• Subjective sensory or psychic phenomena only (*non-motor*)	• Staring into space for 30–60 seconds before recommencing activity	

(Continued)

Table 16.6 (Continued)

Focal onset	Generalised onset	Unknown onset
Focal impaired awareness seizures	Motor	
• Impaired consciousness or awareness	Tonic-clonic seizures	
• Focal seizures may evolve to bilateral, convulsive seizure	• Start of seizure:	
• These seizures can have a *motor* (e.g. myoclonic, tonic) or *non-motor* onset (behaviour arrest, sensory, emotional) (Fisher, 2017)	Person becomes unconscious	
	Muscles become rigid (tonic phase)	
	• During seizure:	
	Person convulses as muscles relax and tighten rhythmically (clonic phase)	
	Breathing might become difficult or sound noisy	
	• After seizure (after convulsions):	
	Person often tired, sleepy and initially may be confused	
	Myoclonic seizures	
	• More common in childhood	
	• Brief but can cluster	
	• Rapid involuntary contractions (jerking) of one or more muscle groups	
	• Common around time of sleep or wakening	
	• Person is conscious	
	Clonic seizures	
	• Rapidly alternating contraction and relaxation of a muscle (clonus)	
	• No tonic phase	
	• Repositioning or restraint does not stop clonus	
	Tonic	
	• Person's muscles suddenly stiffen	
	• Tend to be brief and without warning	
	Atonic	
	• Person's muscles suddenly relax and become flaccid	
	• Tend to be brief, no warning	
	• Differentiate from cataplexy (stimulus-induced sudden loss of muscular tone)	
	• Differentiate from **syncope** (transient, self-limited rapid onset loss of consciousness) caused by transient global cerebral hypoperfusion	

ACTIVITY 16.2: APPLY

Epilepsy and pharmacological treatment

Understanding the pathophysiology of epilepsy will aid comprehension of the main principles of drug treatment. Watch this video to apply this pathophysiology to pharmacological treatment. If you are using the eBook just click on the play button. Alternatively go to
https://study.sagepub.com/essentialpatho/videos

Additionally, you can learn to use the updated (2017) classification of seizures by reading the following article: 'The New Classification of Seizures by the International League Against Epilepsy' (Fisher, 2017).

EPILEPSY AND
PHARMACOLOGY (9:22)

ARTICLE: CLASSIFICATION
OF SEIZURES

APPLY

Phases of a seizure

Seizures have three general phases:

- *Ictus or ictal phase*: the seizure itself; consists of paroxysmal firing of cerebral neurons.
- *Post-ictal phase*: the period after the seizure, with temporary neurological dysfunction.
- *Inter-ictal*: the phase between seizures.

Tonic-clonic seizures are described in four phases:

- *Prodromal*: precedes the seizure (hours/days). It differs from an **aura**, involving symptoms and signs including insomnia, headache, reduced tolerance threshold, increased agitation, low mood and emotional lability.
- *Aura*: can present seconds to minutes before a seizure and is a subjective sensation including experiences from dreamlike feelings, alterations in smells, hearing, vision or other sensation. It marks the beginning of the seizure.
- *Ictus*: in a tonic-clonic seizure this has two distinct sub-phases:

  o *Tonic* - there is increased tone of voluntary muscle and the person may have apnoea. It lasts from 15 to 60 seconds.
  o *Clonic* - violent muscular contractions occur, the person usually hyperventilates, and the eyes roll with the pupils contracting and dilating. This can last for 30 seconds or extend to many minutes.

- *Post-ictal*: the person's breathing will return to a regular, unlaboured pattern. Initially they are likely to be disorientated or confused and will be fatigued and sleepy for some time.

INFLAMMATORY AND INFECTIVE DISORDERS

Encephalitis and meningitis are inflammatory diseases of the brain, spinal cord and surrounding structures caused by bacterial or viral infections. There are other inflammatory and infective disorders but these are the commonest and will be the focus in this chapter.

Encephalitis

Encephalitis is inflammation of the brain parenchyma and presents as diffuse and/or focal. The person may experience obvious neurological deficits but often there is neuropsychological dysfunction. It is more commonly caused by a viral infection causing mild to profound inflammation of the cerebral parenchyma but can be bacterial or fungal in origin. There are two main categories of encephalitis:

- **Primary encephalitis**: the **virus** directly infects the brain and spinal cord. This is the most serious but least common form of encephalitis.
- **Secondary (post-infectious) encephalitis**: the virus first infects another part of the body and secondarily enters the brain. This is the most common form but is less harmful than primary encephalitis.

Interestingly, most people infected with viral encephalitis present with mild or no symptoms, and the illness is short-lived. However, there is a reported 30% mortality from encephalitis and 30% of survivors do so with significant neurological consequences, most notably from Japanese encephalitis (White and Easton, 2008). Numerous **pathogens** may cause encephalitis and while CSF sampling (nucleic acid amplification testing) and brain biopsies are sometimes performed, they are rarely of benefit in identifying the cause; history-taking and thorough, whole-body clinical assessment are the foundations of treatment. Effective antiviral therapy is largely restricted to treating the herpes simplex virus and **HIV** (Tunkel et al., 2008). Indeed, the following are primarily considered the pathogenic causes of encephalitis:

- Herpes simplex virus (HSV-1 and HSV-2)
- Varicella zoster virus
- Cytomegalovirus (CMV)
- Japanese encephalitis virus
- Dengue virus
- Chikungunya virus
- West Nile virus
- Nipah virus
- Enteroviruses (EVs) (Jain et al., 2014)

These pathogens primarily enter the body through the gastrointestinal tract, respiratory tract, from contaminated food or from insect bites. Once in the body, they replicate peripherally before travelling to the CNS through the blood or through neuronal transport mechanisms (Chong and Tan, 2016). In encephalitis, the infected parenchymal tissue develops localised necrotising haemorrhage that becomes generalised as the disease progresses. **Neuropathy** occurs as a direct result of neuronal destruction (Jain et al., 2014) with some viruses targeting specific areas; HSV tends to target neurons of the hippocampus whereas Japanese encephalitis targets the **basal ganglia** (Chong and Tan, 2016). The virus will largely travel through neuronal microtubules, using synapses to move from neuron to neuron. Viral infection, replication and the inflammatory response from **astrocytes**, other glial cells and leucocytes result in inflammation and the death of cells (Chong and Tan, 2016). This is accompanied by oedema and, depending on the location of this disease process in the brain, any form of neurological presentation can occur. Lethargy, confusion and delirium are common presentations.

APPLY

Encephalitis treatment

- Encephalitis can be difficult to treat because the viruses that cause the disease generally do not respond to medications.
- Exceptions are herpes simplex virus and varicella-zoster virus, which respond to the antiviral drug acyclovir (Zovirax™).
- Symptoms can be treated with:

  o anticonvulsants
  o anti-inflammatory drugs
  o multidisciplinary team involvement
  o good fluid intake

Meningitis

Meningitis is infection and inflammation of the membranes (meninges) and fluid (cerebrospinal fluid) surrounding the brain and spinal cord. It is primarily caused by bacteria or viruses with bacterial meningitis usually being the more serious.

Bacterial meningitis

In bacterial meningitis, pathogens usually arrive at the meninges and into the CSF from another part of the body, although they can directly enter the central nervous system as a result of trauma. Bacteria can cross the **blood–brain barrier transcellularly** (penetrate the cell and travel through it), in between cells (**paracellularly**) or via infected phagocytes (Barichello et al., 2013). As bacteria replicate in the CNS, their bacterial products and fragments, which are immunogenic, result in an inflammatory reaction of the meninges, subarachnoid space and parenchymal vessels of the brain (Barichello et al., 2013); the inflammatory response enhances the **infiltration** of **neutrophils** but also allows further pathogens and albumin to infiltrate the CSF and subarachnoid space. Once in the CSF, pathogens can migrate around the brain more quickly through the CSF–ventricular system. This cascade of events further heightens the immune response and the meninges become thickened through inflammation and may develop **adhesions**, resulting in hydrocephalus. Reactive oxygen species and calcium release, resulting from inflammation, lead to the release of apoptosis-inducing factor, resulting in the death of CNS cells. In the subacute phase, degenerative changes to the CNS result from these factors, with glial **proliferation** occurring. The most common bacterial sources of meningitis are *Streptococcus pneumoniae* (pneumococcus), *Haemophilus influenzae*, *Neisseria meningitidis* and *Escherichia coli* and group B streptococci in neonates. Some of these may cause the creation of cerebral abscesses.

Viral meningitis

Viral meningitis, also known as aseptic meningitis, occurs in a pathologically similar way to bacterial meningitis, although it is less severe and the CSF presentation is different (see Apply box below). The source of the virus is often intestinal, and other forms are often associated with mumps or herpes infection. Arboviral (mosquito-borne) disease and **influenza** are also linked with viral meningitis.

APPLY

Signs and symptoms of meningitis

As meningitis causes inflammation of the meninges and surrounding structures, pressure can be placed upon cranial nerves and hydrocephalus may occur. As a result, bacterial meningitis can present with pyrexia, headache, **nuchal** rigidity and cranial nerve deficits, particularly of the 8th cranial nerve. In meningococcal meningitis, a **petechial rash** may appear; this may also occur in other forms of meningitis. Examination of the CSF will reveal if it is cloudy as a result of the infiltration of phagocytes and bacteria, both of which may be raised in CSF cell counts.

APPLY

Cerebrospinal fluid changes in meningitis

In both forms:

- Low glucose
- Presence of micro-organisms

Bacterial

- Appearance: clear, cloudy, or **purulent**
- Opening pressure: elevated (>25 cmH$_2$O)
- Raised WBC
- Glucose level: low (<40% of serum glucose)
- Protein level: elevated (>50 mg/dl)

Viral:

- Appearance: clear
- Opening pressure: normal or elevated
- Low WBC
- Glucose level: >60% serum glucose (may be low in HSV infection)
- Protein level: elevated >50 mg/dl

GO DEEPER

Rarer forms of meningitis

Chronic meningitis

This form of meningitis occurs when slow-growing pathogens, e.g. those that cause **tuberculosis**, invade the meninges and CSF. It develops over weeks with symptoms similar to those of acute forms.

Fungal meningitis

One common fungal form of meningitis is cryptococcal meningitis; this can occur in those who are chronically immunosuppressed. While responsive to antifungal treatments, this form of meningitis is prone to recurrence.

APPLY

Meningitis prevention

The core principles of meningitis prevention are based around:

- Immunisation
- Effective hand washing
- Treatment of infections in the body
- Boosting the immune system through rest, good diet and exercise

NEURODEGENERATIVE CONDITIONS

Neurodegenerative diseases result from the deterioration of neurons. In some cases, the degenerative process stops and starts and in others it continually progresses. Neurodegenerative conditions can be divided into two groups:

- Those affecting memory and cognition
- Those affecting movement

In this chapter we will limit our examination to Alzheimer's disease, motor neuron disease, Parkinson's disease and multiple sclerosis.

Alzheimer's disease

Alzheimer's disease is the leading cause of dementia and a well-documented neurodegenerative condition. In 2015, more than 47 million people globally were estimated to be living with dementia and this is expected to triple by 2050 (WHO, 2015). No cure currently exists, with drug therapies aimed at slowing the pathophysiological processes and managing symptoms associated with the disease. The characteristic pathology involved in Alzheimer's disease is the development of intracellular neurofibrillary tangles and deposits of extracellular amyloidal (beta) protein, leading to plaque formation in the CNS (Kumar and Singh, 2015). These pathophysiological changes result in decreased acetylcholine production, a primary neurotransmitter in the CNS. In Alzheimer's disease, an enzyme (α-secretase) separates amyloid precursor proteins (APP) into fragments (Figure 16.9), the most important being the beta-amyloid protein. These proteins are processed by beta- and gamma-secretases but, in Alzheimer's, their production is greater than their clearance and so an excess accumulates. These are sticky and cling together with other beta-amyloids to eventually form plaques. These result in the production and release of pro-inflammatory **cytokines** from astrocytes which lead to the production of Aβ oligomers; it is the aggregation of these oligomers that causes neuronal and vascular degeneration (Kumar and Singh, 2015).

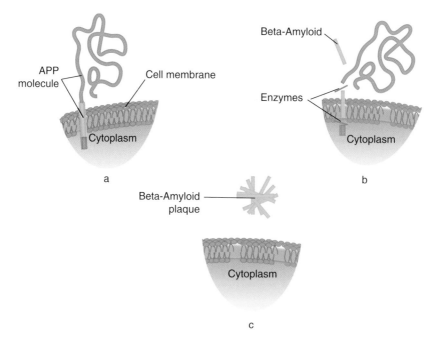

Illustrated by Shaun Mercier © SAGE Publications

Figure 16.9 Formation of beta-amyloid plaques in Alzheimer's disease

---

APPLY

Acetylcholinesterase inhibitors

- Drugs used to treat Alzheimer's disease act by inhibiting acetylcholinesterase activity.
- These drugs block the esterase-mediated metabolism of acetylcholine to choline and acetate. This results in:

   o   increased acetylcholine in the synaptic cleft
   o   increased availability of acetylcholine for postsynaptic and presynaptic nicotinic (and muscarinic) acetylcholine receptors.

Motor neuron disease (MND)

Motor neuron disease (MND), referred to as **amyotrophic lateral sclerosis (ALS)** outside of the UK, occurs when a selective and progressive functional loss in upper and lower motor neurons results in impairment or loss of motor function (Swann, 2011). As the condition is progressive, so is muscle weakening. MND is an umbrella term for a variety of different conditions where the common feature is premature degeneration and death of motor neurons. The prevailing pathophysiology is the focus here.

   In MND, there is progressive injury, degeneration and cell death of lower motor neurons in the spinal cord and brain stem and of upper motor neurons in the motor cortex. The condition demonstrates degraded protein inclusions within motor neuron cell bodies occurring through **ubiquitination**.

This is when a protein has **ubiquitin** (a small protein found in all cells of the body) attached to it. This signals that the protein is to be transported to a **proteasome** for degradation. In addition, there are neurofilament accumulations within motor neuron axons in MND. How this occurs is not fully understood but it is thought to include a complex interrelationship between some of the following:

- Genetic factors: there are approximately 16 mutated DNA/RNA-regulating genes identified in MND (Vucic et al., 2014)
- **Oxidative stress**: an imbalance between the generation and neutralisation (by antioxidants) of free radicals, resulting in toxic levels
- **Excitotoxicity**: over-activation of receptors for the excitatory neurotransmitter glutamate; intracellular organelles are damaged, leading to death of the neuron
- Protein aggregation
- Impaired axonal transport
- Mitochondrial disease/failure.

Interestingly, in MND the pathological process originates in the neuroglia that support the motor neurons and not within the motor neurons themselves. Astrocytes and microglia have been identified as having a primary role in the condition. Astrocytes remove glutamate which is a key component of MND as it is central to excitotoxicity. Failure of the astrocytes to remove it sufficiently is one key area of investigation. Astrocytes produce an enzyme called SOD1 (**superoxide dismutase**) which is an antioxidant needed to prevent oxidative stress in the neighbouring motor neuron. A mutation of the *SOD1* gene in astrocytes is also central to the pathological process (Souza et al., 2016). It appears that motor neurons are specifically sensitive to mutated astrocytes in ways that other neurons in the CNS are not, resulting in motor neuron-related impairments.

GO DEEPER

Variants of MND

There are many variants of MND. These are complex but should you wish to review them access this article, which outlines the pathophysiology of each in brief.

O'Brian, R. and Clabburn, O. (2016) Motor neurone disease/amyotrophic lateral sclerosis: what's in a name? *British Journal of Neuroscience Nursing*, 12 (2): 82-4.

ARTICLE: MOTOR
NEURON DISEASE

Parkinson's disease

Idiopathic Parkinson's disease (primary/classical Parkinson's disease, now commonly referred to as simply Parkinson's) is a progressive neurodegenerative disorder associated with decreased dopamine in parts of the brain, largely due to destruction of the nigrostriatal neurons (in the basal ganglia); other neuronal subtypes also degenerate in Parkinson's (Hirsch et al., 2013). Dopamine is a neurotransmitter that has a significant role in the coordination of motor activity and memory. It is a signaling neurotransmitter that binds to target cells to trigger a cellular action. In Parkinson's, the loss of dopamine results in disordered regulation of movement as there is insufficient dopamine in comparison to the levels of acetylcholine, another neurotransmitter, the effects of which are then heightened as the two oppose each other. Dopamine deficiency results in movement being delayed and uncoordinated.

While considerable research has been undertaken to determine the pathophysiological basis of Parkinson's, the contemporary consensus is that the cellular destruction is as a result of mechanisms that originate from inside and outside of the affected neurons (Hirsch et al., 2013). It is thought that mitochondrial dysfunction is one intraneuronal cause of Parkinson's; an increase in calcium moving into the neuron is thought to result in an increased production of **reactive oxygen species**. These are thought to lead to the damage of **mitochondria**. This would normally lead to the removal of the damaged mitochondria and replacement with healthy ones so that the neuron functions optimally. However, in Parkinson's the effective clearance of these damaged mitochondria is ineffective and results in an accumulation of dysfunctional mitochondria that leads to neuronal dysfunction and eventual destruction of the neuron itself. The processes resulting in the disease from outside of the cell are not yet fully understood but are known to take place as the pathophysiological processes spread to other neuronal populations, facilitated by nonneuronal cells (Hirsch et al., 2013).

A genetic basis for Parkinson's has a focus in understanding its origins. Mutations in the α-synuclein gene *SNCA* and parkin gene *PKN* (genes that create particular proteins) are thought to play a role in the disease being autosomally inherited. α-synuclein is a major component of Lewy bodies which are found to be present in the substantia nigra in those with Parkinson's. However, it is now proposed that Lewy bodies have no role in the pathogenesis of Parkinson's; their presence or absence in neurons does not appear to alter the course of neuronal destruction (Schulz-Schaeffer, 2015). Parkin is a substance with a role in clearing damaged mitochondria from neurons and *PKN* mutation is still considered a viable cause.

A resting tremor, rigidity, **akinesia/bradykinesia** and postural instability occur in Parkinson's as a result of motor cortex dysfunction and dopamine deficit. Within the central nervous system, there is a fine balance of inhibitory and excitatory inputs of the basal ganglia and the cerebellum. Cerebellar output is excitatory and basal ganglia are inhibitory. Apoptosis of **dopaminergic** neurons in the substantia nigra decreases inhibition, causing disruption of signals to the motor cortex via the thalamus. This results in loss of smooth, coordinated movement. Thus, people with Parkinson's are slow to initiate and complete movements and they have difficulty stopping voluntary movements.

APPLY

Reducing the risk of Parkinson's

Caffeine consumption is associated with reduced risk of developing Parkinson's:

- Three cups coffee/day have been shown to decrease risk (Qi and Li, 2014).
- Caffeine antagonises adenosine A_1/A_{2A} receptors in the striatum, protecting against excitotoxic and ischaemic neuronal injury (Simola et al., 2014).

Inverse association with cigarette smoking:

- Nicotine protects mitochondria against oxidative stress (Surmeier, 2014).

Multiple sclerosis

Multiple sclerosis (MS) is a chronic, progressive **autoimmune disease**. It is a combined immune and neurological disorder with multifocal areas of neuronal **demyelination** disrupting the ability of the nerve to conduct action potentials. MS is characterised by chronic inflammation, demyelination, and glutamate (scarring) in the CNS. It is thought to be triggered by a virus in genetically susceptible individuals and a subsequent **antigen**–antibody reaction, leading to demyelination of neuronal axons. There is a loss of myelin and a reduction in **oligodendrocytes**, the cells that produce myelin in the CNS. Instead, a proliferation of astrocytes occurs.

In MS, an autoimmune response is triggered by unconfirmed environmental factors. **Lymphocytes** are activated and adhere to endothelial cells of the blood–brain barrier (BBB) and, along with cytokines, cause the tight junctions of the BBB to relax. Activated T and B lymphocytes can then enter the CNS and have specific actions (Ward-Abel and Burgoyne, 2008):

- Activated T-lymphocytes release pro-inflammatory cytokines (interleukin-2, interferon-gamma and **tumour necrosis factor**). These stimulate and activate **macrophage**s which then attack myelin proteins.
- B-lymphocytes release myelin-specific **antibodies** which target myelin, destroying it. They are also thought to target oligodendrocytes, causing a reduced number, and lead to **oligoclonal bands** (**immunoglobulins**) being present in the CSF of people with MS.

The infiltration of these cells across the BBB results in inflammation, demyelination, **gliosis** and axonal degeneration and creates the lesions seen in MS (Dendrou et al., 2015). These lead to sensory disturbance, motor impairments and, commonly, debilitating fatigue, pain and cognitive impairment. There is no pattern of neurological presentation; the location of lesions can be sporadic and these dictate the signs and symptoms.

Myelin has a role in the conduction of action potentials, but also a role in protecting the axon of the neuron. Thus, demyelination may leave the axon vulnerable to damage, causing destruction of the neuron, although this may not occur early in the disease. Although remyelination can occur in MS, it often does not lead to full functional recovery due to this axonal damage. Additionally, myelin may be replaced by glial scar tissue, formed by astrocytes. There are four primary types of MS (Table 16.7):

Table 16.7 Types of multiple sclerosis

Relapsing-remitting MS (RRMS)

- Affects 85% of people newly diagnosed with MS
- Acute attack is followed by partial or complete recovery as a result of remyelination
- Relapses occur alongside CNS inflammation and demyelination of the white matter
- Symptoms may be inactive for months or years

Secondary-progressive MS (SPMS)

- Occurs in 80% of people with RRMS, 10-20 years post diagnosis
- Presents with occasional relapses but symptoms remain constant without remission; the inflammatory lesions are not characteristic but steady axonal loss results in reduced brain volume (Dendrou et al., 2015)
- Progressive disability late in disease course

Primary-progressive MS (PPMS)

- Approximately 10% of people with MS
- Characterised by slow onset with continuous, progressive worsening. No remyelination occurs

Progressive-relapsing MS (PRMS)

- Rarest form
- Affects approximately 5% of people with MS
- Steady worsening of condition from onset

Influencing factors

There are a number of theories around different influencing factors for MS:

Vitamin D deficiency

Vitamin D_3 receptor is important in immune function; it is present on T regulator cells. **Vitamin D** is a lipophilic vitamin synthesised in the skin by the conversion of 7dehydrocholesterol to vitamin D by ultraviolet radiation from the sun. Studies have shown that higher 25(OH)D levels (representative of vitamin D levels) are associated with reduced MS activity (Fitzgerald et al., 2015). Indeed, low levels of vitamin D increase neonates' risk of developing MS (Nielsen et al., 2017). It is thought that vitamin D induces T cells with immunosuppressive properties which may have a role in preventing the autoimmune response (Correale and Gaitan, 2015).

Epstein–Barr virus (EBV)

The EBV has long been associated with the aetiology of MS. It is thought to activate self-reactive T and B cells, leading to auto-antibody production as well as reducing the **self-tolerance** breakdown threshold while enabling autoreactive B-cells to survive (Correale and Gaitan, 2015). People with MS have higher EBV titres (i.e. antibody levels) than the general population.

HEADACHE

REVISE: A&P RECAP

Physiology of pain

Before reading this section on headache, it is advisable to refresh your memory on the physiology of pain in Chapter 6 of *Essentials of Anatomy and Physiology for Nursing Practice* (Boore et al., 2016).

The pathophysiology of headache is complex and is associated with the trigemino-cervical complex where the trigeminal nerve supplies sensation to the anterior head and face and the upper cervical nerves supply sensation to the posterior head (Jenkins and Tepper, 2011). Many aspects of headache begin distally. Headache pain signals also cause increased activity in the trigeminal ganglia and medulla as they ascend these pathways, particularly in **migraine**. In migraine, however, there is a vascular component to the pathophysiology with activation of the trigemino-vascular pathways, activating the pons (Jenkins and Tepper, 2011). Both central and peripherally generated head pain have a final common pathway along second-order neurons which transmit afferent action potentials to the thalamus where third-order neurons then relay to a variety of areas of the cerebral cortex (Jenkins and Tepper, 2011).

Headache disorders are divided into two distinct categories (Scottish Intercollegiate Guidelines Network (SIGN), 2008):

- *Primary headache disorders* without an associated underlying pathology. **Cluster headaches**, **tension type headaches** and migraine are all forms of primary headache and may be chronic or episodic.
- *Secondary headache disorders* may have a serious underlying pathology (e.g. infection, **neoplasm**).

Migraine

Around 85% of headaches presenting in general practice are related to migraine. This is a severe intermittent disturbance of sensory processing in the CNS with attack-related activation in brain stem structures key for anti-nociception with a concurrent change in cortical serotonin receptor availability (Sprenger and Goadsby, 2010). This results in a failure in full inhibitory pain control with an associated reduction in attentional functional capacity. Key areas of activation are the anterior cingulate cortex (ACC) and the insula (Pro et al., 2014). In migraine, the trigeminal nerve is activated, resulting in the release of neuropeptides that cause neurogenic inflammation of the vasculature of the meninges. Vasodilation is also implicated as part of this process, mediated by calcitonin (Ashina et al., 2012). Oestrogen, monosodium glutamate in the diet and chocolate are thought to be aggravating factors.

Migraine has two classifications: with and without aura. Aura associated with migraine typically includes some transient focal neurological symptoms such as visual and/or language disturbance and/or unilateral **paraesthesia** (Ashina et al., 2012). Aura is thought to be caused by depolarisation of cortical neurons in a spreading wave pattern across the cerebral cortex, ending in a period of suppressed activity (Ashina et al., 2012).

Tension type headache (TTH)

TTH is less well understood and accounts for 10% of headache presentations in general practice. While muscle tension in the scalp and neck were considered causal, generally this is not supported by evidence. The pathophysiology is now thought to be more closely aligned with migraine and TTH may be a variation in the presentation and duration of migraine. Lifestyle factors such as **stress** and mental tension have traditionally been thought of as aggravating factors but again evidence suggests this is not the case (Ashina et al., 2012).

APPLY

Stress and headaches

Richard Jones has suffered from stress in the past and underwent cognitive behavioural therapy to manage his stress. At the time, his stress was also accompanied by tension type headaches which he found to compound his stress. As part of this therapy, he learned how to use mindfulness-based stress reduction techniques and this not only reduced his stress but also reduced the incidence and intensity of the tension type headaches. Omidi and Zargar (2014) found similar results in their research on the impact of mindfulness techniques on tension headaches.

RICHARD JONES
CASE NOTES

Cluster headache

These are the least common form of headache but tend to be very distressing to experience. These are clusters of episodic headaches occurring 1–8 times daily (Braine, 2013) for weeks or months. They are considered one of the most painful experiences a person can have, but the pathophysiology is poorly understood. Pain is unilateral and is thought to occur by activation of the ophthalmic branch of the trigeminal nerve, following the final common pathway and including the hypothalamus. It is experienced in the orbital and temporal regions, has a rapid onset and peaks in 15 minutes, lasting up to

3 hours. Once afferent projections reach the hypothalamus, it is thought that dysregulation occurs (Braine, 2013), resulting in various autonomic symptoms. Cluster headaches are closely associated with **circadian rhythm**s, causing mainly nocturnal symptoms.

ACTIVITY 16.3: APPLY

The lived experience of cluster headaches

Cluster headaches can be horrendous to experience. Watch the following video to get some insight into the experiences of those who endure these headaches. If you are using the eBook just click on the play button. Alternatively go to

https://study.sagepub.com/essentialpatho/videos

CLUSTER HEADACHES (2.59)

Neuralgia

Neuralgia refers to severe, acute experiences of neuropathic pain that are often repetitive. Think of the throbbing pain of toothache and how it travels like lightning. Neuralgia usually has a cutaneous origin, stimulating a spinal or cranial nerve. It is often idiopathic but occasionally has a secondary cause, largely from nerve impingement or damage (e.g. in multiple sclerosis).

Trigeminal neuralgia

The most common form of neuralgia is **trigeminal neuralgia (TN)**. TN occurs largely from compression of the trigeminal nerve or from another structural abnormality that triggers the nerve, for example a pulsating blood supply. There are three branches to the nerve that can be affected and the location of pain can indicate which division is affected (Figure 16.10). Injury to the trigeminal nerve or aggravating stimulation results in hyperexcitable axons that lead to paroxysmal pain discharges (Zakrzewska and McMillan, 2011). Additionally, there is evidence that demyelination and remyelination of the axon may have occurred and this may explain the hyperexcitability. Demyelination is thought to have occurred through mechanical erosion (Zakrzewska and McMillan, 2011). An influx of potassium is thought to eventually end the nervous transmission.

While these mechanical causes are well understood, they are not always present in those with trigeminal neuralgia. An allergic-immune reaction pathogenesis has also been identified as a cause when **mast cell** degranulation and **histamine** release occur due to maxillofacial inflammatory disease (Sabalys et al., 2012).

PERIPHERAL NERVE DISORDERS

Peripheral nerve disorders involve motor and/or sensory neurons of the peripheral nervous system, resulting in muscle weakness and/or atrophy and possibly sensory changes. In peripheral nerve disorders, there is either segmental demyelination of the axon or degeneration of the axon itself. When multiple neurons are involved, there tends to be symmetrical impairments referred to as polyneuropathies. There are various peripheral nerve disorders; here we focus on one of the most well-known, **Guillain-Barré syndrome**. The Go Deeper box identifies further disorders in this category.

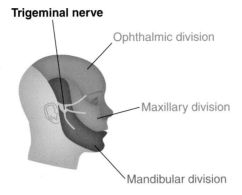

Trigeminal nerve

Ophthalmic division

Maxillary division

Mandibular division

Illustrated by Shaun Mercier © SAGE Publications

Figure 16.10   Divisions of the trigeminal nerve

─────────────── **GO DEEPER** ───────────────

Types of peripheral nerve disorders

Mononeuropathies

- Carpal tunnel syndrome
- Ulnar neuropathy
- Femoral nerve dysfunction
- Radial nerve dysfunction
- Sciatic nerve dysfunction

Polyneuropathies

- Chronic inflammatory demyelinating polyneuropathy (CIPD)
- Guillain-Barré syndrome
- Motor neuron disease (MND)/amyotrophic lateral sclerosis (ALS)
- Diabetic neuropathy
- Diphtheria
- Charcot-Marie-Tooth syndrome
- **Porphyria**

Guillain-Barré syndrome

Guillain-Barré syndrome (GBS) has two distinct presentations: an acute inflammatory demyelinating polyneuropathy or an acute motor axonal neuropathy. The demyelinating form is the most common (90%) in Western society and the axonal form more common in Asia; the axonal type is increasing overall (Yuki and Hartung, 2012).

In the demyelinating form (Figure 16.11), an acute inflammatory response occurs where T cells and macrophages infiltrate and cause segmental demyelination, often resulting in secondary axonal degeneration (Figure 16.12). This can occur in the spinal roots, and motor and sensory neurons, and represents an immune-mediated condition. Recently, T cell involvement has become less clear and a humorally-mediated reaction is considered more accurate (Willison et al., 2016). In this form of GBS, antibodies bind to Schwann cells, depositing activated complement components, causing myelin **vesiculation** (blistering) and macrophage invasion within seven days (Yuki and Hartung, 2012). Epstein–Barr virus is associated with demyelinating EBS but the pathogenesis is not fully understood.

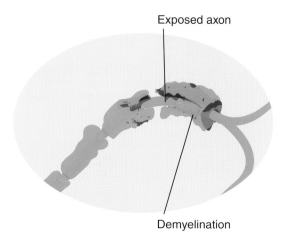

Exposed axon

Demyelination

Illustrated by Shaun Mercier © SAGE Publications

Figure 16.11 Demyelination

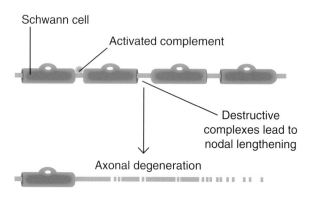

Schwann cell

Activated complement

Destructive complexes lead to nodal lengthening

Axonal degeneration

Illustrated by Shaun Mercier © SAGE Publications

Figure 16.12 Axonal degeneration

In the axonal form (Figure 16.11), IgG and activated complement adhere to the plasma membrane of an axon of motor fibres at the nodes of Ranvier. Complexes that attack the membrane are then formed and result in the destruction of the axon integrity as a result of nodal lengthening (Yuki and Hartung, 2012). *Campylobacter jejuni* (*C. jejuni*) infections are associated with the axonal form in that they are thought to carry substances (lipo-oligosaccharides) that trigger the immune response.

Whether there is axon degeneration or demyelination, the limbs affected will have progressive, ascending muscle weakness that is symmetrical and leads to flaccid paralysis. There may be sensory loss, such as paraesthesia and numbness. Not all paralysis ascends fully up the body but in 30% of people respiratory muscles are affected, requiring ventilatory support. Autonomic involvement can complicate the situation, leading to cardiac arrhythmias, hypotension, urinary retention and diaphoresis (excessive sweating). The condition peaks between 2 and 4 weeks after onset, with a decline in the immune response and the peripheral nerves undergoing endogenous repair (Willison et al., 2016). Remyelination of the peripheral nerve occurs naturally and can fully restore function but axonal regeneration is slow, and potentially irreversible if a large part of the axon is damaged.

Neuromuscular junction disorders

Myasthenia gravis

Myasthenia gravis is an autoimmune disorder with an antibody-mediated reaction at the postsynaptic neuromuscular synapse. There are three distinct forms (Verschuuren, et al. 2013):

- *Antibody obliteration of acetylcholine receptors*: IgG1, IgG3 and anti-acetylcholine receptor antibodies bind complement factors at the postsynaptic membrane, forming a membrane attack complex. Nicotinic acetylcholine receptors are blocked (Figure 16.13), as destroyed or blocked ion channels are prevented from opening in the postsynaptic synapse. This inhibits muscular stimulation and results in fatigue and weakness.
- *Antibody reaction to muscle-specific kinase*: IgG4 antibodies destroy muscle-specific tyrosine kinase, a protein central to normal formation and function of the neuromuscular junction; there is a loss of postsynaptic acetylcholine sensitivity in this form, reducing muscular stimulation as action potentials are being transmitted.
- *Antibody reaction to low-density lipoprotein receptor-related protein 4 (Lrp4)*: Lrp4 has a role in the formation of neuromuscular junctions and is essential in the activation of muscle-specific kinase. In this form of the disease, IgG1 antibodies destroy the Lrp4 with results similar to the second form.

This autoimmune response is largely sporadic, triggered by complex genetic and environmental risk factors; a minority is familial. **Hyperplasia** and neoplasia of the thymus are associated with myasthenia gravis due to the connection between the disease and immunoglobulins (Mestecky, 2013; Verschuuren et al., 2013). Ocular muscles are usually the first affected, followed by generalised muscle weakness (usually proximal muscles more affected in limbs); in the latter half of the condition, speech and respiratory muscles may be affected.

CONGENITAL DISORDERS

Spina bifida

Spina bifida is an open neural tube defect and neuro-developmental disorder that originates during embryogenesis, in the first 30 days after fertilisation (Mohd-Zin et al., 2017). It occurs from

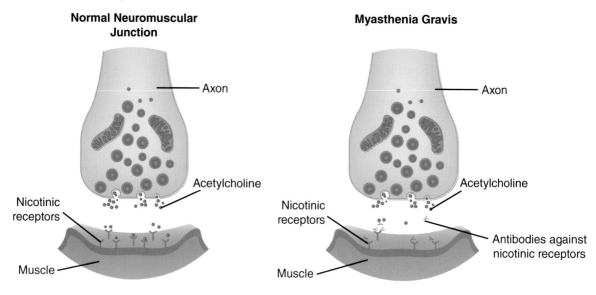

Illustrated by Shaun Mercier © SAGE Publications

Figure 16.13 Blocking of nicotinic receptors in myasthenia gravis

disruption to primary and secondary neurulation (formation of the neural plate). The most severe form (craniorachischisis) occurs when the first fold of the neural plate is disrupted (17–23 days after fertilisation). This results in both the spinal cord and brain being exposed. If disruption to this developmental process occurs between 23 and 26 days after fertilisation, anencephaly occurs; when major portions of the brain, skull and scalp fail to develop. After day 26, disruption to closure of the **caudal neuropore** (the temporary opening at the extreme caudal end of the neural tube) results in a **myelomeningocele**, when failure of closure of the neural tube results in neural tissue exposure, resembling a fluid sac adhered to the back. When there is no neural tissue in the sac, it is called a **meningocele**.

The pathophysiology of this condition is not fully understood, although there are some clear contributing factors that increase risk; most are related to forming nucleic acids, metabolism and exposure to teratogens. Folic acid supplementation can reduce incidence by 70%. Folic acid (folate in its natural form) is central to nucleic acid formation. In addition, homocysteine is **teratogenic** and its level is increased with disruptions in folate metabolism (Mitchell et al., 2004). This is also thought to be how pre-gestational diabetes results in spina bifida and may also be why a raised BMI (above 30) is also a risk. Similarly, low vitamin B$_{12}$ levels are associated with the disease and some anticonvulsant drugs such as valproic acid or carbamazepine are known to be teratogenic, and are implicated in the disease. Smoking is also a known risk factor (Mohd-Zin et al., 2017).

Chiari malformation

Chiari malformation occurs when the cerebellar tonsils descend into the foramen magnum, impairing CSF circulation and affecting cerebellar function (type I malformation: there are four types, Figure 16.14) (Thompson, 2017). While cited as a congenital abnormality, Buell et al. (2015)

highlight that a **foramen magnum decompression** (the removal of sub-occipital bone to increase space and allow CSF to flow) restores pulsatile CSF flow, and therefore disagree that the cause is congenital; they propose that congenital causes would not permit a return of normal CSF flow. The primary causes of a Chiari malformation can be summarised as (Buell et al., 2015):

* Underdevelopment of the bony structures of the posterior fossa
* Tonsillar herniation of the brain as a result of increased intracranial pressure about the foramen magnum
* Cerebellar tonsillar herniation secondary to a drop in spinal intrathecal pressure

This disruption of CSF flow caused by a Chiari malformation may result in formation of a **syrinx**, a CSF-filled sac in either the brain stem or upper spinal cord; syringes (or syrinxes) in these areas are classified as **syringobulbia** and **syringomyelia** respectively. Over time, syringes can expand and compress or destroy the surrounding neural tissue; the goal of treatment is to drain them by shunt to prevent this. This may be implemented alongside repairing the Chiari malformation.

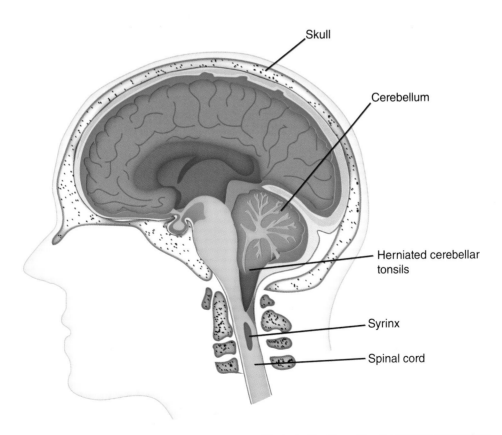

Illustrated by Shaun Mercier © SAGE Publications

Figure 16.14   Chiari malformation

GO DEEPER

Types of Chiari malformations

Type I: Cerebellar tonsillar herniation into the foramen magnum.

Type II: Normally seen in children with hydrocephalus, type II involves both the cerebellum and the brain stem extending into the foramen magnum.

Type III: This is the most severe and rarest form. The cerebellum and brain stem herniate through the foramen magnum and into the spinal cord. It is normally associated with severe neurological impairment.

Type IV: A rare form of Chiari malformation in which there is **cerebellar hypoplasia** (an incomplete or underdeveloped cerebellum).

Cerebral palsy

Cerebral palsy is a group of non-progressive disorders of movement, posture and coordination. It is not always evident at birth, but may become evident over time that the child is not meeting the expected benchmarks of development, e.g. sitting up, walking and having smooth, coordinated movements. Historically, cerebral palsy was largely attributed to a traumatic birth causing hypoxia to the central nervous system. However, despite a six-fold increase in caesarean section births, the incidence of cerebral palsy is unchanged, prompting research into further alternatives. Epidemiological studies demonstrate that causation occurs before labour and it is proposed that hypoxia at birth may exacerbate a pre-existing pathology (MacLennan et al., 2015), if having a role at all. Fourteen percent of cases are possibly due to single-gene mutations. MacLennan et al. (2015) isolated from the literature a variety of risk factors for cerebral palsy:

- Preterm delivery
- Parallel congenital anomaly
- Probable genetic origins
- Intrauterine infection (bacterial and viral)
- Perinatal stroke
- Fetal growth restriction
- Tight nuchal (around the neck) umbilical cord
- Protracted shoulder dystocia
- Placental pathology
- Metabolic disorders

In acknowledging the variety of potential causes of cerebral palsy, it is clear that it is multifactorial and still not fully understood. Marret et al. (2013) highlight that cerebral palsy results from environmental and genetic factors combining to trigger an excitotoxic cascade that disrupts neural development at a vulnerable period during pregnancy. This includes factors resulting in excessive amounts of proinflammatory cytokines and oxidative stress and processes causing a deficiency in maternal growth factor. Essentially, any factor that affects neurological development and impairs movement, posture and coordination may result in this condition; there is also significant variation in presentation and degree of impairment.

CHAPTER SUMMARY

You will now be aware of the complexity of many neurological disorders and how they result in neurological dysfunction. Inflammatory and autoimmune responses feature heavily in these processes. Considering the impact of these disorders on someone's independence, it is easy to see how health-related quality of life can be affected. Understanding the biological basis of these disorders is central to understanding the interventions needed to prevent or treat them, where possible. This understanding is essential for further research for developing more effective treatments. This is a long chapter and this information will be valuable as you meet people with one of the neurological disorders discussed. This is a great opportunity to match the pathophysiology of their condition to their signs and symptoms and their experience of living with the condition. As a person-centred practitioner, it is important to remember that neurological disorders change the life of a person and their family significantly and often for life. Those with degenerative disorders have to cope with deteriorating function and the sense of loss and fear that comes with that. Their families and friends live this experience with them and are equally in need of support. Understanding the conditions leads to better insights into appropriate care and will positively impact on the care received in such challenging times.

KEY POINTS

- Neurological disorders, regardless of origin, have the potential to devastate a person's life and their ability to maintain homeostasis.

- Primary injury is the physical damage that occurs at the time of a trauma, including the microscopic damage that occurs to blood vessels, neurons and neuroglia.

- Secondary injury is the damage that occurs at cellular level resulting from the primary injury, occurs over hours or days and includes ischaemia, hypoxia, infection and raised intracranial pressure.

- The composition of the brain has three main components:
  - blood (10%)
  - CSF (10%)
  - brain tissue (80%)

- An increase in any one of these requires a proportional decrease in one or both of the other two; often this compensation is temporary and cannot be sustained in the long term.

- The location of a brain or spinal injury will determine how it is manifested in signs and symptoms.

- Spasticity is disordered sensorimotor control of the muscles of the body secondary to an upper motor neuron (UMN) lesion, resulting in an intermittent or sustained involuntary activation of those muscles.

- A seizure and epilepsy are not the same thing. A seizure is a single episode of electrical neuronal dysfunction in the brain, resulting in an acute, temporary change in neurological functioning, whereas epilepsy is a seizure disorder characterised by recurrent seizures that occur unprovoked by any systemic or acute neurological event.

- Encephalitis and meningitis are inflammatory diseases of the brain, spinal cord and surrounding structures that are caused by bacterial or viral infections.

- Alzheimer's disease occurs as a result of intracellular neurofibrillary tangles and deposits of extracellular amyloidal (beta) protein, leading to plaque formation in the brain.

- Motor neuron disease (MND) is a selective and progressive functional loss in upper and lower motor neurons, resulting in impairment or loss of motor function; it is associated with neuroglial dysfunction, resulting in neuronal dysfunction because of oxidative stress and excitotoxicity.

- Multiple sclerosis (MS) is a chronic inflammatory, demyelinating disease that has autoimmune characteristics, resulting in destruction of myelin and often the neural axon.

- Guillain–Barré syndrome (GBS) can be caused by either an acute peripheral inflammatory demyelinating polyneuropathy or an acute motor axonal neuropathy.

- Congenital disorders of the nervous system are largely a result of impaired development of the nervous system due to a variety of complex factors including exposure to teratogens, oxidative stress and genetic influences.

REVISE

TEST YOUR KNOWLEDGE

This chapter has introduced you to many neurological disorders and their origins. In order to test your understanding try to answer the questions below.

Answers are available online. If you are using the eBook just click on the answers icon below. Alternatively go to **https://study.sagepub.com/essentialpatho/answers**

1 What type of paralysis occurs in upper motor neuron damage and what happen to muscle tone and size?

2 What type of paralysis occurs in lower motor neuron damage and what happens to muscle tone and size?

3 Identify the different types of multiple sclerosis, their presentation and prognosis.

4 What part of the brain is affected in Parkinson's disease and what is the defect?

5 Briefly describe the two types of abnormal movement that occur in Parkinson's.

6 Briefly describe the stages of tonic–clonic seizures.

7 What is the difference between a seizure and epilepsy?

8 What are the main mechanisms of action of anti-epileptic drugs (AEDs)?

9 What is GABA?

10 What is hydrocephalus?

11 What is meningitis and which type is most dangerous?

12 What cerebrospinal fluid changes occur in meningitis?

13 What is encephalitis?

14 Explain which aspects of the brain control consciousness and how they interrelate.

- Further revision and learning opportunities are available online
- Test yourself away from the book with **Extra multiple choice questions**
- Learn and revise terminology with **Interactive flashcards**

REVISE

**ACE YOUR
ASSESSMENT**

If you are using the eBook access each resource by clicking on the respective icon. Alternatively go to **https://study.sagepub.com/essentialpatho/chapter16**

CHAPTER 16
ANSWERS

EXTRA QUESTIONS

FLASHCARDS

REFERENCES

Allen, B.B., Chiu, Y.L., Gerber, L.M., Ghajar, J. and Greenfield, J.P. (2014) Age-specific cerebral perfusion pressure thresholds and survival in children and adolescents with severe traumatic brain injury. *Pediatric Critical Care Medicine, 15* (1): 62–70.

Ashina, S., Bendtsen, L. and Ashina, M. (2012) Pathophysiology of migraine and tension-type headache. *Techniques in Regional Anesthesia and Pain Management, 16* (1): 14–18.

Barichello, T., Fagundes, G.D., Generoso, J.S., Elias, S.G., Simões, L.R. and Teixeira, A.L. (2013) Pathophysiology of neonatal acute bacterial meningitis. *Journal of Medical Microbiology, 62* (12): 1781–9.

Benevento, B.T. and Sipski, M.L. (2002) Neurogenic bladder, neurogenic bowel, and sexual dysfunction in people with spinal cord injury. *Physical Therapy, 82* (6): 601–12.

Berg, A.T., Berkovic, S.F., Brodie, M.J., Buchhalter, J., Cross, J.H., van Emde Boas, W. et al. (2010) Revised terminology and concepts for organization of seizures and epilepsies: report of the ILAE Commission on Classification and Terminology, 2005–2009. *Epilepsia, 51* (4): 676–85.

Boore, J., Cook, N. and Shepherd, A. (2016) *Essentials of Anatomy and Physiology for Nursing Practice.* London: Sage.

Braine, M.E. (2013) Cluster headache. *British Journal of Neuroscience Nursing, 9* (1): 8–9.

Buell, T.J., Heiss, J.D. and Oldfield, E.H. (2015) Pathogenesis and cerebrospinal fluid hydrodynamics of the Chiari I malformation. *Neurosurgery Clinics of North America, 26* (4): 495–9.

Centers for Disease Control and Prevention (2014) Traumatic brain injury in the United States: Fact sheet. [online]. Available at: www.cdc.gov/traumaticbraininjury/get_the_facts.html (accessed 30 June 2017).

Chin, J.H. and Vora, N. (2014) The global burden of neurologic diseases. *Neurology, 83* (4): 349–51.

Chong, H.T. and Tan, C.T. (2016) Acute viral encephalitis. In R.P. Lisak, D.D. Troung, W.M. Carroll and R. Bhidayasiri (eds), *International Neurology*, 2nd edn. New York: John Wiley & Sons. pp. 305–15.

Correale, J. and Gaitan, M.I. (2015) Multiple sclerosis and environmental factors: the role of vitamin D, parasites, and Epstein–Barr virus infection. *Acta Neurologica Scandinavica, 132* (S199): 46–55.

Dendrou, C.A., Fugger, L. and Friese, M.A. (2015) Immunopathology of multiple sclerosis. *Nature Reviews Immunology, 15* (9): 545–58.

Di Perri, C., Stender, J., Laureys, S. and Gosseries, O. (2014) Functional neuroanatomy of disorders of consciousness. *Epilepsy & Behavior, 30*: 28–32.

Edlmann, E., Giorgi-Coll, S., Whitfield, P.C., Carpenter, K.L. and Hutchinson, P.J. (2017) Pathophysiology of chronic subdural haematoma: inflammation, angiogenesis and implications for pharmacotherapy. *Journal of Neuroinflammation, 14* (1): 108.

Fisher, R.S. (2017) The New Classification of Seizures by the International League Against Epilepsy 2017. *Current Neurology and Neuroscience Reports, 17* (6): 48. Available at: https://link.springer.com/article/10.1007/s11910-017-0758-6.

Fitzgerald, K.C., Munger, K.L., Köchert, K., Arnason, B.G., Comi, G., Cook, S. et al. (2015) Association of vitamin D levels with multiple sclerosis activity and progression in patients receiving interferon beta-1b. *JAMA Neurology, 72* (12): 1458–65.

Greve, M.W. and Zink, B.J. (2009) Pathophysiology of traumatic brain injury. *Mount Sinai Journal of Medicine, 76* (2): 97–104.

Griesdale, D.E., Örtenwall, V., Norena, M., Wong, H., Sekhon, M.S., Kolmodin, L. et al. (2015) Adherence to guidelines for management of cerebral perfusion pressure and outcome in patients who have severe traumatic brain injury. *Journal of Critical Care, 30* (1): 111–15.

Hagen, E.M. (2015) Acute complications of spinal cord injuries. *World Journal of Orthopedics, 6* (1): 17–23.

Henry, T.R. (2012) Seizures and epilepsy: pathophysiology and principles of diagnosis. *Hospital Physician Epilepsy Board Review Manual, 1* (Part 1): 1–26.

Hirsch, E.C., Jenner, P. and Przedborski, S. (2013) Pathogenesis of Parkinson's disease. *Movement Disorders, 28* (1): 24–30.

Huisman, T.A.G.M. and Tschirch, F.T.C. (2009) Epidural hematoma in children: do cranial sutures act as a barrier? *Journal of Neuroradiology, 36* (2): 93–7.

Hunt, R.F., Boychuk, J.A. and Smith, B.N. (2013) Neural circuit mechanisms of post-traumatic epilepsy. *Frontiers in Cellular Neuroscience, 7*: 1–14.

Jain, S., Patel, B. and Bhatt, G.C. (2014) Enteroviral encephalitis in children: clinical features, pathophysiology, and treatment advances. *Pathogens and Global Health, 108* (5): 216–22.

Jazayeri, S.B., Beygi, S., Shokraneh, F., Hagen, E.M. and Rahimi-Movaghar, V. (2015) Incidence of traumatic spinal cord injury worldwide: a systematic review. *European Spine Journal, 24* (5): 905.

Jenkins, B. and Tepper, S.J. (2011) Neurostimulation for primary headache disorders, part 1: pathophysiology and anatomy, history of neuromodulation in headache treatment, and review of peripheral neuromodulation in primary headaches. *Headache, 51* (8): 1254–66.

Johnson, V.E., Stewart, W. and Smith, D.H. (2013) Axonal pathology in traumatic brain injury. *Experimental Neurology, 246*: 35–43.

Keenan, E. (2009) Spasticity management, part 1: an educational approach to person-centred care. *British Journal of Neuroscience Nursing, 5* (6): 260–3.

Kirkman, M.A. and Smith, M. (2014) Intracranial pressure monitoring, cerebral perfusion pressure estimation, and ICP/CPP-guided therapy: a standard of care or optional extra after brain injury? *British Journal of Anaesthesia, 112* (1): 35–46.

Kumar, A. and Singh, A. (2015) A review on Alzheimer's disease pathophysiology and its management: an update. *Pharmacological Reports, 67* (2): 195–203.

Lamar, C.D., Hurley, R.A., Rowland, J.A. and Taber, K.H. (2014) Post-traumatic epilepsy: review of risks, pathophysiology, and potential biomarkers. *Journal of Neuropsychiatry and Clinical Neurosciences, 26* (2): 108–13.

Lee, M., McGeer, E.G. and McGeer, P.L. (2016) Quercetin, not caffeine, is a major neuroprotective component in coffee. *Neurobiology of Aging, 46*: 113–23.

Lin, C.M., Lin, M.C., Huang, S.J., Chang, C.K., Chao, D.P., Lui, T.N. et al. (2015) A prospective randomized study of brain tissue oxygen pressure-guided management in moderate and severe traumatic brain injury patients. *BioMed Research International*, 2015 (Article ID 529580): 1–8.

MacLennan, A.H., Thompson, S.C. and Gecz, J. (2015) Cerebral palsy: causes, pathways, and the role of genetic variants. *American Journal of Obstetrics and Gynecology, 213* (6): 779–88.

Marret, S., Vanhulle, C. and Laquerriere, A. (2013) Pathophysiology of cerebral palsy. *Handbook of Clinical Neurology, 111*: 169–76.

Martini, R.P., Deem, S. and Treggiari, M.M. (2013) Targeting brain tissue oxygenation in traumatic brain injury. *Respiratory Care, 58* (1): 162–72.

Mestecky, A.M. (2013) Myasthenia gravis. *British Journal of Neuroscience Nursing, 9* (3): 110–12.

Mitchell, L.E., Adzick, N.S., Melchionne, J., Pasquariello, P.S., Sutton, L.N. and Whitehead, A.S. (2004) Spina bifida. *The Lancet, 364* (9448): 1885–95.

Modi, N.J., Agrawal, M. and Sinha, V.D. (2016) Post-traumatic subarachnoid hemorrhage: a review. *Neurology India, 64* (7): 8–13.

Mohd-Zin, S.W., Marwan, A.I., Abou Chaar, M.K., Ahmad-Annuar, A. and Abdul-Aziz, N.M. (2017) Spina bifida: pathogenesis, mechanisms, and genes in mice and humans. *Scientifica, 2017*, 1–29. https://doi.org/10.1155/2017/5364827.

Nassar, B.R. and Lippa, C.F. (2016) Idiopathic normal pressure hydrocephalus: a review for general practitioners. *Gerontology and Geriatric Medicine, 2*: 1–6.

Nielsen, N.M., Munger, K.L., Koch-Henriksen, N., Hougaard, D.M., Magyari, M., Jørgensen, K.T. et al. (2017) Neonatal vitamin D status and risk of multiple sclerosis: a population-based case–control study. *Neurology, 88* (1): 44–51.

Omidi, A. and Zargar, F. (2014) Effect of mindfulness-based stress reduction on pain severity and mindful awareness in patients with tension headache: a randomized controlled clinical trial. *Nursing and Midwifery Studies, 3* (3): e21136.

Peeters, W., van den Brande, R., Polinder, S., Brazinova, A., Steyerberg, E.W., Lingsma, H.F. et al. (2015) Epidemiology of traumatic brain injury in Europe. *Acta Neurochirurgica, 157* (10): 1681–96.

Prabhakar, H., Sandhu, K., Bhagat, H., Durga, P. and Chawla, R. (2014) Current concepts of optimal cerebral perfusion pressure in traumatic brain injury. *Journal of Anaesthesiology, Clinical Pharmacology, 30* (3): 318–27.

Prince, M., Bryce, R., Albanese, E., Wimo, A., Ribeiro, W. and Ferri, C.P. (2013) The global prevalence of dementia: a systematic review and metaanalysis. *Alzheimer's & Dementia, 9* (1): 63–75.

Pro, S., Tarantino, S., Capuano, A., Vigevano, F. and Valeriani, M. (2014) Primary headache pathophysiology in children: the contribution of clinical neurophysiology. *Clinical Neurophysiology, 125* (1): 6–12.

Qi, H. and Li, S. (2014) Dose–response meta-analysis on coffee, tea and caffeine consumption with risk of Parkinson's disease. *Geriatrics & Gerontology International, 14* (2): 430–9.

Royal College of Physicians (2015) *Prolonged Disorders of Consciousness: National Clinical Guidelines – Report of a Working Party 2013*. London: RCP.

Sabalys, G., Juodzbalys, G. and Wang, H.L. (2012) Aetiology and pathogenesis of trigeminal neuralgia: a comprehensive review. *Journal of Oral and Maxillofacial Research*, *3* (4)e2: 1–12.

Schlunk, F. and Greenberg, S.M. (2015) The pathophysiology of intracerebral hemorrhage formation and expansion. *Translational Stroke Research*, *6* (4): 257–63.

Schulz-Schaeffer, W.J. (2015) Is cell death primary or secondary in the pathophysiology of idiopathic Parkinson's disease? *Biomolecules*, *5* (3): 1467–79.

Scottish Intercollegiate Guidelines Network (SIGN) (2008) *Diagnosis and Management of Headache in Adults*. Clinical guideline 107. Edinburgh: SIGN.

Seifert, T. and Shipman, V. (2015) The pathophysiology of sports concussion. *Current Pain and Headache Reports*, *19* (8): 36.

Siedler, D.G., Chuah, M.I., Kirkcaldie, M.T., Vickers, J.C. and King, A.E. (2014) Diffuse axonal injury in brain trauma: insights from alterations in neurofilaments. *Frontiers in Cellular Neuroscience*, *8*: 429.

Simola, N., Pinna, A., Frau, L. and Morelli, M. (2014) Protective agents in Parkinson's disease: caffeine and adenosine A2A receptor antagonists. In R. Kostrzewa (ed.), *Handbook of Neurotoxicity*. New York: Springer. pp. 2281–98.

Souza, P.V.S.D., Pinto, W.B.V.D.R., Rezende Filho, F.M. and Oliveira, A.S.B. (2016) Far beyond the motor neuron: the role of glial cells in amyotrophic lateral sclerosis. *Arquivos de neuro-psiquiatria*, *74* (10): 849–54.

Sprenger, T. and Goadsby, P.J. (2010) What has functional neuroimaging done for primary headache … and for the clinical neurologist? *Journal of Clinical Neuroscience*, *17* (5): 547–53.

Stafstrom, C.E. and Carmant, L. (2015) Seizures and epilepsy: an overview for neuroscientists. *Cold Spring Harbor Perspectives in Medicine*, *5* (6): a022426.

Surmeier, D.J. (2014) *Glutamate Signaling and Mitochondrial Dysfunction in Models of Parkinson's Disease*. Chicago, IL: North Western University.

Swann, J. (2011) Motor neurone disease: research, treatment and care. *British Journal of Neuroscience Nursing*, *5* (5): 229–33.

Teasdale, G. and Jennett, B. (1974) Assessment of coma and impaired consciousness: a practical scale. *Lancet*, *2*: 81–4.

Thompson, S. (2017) An introduction to hydrocephalus: types, treatments and management. *British Journal of Neuroscience Nursing*, *13* (1): 36–40.

Tunkel, A.R., Glaser, C.A., Bloch, K.C., Sejvar, J.J., Marra, C.M., Roos, K.L. et al. (2008) The management of encephalitis: clinical practice guidelines by the Infectious Diseases Society of America. *Clinical Infectious Diseases*, *47* (3): 303–27.

Verschuuren, J.J., Huijbers, M.G., Plomp, J.J., Niks, E.H., Molenaar, P.C., Martinez-Martinez, P. et al. (2013) Pathophysiology of myasthenia gravis with antibodies to the acetylcholine receptor, muscle-specific kinase and low-density lipoprotein receptor-related protein 4. *Autoimmunity Reviews*, *12* (9): 918–23.

Vucic, S., Rothstein, J.D. and Kiernan, M.C. (2014) Advances in treating amyotrophic lateral sclerosis: insights from pathophysiological studies. *Trends in Neurosciences*, *37* (8): 433–42.

Ward-Abel, N. and Burgoyne, T. (2008) The importance of the immune response in multiple sclerosis, part 1: pathophysiology. *British Journal of Neuroscience Nursing*, *4* (5): 212–17.

White, S. and Easton, A. (2008) Encephalitis: the broader spectrum. *British Journal of Neuroscience Nursing*, *4* (3): 131–2.

Wilensky, E.M., Bloom, S., Leichter, D., Verdiramo, A.M., Ledwith, M., Stiefel, M. et al. (2005) Brain tissue oxygen practice guidelines using the LICOX (R) CMP monitoring system. *Journal of Neuroscience Nursing*, *37* (5): 278–88.

Willison, H.J., Jacobs, B.C. and Van Doorn, P.A. (2016) Guillain–Barré syndrome. *The Lancet*, *388* (10045): 717–27.

World Health Organisation (WHO) (2005) *Neurological Disorders: Public Health Challenges.* Geneva: WHO.

World Health Organisation (WHO) (2015) *World Report on Ageing and Health.* Geneva: WHO.

Xu, W., Tan, L., Wang, H.F., Jiang, T., Tan, M.S., Tan, L. et al. (2015) Meta-analysis of modifiable risk factors for Alzheimer's disease. *Journal of Neurology, Neurosurgery and Psychiatry, 86* (12): 1299–306.

Yilmazlar, S., Kocaeli, H., Dogan, S., Abas, F., Aksoy, K., Korfali, E. et al. (2005) Traumatic epidural haematomas of nonarterial origin: analysis of 30 consecutive cases. *Acta Neurochirurgica, 147* (12): 1241–8.

Yuki, N. and Hartung, H.P. (2012) Guillain–Barré syndrome. *New England Journal of Medicine, 366* (24): 2294–304.

Zakrzewska, J.M. and McMillan, R. (2011) Trigeminal neuralgia: the diagnosis and management of this excruciating and poorly understood facial pain. *Postgraduate Medical Journal, 87* (1028): 410–16.

DISORDERS OF ENDOCRINE REGULATION

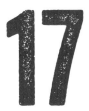

17

UNDERSTAND: CHAPTER VIDEOS

Watch the following videos to ease you into this chapter. If you are using the eBook just click on the play buttons. Alternatively go to **https://study.sagepub.com/essentialpatho/videos**

ENDOCRINE SYSTEM 1 (9:36)

ENDOCRINE SYSTEM 2 (5:07)

REVISE: A&P RECAP

The endocrine system

You will find it helpful to review the content of Chapter 7 in *Essentials of Anatomy and Physiology for Nursing Practice* (Boore et al., 2016) to refresh your knowledge of the endocrine system.

LEARNING OUTCOMES

When you have finished studying this chapter you will be able to:

1. Understand the disorders affecting the major organs of regulation of the endocrine system, i.e. the hypothalamus and the pituitary gland.
2. Recognise the implications of disordered function of the adrenal cortex.
3. Understand the effects of disordered adrenal medullary function and its relationship to the sympathetic branch of the autonomic nervous system.

Disorders of some hormone functions are considered in the following chapters of this book:

Chapter 11. Disorders of Fluid, Electrolyte and Acid–Base Balance and Urine Elimination
Chapter 13. Disorders of Metabolism (thyroid hormones)
Chapter 16. Disorders of Neurological Control
Chapter 18. Disorders of the Female Reproductive System
Chapter 19. Disorders of the Male Reproductive System

INTRODUCTION

In this chapter, you will consider disorders of endocrine regulation of bodily functions. This will build on earlier chapters in this book and links to later chapters (see above); it will examine the cause and effects of the major disorders of the endocrine system. In this chapter, we are dealing with growth hormone and hormones of the adrenal gland. Additionally, you will also consider the emotional/psychological and social implications of such pathophysiological changes, a central component of person-centred nursing. Adequate endocrine function is crucial throughout the different stages of life and the Bodie family give some good examples of how endocrine regulation adjusts function and how altered secretion can alter physiology.

—— PERSON-CENTRED CONTEXT: THE BODIE FAMILY ——

BODIE FAMILY
CASE NOTES

Throughout life, changes in endocrine function alter the rate of growth and development. As a baby and throughout childhood, Danielle is and will continue growing under the influence of growth hormone (somatotrophin) secreted from the anterior pituitary gland until puberty. She will pass through two periods of accelerated growth, the first before and shortly after birth (the infant growth spurt) and the second (the adolescent growth spurt) taking place around puberty, a few years earlier in girls than boys (generally resulting in women being shorter than men) (Cooke et al., 2011). Growth can be inhibited by **stress**, as occurred with Michelle due to illness when she was 10, resulting in her height being two inches shorter than her identical twin sister, Margaret.

A number of changes occur during later stages of life, many of which are related to endocrinological alterations. The menopause is diagnosed retrospectively by 12 months of **amenorrhoea** and can occur at varying ages; around 50 years is not uncommon. It is the period of life during which reduced secretion of ovarian hormones occurs and causes reduced activity of the female reproductive system and infertility. During this stage a number of unpleasant symptoms may occur, including hot flushes, depression and urogenital disturbances. Hormone replacement therapy (HRT) can reduce these symptoms; Sarah has recently stopped taking HRT after 2½ years and Hannah is still applying HRT patches. Lamberts (2011) noted that there are comparable endocrine changes that occur in men during the andropause.

It is also common for the bones of older adults to become frailer with the chance of developing osteoporosis (see Chapter 10) due to the reduced secretion of growth hormone and hormones involved in calcium metabolism. This can result in vertebral compression due to micro-fractures and curving of the thoracic vertebrae, causing a dowager's hump. Maud is now about two inches shorter than she used to be. In addition, thyroid dysfunction, resulting in a reduction in thyroid hormones (**hypothyroidism**, see Chapter 13), is relatively common in elderly people and Maud has been diagnosed with hypothyroidism and is receiving treatment with Levothyroxine, a manufactured form of thyroxine. She is in generally good health.

Hormones from the adrenal cortex are secreted as part of the stress response and Richard suffered from stress in the past, treated by cognitive behavioural therapy. This illustrates the link between physiological and psychological functioning. However, these hormones are also important in the treatment of allergic conditions, as with Derek who uses a steroid inhaler to control his asthma symptoms.

Concerning Thomas, the airline pilot, the secretion of melatonin from the pineal gland is important in regulating his **circadian rhythm** and enabling him to function fully in carrying out his role (Low, 2011).

DISORDERS OF THE HYPOTHALAMUS AND PITUITARY GLAND

We will now go on to consider what can go wrong with the major control centres of the endocrine system. The activity of the pituitary gland is controlled by the **hypothalamus** and thus disorders of the hypothalamus often present as altered function of the pituitary gland.

ACTIVITY 17.1 UNDERSTAND

Central regulation of endocrine

Watch the following video for a review of the normal central regulation of the endocrine system. If you are using the eBook just click on the play button. Alternatively go to

https://study.sagepub.com/essentialpatho/videos

(▷)

ENDOCRINE REGULATION (6:34)

The disorders that occur are due to increased pituitary secretion (**hyperpituitarism**) or decreased pituitary secretion (**hypopituitarism**). The pituitary gland is, in reality, two glands – anterior and posterior, but only anterior pituitary hormones are dealt with here. Disordered secretion from the posterior pituitary gland is considered elsewhere:

* Anti-diuretic hormone (ADH) in Chapter 11
* Oxytocin in Chapter 18

Hyperpituitarism

The most common cause of hyperpituitarism is an **adenoma** (-oma implies a benign growth derived from the tissue indicated by the first part of the name) in the anterior pituitary gland. It is a neoplasm (i.e. a new growth) derived from epithelial glandular tissue resulting in a benign **tumour**. Other causes include **hyperplasia** and malignant tumours of the anterior pituitary, hormonal secretion by tumours elsewhere in the body, or **lesions** in the hypothalamus (Melmed and Kleinberg, 2011).

Pituitary adenomas

Pituitary adenomas may vary in size from small (microadenomas, <1 cm size) to large (macroadenomas, >1 cm size) and can erode the bone and other tissues surrounding the pituitary gland and result in compression of the optic chiasma (where the optic nerves cross over), thereby impairing vision. The signs and symptoms that may occur are due to functional tissue which secretes the hormones normally produced by the type of cells forming the adenoma, and non-functional tissue which has effects due to pressure caused by expansion of the growth (Porth, 2015) (see Table 17.1).

Table 17.1 Signs and symptoms of anterior pituitary adenomas

Endocrine abnormalities	*Lactotrophic adenoma*: Prolactin producing. Inhibits **luteinising hormone** secretion and thus ovulation, causing **amenorrhoea**, **galactorrhoea**, infertility in women. In men, vague symptoms including impotence and loss of libido
	Somatotrophic adenoma: Growth hormone-secreting (see below)
	Corticotrophic adenoma: Stimulates ACTH secretion and increases secretion of **cortisol** from adrenal cortex (see below)
	Less common:
	Gonadotrophic adenoma: LH and FSH secretion. Less easy to diagnose
	Thyrotrophic adenoma: Rare cause of **hyperthyroidism**
Mass effects of expansion	Pressure on optic nerves and chiasma cause abnormalities of visual field
	Expanding mass leads to increased intracranial pressure, causing: headache, **nausea** and **vomiting**
	Further expansion can lead to: **seizures** and obstructive **hydrocephalus**
	Acute haemorrhage into adenoma produces rapid enlargement of pituitary

Prolactinomas are the most common form of pituitary tumours (more common in women than in men); they are non-malignant and produce prolactin. The effects are due to excessive prolactin or pressure on the surrounding tissues (Table 17.1). As prolactin influences milk production, it is to be expected that such a growth has significant effects during pregnancy. Treatment aims to:

* return prolactin secretion to normal levels
* reduce the size of the pituitary tumour and restore normal function
* eliminate the effects of tumour pressure, such as headaches or vision problems
* improve quality of life.

GO DEEPER

Prolactinomas

A prolactinoma can result in infertility and changes in menstruation, as well as disturbed vision. It is diagnosed by measuring prolactin levels and carrying out an MRI (magnetic resonance imaging) scan to determine the presence of a pituitary tumour. It can be treated medically and/or surgically. Medications include bromocriptine and cabergoline (NIH, 2012), which decrease prolactin production and may shrink the tumour.

A small prolactinoma may not disrupt a pregnancy. A woman aiming to become pregnant is usually advised to stop taking medications as their safety for the fetus is not yet clear. The woman will be monitored carefully as a large prolactinoma may grow up to 30% and cause symptoms including headaches, visual changes, nausea and vomiting, thirst and excessive urination, or lethargy (Mayo Clinic, 2018a).

Hypopituitarism

Hypopituitarism refers to decreased secretion of the pituitary hormones due to either hypothalamic or pituitary dysfunction, with most cases involving the anterior pituitary gland. There is a deficiency of growth hormone (GH), **luteinising hormone** (LH), **follicle stimulating hormone** (FSH), **adrenocorticotrophic hormone** (ACTH), thyroid stimulating hormone (TSH) and **antidiuretic hormone** (ADH). Deficiencies of these hormones have far-reaching consequences on the body's ability to maintain normal function and thus homeostasis. The range of possible causes are indicated in Table 17.2.

Table 17.2   Causes of hypopituitarism

Tumours and other masses	Adenomas and other benign and malignant lesions can cause damage by pressure on adjacent cells
Traumatic brain injury and **subarachnoid haemorrhage**	Most common causes, damage and pressure cause pituitary hypofunction
Pituitary **surgery** or radiation	Surgery can extend beyond growth and radiation and can damage non-adenomatous tissue
Pituitary apoplexy (haemorrhage into pituitary gland)	A neurosurgical emergency. Sudden haemorrhage causes severe headache, diplopia, hypopituitarism, cardiovascular collapse, unconsciousness, sudden death
Ischaemic **necrosis** of pituitary and **Sheehan syndrome**	Anterior pituitary enlarges to twice its size during pregnancy Without increase in blood supply there is relative **hypoxia** Ischaemic area is reabsorbed and replaced by fibrous tissue
Rathke cleft cyst	These cysts can accumulate protein-rich fluid and expand, compromising the normal gland
Empty sella **syndrome**	Any condition/treatment destroying part of gland leads to empty sella or a mass enlarges sella and removal or **infarction** leads to reduced function of pituitary gland
Hypothalamic conditions	Hypothalamic lesions can interfere with hypothalamic hormones
Inflammatory disorders and infections	e.g. Sarcoidosis or tuberculous **meningitis** of hypothalamus can cause deficiencies in pituitary hormones
Genetic defects	**Congenital** deficiencies in factors for normal pituitary function is a rare cause of hypopituitarism

Growth disorders

Growth disorders fall into two main groups – reduced growth and increased growth – and can occur in adults or children.

Short stature in children

Short stature in children can be due to a range of different factors, indicated in Table 17.3. In most of these, there will be a diminished secretion of hormones that influence growth. Those with this condition are described as being of restricted growth (dwarfism – a term that is considered politically incorrect by many), which may be:

* proportionate, in which the different parts of the body are in proportion to each other; occurs in growth hormone deficiency (used to be known as pituitary dwarfism), or

- disproportionate, in which the parts of the body are not in proportion, for example in **achondroplasia**:
  1. The trunk is normal length but the long bones of the extremities are short.
  2. The head is large with flat nasal bridge and prominent forehead.
  3. Hands and feet are short and wide.
  4. Fingers and toes are short.

Table 17.3   Causes of short stature

Endocrine disorders	Growth hormone deficiency or inactivity
	Hypothyroidism
	Diabetes mellitus (poorly controlled)
	Corticosteroid excess (**Cushing's syndrome**)
Genetic factors	Chromosomal abnormalities, e.g. Turner syndrome; Down syndrome
	Skeletal disorders, e.g. achondroplasia
Medical conditions and treatment	**Chronic illnesses**, e.g. renal disease, **asthma**, heart disease
	Malabsorption syndrome
	Corticosteroid treatment
	Nutritional deprivation
Small at birth	Familial short stature (genetic influence) within normal limits; growth delay
	Growth retarded due to uterine conditions
Psychosocial factors	Early life deprivation
	Institutional deprivation/emotional deprivation

Source: Adapted from Johnson et al., 2010; Krishna et al., 2015

Growth hormone (GH) or insulin-like growth factor 1 (IGF-1) deficiency

GH or IGF-1 deficiencies may be due to a variety of causes. Idiopathic GH deficiency is when growth hormone releasing hormone (GHRH) normally formed and secreted from the hypothalamus is missing, but the somatotropes (GH-secreting cells) in the pituitary gland are present and functioning. However, a child may have some condition (e.g. a tumour or pituitary tissue without somatotropes) resulting in lack of growth hormone secretion.

Babies with congenital GH deficiency are short at birth and grow slowly. The signs and symptoms are:

- Proportionate restricted growth
- Normal intelligence
- **Obesity** and immature facial features
- Delayed maturation of skeletal system
- Delayed puberty and males may have a small penis
- In the newborn, **hypoglycaemia** can result in seizures

Growth hormone deficiency (GHD) in adults

In adults, there are two groups of GH deficiencies: those that continue from childhood and those that develop in adult life from, for example, a pituitary tumour or its treatment, causing hypopituitarism. GH deficiency can also occur in elderly people. Other conditions have been identified as causes of GH deficiency, including traumatic brain injury (Klose and Feldt-Rasmussen, 2015).

Anti-pituitary antibodies (APA) at high titres have been found in the blood of rare individuals with apparently idiopathic GHD; this may indicate an autoimmune involvement with the pituitary (De Bellis et al., 2016).

The effects of GHD in adults are primarily metabolic, affecting body composition including: reduced lean body mass, hyperlipidaemia, a fall in bone density, reduced exercise ability and well-being. The effects are similar to **metabolic syndrome** (Attanasio et al., 2010), associated with diabetes mellitus and discussed in Chapter 13. In addition, a link between GHD and a diminution in cognitive ability has been demonstrated and GH treatment has a beneficial effect (Falleti et al., 2006). GHD in adults is treated with long-term GH replacement which improves the bone and metabolic disturbances as well as enhancing the quality of life (Jørgensen et al., 2011).

Gender differences in GH and IGF-1 occur, with females producing about three times as much GH as men, although IGF-I is similar; it appears that women are less responsive to GH than men. In treating adults with GHD, this difference needs to be taken into account (Span et al., 2000).

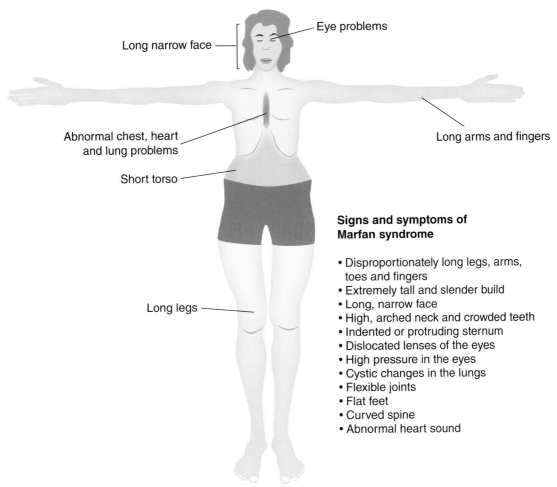

Long narrow face —
Eye problems

Abnormal chest, heart and lung problems

Long arms and fingers

Short torso —

Long legs —

Long legs

Signs and symptoms of Marfan syndrome

- Disproportionately long legs, arms, toes and fingers
- Extremely tall and slender build
- Long, narrow face
- High, arched neck and crowded teeth
- Indented or protruding sternum
- Dislocated lenses of the eyes
- High pressure in the eyes
- Cystic changes in the lungs
- Flexible joints
- Flat feet
- Curved spine
- Abnormal heart sound

Illustrated by Shaun Mercier © SAGE Publications

Figure 17.1 Marfan syndrome

Growth hormone excess in children

People can only become excessively tall if their bones grow faster and further than in their peers. Growth in height will stop when the epiphyses of the long bones, where bone growth takes place, fuse.

Children can become excessively tall for a few main reasons:

- Constitutional tall stature: children with particularly tall parents tend to be taller than other children.
- Genetic causes: Marfan syndrome (Figure 17.1) is an autosomal dominant condition which results in very tall individuals.

Excessive GH secretion before puberty and fusion of epiphyses of the long bones cause the development of gigantism. This condition is uncommon because the causative adenoma is usually recognised and treated early.

ACTIVITY 17.2: APPLY

Acromegaly in practice

Watch these two videos. The first video summarises **acromegaly** and approaches to treatment. The second one indicates how someone lives with this condition. If you are using the eBook just click on the play button. Alternatively go to **https://study.sagepub.com/essentialpatho/videos**

$\triangleright$

$\triangleright$

WHAT IS ACROMEGALY?
(2:38)

LIVING WITH
ACROMEGALY (3:29)

GO DEEPER

Gigantism

This video shows an example of gigantism: 'World's TALLEST MAN to have ever lived! (Robert Pershing Wadlow)'. If you are using the eBook just click on the play button. Alternatively go to **https://study.sagepub.com/essentialpatho/videos**

In October 2016 BBC NI News reported that an area in Northern Ireland had been identified as a 'giant hotspot' by scientists studying a gene defect which causes people to grow abnormally tall. One in 150 people in Mid Ulster carry the gene, compared to one in 1,000 in Belfast and one in 2,000 in the rest of the UK. The gene (*AIP*, but known as the 'giant gene') can result in too much growth hormone, produced and released by the pituitary gland. The excessive production occurs from a non-**cancer**ous tumour in the gland. The study found the genetic **mutation** in more than 400 people, and at least 15 families in Northern Ireland are carriers. According to Dr Steven Hunter, an endocrinologist at the Royal Victoria Hospital in Belfast, only 20% of carriers will develop symptoms:

'It can present with tall stature and people growing excessively tall at a young age. It can cause problems with growth of hands and feet in older people and is related to headaches because of the growing tumour in the brain and affects eyesight. We've seen people with other hormonal problems and infertility. It can be life-threatening, but is often disfiguring.'

There are effective treatments and the emphasis is on early diagnosis.

The gene caused Charles Byrne, born in 1761 near Cookstown and known as the 'Irish giant', to grow to more than 7 ft 6 in (2.3 m) tall. He became an object of curiosity after travelling to London to seek his fortune before his death in 1783. Mr Byrne and the living carriers of the gene shared a common ancestor who lived about 2,500 years ago. Brendan Holland, from Dungannon, who is 6 ft 9 in (2.1 m) tall and a distant relative of Byrne, told the BBC:

'It may not please the romantic in some people, but those afflicted with this condition probably won't object to the end of it. I've been lucky, I've been cured and had the best treatment available. My mother passed the gene to me and she never knew that and many people still are passing the gene on without knowing.'

Belfast clinical genetics consultant Professor Patrick Morrison said most people believe the giants are 'very fit and athletic and would make great basketball players', but 'it's a miserable life for a giant, actually. If you're nearly 7 ft (2.1 m) in height your heart doesn't work so well, you can have **heart failure**. Your pituitary gland can cause vision problems, you're actually quite weak. Maybe by your mid to late 20s you've a lot of problems and a lot of these giants will die in their late 20s if not treated.'

The research into the population screening in Mid Ulster was led by Marta Korbonits, Professor of Endocrinology at Barts and the London School of Medicine Queen Mary. She discovered the genetic link for the mutation of the Irish giant gene. The scientists hope their work will help to identify those at risk of passing on the gene and lead to earlier diagnosis.

Source: Adapted from Fowler, 2016

GIGANTISM (3:18)

Precocious puberty

Central precocious puberty is the early activation of the hypothalamic–pituitary–gonadal axis. It causes the same effects as normal puberty, resulting in the development of secondary sexual characteristics and fertility, but before 8 years in girls and 9 years in boys. The cause is unclear but may be due to malformation or cerebral damage, or genetic abnormalities (Latronico et al., 2016).

Indications of puberty differ between boys and girls (NHS Choices, 2016):

- Girls: average age for girls to start puberty is 11, between 8 and 13. Breast development and the menarche (first menstrual periods) begin.
- Boys: average age is 12, between 9 and 14, development of a larger penis and testicles, a deeper voice and a more muscular appearance.

Early or delayed puberty could indicate an underlying condition needing treatment but it may just run in the family. However, it may be caused by:

- a brain disorder, e.g. a tumour
- brain trauma due to infection, surgery or **radiotherapy**
- some abnormality of the ovaries or thyroid gland
- a genetic disorder.

Early puberty is more common in girls, whilst in boys it is more likely to be associated with an underlying problem. To achieve a diagnosis, measurement of blood hormone levels, a hand X-ray (to help to predict adult height) and an MRI scan (to check for tumours) are all required. Early puberty can be managed, if it is likely to cause physical or psychological problems, by treating any underlying cause and prescribing medication to put puberty on hold for a few years by reducing hormone levels.

Growth hormone excess in adults

Secretion of GH excess continuing after fusion of the epiphyses of the long bones results in acromegaly. As growth of the long bones occurs at the epiphyseal cartilage between the main long bones and the ends where the joints are between bones, growth in length cannot happen after the cartilage has become ossified and can no longer grow. However, growth of the ends of the long bones continues and the extremities become enlarged. This is a condition that develops slowly, usually due to GH secreting adenoma at around 40–45 years, and often takes some time to be diagnosed. The signs and symptoms fall into a number of groups and may vary somewhat between individuals (Chapman, 2017):

- Enlarged tissues:
  - Enlargement of small bones of the hands and feet results in needing larger shoe sizes, and having problems with wearing rings.
  - Nerve entrapment, e.g. carpal tunnel syndrome, can lead to the development of paraesthesia.

- Increased growth of other bones can cause various changes:
  - Vertebral changes leading to **kyphosis** (hunchback), degenerative **arthritis** (**inflammation** of joints) and **arthralgia** (joint pain) of the spine, hips and knees, leading to pain and limited joint mobility.
  - Soft tissues continue to grow, causing characteristic enlarged facial features, including an enlarged nose, thickened lips, teeth that develop increased space between them and outward inclination, and a protruding lower jaw and brow. The skin often becomes coarse, oily and thickened.
  - Larynx and respiratory tract enlargement leads to a deepened, husky voice with some obstruction of the upper airway, sometimes causing snoring and sleep apnoea.
  - Most bodily organs increase in size and an enlarged heart and related **atherosclerosis** can lead to early death. There is an enlarged tongue, enlarged liver, heart, kidneys, spleen and other organs. The chest size increases, causing barrel chest.

- Metabolic disturbances involving altered fat and carbohydrate **metabolism**, often causing fatigue and muscle weakness:
  - Increased level of free fatty acids released from adipose tissue into body fluids and moderate weight gain.
  - Disturbed glucose metabolism includes reduced uptake into muscle and adipose tissues, resulting in increased glucose release from the liver and increased insulin secretion. In addition, insulin resistance can lead to impaired glucose tolerance and diabetes mellitus. The incidence of diabetes mellitus is significantly higher in those with acromegaly (Dreval et al., 2014). Those patients with acromegaly and diabetes are reported as having a higher incidence of malignancy and reduced survival (Wen-Ko et al., 2016).

- Other changes:
  - Excessive sweating and unpleasant body odour, oily skin and heat intolerance may occur.
  - Endocrine disturbances may lead to a decreased libido and menstrual irregularities in women or **erectile dysfunction** in men.
  - Headaches and impaired vision (in particular, hemianopia, i.e. loss of half the visual field) may occur due to pressure on the optic chiasm/chiasma from the growing tumour.

Management of someone with this condition aims to correct any metabolic disturbances, and, if possible, remove the tumour or minimise its effect by radiation (Mayo Clinic, 2018b, 2018c).

DISORDERS OF THE ADRENAL GLAND

The two adrenal glands are positioned on the top of the two kidneys. In essence, each adrenal gland consists of two glands, the adrenal cortex and adrenal medulla, which are functionally quite distinct.

REVISE: A&P RECAP

The adrenal glands

The structure and function of the adrenal glands can be revised from Chapter 7, The Endocrine System, in *Essentials of Anatomy and Physiology for Nursing Practice* (Boore et al., 2016). Figure 7.7 may be particularly helpful.

The adrenal cortex

The different layers of the adrenal cortex produce three types of hormones, although all are **corticosteroids** (i.e. derived from **cholesterol**, composed of a steroid nucleus but with various additions):

*   **Zona glomerulosa** (outer layer) produces primarily mineralocorticoids (mainly aldosterone) controlling fluid and electrolyte balance.
*   **Zona fasciculata**, and to a lesser extent **zona reticularis**, produce **glucocorticoids** (principally cortisol) involved in glucose metabolism.
*   Zona fasciculata produces sex hormones (oestrogens and **androgens**).

The disorders of the adrenal cortex fall into two main groups: hyperfunction and hypofunction (Maitra, 2015).

Adrenocortical hyperfunction

Adrenocortical hyperfunction results in the hypersecretion of the three types of corticosteroid hormones.

Cushing's syndrome (hypercorticalism)

This condition results from elevated levels of glucocorticosteroid hormones. The majority are exogenous (**iatrogenic**) in nature, occurring due to medical intervention with corticosteroid hormones which may be used in the treatment of a number of different conditions (Decani et al., 2014).

Table 17.4 Cushing's syndrome: endogenous causes

Cause	Relative frequency	Ratio F to M
ACTH-dependent		
Cushing disease (ACTH-secreting pituitary tumour)	70	3.5 : 1
Secretion of ectopic ACTH by non-pituitary tumours	10	1 : 1
ACTH-independent		
Adrenal adenoma	10	4 : 1
Adrenal carcinoma	5	1 : 1
Other uncommon causes of hyperplasia	<2 each	1 : 1

Long-term corticosteroid treatment, or frequent short courses of such therapy, can result in suppression of the **hypothalamic–pituitary–adrenal (HPA) axis** and will require careful management (Stewart and Krone, 2011). People taking large enough doses to cause HPA suppression will develop iatrogenic Cushing's syndrome in 3–4 weeks (Hopkins and Leinung, 2005).

Endogenous Cushing's syndrome falls into two categories, ACTH-dependent and ACTH-independent, with examples shown in Table 17.4.

Those affected with Cushing's syndrome tend to gain weight and develop **hypertension** early in development of the condition with additional signs and symptoms developing later (Figure 17.2). These may include:

- Altered fat metabolism, resulting in obesity/weight gain, protruding abdomen with the appearance of stretch marks, buffalo hump on the shoulders, rounded (moon) face
- Increased protein breakdown, causing muscle weakness, thinning of the limbs with muscle wasting
- Alterations in calcium metabolism and bone proteins, leading to osteoporosis that may cause back pain, compression of vertebrae (Dowager's hump), rib **fractures** and possibly the development of renal calculi
- Disturbed glucose metabolism, sometimes resulting in diabetes mellitus
- Increased gastric acid secretion
- **Hirsutism** (excessive body hair in men; in women there is excessive hair on parts of the body where hair is normally absent or minimal, e.g. the chin, chest, face), mild acne, menstrual irregularities, decreased libido
- Inflammatory and immune responses are inhibited, bruising
- Mental health changes, ranging from mild euphoria to psychosis

Increased cortisol secretion is central to the diagnosis, but the normal circadian rhythm may be disrupted so that overnight levels are particularly high.

ACTIVITY 17.3: APPLY

Living with Cushing's syndrome

Watch the following video to gain insight into the lived experience of someone with Cushing's syndrome. If you are using the eBook just click on the play button. Alternatively go to
https://study.sagepub.com/essentialpatho/videos

CUSHING'S SYNDROME (4:19)

Hyperaldosteronism

Hyperaldosteronism is excess secretion of mineralocorticoids due to aldosterone-secreting adenomas or hyperplasia (an enlargement of tissues due to increased cellular reproduction). Hypertension is the main change, which occurs due to increased sodium reabsorption which retains water, resulting in expansion of the extracellular fluid volume and thus raising **cardiac output. Hypokalaemia** also often occurs, leading to weakness, paraesthesia and visual disturbances (Maitra, 2015).

The three main (primary) causes are:

- Bilateral idiopathic **hyperaldosteronism**: commonest cause and those affected tend to be older and have less severe hypertension than those with neoplasms.

- Adrenocortical neoplasm: can be benign (adenoma) or malignant (carcinoma). Conn syndrome is when the person affected has a single aldosterone-secreting adenoma. Multiple adenomas occur occasionally.
- Glucocorticoid-remediable hyperaldosteronism: uncommon cause of familial condition.

In secondary hyperaldosteronism, aldosterone is secreted in response to the **renin**–angiotensin system (see Chapter 11).

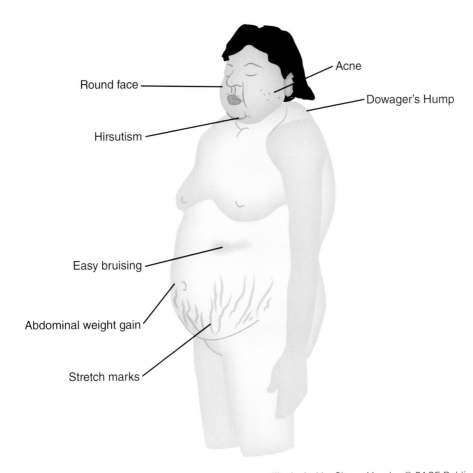

Illustrated by Shaun Mercier © SAGE Publications

Figure 17.2   Signs and symptoms of Cushing's syndrome

Adrenogenital syndromes (congenital adrenal hyperplasia)

These are caused by a number of different autosomal recessive conditions in which there is a deficiency in one of the enzymes involved in the formation of corticosteroids. This results in a redirection of the normal pathway and leads to an increased secretion of androgens. Signs and symptoms may occur early or later depending on the specific nature of the disorder. For example, females may show signs of masculinisation (clitoral **hypertrophy** and other indicators of male genitalia) as infants, or **oligomenorrhea** (infrequent or very light menstruation), hirsutism (unwanted, male-pattern hair growth in women) and acne after puberty. Males may show precocious puberty. Ambiguous genitalia should lead to investigations for these conditions. These disorders of the secretion of androgens (male sex hormones) are more commonly due to carcinomas than adenomas.

There are three main disturbances which occur, shown in Table 17.5.

Table 17.5 Adrenogenital syndromes

Salt-wasting syndrome	A block in synthesis of mineralocorticoids and deficient cortisol secretion. Leads to salt wasting, **hyponatraemia** and hyperkalaemia, resulting in **acidosis**, hypotension and cardiovascular collapse (possibly death)
	Females – recognised at birth, males – at 5–15 days
Simple virilising adrenogenital syndrome without salt wasting	Enough mineralocorticoids to prevent salt wasting. Lack of ACTH feedback leads to increased level of testosterone. Progressive virilisation occurs
Non-classic or late onset adrenal virilism	Only a partial deficiency, thus mild symptoms occur: hirsutism, acne, menstrual irregularities

Adrenal cortical insufficiency

These conditions can be due to adrenal disease itself or a deficiency of ACTH due to hypothalamic or pituitary disturbances. Table 17.6 shows a range of causes of these conditions.

Table 17.6 Some causes of adrenocortical insufficiency

PRIMARY INSUFFICIENCY	
Loss of cortical cells	**Metabolic failure in hormone production**
Congenital adrenal **hypoplasia**	**Congenital adrenal hyperplasia** (cortisone and aldosterone insufficiency with virilisation)
Autoimmune adrenal insufficiency or other endocrine syndrome	Drug or steroid-induced inhibition of ACTH or cortical cell function
Infection: AIDS, tuberculosis, fungi	
Amyloidosis, sarcoidosis, haemochromatosis	
Metastatic carcinoma	

SECONDARY INSUFFICIENCY	
Hypothalamic pituitary disease	**Hypothalamic pituitary suppression**
Neoplasm, inflammation (sarcoidosis, tuberculosis, **pyogenes**, fungi)	Long-term steroid administration
	Steroid-producing neoplasms

Primary adrenal cortical insufficiency

This is when there is insufficient production of cortisol from the adrenal cortex. There may also be insufficient aldosterone production. This can be acute or chronic in nature:

- *Acute*: there are three main causes:
    1. A crisis when an individual is unable to respond to a stressor by secreting extra steroid hormones due to chronic corticosteroid insufficiency. The symptoms come on rapidly when even a minor illness or stressor can precipitate nausea, vomiting, muscular weakness, **hypotension**, dehydration and vascular collapse. It is treated with fluid replacement and glucocorticosteroid therapy.
    2. Rapid withdrawal of prescribed corticosteroids or insufficient increase in the prescribed dose in response to stress.
    3. Acute adrenal cortex damage secondary to adrenal haemorrhage, trauma and hypoxia in neonates, anticoagulant treatment, **disseminated intravascular coagulation**, and

overwhelming bacterial infection. **Waterhouse-Friderichsen syndrome** is a potentially catastrophic condition resulting from this last cause (Agrawal et al., 2014).

- *Chronic*: known as **Addison's disease**. This is relatively uncommon and develops slowly, only being diagnosed when the circulating hormones have reached a significantly low level. It occurs due to progressive destruction of the adrenal cortex. Initially it is non-specific with the person concerned suffering from weakness, becoming readily fatigued and having gastrointestinal symptoms, e.g. nausea, vomiting, diarrhoea or **constipation**. Some may develop hyperpigmentation of exposed area and places where there is friction (Figure 17.3).

ACTIVITY 17.4: UNDERSTAND

Characteristics of Addison's disease

Watch this video to clarify the characteristics of Addison's disease. If you are using the eBook just click on the play button. Alternatively go to
https://study.sagepub.com/essentialpatho/videos

ADDISON'S DISEASE
(7:21)

Secondary adrenal cortical insufficiency

Disorders of the hypothalamus and pituitary that cause a reduction in ACTH result in a hypoadrenalism that is very similar to Addison's disease, but does not cause the hyperpigmentation mentioned above. The key difference from primary adrenal cortical insufficiency is that cortisol and androgen secretion are reduced but aldosterone is minimally altered, thus hyponatraemia and hyperkalaemia do not occur.

Disorders of the adrenal medulla

Excessive mineralocorticoid/catecholamine secretion

The adrenal medulla is functionally part of the sympathetic nervous system and the secretion of **catecholamines** (adrenaline and noradrenaline) is regulated by the nerve impulses transmitted from the sympathetic ganglionic chain. The major diseases of the adrenal medulla are neoplasms. There are two types:

- Neuronal neoplasms (neuroblastic tumours) (see Chapter 9)
- **Phaeochromocytomas**. These are formed from chromaffin cells which synthesise and secrete catecholamines. About 10% of these are malignant. There are at least six known gene mutations which can cause up to 25% of these tumours.

Phaeochromocytomas

These are tumours that secrete catecholamines, e.g. adrenaline, noradrenaline, and are a cause of surgically treatable hypertension and so are important to identify. The main characteristic of the condition is hypertension, occurring in 90% of individuals with about two-thirds having paroxysmal (occasional) episodes. When these happen, the person concerned presents with (Maitra, 2015):

- Sudden, rapid rise in blood pressure
- **Tachycardia**, palpitations, headache, sweating, tremor, apprehension
- Abdominal or chest pain, nausea and vomiting.

Most of those with phaeochromocytomas have continually raised blood pressure interspersed with paroxysmal events which can be precipitated by a number of different situations such as stress, exercise etc. These can initiate cardiac disturbances such as **myocardial infarction**, **congestive heart failure**, etc., or stroke. Single tumours can be removed surgically with the associated adrenergic blocking drugs. Those with more sites of secretion need long-term treatment of hypertension.

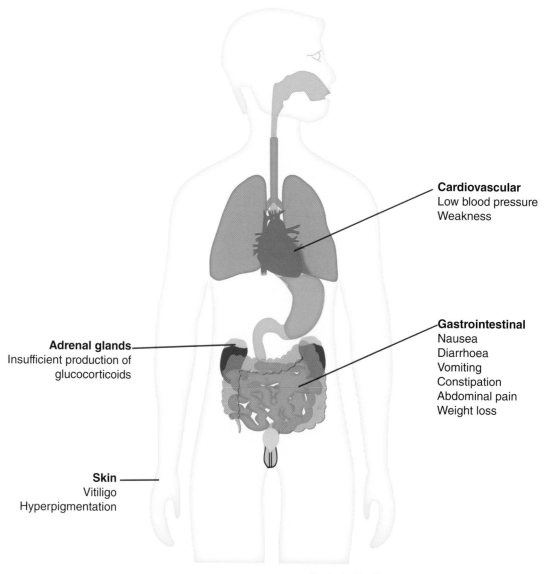

Illustrated by Shaun Mercier © SAGE Publications

Figure 17.3 Signs and symptoms of Addison's disease

ACTIVITY 17.5: UNDERSTAND

Phaeochromocytoma

Watch this video for an explanation of phaeochromocytoma. If you are using the eBook just click on the play button. Alternatively go to
https://study.sagepub.com/essentialpatho/videos

PHAEOCHROMOCYTOMA (3:01)

CHAPTER SUMMARY

This chapter has examined some of the major disorders of the endocrine system, in particular those of the hypothalamus and pituitary gland and the adrenal glands. Numerous other endocrine glands are included in the relevant chapters in this book. The conditions considered have significant implications for those with these conditions and the importance of person-centred care is paramount. In addition, consideration of the possible effects on family members must also be taken into account.

KEY POINTS

- The endocrine system has a major role in controlling body function, with the hypothalamus and pituitary gland playing central roles in regulating the overall function of the endocrine system.

- Hyperpituitarism is mainly caused by secretions from pituitary adenomas which cause two types of disturbed function: due to endocrine secretion abnormalities and due to the effects of expansion of the tissues of the pituitary.

- There are numerous causes of short stature in children with a deficiency in growth hormone, causing proportionate short stature but normal intelligence and certain other visible characteristics. In adults, a deficiency in growth hormone has predominantly metabolic alterations similar to metabolic syndrome (Chapter 13).

- Certain genetic abnormalities result in excess growth hormone secretion in childhood when the bones are still growing, resulting in gigantism with excessive height. Extra strain is placed on the cardiovascular system and other organs and tissues involved in metabolism.

- The adrenal gland is really two glands: the adrenal cortex and the adrenal medulla. The cortex produces three groups of hormones – mineralocorticoids, glucocorticoids and sex hormones – and can have altered levels of all of these hormones.

- Cushing's syndrome is hypersecretion or excessive administration of glucocorticoid hormones. Those with this condition tend to gain weight and develop hypertension, as well as developing alterations in the metabolism of tissues.

- Hyperaldosteronism is excessive secretion of mineralocorticoids which results in increased sodium and water retention, resulting in raised blood pressure.

- Adrenal cortical insufficiency results in an inability to respond to stress and may present with nausea, vomiting, muscular weakness, hypotension, dehydration and vascular collapse.

- Adrenal medullary hypersecretion can occur with phaeochromocytoma, with the major disturbance being hypertension.

REVISE

TEST YOUR KNOWLEDGE

The content of this chapter will help you understand the implications of the endocrine disorders which may be mentioned in other chapters as well as understand the conditions considered here. Revise the sections in turn then try to answer the questions.

Answers are available online. If you are using the eBook just click on the answers icon below. Alternatively go to **https://study.sagepub.com/essentialpatho/answers**

1 Outline the changes in endocrine control that occur throughout life.

2 Explain the commonest cause of anterior hyperpituitarism. Outline the groups of signs and symptoms that may occur.

3 What are the groups of causes of short stature in children? Give at least one example in each group. Describe the main signs and symptoms of growth hormone deficiency in babies and children.

4 Name the condition that occurs with excess growth hormones in adults. Outline the main signs and symptoms of this condition.

5 What is Cushing's syndrome? Describe the presentation of this condition.

6 What is hyperaldosteronism? How does it present?

7 What are the three main causes of acute primary adrenal cortical insufficiency?

8 What is a phaeochromocytoma and how does it present?

REVISE

ACE YOUR ASSESSMENT

- Further revision and learning opportunities are available online

- Test yourself away from the book with **Extra multiple choice questions**

- Learn and revise terminology with **Interactive flashcards**

If you are using the eBook access each resource by clicking on the respective icon. Alternatively go to **https://study.sagepub.com/essentialpatho/chapter17**

CHAPTER 17
ANSWERS

EXTRA
QUESTIONS

FLASHCARDS

REFERENCES

Agrawal, A., Jasdanwala, S., Agarwal, A. and Eng, M. (2014) Fatal Waterhouse–Friderichsen syndrome due to Serotype C *Neisseria meningitidis* in a young HIV negative MSM (men who have sex with men). *Gut BMJ Case Reports*. Epub 29 September. doi: 10.1136/bcr-2014-206295.

Attanasio, A.F., Mo, D., Erfurth, E.V., Tan, M., Ho, K.Y., Kleinberg, D. et al. (2010) Prevalence of metabolic syndrome in adult hypopituitary growth hormone (GH)-deficient patients before and after GH replacement. *Journal of Clinical Endocrinology and Metabolism*, 95 (1): 74–81.

Boore, J., Cook, N. and Shepherd, A. (2016) *Essentials of Anatomy and Physiology for Nursing Practice*. London: Sage.

Chapman, I.M. (2017) Gigantism and acromegaly. MSD Manual Professional Version Endocrine and Metabolic Disorders. [online]. Available at: www.msdmanuals.com/en-gb/professional/endocrine-and-metabolic-disorders/pituitary-disorders/gigantism-and-acromegaly (accessed 21 June 2018).

Cooke, D.W., Divall, S.A. and Radovick, S. (2011) Normal and aberrant growth. In S. Melmed, K.S. Polonsky, P.R. Larsen and H.M. Kronenberg (eds), *Williams Textbook of Endocrinology*, 12th edn. Philadelphia, PA: Elsevier Saunders. Ch. 24.

De Bellis, A., Bestella, G., Maiorino, M.I., Aitella, E., Lucci, E., Cozzolino, D. et al. (on behalf of the Italian Autoimmune Hypophysitis Network Group) (2016) Longitudinal behavior of autoimmune GH deficiency: from childhood to transition age. *European Journal of Endocrinology*, 174: 381–7.

Decani, S., Federighi, V., Baruzzi, E., Sardella, A. and Lodi, G. (2014) Iatrogenic Cushing's syndrome and topical steroid therapy: case series and review of the literature. *Journal of Dermatological Treatment*, 25 (6): 495–500.

Dreval, A.V., Trigolosova, I.V., Misnikova, I.V., Kovalyova, Y.A., Tishenina, R.S., Barsukov, I.A. et al. (2014) Prevalence of diabetes mellitus in patients with acromegaly. *Endocrine Connections*, 3 (2): 93–8.

Falleti, M.G., Maruff, P., Burman, P. and Harris, A. (2006) The effects of growth hormone (GH) deficiency and GH replacement on cognitive performance in adults: a meta-analysis of the current literature. *Psychoneuroendocrinology*, 31 (6): 681–91.

Fowler, J. (2016) Mid Ulster identified as 'giant hotspot' by scientists. *BBC News NI*, 12 October 2016. Available at: www.bbc.co.uk/news/uk-northern-ireland-37622249 (accessed 21 December 2018).

Hopkins, R.L. and Leinung, M.C. (2005) Exogenous Cushing's syndrome and glucocorticoid withdrawal. *Endocrinology and Metabolism Clinics of North America*, 34: 371–84.

Johnson, D.E., Guthrie, D., Smyke, A.T., Koga, S.F., Fox, N.A., Zeanah, C.H. et al. (2010) Growth and relations between auxology, caregiving environment and cognition in socially deprived Romanian children randomized to foster vs. ongoing institutional care. *Archives of Pediatrics and Adolescent Medicine*, 164 (6): 507–16.

Jørgensen, A.P., Fougner, K.J., Ueland, T., Gudmundsen, O., Burman. P., Schreiner, T. et al. (2011) Favorable long-term effects of growth hormone replacement therapy on quality of life, bone metabolism, body composition and lipid levels in patients with adult-onset growth hormone deficiency. *Growth Hormone and IGF Research*, 21 (2): 69–75.

Klose, M. and Feldt-Rasmussen, U. (2015) Hypopituitarism in traumatic brain injury – a critical note. *Journal of Clinical Medicine*, 4 (7): 1480–97.

Krishna, A., Oh, J., Lee, J-k., Lee, H-Y., Perkins, J.M., Heo, J. et al. (2015) Short-term and long-term associations between household wealth and physical growth: a cross-comparative analysis of children from four low- and middle-income countries. *Global Health Action*: 8 (1). Available at: www.tandfonline.com/doi/full/10.3402/gha.v8.26523?scroll=top&needAccess=true (accessed 22 January 2018).

Lamberts, S.W.J. (2011) Endocrinology and aging. In S. Melmed, K.S. Polonsky, P.R. Larsen and H.M. Kronenberg (eds), *Williams Textbook of Endocrinology*, 12th edn. Philadelphia, PA: Elsevier Saunders. Ch. 27.

Latronico, A.C., Brito, V.N. and Carel, J.C. (2016) Causes, diagnosis, and treatment of central precocious puberty. *The Lancet Diabetes & Endocrinology, 4* (3): 265–74.

Low, M.J. (2011) Neuroendocrinology. In S. Melmed, K.S. Polonsky, P.R. Larsen and H.M. Kronenberg (eds), *Williams Textbook of Endocrinology*, 12th edn. Philadelphia, PA: Elsevier Saunders. Ch. 7.

Maitra, A. (2015) The endocrine system. In V. Kumar, A.K. Abbas and J.C. Aster (eds), *Robbins and Cotran Pathologic Basis of Disease*. Philadelphia, PA: Elsevier Saunders.

Mayo Clinic (2018a) Prolactinoma. [online]. Available at: www.mayoclinic.org/diseases-conditions/prolactinoma/symptoms-causes/syc-20376958 (accessed 21 June 2018).

Mayo Clinic (2018b) Acromegaly: symptoms and causes. [online]. Available at: www.mayoclinic.org/diseases-conditions/acromegaly/symptoms-causes/syc-20351222 (accessed 21 June 2018).

Mayo Clinic (2018c) Acromegaly: diagnosis and treatment. [online]. Available at: www.mayoclinic.org/diseases-conditions/acromegaly/diagnosis-treatment/drc-20351226 (accessed 21 June 2018).

Melmed, S. and Kleinberg, D. (2011) Pituitary masses and tumors. In S. Melmed, K.S. Polonsky, P.R. Larsen and H.M. Kronenberg (eds), *Williams Textbook of Endocrinology*, 12th edn. Philadelphia, PA: Elsevier Saunders.

NIH (National Institutes of Health) (2012) *Prolactinoma*. National Institute of Diabetes and Digestive and Kidney Diseases. Bethesda, MA: NIH.

NHS Choices (2016) Early or delayed puberty. [online]. Available at: www.nhs.uk/conditions/early-or-delayed-puberty/ (accessed 25 January 2018).

Porth, C.M. (2015) *Essentials of Pathophysiology: Concepts of Altered Health States*, 3rd edn. Philadelphia, PA: Wolters Kluwer/Lippincott Williams & Watkins.

Span, J.P.T., Pieters, G.F.F.M., Sweep, C.G.J., Hermus, A.R.M.M. and Smals, A.G.H (2000) Gender difference in insulin-like growth factor I response to growth hormone (GH) treatment in GH-deficient adults: role of sex hormone replacement. *Journal of Clinical Endocrinology and Metabolism, 85* (3): 1121–5.

Stewart, P.M. and Krone, N.P. (2011) The adrenal cortex. In S. Melmed, K.S. Polonsky, P.R. Larsen and H.M. Kronenberg (eds), *Williams Textbook of Endocrinology*, 12th edn. Philadelphia, PA: Elsevier Saunders.

Wen-Ko, C., Chen Szu-Ta, C., Feng-Hsuan, L., Chen-Nen, C., Ming-Hsu, W. and Jen-Der, L. (2016) The impact of diabetes mellitus on the survival of patients with acromegaly. *Endokrynologia Polska, 67* (5): 501–6. doi: 10.5603/EP.a2016.0031.

DISORDERS OF THE FEMALE REPRODUCTIVE SYSTEM

18

UNDERSTAND: CHAPTER VIDEOS

Watch the following videos for a recap of the structure and function of the female reproductive system. If you are using the eBook just click on the play buttons. Alternatively go to

https://study.sagepub.com/essentialpatho/videos

FEMALE REPRODUCTIVE
SYSTEM 1 (5:00)

FEMALE REPRODUCTIVE
SYSTEM 2 (5:32)

FEMALE INFERTILITY
(3:47)

LEARNING OUTCOMES

When you have finished studying this chapter you will be able to:

1. Understand the development of the female reproductive system through the life cycle and how some of these changes cause pathophysiological disturbances.
2. Outline some of the developmental anomalies that can occur.
3. Describe the infectious disorders of the female reproductive system and how these influence the normal function of the system.
4. Discuss the implications for those affected by the main disorders of the female reproductive system.
5. Specify the complications which can occur during pregnancy and the effects on the woman and her offspring.
6. Identify causes of infertility and discuss approaches to managing this situation.
7. Discuss the disorders of the breast.

INTRODUCTION

This chapter will examine the major disorders of the female reproductive system and their effect on the individual concerned and, where appropriate, their partners and babies. Some of these disorders, in particular infertility, have a major influence on the relationship between couples and, in this chapter, approaches to dealing with this are considered.

Following the introduction, including changes in the reproductive system through the life span, this chapter falls into five main areas:

- Infections and their effects on the female reproductive system
- **Benign** and **malignant** disorders of the female reproductive system
- Disturbances that occur in relation to gestation, including pregnancy, labour and postpartum problems
- Infertility and its management
- Disorders of the breast

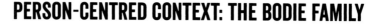

PERSON-CENTRED CONTEXT: THE BODIE FAMILY

BODIE FAMILY
CASE NOTES

Within the Bodie family, there are a number of females of different ages who exemplify the normal physiological changes that occur throughout the life cycle. These changes underpin the pathophysiological disturbances which may occur in relation to the reproductive system.

Danielle, the youngest member of the family, is at the beginning of her life and will grow and develop into her adult body over time. She is likely to commence puberty around 10-11 years with menarche (the first menstrual period) and complete it between 15 and 17 by which time she will have a fully mature female body (Euling et al., 2008). There is some evidence that a raised body mass index (a rise in body weight in relation to height demonstrated as **obesity**) is related to a fall in the age of puberty (Biro et al., 2012).

REVISE: A&P RECAP

Stages of puberty

You can review the stages of puberty in females (and males) as described by Tanner in Chapter 17, Development through the Life Span, in *Essentials of Anatomy and Physiology for Nursing Practice* (Boore et al., 2016).

Michelle has recently been through pregnancy and delivered Danielle 2 months ago. She was well during her pregnancy and had no complications during labour and delivery, although she needed a few perineal stitches to aid healing. During the 6-week post-partum period (or puerperium) her reproductive organs have returned to their normal state and she is currently breast-feeding Danielle. Her breasts have responded to the stimulation by prolactin produced by the anterior pituitary gland by growing in size and she is producing enough breast milk to feed Danielle.

Two of the women in the family, Sarah and Hannah, have recently or are currently going through the menopause and have been taking HRT (hormone replacement therapy) by one route or another to minimise the symptoms. A number of factors influence the age a woman starts the menopause, including socioeconomic factors, nationality and geography as well as health- and treatment-related issues. Endocrine changes begin at around 45 years and in Caucasian women in industrialised countries menopause usually starts at between 50 and 52 years (Gold, 2011). It usually begins with a change in the pattern of menstruation which may become irregular and be lighter or heavier than usual, but is diagnosed in retrospect after 12 months without a period. There are a number of additional symptoms and women vary in their experiences. These include (NHS Choices, 2015a):

* Hot flushes and night sweats – hot flushes that occur at night
* Difficulty with sleeping, which may result in tiredness and irritability during the day, and reduced libido
* Vaginal dryness and pain, itching or discomfort during sex
* Recurrent urinary tract infections (UTIs), such as **cystitis**
* Palpitations – heartbeats become more noticeable
* Mood changes, such as low mood or anxiety, and headaches
* Problems with memory and concentration
* Joint stiffness, aches and pains, reduced muscle mass
* Osteoporosis becomes more common.

Maud is the eldest of the women in the Bodie family and is showing many of the physical changes that occur with ageing. Osteoporosis often develops due to the reduced oestrogen secreted following the menopause. Therefore, older women are at increased risk of **fractures**. They also often develop a degree of **kyphosis** (bowed spine) and become shorter as the vertebrae shrink.

ACTIVITY 18.1: APPLY

The menopause

Two members of the Bodie family have been going through the menopause and have been coping with the symptoms involved. The videos below will help you to understand some of the experiences. If you are using the eBook just click on the play button. Alternatively go to

https://study.sagepub.com/essentialpatho/videos

⊳   ⊳

MENOPAUSE SYMPTOMS   MENOPAUSE DEPRESSION
(11:31)   (2:29)

DEVELOPMENTAL ANOMALIES

Some anatomical or physiological abnormalities can occur during development, and **congenital adrenal hyperplasia** has already been discussed in Chapter 17. In this condition, there is increased secretion of **androgens**, resulting in **hypertrophy** of the clitoris in a female baby which then looks similar to a penis in a male infant. Other signs of masculinisation of the child occur during development, including greater growth than usual, **hirsutism** (i.e. excessive body hair), acne and ovarian dysfunction (White and Speiser, 2000).

Another anomaly that occurs uncommonly develops during gender differentiation (Boore et al., 2016). In females, the two Müllerian ducts (these develop in the embryo from specialised ridges of tissue) normally differentiate into the female reproductive tracts, forming the oviducts (Fallopian tubes), and then

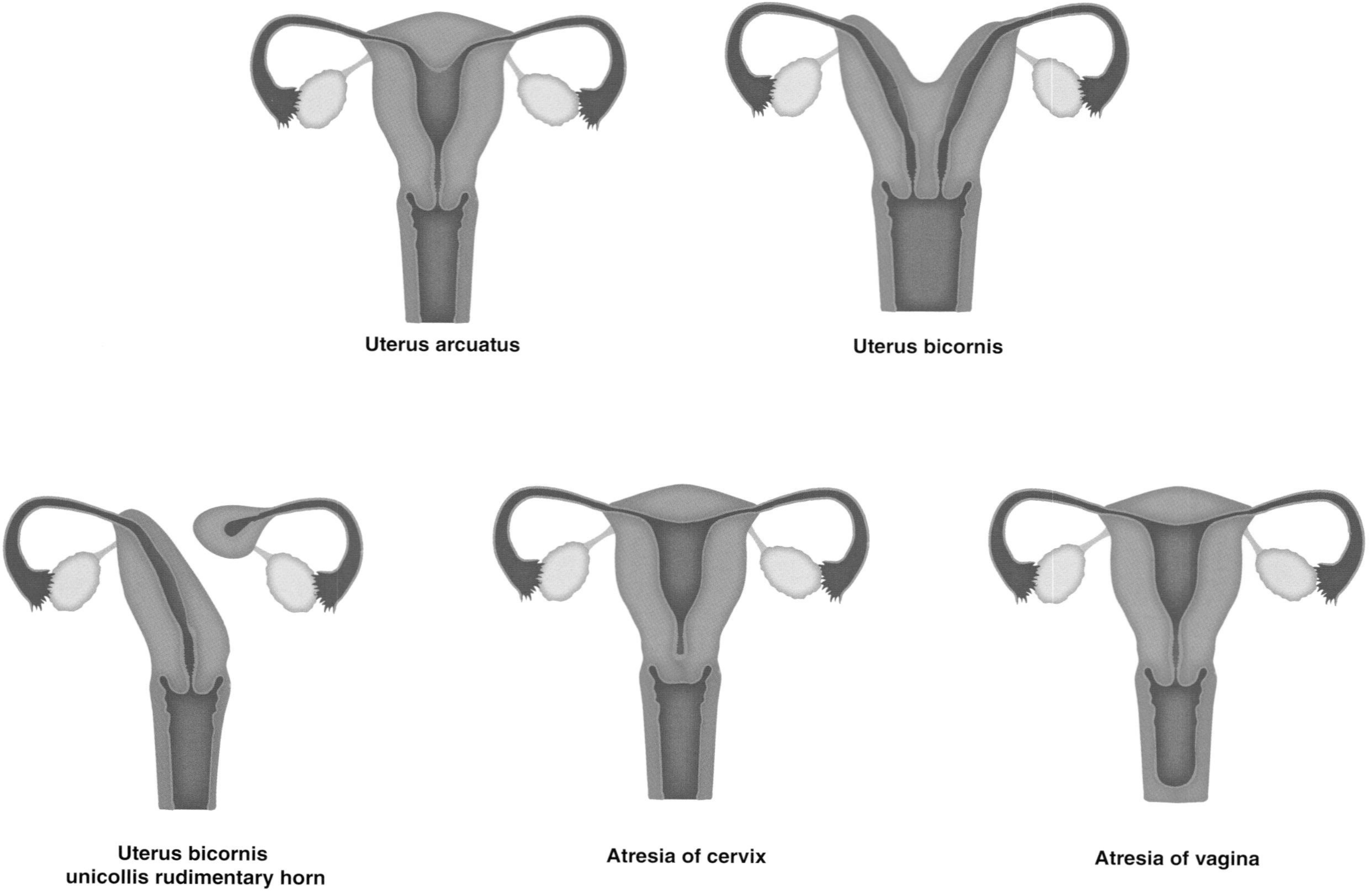

Uterus arcuatus

Uterus bicornis

Atresia of cervix

Atresia of vagina

Uterus bicornis unicollis rudimentary horn

Illustrated by Shaun Mercier © SAGE Publications

Figure 18.1 Malformations of the uterus

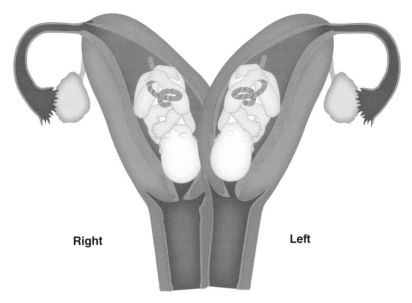

Right   **Left**

Illustrated by Shaun Mercier © SAGE Publications

Figure 18.2   Double uterus (uterus didelphys)

fusing and forming the uterus and upper part of the vagina. However, fusion does not always happen normally and abnormalities of the uterus occur, including uterus didelphys (or double uterus), often with two cervices and sometimes with a double vagina. Each horn of the double uterus connects to one fallopian tube (Figures 18.1, 18.2). Such abnormalities can be due to genetic factors, exposure to diethyl-stilboestrol (DES) during fetal development, or other causes.

INFECTIONS OF THE FEMALE REPRODUCTIVE TRACT

There are a considerable number of different microorganisms which infect the female reproductive system and fall into the following categories, many of which are sexually transmitted:

- Some cause **inflammation** and discomfort and are common causes of **vaginitis** but do not result in serious effects, e.g. *Candida albicans, Trichomonas vaginalis.*
- Some are causes of infertility or preterm deliveries, e.g. *Neisseria gonorrhoeae, Chlamydia* infections (female infertility), *Ureaplasma urealyticum, Mycoplasma hominis* (premature deliveries).
- **Viruses** include:
  - herpes simplex viruses (HSVs), which lead to painful genital ulcers (non-malignant)
  - human papilloma virus (HPV), which contributes to the development of **cancers** of the cervix, vagina and vulva (Ellenson and Pirog, 2015).

Infections of the lower genital tract

There are a number of different causes of infections of the lower genital tract, some of which are indicated in Table 18.1.

Other infections of the reproductive tract

Pelvic inflammatory disease (PID)

This condition usually starts in the vulva or vagina and spreads upwards, involving most of the organs of the female reproductive system, causing pelvic pain, adnexal tenderness (i.e. tenderness of the structures closely related to the uterus, such as the ovaries, Fallopian tubes and related ligaments), fever and vaginal discharge. *Neisseria gonorrhoeae* and *Chlamydia trachomatis* are both common causes of PID with *gonococcal* infections causing inflammatory changes 2–7 days after infection. **Puerperal** (i.e. related to the period after childbirth) infections after delivery (normal or abnormal) or abortion (spontaneous or induced) are important causes of PID.

Table 18.1 Examples of female lower genital tract infections

HSV (herpes simplex viruses)	Common and involve cervix, vagina and vulva. Symptoms include: • Systemic: e.g. fever, general **malaise**, inflamed inguinal lymph nodes • **Lesions**: red **papules** develop into **vesicles**, and merge to ulcers. On vulva - readily visible. In cervix and vagina - **purulent** vaginal discharge, pain in pelvis. Around urethra - pain on urination and urinary retention Virus can establish infectious source in lumbosacral ganglia from which virus reactivation and recurrence of signs and symptoms can occur with **immunosuppression** or hormonal changes Readily transmitted between partners, or to babies during delivery
Poxvirus (molluscum contagiosum)	Four types exist: MCV-1 most common, MCV-2 most sexually transmitted Can cause infections in children through direct contact. Adults: usually affect genitals, lower abdomen, buttocks and inner thighs and consist of dome-shaped papules, 1-5 cm diameter
Fungal infections (e.g. *Candida albicans*)	Candida: yeast is common component of reproductive microbiota Can result in symptomatic candidiasis when microbial environment is disturbed by, e.g. diabetes, antibiotics, pregnancy, immunosuppression. Not a STI (**sexually transmitted infection**) Symptoms: vulvovaginal pruritus, swelling, discharge, erythema (redness). Severe infection → mucosal ulcers
Trichomonas vaginalis	Large flagellated oval protozoan, sexually transmitted, develops over 4 days to 4 weeks. Asymptomatic or symptoms of yellow frothy vaginal discharge, vulvovaginal discomfort, **dysuria**, **dyspareunia**
Gardnerella vaginalis	Gram-negative bacillus which is the main cause of bacterial vaginosis within changes in the normal vaginal microflora. Symptoms: thin, grey-green, fishy vaginal discharge. Implicated in premature labour
Chlamydia trachomatis	STI: mainly affects cervix. Can ascend to uterus and Fallopian tubes and can cause **pelvic inflammatory disease** (PID)
Bartholin cyst	The two Bartholin's glands are positioned slightly behind and to the right and left of the vaginal opening. These can become infected and become 3-5 cm in diameter, causing local discomfort and pain

Source: Adapted from Ellenson and Pirog, 2015

Acute complications of PID include peritonitis and **bacteraemia**, which can result in suppurative **arthritis**, endocarditis and **meningitis**. Chronic complications occur due to **adhesions** between the pelvic and bowel organs, resulting in tubal adhesions and causing obstruction of the Fallopian tubes and infertility, **ectopic pregnancy**, pelvic pain and **intestinal obstruction**.

Salpingitis

Infections of specific organs can also occur and gonococcal infection causes acute inflammation of mucousal surfaces. **Salpingitis** is an inflammatory condition of the Fallopian tubes and several variants can present including:

- *Acute suppurative salpingitis*: If the **mucosa** of the tubules becomes congested and infiltrated by various cells involved in the immune response, the **epithelium** becomes injured and the folds (**plicae**) slough off and the lumen fills with purulent exudate. This can ooze out of the fimbriated end of the Fallopian tubes and spread to the ovaries to cause salpingo-oophoritis which may result in:
  - *tubo-ovarian abscesses* from pockets of pus accumulating in the ovaries
  - *pyosalpinx*: the accumulation of pus in the lumen of the tubes.
- *Chronic salpingitis*: Scarring of the Fallopian tube may prevent oocytes passing and result in infertility or ectopic pregnancy.
- *Hydrosalpinx*: Fused fimbriae can block a Fallopian tube at the ovarian end. Initially the tube fills with serous or clear fluid but pus can develop and accumulate, distending the tube (Figure 18.3).

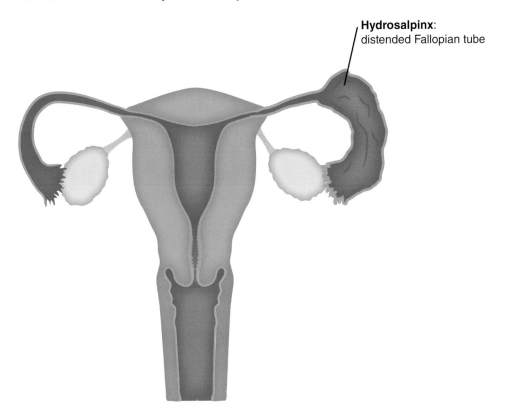

Hydrosalpinx:
distended Fallopian tube

Illustrated by Shaun Mercier © SAGE Publications

Figure 18.3 Hydrosalpinx

CELLULAR DISTURBANCES OF THE FEMALE REPRODUCTIVE TRACT

The organs comprising the reproductive system are formed of different tissues, any of which can develop different cellular disturbances, some benign and some malignant. The cavities and surfaces of the different organs of the reproductive system are lined with epithelium and glands within this system are also formed of epithelial tissue with the **myometrium** or smooth muscle tissue forming the middle layer of the uterus. In addition to the main organs of the female reproductive system, the uterosacral ligaments are important in providing support and maintaining these organs in their correct positions.

Vulva

The external genitalia are similar to the skin of the body, covered with squamous epithelium. It is susceptible to a number of disorders, neoplastic and benign, which are discussed below.

Non-neoplastic epithelial disorders

This term refers to a number of disorders that can affect the vulva. We will look at two in this section:

Lichen sclerosus

Lichen sclerosus (or sclerosis) is a condition in which the vulva is inflamed with areas of very thin epithelium and superficial ulcers due to scratching because of itching. It is an autoimmune disorder and may be associated with other **autoimmune diseases**. The skin becomes white, thin and crinkly but may also show signs of **squamous cell hyperplasia** (see below). Tissues become atrophied and stenosed and dyspareunia can result. These changes develop slowly and progress, with 2–5% developing into a squamous cell carcinoma. A biopsy is needed to achieve a diagnosis. Treatment with a topical steroid cream is usually needed (Burton, 2014).

ACTIVITY 18.2: UNDERSTAND

Treatment of lichen sclerosus

The following video will help you understand this condition and its management. If you are using the eBook just click on the play button. Alternatively go to
https://study.sagepub.com/essentialpatho/videos

LICHEN SCLEROSUS (8:58)

Squamous cell hyperplasia

This is a thickened plaque with an irregular surface resulting from pruritus and leading to rubbing or scratching. Causation is unclear: it is thought to be due to some irritant, but is only diagnosed after HPV, fungal infections and other possible causes have been eliminated.

Premalignant and malignant tumours

These are uncommon **tumours**, causing only 3–5% of cancers of the female reproductive system. There are two main types:

* Carcinomas due to infection with HPV (30% of cases). Risk factors are similar to those for carcinoma of the cervix (Ca cervix)
* Keratinising squamous cell carcinoma, not due to HPV (70%)

Any growing vulval lesion should be biopsied for diagnosis.

Vulvodynia

Vulvodynia is vulval pain or burning sensation without visible lesions and has been described as:

> burning pain occurring in the absence of relevant visible findings or a specific clinically identifiable, neurological disorder (Haefner et al., 2005: 41).

The cause of this condition is not clear, with a number of conditions eliminated, including infection, neoplasia and neurological disorders. Possible causes include developmental abnormalities, increased **urinary oxalates** (a chemical in urine which can form kidney stones), genetic or immune factors, infection, neuropathic changes or a combination of these (Haefner et al., 2005).

Vaginal disorders

The normal flora of the vagina plays a protective role against infection. Causes of infection have been discussed above. In this section we will concentrate on other vaginal disorders.

Vaginitis

This inflammation of the vagina with discharge, itching, burning, redness and swelling, and pain can be caused by chemicals, foreign bodies or infection (see earlier); the most common cause being a change in the normal balance of vaginal bacteria. After the menopause, the fall in oestrogen levels results in a thinning of the **endothelium** and can cause atrophic vaginitis.

Cancer of the vagina

Primary cancer of the vagina is very rare, with similar causes as Ca cervix (see below), occurring mainly in older women (usually at 75+ years) (Cancer Research UK, 2018). The risk is increased by smoking and HIV (**human immunodeficiency virus**) (Diarra and Botha, 2017). The different types of cancer that occur are: squamous cell carcinoma 70%; adenocarcinomas 15%; malignant melanoma 9%; sarcomas <4%. Abnormal vaginal bleeding is the most common symptom, with palpable mass and dyspareunia also occurring. These cancers spread readily. Routine Papanicolaou (Pap) smears (named after Georgios Nikolaou Papanikolaou – a Greek pioneer in cytology) play an important role in identifying these cancers, which are treated by surgery or **radiotherapy**.

Cervix

Premalignant and cancerous lesions of the cervix

HPV (human papillomavirus) is the cause of the majority of instances of cervical cancer. There are over 100 types of HPV and two of these (16 and 18) cause 70% of cases (World Health Organisation, 2016); vaccines for these two types are now available for use in many countries. It can take 15–20 years for cervical cancer to develop, or less time in someone with a poor immune system. Risk factors are: early first sexual intercourse, many sexual partners, smoking and immunosuppression. HPV infections start in the deepest layers of the skin and cause increased division of skin cells which then form new virus particles.

In some people, the DNA of the cells is damaged by the virus and stimulates cell division and uncontrolled growth, leading to cancer.

If not identified early by screening, symptoms will eventually occur, which may include:

* Irregular, intermenstrual or abnormal vaginal bleeding after sexual intercourse
* Back, leg or pelvic pain
* Fatigue, weight loss, loss of appetite
* Vaginal discomfort or malodorous discharge
* Unilateral lower limb oedema

More severe symptoms may arise at advanced stages.

Uterus

Endometriosis

This is a condition in which functional endometrial tissue, normally within the uterine cavity, is found in sites outside the uterus, usually the ovaries, fallopian tubes, other organs of the reproductive system, uterosacral ligaments, intestines and pelvic organs. This is referred to as ectopic endometrial **stroma** and epithelium (Anglesio et al., 2017). Although the specific cause of these abnormal positions is not clear, there are certain factors related to the condition: genetic predisposition, oestrogen dependence, progesterone resistance and inflammation with **retrograde** menstruation (i.e. menstrual blood flowing back into the body during menstruation, cause unknown) physically moving endometrial fragments (Burney and Giudice, 2012).

The main symptoms are:

* Chronic pelvic pain. **Endometriosis** is associated with severe **dysmenorrhea** (period-related pain) affecting daily activities and quality of life in 50% of cases (Fauconnier and Chapron, 2005)
* Deep pain during or after sexual intercourse
* Period-related or cyclic gastrointestinal symptoms, particularly painful bowel movements
* Period-related or cyclic urinary symptoms, particularly pain passing urine or haematuria
* Infertility in association with one or more of the above

Abdominal and pelvic examinations are performed to identify additional signs of pelvic changes and endometrial lesions (NICE, 2017). Endometriosis is usually identified during reproductive life as the ectopic **endometrium** behaves like the normal endometrium and proliferates and bleeds in response to the endocrine changes of the menstrual cycle. The effects are as identified above and pelvic adhesions can occur, which often result in infertility. This is a condition affecting 6–10% of women, mainly in the reproductive stage of life. Treatment consists of three main approaches: pain management, hormonal therapy to suppress endometrial bleeding, and surgery (NHS Choices, 2015b). In addition, psychological support for those affected emotionally by infertility will be important.

Leiomyomas

These are benign growths derived from smooth muscle and are the most common type of female reproductive tumours, known as **fibroids**. They are in different positions in the uterus, illustrated in Figure 18.4.

They develop from excessive growth of the smooth muscle and **connective tissue** comprising the uterus, stimulated by the female hormones of oestrogen and progesterone, which regulate the menstrual cycle. The tissue-forming fibroids tend to have more receptors for these hormones than normal tissue, possibly due to a genetic predisposition. Some other growth factors may be involved. After the menopause, these growths often shrink in size but a hysterectomy may be performed if they cause distress.

Leiomyomas are asymptomatic about 50% of the time. However, **menorrhagia** (excessive menstrual flow) may cause **anaemia**, and growth of the **neoplasm** may result in frequency of urination, **constipation**, abdominal swelling and, occasionally, pain (Mayo Clinic, 2018). Fibroids may grow during pregnancy or where oestrogen levels are raised by, for example, oral contraceptives or oestrogen replacement during the menopause (NHS Choices, 2015c).

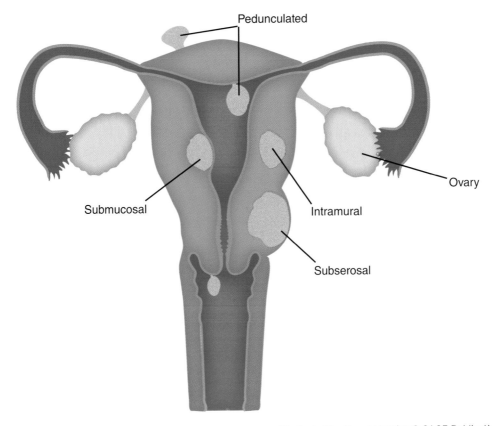

Illustrated by Shaun Mercier © SAGE Publications

Figure 18.4 Types of leiomyomas (fibroids)

Endometrial cancer

This develops from the abnormal growth of cells in the endometrium of the uterus which are able to **metastasise** (i.e. spread to other parts of the body and produce additional growths at those sites). It occurs most often in postmenopausal women, with 2–5% of cases related to inherited characteristics (Kong et al., 2012), and is the fourth commonest cancer in women in developed countries (Colombo et al., 2013).

A number of aetiological factors (Colombo et al., 2013) are involved in this condition, including:

- Obesity: a BMI (body mass index) >30 causes a 3–4-fold increase
- Prolonged raised oestrogen levels, prescribed or endogenous (e.g. from polycystic ovaries)
- **Hypertension**

- **Diabetes mellitus**
- Genetics

Two main types of endometrial carcinoma are identified:

- Type I – oestrogen-dependent: women with excess oestrogen before and during the menopause make up 80% of cases. In addition to raised oestrogen levels, other risk factors are obesity, diabetes, no child-bearing, early menarche and late menopause.
- Type II – oestrogen-independent: this occurs at an older age without increased oestrogen levels and some **atrophy** of the endometrial lining. This has a worse prognosis than Type I.

In addition, these carcinomas can be classified according to the cellular characteristics (histology) identified in Table 18.2.

Table 18.2   Cellular characteristics of different endometrial cancers

Cell type	Characteristics
Carcinomas (i.e. adenocarcinoma)	Originate from single layer of epithelial cells lining endometrium
	Type I: low-grade, minimally invasive, oestrogen-dependent; plus risk factors referred to in the text
	Type II: High-grade, at older age, invasive into uterine wall, poor prognosis
Endometrioid adenocarcinoma	Cells grow in patterns of normal endometrium, new glands with some abnormal nuclei
	Low-grade: cells well differentiated, not invasive of myometrium, next to endometrial hyperplasia
	High-grade: less well differentiated, solid sheets of tumour cells, atrophied endometrium
	Certain genetic **mutations** associated with abnormal cell function
Serous carcinoma	5-10% of these cancers. Common in post-menopausal women with atrophied endometrium, and in black women
	Aggressive, often invades myometrium, metastasises within peritoneum
	Atypical nuclei and cells
Clear cell carcinoma	See Type II above
	Has clear cytoplasm when stained. More common in post-menopausal women. P53 cell signalling system not active
Mucinous carcinoma	Rare – <1-2% of endometrial cancer. Usually well-differentiated columnar cells organised in glands containing mucin
	Need differentiation from adenocarcinoma. Good prognosis

Source: Adapted from Colombo et al., 2013; Murali et al., 2014

Diagnosis and treatment

The main symptom that calls for further investigation is abnormal painless bleeding or vaginal discharge. There are four approaches to diagnosis, with the last three of those below able to be carried out at the same time:

- Ultrasound can be used for measuring the thickness and characteristics of the endometrium. If the endometrium is less than 4 mm thick and is smooth, it is unlikely that cancer is present (Crawford, 2014).
- Biopsy of the endometrium in which a small piece of tissue is taken from the uterine wall by access through the cervix enables the type of tissue to be identified.

- Dilatation and **curettage** (D & C) is performed under general **anaesthesia**.
- **Hysteroscopy** is when the cavity of the uterus is viewed directly through a hysteroscope (a fine telescope).

Before treatment begins, various tests will be performed. These can include: chest X-ray, ultrasound, MRI (magnetic resonance imaging) to identify physical evidence of metastases, and liver function tests will show reduced biochemical function due to the spread of cancer, affecting **metabolism**.

Treatment is mainly by surgical intervention, with the precise nature and extent depending on the depth and spread of development of the malignancy. The possible surgery can include hysterectomy and bilateral **salpingo-oophorectomy** (removal of the uterus and the Fallopian tube and ovary from both sides of the uterus). In addition, there is a possibility of removal of some lymph nodes, depending on the degree of spread. **Adjuvant therapy** (i.e. given in addition to the primary treatment) may be given as radiotherapy, and less commonly as **chemotherapy**, to limit recurrence of the cancer.

Disorders of uterosacral ligaments

These ligaments provide the necessary support to hold the uterus and other pelvic organs in the correct position. Pregnancy and the process of childbirth can stretch them and as women approach their 60s and 70s these ligaments and related muscles weaken and lose elasticity. These changes result in a reduction of the support for the pelvis and its contents. A number of conditions (Figure 18.5) can develop because of this (Ramsay, 2014):

- *Urethrocele and cystocele*: A urethrocele occurs when part of the vaginal wall fused to the urethra descends and causes disruption of continence. This can be linked with a cystocele when the support of the bladder base is weakened, the bladder falls below the uterus and the bladder wall causes the anterior vagina wall to bulge. The bladder also herniates into the vagina, particularly when coughing, lifting and defaecating. The individual affected has a frequency and urgency of micturition, difficulty in urinating and feels a 'bearing-down' sensation.
- *Rectocele and enterocele*: Rectocele develops in a similar way to cystocele but it is the posterior vaginal wall that is weakened and permits the rectum to bulge forward. Defaecation becomes difficult, and the person concerned has discomfort, a 'dragging' sensation and possibly a low backache. An enterocele occurs when a portion of the small bowel descends into the space between the posterior surface of the vagina and the anterior surface of the rectum.
- *Uterine prolapse*: This happens when the main supportive ligaments for the uterus are stretched and the uterus bulges down into the vagina. The different stages of uterine prolapse are classified in Table 18.3 and illustrated in Figure 18.6.

Treatment is either surgical or the use of a pessary which fits into the vagina and supports the uterus, or other organs (bladder, rectum, vagina) which are out of position (Doshani et al., 2007).

Table 18.3 The stages of uterine prolapse

Stage 0	No prolapse
Stage 1	The furthermost part of the prolapse is more than 1 cm above the introitus (the opening into the vaginal canal)
Stage 2	The furthermost part of the prolapse is equal to or less than 1 cm above the introitus
Stage 3	The furthermost part of the prolapse is more than 1 cm below the introitus, but protrudes no more than 2 cm less than the length of the vagina
Stage 4	Complete eversion of the vagina, i.e. the whole of the uterus is outside the introitus of the vagina, known as procidentia

Source: Doshani et al., 2007

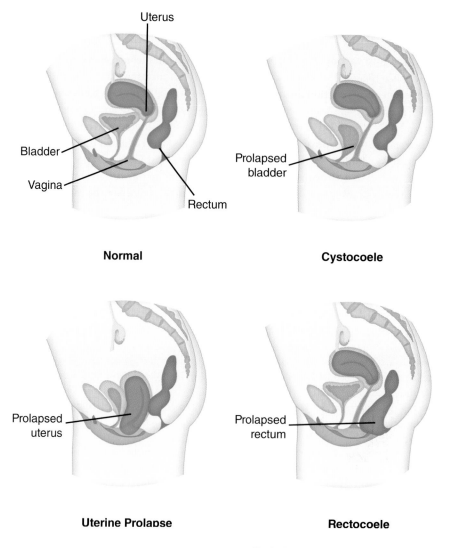

Figure 18.5 Effects of disorders of uterosacral ligaments

Illustrated by Shaun Mercier © SAGE Publications

Fallopian tube disorders

Disorders of the Fallopian tubes are obstructions or epithelial dysfunctions that impede movement along the tube by sperm, ova or zygotes. A number of causes have been identified:

- Infections due to:
  - ○ pelvic inflammatory disease (PID)
  - ○ chlamydia asymptomatically infecting the Fallopian tubes which can permanently damage and block them by forming scar tissue
  - ○ an intrauterine device
  - ○ ruptured appendix

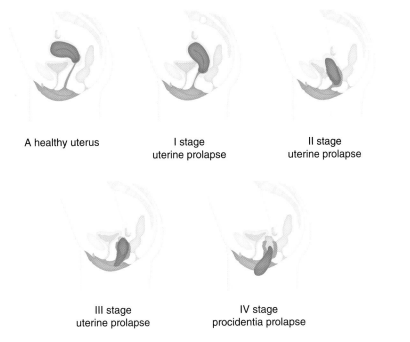

A healthy uterus

I stage
uterine prolapse

II stage
uterine prolapse

III stage
uterine prolapse

IV stage
procidentia prolapse

Illustrated by Shaun Mercier © SAGE Publications

Figure 18.6 Stages of uterine prolapse

- Inflammation or other damage to the Fallopian tubes:
    - pelvic or lower abdominal surgery, resulting in pelvic adhesions
    - ectopic pregnancy in the fallopian tubes. (Rebar, 2017)

The major outcome of damage to the Fallopian tubes is infertility, so assisted reproductive technology may be used to overcome what may be a major personal concern for the individual or couple.

Ovarian disorders

Menstrual and fertility disturbances can occur due to ovarian disorders which can be due either to a lesion of the ovaries themselves or to **hypothalamus**, pituitary or adrenal dysfunction. They include benign cysts and tumours as well as malignant tumours, and classification is difficult because often they cannot be differentiated without histological (using a microscope) examination (Oats and Abraham, 2010).

Benign ovarian tumours and cysts

Cystic ovaries

Cysts are the most common cause of disrupted ovarian function and most of these are benign. Many are derived from ovarian follicles which continue to grow, and develop into cavities that fill with fluid. Many of these cysts are asymptomatic, unless they grow excessively or bleeding occurs into the cysts. Some will cause discomfort or a dull ache and some may burst into the abdominal cavity. Many regress spontaneously.

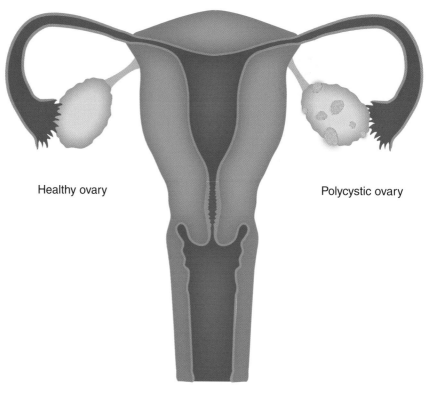

Healthy ovary   Polycystic ovary

Illustrated by Shaun Mercier © SAGE Publications

Figure 18.7 Polycystic ovary

Polycystic ovary syndrome

Polycystic ovary syndrome (PCOS) (Figure 18.7) occurs in 5–10% of women in the reproductive age range, usually starting at menarche. It is considered a heritable disorder with a number of genes identified as indicating susceptibility and probable development even before humans left Africa. Reproductive conditions, including PCOS, are more common in women with **epilepsy** and are possibly linked to the medication used in treatment (Sirmans and Pate, 2014). PCOS often occurs in combination with obesity and signs of **metabolic syndrome** (discussed in Chapter 13), including **insulin** resistance. Diabetes, **cardiovascular disease** and other chronic health conditions are related to this syndrome, including an increased risk of endometrial cancer (Goodarzi et al., 2011).

The major characteristics of **anovulation** (when ovaries do not release an oocyte during a menstrual cycle) and androgen excess occur in this condition. Diagnosis can be difficult as signs and symptoms can vary with time. However, they usually have a disturbed secretion of gonadotrophins linked with fewer than normal menstrual periods (Ehrmann, 2005). The major presenting signs and symptoms are: infertility, irregular uterine bleeding and pregnancy loss (Bulun, 2011). In addition, hirsutism (excessive body hair in men and women on body parts where hair is normally absent or minimal) and enlarged polycystic ovaries are common (Sirmans and Pate, 2014).

Treatment aims to minimise the development of the effects mentioned, mainly by patient education for modification of lifestyle in aiming to lose weight, which improves many of the symptoms. The main areas of treatment fall into three main categories (Sirmans and Pate, 2014):

- *CHCs (Combined hormonal contraceptives)* are useful for those with hirsutism and menstrual irregularities and those who do not wish to become pregnant. Menstruation related disorders can increase the risks of endometrial hyperplasia and carcinoma. Low-dose CHCs are commonly recommended for PCOS related menstrual irregularities.

- Androgen-related symptoms: are treated by anti-androgens such as spironolactone which block androgen receptors; metformin and thiazolidinedione act as insulin-lowering drugs and also decrease androgen levels.
- Infertility: a focus on reducing weight is important. In addition, various approaches on management of infertility are used, some of which discussed at the end of this chapter.

Ovarian tumours - benign

About 80% of ovarian tumours are benign and occur mainly in women of reproductive age. Risk factors tend to be lack of previous pregnancies and **gonadal dysgenesis** (loss of germ cells). Most of these tumours are non-functional and usually grow very slowly, producing minimal symptoms unless they become very large. However, some do secrete hormones and may disturb the menstrual cycle and cause infertility problems (Herrington, 2014).

There are three main types of tumours:

- **Benign cystic teratomas**: derived from all germ cell layers but mainly ectoderm (also called dermoid cysts)
- **Fibromas**: slow-growing tumours and usually <7 cm in diameter. Fibromas may lead to **ascites** (fluid in the abdomen)
- **Cystadenomas**: most commonly serous or mucinous. (McNeeley, 2017)

Ovarian cancer

The ovarian cancer rate increases with age, being most common between 45 and 60 years, possibly due to a high level ovulation over time. Both pregnancy and taking birth control pills reduce the risk of developing ovarian cancer, both of which reduce the number of ovulations. It has been suggested that there is a link between the number of ovulations and the risk of ovarian cancer (Purdie et al., 2003). A key characteristic is that diagnosis is difficult, partly due to the late development of symptoms and the necessity for histological differentiation, thus the survival rate is low. Ovarian cancers fall into three types based on:

- *Epithelial cell tumours*: these comprise about 90% of ovarian cancers. They are usually found in older women, discovered late and with a high mortality rate. They begin in the epithelial (surface) layer covering the ovary. There are several types of these cancers deriving from different cell types, but serous are the commonest, comprising about two-thirds of the total. They may start at the end of the Fallopian tube and spread to the ovary. About 10% of the total is undifferentiated or unclassifiable.

The other two types occur in younger women, are identified earlier and have better survival rates:

- *Germ cell tumours*: these are derived from the germ cells which form the eggs in the ovaries. There are several types of these (one being **teratomas**) and they often contain cells of different tissues, e.g. skin, muscles, hair, bone. Each type is quite rare, with the total comprising only about 5% of ovarian tumours.
- *Gonadal stromal cell tumours* (also known as ovarian granulosa cell tumours – GCT), i.e. formed from the stromal (connective tissue) cells of the ovary. These are rare, at only about 2–5% of ovarian cancers, but they can secrete some hormones. There are two groups of these tumours, depending on the age of those affected (Li, *et al*. 2018):
  - AGCT (adult granulosa cell tumour): 95% of those with the condition. It is probably due to a mutation but the cause is not clear.
  - JGCT (juvenile granulosa cell tumour).

The most common treatment is surgery. In addition, hormone, growth factors and signalling pathways are used and contribute to GCT cell proliferation, apoptosis, or angiogenesis.

These tumours often have a very non-specific presentation, making diagnosis more difficult and often fairly late. Symptoms may include: abdominal bloating (possibly due to ascites), feeling 'full' early in a meal, indigestion, and sometimes abdominal or pelvic pain.

There are a number of risk factors for ovarian cancer. Some that are supported by convincing evidence include:

- Asbestos
- Hormone replacement therapy (HRT) (oestrogen-only)
- Tobacco smoking
- Adult-attained height (as a marker for genetic, environmental, hormonal, nutritional factors affecting growth) from preconception to completion of linear growth (WCRF International, 2014)
- Excess body fat
- Genetic predisposition: About 20% of ovarian tumours occur in women with a genetic predisposition to their development. In around 65–85% of these they carry the *BRCA* (*BR*east *CA*ncer genes) with a mutation which increases the risk of developing breast cancer (and ovarian cancer). There are also additional genes which are associated with the development of ovarian cancer (Toss et al., 2015).

Some with limited evidence include:

- Perineal use of talc-based body powder
- X-radiation, gamma radiation (Cancer Research UK, 2016)

Treatment

The treatment provided to those identified with ovarian cancer depends on a number of factors:

- Exactly where the malignancy is positioned and the stage of growth it has reached
- The type of malignancy it is linked with and how the cells appear under a microscope
- The general state of health and fitness of the person concerned. (Cancer Research UK, 2016)

GESTATIONAL DISORDERS

There are numerous conditions related to pregnancy which can result in fetal or maternal **morbidity** and/or mortality.

The potential outcomes of disorders considered here include:

- Intrauterine fetal or perinatal death
- Congenital malformations
- Growth retardation in utero
- Maternal death

───────────── **REVISE: A&P RECAP** ─────────────

Gestational disorders

Before reading this chapter it will be helpful to review Part 5, The Next Generation, in *Essentials of Anatomy and Physiology for Nursing Practice* (Boore et al., 2016), which includes two chapters:

- Chapter 16, The Reproductive Systems
- Chapter 17, Development through the Life Span

Both of these include content relevant to this section of this chapter, including stages of pregnancy, structure and function of the placenta and maternal post-partum changes.

Disorders in early pregnancy

Spontaneous abortion ('miscarriage')

The spontaneous loss of a pregnancy before 20 weeks of gestation, with the fetus not normally judged as viable, is known as an abortion. Most occur before 12 weeks of pregnancy. A number of causes of **spontaneous abortion** have been identified, including (Ellenson and Pirog, 2015):

- Fetal chromosomal abnormalities: see Chapter 5, Genetic Disorders
- Maternal endocrine factors, including poorly controlled diabetes mellitus, defects in the luteal phase (first 14 days) of the menstrual cycle when lack of progesterone inhibits preparation of the uterine lining for implantation of the fertilised ovum, and other endocrine disorders
- Physical abnormalities of the uterus, including: submucosal leiomyomas (fibroid), polyps, malformations of the uterus, any of which may prevent implantation of the **blastocyst**
- Maternal disorders such as hypertension or abnormalities of coagulation can cause reduced blood flow to the uterus, causing placental **infarction** and leading to fetal **hypoxia**
- Infections with various **protozoa**, bacteria or viruses can cause fetal malformations or irritability of the uterus.

Ectopic pregnancy

This is when the fertilised ovum becomes implanted somewhere outside the uterus (Figure 18.8). The most common site, where 90% occur, is within the Fallopian tube, before the blastocyst reaches the uterus. However, it can also implant in the ovary, the abdominal cavity or the intrauterine section of the Fallopian tube. An ectopic pregnancy in the Fallopian tube can result in rupture of the tube, resulting in abdominal pain (moderate to severe) and vaginal bleeding at 6–8 weeks after the last menstrual period (Ellenson and Pirog, 2015).

Late pregnancy and placental disorders

Many of the conditions that occur during the third trimester of pregnancy are related to the placenta and its complexity. Anything preventing blood flow though the umbilical cord from the placenta to the fetus may cause fetal death due to lack of oxygen. Loss of maternal blood due to partial or total placental separation of the placenta from the uterine wall puts the mother at risk of severe blood loss.

Twin pregnancy

There are several different types of placenta that can occur with monozygotic (from one ovum that has split) and dizygotic (from two separate eggs) twins (Figure 18.9).

Twins with a single **chorion** and shared placenta (who are monozygotic) are at risk of a condition called twin–twin transfusion syndrome which occurs in approximately 10–15% of monochorionic twins. In this condition, blood shifts from the circulation of one twin (the donor) to the other (the recipient). As you would expect, the donor becomes anaemic, growth is restricted and the amniotic fluid volume is reduced. In contrast, the recipient becomes swollen with blood and reddened (plethora), and may develop congestive cardiac failure and cardiomegaly, with **polyhydramnios** (increased amniotic fluid). Untreated, this condition has a very high mortality rate, as much as 80%. One approach to treatment is the removal of excess amniotic fluid from the recipient (Mari et al., 2001).

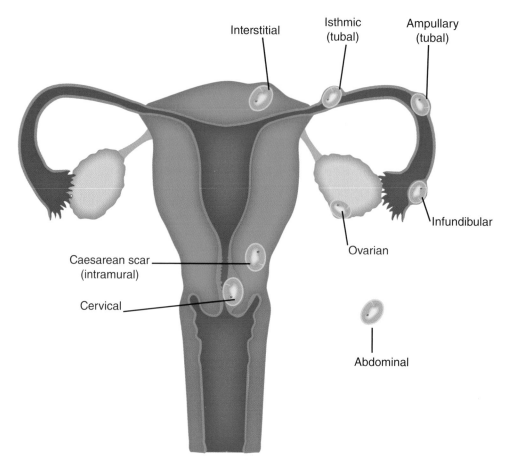

Figure 18.8 Sites of ectopic pregnancies

Abnormalities of implantation of the placenta

Placenta praevia

This is a situation where the placenta has implanted in the lower part of the uterus or cervix. A complete **placenta praevia** totally covers the **internal cervical os** (opening of cervix into the uterus) and thus prevents a normal delivery; a Caesarean section (C-section) is necessary for a safe delivery of the baby. A partial placenta praevia may cause severe bleeding as the cervical os dilates and part of the placenta comes away from the uterine wall; often a C-section will be needed to minimise blood loss.

Placenta abruptio

In **placenta abruptio** the placenta comes away from the lining of the uterus before delivery of the baby occurs, most commonly at around 25 weeks of gestation. The cause is not entirely clear although a number of risk factors have been identified. Some not linked to the pregnancy include cigarette smoking, alcohol and drug abuse, chronic hypertension and blood-clotting disorders. Some risk factors associated with pregnancy include **multiparity** (i.e. has had a number of children), older age (≥35 years), abdominal trauma during pregnancy, hypertension and **pre-eclampsia** during pregnancy. It may develop because of difficulties during placental implantation early in pregnancy (DeRoo et al., 2016).

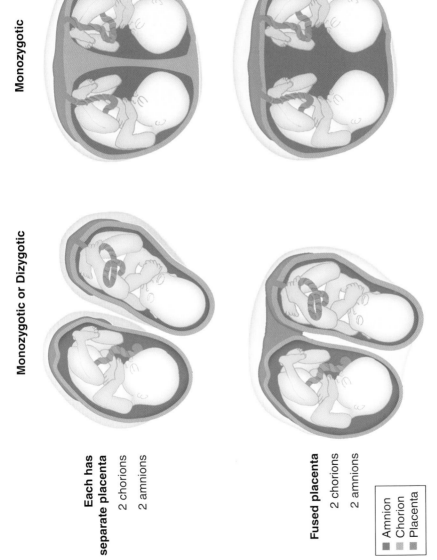

Monozygotic or Dizygotic

Monozygotic

Single placenta

1 chorion

2 amnions

Single placenta

1 chorion

1 amnion

Each has separate placenta

2 chorions

2 amnions

Fused placenta

2 chorions

2 amnions

Amnion
Chorion
Placenta

Illustrated by Shaun Mercier © SAGE Publications

Figure 18.9 Types of placentae with twin pregnancies

Placenta abruptio can result in:

*   vaginal bleeding from the centre of the placenta, which is likely to be maternal in origin and arterial in nature, resulting in severe symptoms, or venous at the placental periphery from the fetal circulation with much less serious effects
*   lower abdominal pain
*   low blood pressure.

The mother may develop disseminated intravascular coagulopathy, a condition in which blood clots form throughout the body, block small blood vessels and the blood clotting factors are used up. It can be caused by infection resulting in inflammation or by obstetric complications such as amniotic fluid entering the bloodstream. Initially a range of symptoms occur, including chest pain, leg pain and symptoms of blood clots in the brain (speech and movement difficulties), but these may be followed by bleeding from various sites such as the vagina, or in urine, faeces or the skin (Franchini et al., 2006). Organ failure may develop. Damage to the uterine wall may result in the placenta becoming disrupted.

Similarly, the baby may suffer in several ways, including:

*   fetal distress, when there is decreased movement felt, cardiac function is disturbed (**tachycardia** or **bradycardia**), meconium-stained amniotic fluid appears, **acidosis**
*   the baby has a low birthweight and birth may occur early (preterm)
*   the baby may be stillborn.

The cause of placenta abruptio is not always clear, but there are a number of risk factors including: pre-eclampsia or hypertension, trauma during pregnancy or to the abdomen, cocaine use, smoking, uterine scarring due to previous caesarean section or placenta abruptio or other uterine abnormalities, over 35 years, pregnant with twins or triplets. A number of these situations can loosen the link between the placenta and the uterine wall (American Pregnancy Association, 2017).

Placental infections

Infection of the placenta may produce cloudy amniotic fluid due to pus production, and the membranes surrounding the fetus may be oedematous and infiltrated with **neutrophils**. This usually develops due to ascending infection often by vaginal bacteria such as *Escherichia coli*, group B streptococci and anaerobic bacteria, and occasionally by crossing the placenta from the maternal circulation. Infection of the membranes often results in premature rupture of the membranes and preterm delivery.

Hypertension during pregnancy

There are four main causes of hypertension during pregnancy with complications resulting in 5–8% of pregnancies: **gestational hypertension**, pre-eclampsia, **eclampsia**, chronic hypertension, and, in addition, there is renal disease in pregnancy (Mammaro et al., 2009; Oats and Abraham, 2010).

Gestational hypertension

This is hypertension that occurs after 20 weeks of gestation but there are no other signs of pre-eclampsia and it disappears within 3 months of delivery. If B/P rises above 140/90 then therapy is instigated to maintain the systolic level between 110 and 140 mmHg and the diastolic between 80 and 90 mmHg.

Pre-eclampsia

Pre-eclampsia is a maternal syndrome that occurs during pregnancy and apparently has a genetic component as other family members also have an increased risk. In addition, those with insulin resistance and central obesity are at higher risk, as are those with some connective tissue disorders which may be due to autoimmune changes and some other conditions. There appears to be a connection between metabolic, immunological and coagulation disturbances, possibly linked by endothelial dysfunction of the blood vessels. There are two phases to pre-eclampsia (Ellison, 2014):

- *Phase 1*: consists of abnormal placental development with inadequate **trophoblasts** cell (which form the outer layer of the blastocyst) invading the maternal arteries, causing inadequate blood supply to the placenta. It is suggested that the abnormalities which occur are due to immunological disruptions, possibly due to maternal rejection of **antigens** from the father.
- *Phase 2*: consists primarily of endothelial damage and disordered function. There is an excessive inflammatory response in the mother with additional activity of **leucocytes**, platelets and coagulation. Overall there is diminished **perfusion** of organs. Metabolic changes with raised lipid levels may contribute to the endothelial damage. Altered platelet function and increased response to vasoconstrictors occur. All these changes lead to vasoconstriction and hypertension. The placenta plays a key role in the development of pre-eclampsia as indicated by the rapid disappearance of symptoms after delivery of the placenta. Various microscopic changes in the placenta occur, including vascular damage and **ischaemia**, resulting from infarcts, **haematomas** and abnormal blood vessels.

The woman develops hypertension, **oedema** and **proteinuria**, usually during the last trimester of pregnancy, and more commonly if having her first baby. Management of women with this unpredictable condition depends on the gestational age of the fetus and the severity of the disease. If the pre-eclampsia is mild then careful monitoring of the mother and baby may allow the pregnancy to continue. The aim of care during the different stages is to control hypertension and prevent the development of eclampsia. Pre-eclampsia is determined by the stage of pregnancy when it is diagnosed:

- Diagnosed before week 32: aim to maintain the pregnancy until week 35, with regular monitoring.
- Between 32 and 35 weeks: managed as earlier in pregnancy. If fetal or maternal state indicates need to end pregnancy then induction of labour or C-section carried out.
- After 35 weeks: condition controlled rapidly and C-section or induction of labour is carried out depending on the condition of the fetus and the cervix (i.e. it becomes softer and more stretchable).

However, severe pre-eclampsia, eclampsia or fetal distress are all indications for delivery at any stage of pregnancy. If the pregnancy is near or at term, then induction of labour or a caesarean section, depending on the condition of the baby, is indicated.

Eclampsia

Some of those affected develop eclampsia in which they become seriously ill and have **convulsions**. The management of pre-eclampsia is to prevent the development of eclampsia and enable the delivery of a live baby. Headaches and visual disturbances indicate severe pre-eclampsia and delivery is often initiated in this situation. Someone with eclampsia has neurological disturbances with convulsions and possibly **coma**. Most of those who develop eclampsia already have pre-eclampsia or have developed proteinuria or chronic hypertension, although 10–30% of them develop eclampsia without any warning. The incidence of eclampsia has diminished in industrialised countries to about 1 in 2000, but it is higher in developing countries.

The physiological changes leading to eclampsia develop from those of pre-eclampsia. Severe **vasospasm** results in tissue hypoxia, urinary volume diminishes and water retention can limit cell metabolism and cause **cerebral oedema**. Coagulation can become impaired. A person affected becomes disorientated and then moves into a convulsion, or convulsions, followed by passing into a coma. The pattern of convulsions and coma can vary and it can occur in late pregnancy, during labour, or after delivery. The aim of treatment is to control convulsions, reduce blood pressure and to deliver the baby (Oats and Abraham, 2010). Magnesium sulphate is injected IV or IM to reduce the convulsions and antihypertensive drugs are administered to lower the blood pressure (Peres et al., 2018). With pre-eclampsia, **corticosteroids** may be administered to stimulate development of the fetal lungs.

Chronic hypertension

This will have been diagnosed in most women before they are identified as pregnant. A raised blood pressure before the 20th week is indicative of **essential hypertension** but it may be missed because of the small fall in B/P early in pregnancy. However, later in pregnancy, the B/P may be raised but the maternal blood flow is reduced and may lead to a decrease in fetal growth. If it is accompanied by proteinuria it appears the same as pre-eclampsia. The treatment aims to maintain blood flow to the uterus, minimise the rise in B/P and promote delivery of the baby if growth is reduced (Oats and Abraham, 2010).

Renal disease in pregnancy

This may also be a cause of hypertension during pregnancy although the diagnosis may have been known beforehand. If serum **creatinine** levels rise, indicating impaired renal function, and fetal growth is poor, then labour should be induced or renal dialysis used. If the woman's condition is well controlled there is a good chance of a successful outcome (Oats and Abraham, 2010).

Gestational trophoblastic disease

There are a number of tumours and similar conditions which develop from placental tissue, and the two major ones are identified below.

Hydatidiform mole

Hydatidiform mole is commonest at the two ends of reproductive life (teenagers and women of 40–50 years). The genetic structure is abnormal due to abnormal fertilisation of the ovum. Most complete moles are derived from an egg that has lost its **chromosomes** and its DNA is entirely from the sperm. Fertilisation by two sperm results in a partial mole. These growths are clearly abnormal; the complete mole is a fragile mass of abnormal cells in grapelike structures and no fetus, while in a partial mole an abnormal fetus begins to develop but cannot develop into a baby.

Most women with these conditions will spontaneously abort or are diagnosed early and undergo a D & C (dilatation and curettage of the uterus) where the contents of the uterus are evacuated via the cervix. Sometimes the mole will develop into a malignant **choriocarcinoma**.

Choriocarcinoma

This is a malignant growth of cells derived from a normal or abnormal pregnancy, e.g. an ectopic pregnancy, hydatidiform mole, previous abortions or normal pregnancy; occasionally it develops from ovarian germ cells. Human growth hormone levels may be raised and vaginal discharge occurs but it might not be diagnosed until some time after the pregnancy. Metastases are common. Treatment consists of removal of the growth and chemotherapy, and usually has very good results.

Problems related to labour and delivery

There are a number of disturbances that can arise in relation to labour and delivery which may result in problems for the mother or baby or both (Moldenhauer, 2016a).

Timing of labour

Theoretically, delivery is expected to occur at 40 weeks' gestation or within one or two weeks either side of that. The risks to the fetus and the mother increase as labour moves further away from the 40 weeks. Premature rupture of membranes increases the risk of labour beginning and preterm labour and delivery, with increased risk to the infant. If it occurs before 37 weeks, there may be some delay before labour begins and there is an increased risk of infection ascending to the uterus.

A post-term pregnancy lasts 42 weeks or more, and the risks to the woman and the fetus increase. Fetal risks include post-maturity, when the placenta can no longer support the fetus through normal growth and development because the increased length of the pregnancy has put excessive strain on the placenta. The signs of post-maturity include:

- Dry, peeling skin, overgrown nails, a large amount of scalp hair, marked creases on the palms and soles, lack of fat deposition, and skin that is stained green or yellow by meconium (contents of the fetal bowel) (Moldenhauer, 2016b)
- Abnormal fetal growth, **oligohydramnios** (reduced amniotic fluid), meconium-stained amniotic fluid (greenish first faeces of baby, released before birth into the amniotic fluid)
- Fetal and/or neonatal death

Maternal risks include:

- Abnormal or difficult labour, which may be longer than normal because the fetus has grown until it has difficulty getting through the mother's pelvis or because uterine contractions are weak or infrequent
- Assisted delivery by, for example, vacuum extraction with damage to the perineum requiring suturing
- **Postpartum haemorrhage (PPH)**: this is the loss of 500 ml of blood within 24 hours of delivery. It can be minor (500–1000 ml) or major (more than 1000 ml) (RCOG, 2016)
- Risks associated with surgery, i.e. Caesarean section

Fetal problems during labour

A number of issues related to the fetus can also cause concern in relation to a safe delivery, including:

- More than one fetus requires extra effort from the mother; the maternal blood volume and her cardiovascular burden are increased (also see earlier).
- Abnormal fetal presentation, including breech (when the baby is positioned in the uterus so that the buttocks or feet arrive first) or with the shoulder positioned so that it cannot pass below the symphysis pubis without considerable manipulation.

- Prolapse of the umbilical cord, which can then get trapped between the baby and the pelvis and the blood flow can be cut off.
- The umbilical cord gets caught around the neck of the baby, with a risk of strangulation.

Postpartum disturbances

These tend to occur shortly after delivery of the baby with the delivery of the placenta and include:

- Postpartum haemorrhage, discussed earlier.
- Uterine damage, including inverted uterus or uterine rupture. An inverted uterus can occur when the placenta is retained and excessive cord traction used to remove it, pulling the uterus inside out. A woman who has had previous surgery (e.g. C-section) is at increased risk of a ruptured uterus (Moldenhauer, 2016c).
- **Amniotic fluid embolism** occurs when some amniotic fluid enters the maternal circulation and results in a serious reaction which may result in cardiorespiratory collapse and serious bleeding.
- Post-natal depression. Between 30 and 80% of women have some mood changes after having a new baby, commonly known as 'baby blues', which usually disappear after a short period of time. However, post-natal depression occurs in 9–21% of new mothers who need support from their family, friends and midwife or health visitor. A woman with post-natal depression has similar symptoms to depression, including low mood and lack of interest, fatigue and low energy, loss of concentration and worrying. She may also sleep poorly and have appetite changes. Some new mothers think about harming their baby, but rarely do so. Puerperal psychosis can occur post-partum when psychotic symptoms including auditory or visual hallucinations can occur (Mental Health Foundation, n.d.).

Puerperal fever

Puerperal fever is any form of bacterial infection of the female reproductive tract following childbirth or miscarriage. This sometimes occurs due to infection in the uterus, causing:

- pain in the lower abdomen or pelvis caused by a swollen uterus; foul-smelling vaginal discharge
- feelings of discomfort or illness, headache, loss of appetite
- elevated temperature, chills
- pale skin, which can be a sign of large-volume blood loss.

GO DEEPER

Aseptic surgery

- While working as a doctor in obstetric care in Vienna General Hospital, Ignaz Semmelweis noticed that the mortality rate varied enormously between two maternity units. One unit was used for the training of midwives; the other was used for training medical students. The unit where medical students were trained had a mortality rate from puerperal fever of 13-18%, several times greater than in the unit where midwives trained. On further investigation he found that medical students carried out postmortems (which the midwives did not) and went straight from this activity to delivering babies. Handwashing was not part of the routine. Semmelweis introduced hand-washing with a 'chloride of lime solution' and the mortality rate dropped to about 2% - the same as in the unit with midwives carrying out the deliveries.

- Unfortunately, the results from Semmelweis' work were not accepted by his medical colleagues, his contract was not renewed, and he returned to his home in Budapest where he worked for some years before he died in an insane asylum in 1865 at the age of 47. However, later his work was recognised and he is now considered one of the founders of aseptic surgery (Best and Neuhauser, 2004).
- Puerperal fever is now much less common as hand-washing is a routine part of care and **asepsis** and antisepsis are practised in maternity care.

DISORDERS OF THE BREAST

The breasts play an important role in infant nutrition but are also significant in a woman's body image.

REVISE: A&P

The breast

You may wish to review the structure of the breast in Chapter 16, The Reproductive Systems, in *Essentials of Anatomy and Physiology for Nursing Practice* (Boore et al., 2016).

There are a number of disorders of the breast that can cause discomfort and these fall into various categories. There are a variety of non-specific symptoms which lead women to consult a doctor about a breast disorder. These are:

- Pain: may be cyclic coinciding with menstrual periods due to premenstrual oedema or non-cyclic, often in one part of the breast due to some specific lesion. Most painful masses are benign but 10% of malignant breast tumours present with pain.
- A palpable mass (i.e. that can be felt) needs to be differentiated from the normal 'lumpiness' of the breast. The most common masses are cysts, **fibroadenomas** and invasive carcinomas. Only 10% of breast masses in women under 40, but 60% of those in women over 50, are malignant. However, benign breast lesions may begin in the teens and reach a peak between 30 and 50 years, diminishing after the menopause (Guray and Sahin, 2006).
- Nipple discharge is less common but more likely to be associated with malignancy, although there are other causes.

Mammography and sonography, supported by biopsy, are now the commonest means of diagnosing breast lesions, even when they are small, non-palpable and asymptomatic (Lester, 2015).

Benign disorders of the breast

These disorders can be grouped as developmental, inflammatory, fibrocystic, stromal and neoplastic in nature (Guray and Sahin, 2006).

Developmental abnormalities

These fall into two main groups:

- Ectopic breast tissue occurring outside the normal breast tissue is the most common such disorder. Such abnormalities usually consist of the range of normal breast tissues and can present with similar disorders.

- Underdevelopment of the breast can also occur, mainly associated with certain genetic disorders such as Turner's syndrome.

Inflammatory disorders

These make up less than 1% of breast disorders but include the following:

Mastitis

This consists of inflammatory changes which may be due to varying causes, some of which are unclear. The most common types are:

- *Acute mastitis.* This usually occurs early (first month) during breast-feeding due to a bacterial infection in lesions that develop in the nipples and spread into the breast which becomes inflamed and painful and the woman develops a raised temperature. Inadequate treatment enables further spread through the breast, developing **abscesses** (*Staphylococci*) or cellulitis (*Streptococci*). Antibiotics and expression of milk normally control the infection.
- *Granulomatous mastitis.* This can be due to a variety of different organisms but some are idiopathic (i.e. of unknown cause) and autoimmune reactions have been proposed. **Granuloma** is an inflammation including a collection of **macrophage**s where the immune system tries to wall off substances identified as foreign but which cannot be eliminated. Such substances include organisms like bacteria and **fungi**. Foreign bodies of materials such as silicone used in reconstructive surgery and suture fragments can cause similar reactions.

Mammary duct ectasia

In this condition, the **lactiferous duct** becomes dilated and chronic inflammation develops in the surrounding tissues. It is commonest in middle-aged to elderly women who have had children. The aetiology is unclear but the epithelium lining the duct becomes thinned with thickening of the wall due to plasma cells and **lymphocytes** infiltrating it. Foamy macrophages may be in the duct and discharge from the nipple. The nipple discharge with inflammation and pain can occur if the duct becomes blocked with whitish material due to stasis of secretions, possibly stagnant **colostrum** (the first milk produced after delivery of the baby). The duct may become fibrosed with some calcification. Nipple inversion and discharge can occur (Pinder et al., 2014).

Fat necrosis

This is an inflammatory process following injury or surgery to the breast which is benign and non-suppurative (not pus-forming). After **adipocytes** have been injured or have died, haemorrhage can occur followed by **phagocytosis** of the debris by macrophages which may collect as a liquid within a cyst. Inflammation and scar tissue may develop, resulting in a hard mass that resembles breast cancer, except that it is very tender and is readily differentiated by a mammogram (Pinder et al., 2014).

Fibrocystic changes

Fibrocystic changes are the most common benign breast lesions, mainly occurring in women of 20–50 years old. The causes are not entirely clear but hormonal imbalance is often involved, particularly oestrogen and progesterone but also other hormones such as prolactin, growth factor, insulin and thyroid hormone. These conditions are diagnosed by physical examination, mammography, ultrasound and biopsy. Sometimes the increased density of the breast tissue makes it difficult to differentiate between benign and malignant growths by mammography, however ultrasonography can distinguish between a solid mass and cysts. The types of condition fall into three main groups: nonproliferative lesions, proliferative lesions without **atypia** and proliferative lesions with atypia (Guray and Sahin, 2006).

Nonproliferative lesions

These conditions include a number of types of lesions including cysts (large and small) and solid growths, increased fibrous tissue and variable increases in epithelial tissue in the terminal of the lactiferous duct. The breast lumps are not malignant but can cause discomfort, sometimes in synchrony with hormonal changes related to menstruation. These are nodular breast masses that are most prominent during the progesterone stage of the menstrual cycle and cause pain varying from 'heaviness to exquisite tenderness depending on the degree of vascular **engorgement** and cystic distension' (Porth, 2015: 1043).

Proliferative lesions

There is a range of proliferative lesions from duct or lobular epithelium, some with (**atypia** – not typical of the tissue) and some without such cells, which are not typical for the breast tissue. These all need examination, and often histological study, to determine whether there are any signs of malignancy developing.

- *Without atypia*: These lesions of typical cells include:
    - *epithelial hyperplasia*: cells of ducts and lobules in the breast multiply and stretch the tissues, leading to tissue masses
    - *sclerosing adenosis*: increasing fibrosis causes compression and distortion of the epithelium and **acini** (small sacs within the glandular tissue)
    - *intraductal papillomas*: these are growths within the lactiferous ducts made up of supporting tissue, cells lining the lumen and myoepithelial cells (immediately below luminal cells with muscular function). Many (80%+ of) large duct papillomas produce a discharge, sometimes bloodstained, from the nipple (Lester, 2015).
- *With atypia*: The other lesions are of cells which are similar to the cells of carcinoma in situ, i.e. atypical of the normal breast cells. The two types are:
    - *atypical ductile hyperplasia* (similar to DCIS – ductile carcinoma in situ)
    - *atypical lobular hyperplasia* (similar to LCIS – lobar carcinoma in situ).

Both these conditions need careful follow-up to identify and treat carcinoma if it should develop.

Stromal lesions

Stromal lesions arise from the supportive-connective tissues within the breast and consist of two main types:

- **Diabetic fibrous mastopathy**: is associated with severe microvascular complications of type 1 diabetes mellitus. The cause is unknown but may be related to an immune response to abnormal extracellular tissue.
- **Pseudoangiomatous stromal hyperplasia**: is a benign proliferation of **myofibrils** in the stroma. The cause is unclear.

Neoplasms

These are non-malignant new growths arising from a number of different tissues, including:

* Fibroadenoma: commonest breast lesion; composed of epithelial and mesenchymal (circulatory and lymphatic) tissues
* **Lipoma**: composed of mature fat cells
* **Adenoma**: formed from epithelial cells; can become lactating or tubular adenoma
* **Hamartoma**: uncommon tumour of varying amounts of glandular, adipose and fibrous tissue
* **Granular cell tumour**: originates from Schwann cells of peripheral nervous system

The treatment is usually surgical.

Breast cancer

This is the most common form of cancer in women with about 1 in 8 of women in the UK developing it at some time in their life, arising from the tissues of the duct system. A distinction used to be made between the origins of ductal and lobular carcinomas. However, it is now thought that initially the malignancy begins within the terminating section of the lobule and remains within the duct as ductal carcinoma in situ (DCIS) but then invades the breast tissue, becoming more widely invasive (Pinder et al., 2014).

There are two main groups of breast cancer to be considered: carcinoma in situ and invasive carcinoma. DCIS is usually limited to one duct system in the breast and is usually a readily felt mass which is easily differentiated by mammography. It is normally treated by surgical excision and adjunct radiotherapy. The tumour size, degree of spread of malignant cells into the lymph nodes and the histological grading of the cells (Table 18.4) all contribute to the prognosis.

Table 18.4 Histological grading of breast cancer cells

Grade 1 or low grade (sometimes called well differentiated)	They look a little different from normal cells. They grow in slow, well-organised patterns. Not many cells are dividing to make new cancer cells
Grade 2 or intermediate/moderate grade (moderately differentiated)	They do not look like normal cells. They are growing and dividing a little faster than normal
Grade 3 or high grade (poorly differentiated)	They look very different from normal cells. They grow quickly in disorganised, irregular patterns, with many dividing to make new cancer cells

There are a number of different cell groups involved in breast cancer. The duct-lobular units are lined by two main types of cells. These are inner luminal secretory cells which are ER (Oestrogen Receptor) positive and divided into two types – luminal A and luminal B, and basal-like tumours which are hormone negative, particularly HER2 (human epidermal growth factor receptor 2) negative.

Main types of breast cancer

There are five main intrinsic or molecular subtypes of breast cancer that are based on the genes that a cancer expresses (Changavi et al., 2015):

- *Luminal A* breast cancer is hormone-receptor-positive (oestrogen-receptor (ER+) and/or progesterone-receptor-positive (PR+), HER2-negative, and has low levels of the protein Ki-67. This is a nuclear protein that is associated with promoting cell growth and division through **mitosis**, and with ribosomal RNA transcription. Thus, increased Ki-67 results in increased multiplication of the cancer cells. Luminal A cancers are low-grade, tend to grow slowly and have the best prognosis.
- *Luminal B* breast cancer is hormone-receptor-positive (ER+ and/or PR+), and either HER2+ or HER2– with high levels of Ki-67. Luminal B cancers generally grow slightly faster than luminal A cancers and their prognosis is slightly worse.
- *Triple-negative/basal-like* breast cancer is hormone-receptor-negative (ER– and/or PR–), HER2– and low Ki-67. This type of cancer is more common in women with *BRCA1* gene mutations. *BRCA1* and *BRCA2* are genes that normally help to prevent breast cancer and are known as tumour suppressor genes but mutations greatly increase the risk (NIH, 2018).) It is not clear why, but this type of cancer is more common among younger and African-American women. These cells may grow more slowly and are less likely to recur or spread to other parts of the body than cancer cells that have a large amount of HER2 on their surface. These tumours are more aggressive than luminal tumours.
- *HER2-enriched* breast cancer is hormone-receptor-negative (ER– and PR–) and HER2+. HER2-enriched cancers tend to grow faster than luminal cancers and can have a worse prognosis, but they are often successfully treated with targeted therapies aimed at the HER2 protein.
- *Normal-like* (or unclassified) breast cancer is similar to luminal A disease: hormone-receptor-positive (ER+ and/or PR+), HER2-negative, and low levels of Ki-67. Still, while normal-like breast cancer has a good prognosis, it is slightly worse than luminal A cancer's prognosis.

Invasive cancer

Invasive carcinoma falls into a number of types, outlined in Table 18.5.

Table 18.5 Types of invasive carcinoma

Invasive breast cancer of No Special Type (NST)	Over 50% of invasive cancers. 10-40 mm diameter. Cords and sheets of epithelial cells variable in size and shape
Invasive lobular carcinoma	10-15% of invasive cancers. Small-moderate-sized cells, ill-defined outline, cords of cells within fine **collagen** bands
Tubular carcinoma	2% of invasive cancers. Small lesions, <10 mm in diameter, firm. Tubules lined by regular epithelial cells
Medullary-like carcinoma	Rare, 10-40 mm diameter, **syncetium** (fusion of several cells) of large epithelial cells. Variable in shape with obvious mitoses. Found in *BRCA1* carriers
Mucinous carcinoma	<1% well-defined gelatinous jelly-like appearance. Small clumps of cells within lakes of mucin
Mixed type of carcinoma	<1%. Less than 90% pure cells. May be different mixes of types of cells

Source: Pinder et al., 2014

The majority of these cancers have no special features. About 10% are invasive lobular carcinoma and begin in the lobules of the breast, and a few are even rarer types. It is about 100 times commoner in women than men, and most of the women are post-menopausal, with only about 20% being under 50 years of age (Cancer Research UK, 2017a). There are a number of factors which modify the risk of developing breast cancer (Table 18.6).

Treatment

If treatment is effective, then prognosis can be very good. A number of different types of treatment are used to cure or alleviate cancerous growths. The programme of treatment or treatments used is planned with care depending on the type of growth and response to different interventions (Cancer Research UK, 2017b).

Surgery

There are various types of surgery from which to choose, taking into account: the size of the tumour, position of the tumour, breast size and wishes of the person involved (Cancer Research UK, 2017c). These are:

- *Lumpectomy*: in which only the tumour and a small area of healthy tissue around it are removed. This works for small tumours which are in an accessible position in the breast. Lumpectomy is usually followed by radiotherapy to kill any remaining malignant cells.

Table 18.6 Risk factors for breast cancer

Genetic factors	Family members with breast cancer
	Breast cancer genes, particularly *BRCA1* and *BRCA2* genes:
	• Rare but 45–90% of those with one of these develop breast cancer at some time
	• Ovarian and male breast or **prostate cancer** increased
Lifestyle factors	Overweight or obesity after menopause increases the risk
	Alcohol intake slightly increases risk; recommended intake was 14 units a week, but recommendations are variable
Hormonal factors	Hormone replacement therapy increases risk while on HRT + 5 years after
	Contraceptive pill: very small increased risk while taking it + 10 years after
	Women with children have slightly lower risk of breast cancer than others. Younger the age when having first child, the lower the risk
	Sex hormones and other hormones:
	• Levels of oestrogen, and testosterone, affect the risk
	• Post-menopause, higher levels of prescribed oestrogen and testosterone increase the risk
	• Higher levels of testosterone before menopause increase the risk
Individual factors	Getting older: breast cancer is mainly in over 50s and rare in under 40s
	Mammograms used: national breast screening programme from 47 to 73 years
	Age when menstruation started and stopped: increased risk of breast cancer if started before 12 and finished after 55
	Height: women who are taller than average have slightly increased risk after the menopause. Possibly due to different hormone levels in taller women
	Ethnicity: risk higher in white women than other groups. Possibly due to lifestyle factors
Medical history	Factors increasing risk: X-rays and radiotherapy: exposure to radiation
	Other conditions: diabetes, autoimmune thyroiditis, high bone density
	Previous cancer: previous breast cancer increases risk of getting another
	Previous other cancers, melanoma skin cancer, lung cancer, bowel cancer, uterine cancer, chronic lymphocytic leukaemia can also increase the risk
	Radiotherapy treatment to chest (Hodgkin lymphoma) increases the risk
Previous breast disorders	DCIS/LCIS: double risk of breast cancer than in normal breast
	Benign breast disease: increased risk with some types
	Dense breast tissue: risk higher with more dense breast tissue

Source: Cancer Research UK, 2017a

- *Mastectomy*: in which the whole breast is removed. This includes the breast tissue, the skin and nipple, and tissues over the chest wall. If necessary, the chest wall muscles and, if malignant cells have spread, the lymph nodes near the breast in the axilla will be removed. This approach is used when the tumour is large, in the centre of the breast, or is spreading through the breast or to any adjacent tissues, or there are other lesions or radiotherapy have been administered previously. A course of radiotherapy may be used to minimise the risk of recurrence (NHS Choices, 2015d).

Lymphoedema often occurs following surgery for breast cancer, particularly if lymph nodes were also removed and thus the lymph drainage system is disrupted and lymph accumulates in the tissue, causing swelling.

ACTIVITY 18.3: UNDERSTAND

Lymphoedema

Watch this video which explains the mechanism of lymphoedema development. If you are using the eBook just click on the play button. Alternatively go to
https://study.sagepub.com/essentialpatho/videos

LYMPHOEDEMA (3:38)

It is important to take care of the arm with lymphoedema to prevent further development. The main aim of management is to protect the arm from any action that might increase the risk of swelling. This includes preventing infection by: avoiding damage to the skin, minimising heat and sunburn; reducing the swelling by exercises to promote fluid drainage, using an elasticated sleeve or bandage, and specialised massage; laying the arm in a supported position when sitting (NHS Health A–Z, 2016).

- *Breast reconstruction*: This is carried out after a mastectomy to provide a breast similar in appearance to the one removed. There are a few different ways this can be carried out, depending on the amount of tissue removed and skin remaining. An implant usually provides a structural framework. Additional surgery may replace a nipple. Breast reconstruction may have to be delayed until additional treatments have been completed.
- *Removal of lymph nodes*: If malignant cells have spread into the nearby lymph nodes, then most or all of the nodes under the arm may be removed at the same time or in a separate operation. Sometimes these nodes are treated with radiotherapy.

Radiotherapy and chemotherapy

These forms of treatment are discussed in Chapter 3.

Hormone therapy

These treatments are effective on cells with oestrogen receptors and aim to prevent the action of oestrogen or progesterone by lowering their level or blocking their effects. It is usually used as adjuvant (or neo-adjuvant) treatment before or after surgery or chemotherapy, or combined with radiotherapy. It can also be used alone and may control the cancer for 18 months to 2 years, if necessary, followed by another type of hormone therapy. There are a number of different treatments including tamoxifen (an antioestrogen medication) or other drugs or removal of the ovaries. A number of side-effects similar to those of the menopause may occur.

Targeted cancer drugs

There are certain drugs which act on specific receptors on some malignant breast cells and help the body to control their growth. These are **monoclonal antibodies** (see Chapter 7 on the immune system). Some of the side-effects include: 'an increased risk of infection, hot flushes and sweats, **diarrhoea**, joint or muscle pain, tiredness, an **allergic reaction**' (Cancer Research UK, 2017d). Some examples which target HER2 receptors on the breast cancer cells and stop growth and division of the cells include the following: Herceptin (chemical name: trastuzumab), Perjeta (chemical name: pertuzumab) and Tykerb (chemical name: lapatinib) target both HER2 and EGFR. Docetaxel has been combined with other drugs in such treatments and enhances the anti-cancer effect by diminishing mitosis and reducing cell multiplication (Yamashita-Kashima et al., 2017). Patients with HER2-positive metastatic breast cancer showed a considerable mean increase in survival (an additional 15.7 months up to 56.5 months) over a control group when treated with docetaxel in combination with trastuzumab and pertuzumab (Swain et al., 2015).

INFERTILITY

Infertility is identified as a lack of conception occurring following 12 months of unprotected intercourse timed to coincide with ovulation. This is an issue which can result in considerable emotional disturbance in a couple who have assumed that they will have no difficulty in having a child within a reasonable time span, and then discover that this will not be so. This chapter will largely focus on female aspects of infertility. A number of causes of female infertility have already been mentioned in earlier parts of this chapter but a summary of causes is shown in Table 18.7.

Table 18.7   Identified causes of female infertility

Ovulation problems	Polycystic ovary syndrome (PCOS) in which periods may be absent or irregular associated with no or irregular ovulation
	Under- or over-active thyroid glands may prevent ovulation
	Premature failure of ovaries – before age 40
Surgery	Pelvic surgery can result in scarring of Fallopian tubes
	Cervix can be scarred by surgery
Cervical **mucus**	Cervical mucus not thinning at ovulation may make it difficult for sperm to swim through
Fibroids	May prevent fertilised egg attaching to uterine lining or may block Fallopian tube
Endometriosis	Can damage Fallopian tubes and prevent passage of ovum
Pelvic inflammatory disease	Infection of the genital tract, including uterus, fallopian tubes, ovaries. Infection can damage and scar Fallopian tubes
Certain drugs	Non-steroidal anti-inflammatory drugs
	Chemotherapy
	Antipsychotic medications
	Spironolactone (a diuretic)
	Illegal drugs (e.g. marijuana, cocaine)

Source: Adapted from NHS Choices, 2017a

However, there are also instances of infertility for which there is no explanation. Up to 30% of couples unable to conceive are identified as having unexplained infertility and referred for additional investigation and management (Ray et al., 2012).

An additional possible cause of infertility is a substantial and mixed group of chemicals known as endocrine disruptors (EDs). This group includes industrial lubricants and solvents and by-products such as plastics, plasticisers, pesticides, DDT (dichlorodiphenyltrichloethane) and numerous others. ED residues have been found in serum and in fluids in ovaries and testes and it is thought that these substances are influencing human fertility through their effect on reproductive functioning. It is considered that the major route for exposure to these substances is through food (vegetables, meat, fish, dairy products) and drink (water and other fluids). It is also thought that plastics used in packaging are important sources of EDs (Marques-Pinto and Carvalho, 2013).

A couple discovering that they are infertile will move through the experience together and will have to decide how they want to go forward. Research on the psychosocial aspects of infertility has been developing along two lines. One group is focusing on the psychological aspects, aiming to assess the need and provide appropriate service intervention to meet the need for psychological counselling. Other researchers are focusing on finding out about how infertile individuals and couples experience the socio-cultural context and integrate their lives within that context (Greil et al., 2010). Together these support the decision-making about various interventions to achieve their own child, or to accept being childless, or to achieve a situation where they become a family and have a child or children in their life through adoption or fostering.

For a couple who desires their own child, the next stage is treatment determined by the problem causing the infertility and what is available in their area. There are three main types of treatment available: medication, surgery and assisted conception (NHS Choices, 2017b).

Medication

Medicines can be given to women, and sometimes to men, to enhance their fertility. These are mostly used to deal with problems of ovulation and include:

* Drugs that encourage monthly ovulation, e.g. clomifene, tamoxifen.
* Something particularly useful for those with polycystic ovary syndrome (PCOS) is metformin, which helps to control the effect of insulin resistance, a characteristic metabolic change in PCOS, and improves metabolic disturbances, thus helping to normalise the menstrual cycle and improve the chance of pregnancy (Lashen, 2010).
* Gonadotrophins, which encourage ovulation and sometimes enhance male fertility.
* Other medicines that encourage ovulation.

These are only used when the cause of infertility is understood.

Surgery

Procedures which may help to correct female infertility include:

* Repair of Fallopian tubes by removing scarring or blockage
* Removal of abnormal tissue in endometriosis, fibroids, PCOS.

These can often be carried out through a laparoscopy.

Assisted conception

Assisted conception refers to some method of introducing gametes or a fertilised embryo into the female reproductive tract. Various procedures are available (NHS Choices, 2015e):

- Intrauterine insemination: sperm are collected and introduced though a fine tube through the cervix into the uterus.
- In vitro fertilisation (IVF): the women takes medication to stimulate greater than usual egg production and these are removed from the ovaries. These are then fertilised in a laboratory and the viable embryo(s) inserted into the uterus to embed into the uterine wall and develop.
- Egg and sperm donation: an egg or sperm can be provided by a donor(s) and fertilisation performed by IVF. In the UK, at the age of 18 a child derived from donated germ cells is entitled to know who their biological parents are.

CHAPTER SUMMARY

This chapter has examined the main pathophysiological conditions affecting the female reproductive organs. A range of conditions affect females at different stages in the life cycle and many will cause difficulties with reproduction and result in difficulties for mother and fetus.

KEY POINTS

- Infections of the reproductive system can be due to a number of different organisms, some of which cause inflammation and others infertility or premature deliveries. Human papilloma virus (HPV) can contribute to the development of carcinoma of parts of the reproductive system. Pelvic inflammatory disease (PID) can result in a range of complications, including peritonitis and bacteraemia.

- All the different organs of the reproductive system can develop disorders of the different tissues; some lesions are benign and some malignant. Some of the major malignant disorders are carcinoma of the cervix (HPV), the endometrium, the ovary and that developed from placental tissue.

- Common benign uterine disorders include endometriosis, where endometrial tissue is found in sites outside the uterus, and fibroids (leiomyomas).

- A group of conditions that usually result from pregnancy and delivery are disorders of the uterosacral ligaments, which can result in cystocele, rectocele and uterine prolapse.

- Polycystic ovary syndrome and ovarian tumours (benign and malignant) are important conditions of the ovary which can have deleterious effects on health.

- During pregnancy, a number of conditions can occur which have serious implications for maternal and/or fetal morbidity and mortality. Some of these include disorders of the placenta or are tumours derived from placental tissue, pre-eclampsia and eclampsia, postpartum disturbance and puerperal fever.

- Breasts play an important role in infant nutrition. There are a number of benign and malignant disorders which can be treated using several approaches.

- There are a number of causes of infertility in women and three main approaches to facilitate conception.

There are numerous disorders affecting the female reproductive system and at some point in your career you may well be caring for someone with one of these. The following questions will help to guide your revision.

1   Identify two types of developmental anomalies and briefly describe their cause.

2   Identify four microbes that cause infections of the female reproductive tract and the disorders which they cause.

3   What are the signs and symptoms of pelvic inflammatory disease and what complications can occur?

4   What is endometriosis? What are the main symptoms?

5   What is a leiomyoma and what are the different types?

6   What are the three conditions that occur with disorders of the uterosacral ligaments? What are the four stages of one of these conditions?

7   What are the major signs and symptoms of polycystic ovary syndrome? Name some other chronic health conditions associated with it.

8   What are the risk factors for ovarian cancer?

9   What is an ectopic pregnancy? How does it usually present?

10 What are the signs and symptoms and possible effects of pre-eclampsia?

11 What is a post-term pregnancy? Outline the potential risks to mother and baby.

12 What is puerperal fever and what are the symptoms?

13 What are the non-specific symptoms of breast problems which lead a women to consult her doctor?

14 Discuss the risk factors for breast cancer.

15 Identify the main approaches to the treatment of breast cancer.

16 Name four causes of female infertility.

17 Briefly explain the three main approaches to managing infertility.

REVISE

ACE YOUR ASSESSMENT

- Further revision and learning opportunities are available online
- Test yourself away from the book with **Extra multiple choice questions**
- Learn and revise terminology with **Interactive flashcards**

If you are using the eBook access each resource by clicking on the respective icon. Alternatively go to **https://study.sagepub.com/essentialpatho/chapter18**

CHAPTER 18 ANSWERS   EXTRA QUESTIONS   FLASHCARDS

REFERENCES

American Pregnancy Association (2017) Placental abruption. [online] americanpregnancy.org/pregnancy-complications/placental-abruption/Feedback (accessed 24 April 2018).

Anglesio, M.S., Papadopoulos, N., Ayhan, A., Nazeran, T.M., Noë, M., Horlings, H.M. et al. (2017) Cancer-associated mutations in endometriosis without cancer. *New England Journal of Medicine, 376* (19): 1835–48.

Best, M. and Neuhauser, D. (2004) Ignaz Semmelweis and the birth of infection control. *Quality and Safety in Health Care, 13* (3): 233–4.

Biro, F.M., Greenspan, L.C. and Galvez, M.P. (2012) Puberty in girls of the 21st century. *Journal of Pediatric and Adolescent Gynecology, 25* (5): 289–94.

Boore, J., Cook, N. and Shepherd, A. (2016) *Essentials of Anatomy and Physiology for Nursing Practice.* London: Sage. Chs 16, 17.

Bulun, S.E. (2011) Physiology and pathology of the female reproductive axis. In S. Melmed, K.S. Polonsky, P.R. Larsen and H.M. Kronenberg (eds), *Williams Textbook of Endocrinology,* 12th edn. Philadelphia, PA: Elsevier Saunders.

Burney, R.O. and Giudice, L.C. (2012) Pathogenesis and pathophysiology of endometriosis. *Fertility and Sterility, 98* (3): 511–19.

Burton, K. (2014) Disorders of the vulva. In B.A. McGowan, P. Owen and A. Thomson (eds), *Clinical Obstetrics and Gynaecology,* 3rd edn. Edinburgh: Elsevier Saunders. Ch. 22.

Cancer Research UK (2016) Ovarian cancer. [online]. Available at: www.cancerresearchuk.org/about-cancer/ovarian-cancer) (accessed 22 June 2018).

Cancer Research UK (2017a) Breast cancer – risk factors. [online]. Available at: www.cancerresearchuk.org/about-cancer/breast-cancer/risks-causes/risk-factors) (accessed 10 February 2018).

Cancer Research UK (2017b) Breast cancer – Treatment. [online]. Available at: www.cancerresearchuk.org/about-cancer/breast-cancer/treatment (accessed 10 February 2018).

Cancer Research UK (2017c) Surgery for breast cancer. [online]. Available at: www.cancerresearchuk.org/about-cancer/breast-cancer/treatment/surgery (accessed 11 February 2018).

Cancer Research UK (2017d) About targeted cancer drugs. [online]. Available at: www.cancerresearchuk.org/about-cancer/breast-cancer/treatment/targeted-cancer-drugs/about-targeted-cancer-drugs (accessed 11 February 2018).

Cancer Research UK (2018) Vaginal cancer incidence statistics. [online]. Available at: www.cancerresearchuk.org/health-professional/cancer-statistics/statistics-by-cancer-type/vaginal-cancer/incidence (accessed 20 April 2018).

Changavi, A.A., Ramji, A.S. and Shashikala, A. (2015) Epidermal growth factor receptor expression in triple negative and nontriple negative breast carcinomas. *Journal of Laboratory Physicians*, *7* (2): 79–83.

Colombo, N., Pretin. E., Landoni, F., Carinelli, S., Colombo, A., Marini, C. et al. (on behalf of the ESMO Guidelines Working Group) (2013) Endometrial cancer: ESMO Clinical Practice Guidelines for diagnosis, treatment and follow-up. *Annals of Oncology*, *24* (Suppl 6): vi33–vi38.

Crawford, S. (2014) Uterine neoplasia. In B.A. McGowan, P. Owen and A. Thomson (eds), *Clinical Obstetrics and Gynaecology*, 3rd edn. Edinburgh: Elsevier Saunders. Ch. 20.

DeRoo, L, Skjærven, R., Wilcox, A., Klungsøyr, K., Wikström, A-K., Morken, N-H. et al. (2016) Placental abruption and long-term maternal cardiovascular disease mortality: a population-based registry study in Norway and Sweden. *European Journal of Epidemiology*, *31* (5): 501–11.

Diarra, A. and Botha, H. (2017) Invasive cervical cancer and human immunodeficiency virus (HIV) infection at Tygerberg Academic Hospital in the period 2003–2007: demographics and characteristics. *Southern African Journal of Gynaecological Oncology*, *9* (1): 1–5.

Doshani, A., Teo, R.E.C., Mayne, C.J. and Tincello, D.G. (2007) Uterine prolapse. *British Medical Journal*, *335* (7624): 819–23.

Ehrmann, D.A. (2005) Polycystic ovary syndrome. *New England Journal of Medicine*, *352* (12): 1223–36.

Ellenson, L.H. and Pirog, E.C. (2015) The female genital tract. In V. Kumar, A.K. Abbas and J.C. Aster (eds), *Robbins and Cotran Pathologic Basis of Disease*, 9th edn. Philadelphia, PA: Elsevier Saunders. Ch. 22.

Ellison, J. (2014) Hypertensive disorders in pregnancy. In B.A. McGowan, P. Owen and A. Thomson (eds), *Clinical Obstetrics and Gynaecology*, 3rd edn. Edinburgh: Elsevier Saunders. Ch. 36.

Euling, S.Y., Herman-Giddens, M.E., Lee, P.A. et al. (2008) Examination of US puberty-timing data from 1940 to 1994 for secular trends: panel findings. *Pediatrics*, *121* (Suppl 3): S172–S191.

Fauconnier, A. and Chapron, C. (2005) Endometriosis and pelvic pain: epidemiological evidence of the relationship and implications. *Human Reproduction Update*, *11* (6): 595–606.

Franchini, M., Lippi, G. and Manzato, F. (2006) Recent acquisitions in the pathophysiology, diagnosis and treatment of disseminated intravascular coagulation. *Thrombosis Journal*, *4*: 4.

Gold, E.B. (2011) The timing of the age at which natural menopause occurs. *Obstetrics and Gynecology Clinics of North America*, *38* (3): 425–40.

Goodarzi, M.O., Dumesic, D.A., Chazenbalk, G. and Azziz, R. (2011) Polycystic ovary syndrome: etiology, pathogenesis and diagnosis. *Nature Reviews Endocrinology*, *7* (4): 219–31.

Greil, A.L., Slauson-Blevins, K. and McQuillan, J. (2010) The experience of infertility: a review of recent literature. *Sociology of Health and Illness*, *32* (1): 140–62.

Guray, M. and Sahin, A.A. (2006) Benign breast diseases: classification, diagnosis, and management. *The Oncologist*, *11* (5): 435–49.

Haefner, H.K., Collins, M.E., Davis, G.D., Edwards, L., Foster, D.C., Hartmann, E.H. et al. (2005) The Vulvodynia Guideline (American Society for Colposcopy and Cervical Pathology). *Journal of Lower Genital Tract Disease*, *9* (1): 40–51.

Herrington, C.S. (2014) The female reproductive system. In C.S. Herrington (ed.), *Muir's Textbook of Pathology*, 15th edn. London: CRC Press, Taylor and Francis. Ch. 14.

Kong, A., Johnson, N., Kitchener, H.C. and Lawrie, T.A. (2012) Adjuvant radiotherapy for stage I endometrial cancer. *Cochrane Database of Systematic Reviews*, *4*, CD003916. http://doi.org/10.1002/14651858.CD003916.pub4.

Lashen, H. (2010) Role of metformin in the management of polycystic ovary syndrome. *Therapeutic Advances in Endocrinology and Metabolism*, *1* (3): 117–28.

Lester, S.C. (2015) The breast. In V. Kumar, A.K. Abbas and J.C. Aster (eds), *Robbins and Cotran Pathologic Basis of Disease*. Philadelphia, PA: Elsevier Saunders. Ch. 23.

Li, J., Bao, R., Peng, S. and Zhang, C. (2018) The molecular mechanism of ovarian granulosa cell tumors. *Journal of Ovarian Research*, 11: 13.

Mammaro, A., Carrara, S., Cavaliere, A., Emito, S., Dinatale, A., Pappalardo, E.M. et al. (2009) Hypertensive disorders in pregnancy. *Journal of Prenatal Medicine*, 3 (1): 1–5.

Mari, G., Roberts, A., Detti, L., Kovanci, E., Stefos, T., Bahado-Singh, R.O. et al. (2001) Perinatal morbidity and mortality rates in severe twin-twin transfusion syndrome: results of the International Amnioreduction Registry. *American Journal of Obstetrics and Gynecology*, 185 (3): 708–15.

Marques-Pinto, A. and Carvalho, D. (2013) Human infertility: are endocrine disruptors to blame? *Endocrine Connections*, R16–R29.

Mayo Clinic (2018) Uterine fibroids. [online]. Available at: www.mayoclinic.org/diseases-conditions/uterine-fibroids/symptoms-causes/syc-20354288 (accessed 9 October 2018).

McNeeley, S.G. (2017) Benign ovarian masses. MSD Manual Professional Version Gynecology and Obstetrics. [online]. Available at: www.msdmanuals.com/en-gb/professional/gynecology-and-obstetrics/benign-gynecologic-lesions/benign-ovarian-masses (accessed 22 June 2018).

Mental Health Foundation (n.d.) Postnatal depression. [online]. Available at: www.mentalhealth.org.uk/a-to-z/p/postnatal-depression (accessed 10 October 2018).

Moldenhauer, J.S. (2016a) Introduction to abnormalities and complications of labor and delivery. MSD Manual Professional Version Obstetrics and Gynecology. [online]. Available at: www.merckmanuals.com/professional/gynecology-and-obstetrics/abnormalities-and-complications-of-labor-and-delivery/introduction-to-abnormalities-and-complications-of-labor-and-delivery (accessed 9 February 2018).

Moldenhauer, J.S. (2016b) Postterm pregnancy. MSD Manual Professional Version Obstetrics and Gynecology. [online]. Available at: www.merckmanuals.com/professional/gynecology-and-obstetrics/abnormalities-and-complications-of-labor-and-delivery/postterm-pregnancy (accessed 9 February 2018).

Moldenhauer, J.S. (2016c) Inverted uterus. MSD Manual Professional Version/Obstetrics and Gynecology. [online]. Available at: www.msdmanuals.com/en-gb/professional/gynecology-and-obstetrics/abnormalities-and-complications-of-labor-and-delivery/inverted-uterus (accessed 25 April 2018).

Murali, R., Soslow, R.A. and Weigelt, B. (2014) Classification of endometrial carcinoma: more than two types. *The Lancet Oncology*, 15 (7): 667–774.

NHS Choices (2015a) Menopause. [online]. Available at: www.nhs.uk/conditions/menopause/ (accessed 1 February 2018).

NHS Choices (2015b) Endometriosis. [online]. Available at: www.nhs.uk/conditions/endometriosis/ (accessed 14 February 2018).

NHS Choices (2015c) Fibroids. [online]. Available at: www.nhs.uk/conditions/fibroids/ (accessed 14 February 2018).

NHS Choices (2015d) Radiotherapy. [online]. Available at: www.nhs.uk/conditions/radiotherapy/side-effects/ (accessed 10 February 2018).

NHS Choices (2015e) IVF overview. [online]. Available at: www.nhs.uk/conditions/ivf/ (accessed 26 February 2018).

NHS Choices (2017a) Infertility – Causes. [online]. Available at: www.nhs.uk/conditions/infertility/causes/ (accessed 26 February 2018).

NHS Choices (2017b) Infertility – Treatment. [online]. Available at: www.nhs.uk/conditions/infertility/treatment/ (accessed 26 February 2018).

NHS Health A–Z (2016) Treatment lymphoedema. [online]. Available at: www.nhs.uk/conditions/lymphoedema/treatment/ (accessed 10 February 2018).

NICE (2017) Endometriosis: diagnosis and management. National Institute for Health and Care Excellence. NICE guideline [NG73]. [online]. Available at: www.nice.org.uk/guidance/ng73 (accessed 12 February 2018).

NIH (National Institutes of Health) (2018) *BRCA Mutations: Cancer Risk and Genetic Testing*. National Cancer Institute. Bethesda, MA: National Institutes of Health.

Oats, J. and Abraham, S. (2010) *Llewellyn-Jones Fundamentals of Obstetrics and Gynaecology*. Edinburgh: Elsevier Mosby.

Peres, G.M., Mariana, M. and Cairrão, E. (2018) Pre-eclampsia and eclampsia: an update on the pharmacological treatment applied in Portugal. *Journal of Cardiovascular Development and Disease, 5* (3): (accessed 25 April 2018).

Pinder, S.E., Lee, A.H.S. and Ellis, I.O. (2014) The breasts. In C.S. Herrington (ed.), *Muir's Textbook of Pathology*, 15th edn. London: CRC Press, Taylor and Francis. Ch. 15.

Porth, C.M. (2015) Disorders of the female genitourinary system. In *Essentials of Pathophysiology: Concepts of Altered Health States*, 3rd edn. Philadelphia, PA: Wolters Kluwer Health/Lippincott Williams and Wilkins. Ch. 40.

Purdie, D.M., Bain, C.J., Siskind, V., Webb, P.M. and Green, A.C. (2003) Ovulation and risk of epithelial ovarian cancer. *International Journal of Cancer, 104*: 228–32.

Ramsay, I.N. (2014) Genital prolapse. In B.A. McGowan, P. Owen and A. Thomson (eds), *Clinical Obstetrics and Gynaecology*, 3rd edn. Edinburgh: Elsevier Saunders. Ch. 16.

Ray, A., Shah, A., Gudi, A. and Homburg, R. (2012) Unexplained infertility: an update and review of practice. *Reproductive Biomedicine Online, 24* (6): 591–602.

RCOG (2016) Postpartum haemorrhage, prevention and management. Royal College of Obstetricians and Gynaecologists. Green-top Guideline No. 52. [online]. Available at: www.rcog.org.uk/en/guidelines-research-services/guidelines/gtg52/ (accessed 14 February 2018).

Rebar, R.W. (2017) Tubal dysfunction and pelvic lesions. MSD Manual Professional Version Gynecology and Obstetrics. [online]. Available at: www.msdmanuals.com/en-gb/professional/gynecology-and-obstetrics/infertility/tubal-dysfunction-and-pelvic-lesions (accessed 11 February 2018).

Sirmans, S.M. and Pate, K.A. (2014) Epidemiology, diagnosis, and management of polycystic ovary syndrome. *Clinical Epidemiology, 6*: 1–13.

Swain, S.M., Baselga, J., Kim, S-B., Ro, J., Semiglazov, V., Campone, M. et al. (for the CLEOPATRA Study Group) (2015) Pertuzumab, trastuzumab, and docetaxel in HER2-positive metastatic breast cancer. *New England Journal of Medicine, 372*: 724–34. [A complete list of investigators in the Clinical Evaluation of Pertuzumab and Trastuzumab (CLEOPATRA) study is provided in the Supplementary Appendix, available at NEJM.org.]

Toss, A., Tomasello, C., Razzaboni, E., Contu, G., Grandi, G., Cagnacci, A. et al. (2015) Hereditary ovarian cancer: not only *BRCA* 1 and 2 genes. *BioMed Research International*, 2015, Article ID 341723. http://doi.org/10.1155/2015/341723.

WCRF International (2014) Ovarian cancer. World Cancer Research Fund International. [online]. Available at: www.wcrf.org/int/research-we-fund/continuous-update-project-findings-reports/ovarian-cancer (accessed 13 February 2018).

White, P.C. and Speiser, P.W. (2000) Congenital adrenal hyperplasia due to 21-hydroxylase deficiency. *Endocrine Reviews, 21* (3): 245–91.

World Health Organisation (WHO) (2016) Human papillomavirus (HPV) and cervical cancer. [online]. Available at: www.who.int/mediacentre/factsheets/fs380/en/ (accessed 11 February 2018).

Yamashita-Kashima, Y., Shu, S., Yorozu, K., Moriya, Y. and Harada, N. (2017) Mode of action of pertuzumab in combination with trastuzumab plus docetaxel therapy in a HER2-positive breast cancer xenograft model. *Oncology Letters, 4* (4): 4197–205.

DISORDERS OF THE MALE REPRODUCTIVE SYSTEM

19

UNDERSTAND: CHAPTER VIDEOS

Watch the following videos to ease you into this chapter. If you are using the eBook just click on the play buttons. Alternatively go to **https://study.sagepub.com/essentialpatho/videos**

TESTICULAR
TORSION (11:00)

HYPOGONADISM
(2:13)

BENIGN PROSTATIC
HYPERPLASIA (16:59)

LEARNING OUTCOMES

When you have finished studying this chapter you will be able to:

1. Discuss the causes of low sperm count (oligozoospermia), including cryptorchidism, epididymitis, hydrocele, varicocele and hypogonadism.
2. Describe the pathophysiological processes involved in erectile and ejaculatory dysfunction.
3. Relay the pathophysiological processes involved in testicular and prostatic cancer.
4. Describe the impact of altered physiology of the male reproductive system on the person and their family.

INTRODUCTION

In this chapter, you will examine the causes and effects of disorders of the male reproductive system. Additionally, you will also consider the emotional/psychological and social implications of such pathophysiological changes, a particularly important element of providing person-centred care.

In this chapter we are going to focus on male reproductive issues across the life span. While these are largely focused upon the physical issues, it is important to consider the impact on the person and their family across the life span in order that, as nurses, we view people from a person-centred context and work with their values and beliefs.

REVISE: A&P RECAP

The male reproductive system

We recommend that you revise the anatomy and physiology of the male reproductive system by reading Chapter 16, The Reproductive Systems, in *Essentials of Anatomy and Physiology for Nursing Practice* (Boore et al., 2016) before reading this chapter.

PERSON-CENTRED CONTEXT: THE BODIE FAMILY

BODIE FAMILY
CASE NOTES

The connection between sexuality and personhood is well established. How we live and express ourselves as sexual beings is fundamentally connected to our quality of life; it underpins our goals to have meaningful intimate relationships with others and to have a family should we so desire. Sexual function is also associated with our self-identity and self-esteem. Considering the importance of these aspects of our lives and health, disorders of the male reproductive system can impact not only physically upon the person, but also psychologically. It also extends wider than the person affected as it can affect relationships and have an influence on wider family issues.

For example, Jack Garcia is vigilant in performing testicular self-examination as a result of his father having had testicular cancer. Disorders of male reproduction can also stem from other disorders; for example, Richard Jones has a history of type 2 diabetes which is a known risk factor for erectile and **ejaculatory dysfunction**. While he may never develop these, optimal management of his diabetes may influence this likelihood and both conditions can have a significant impact on self-esteem. Martins et al. (2016) highlight that men with reproductive issues may present with anxiety, **depression** and challenges in managing their relationships with their partner. Additionally, they may adopt avoidance coping mechanisms, catastrophise the situation or use religion (e.g. God's will) as maladaptive behaviours. These issues are equally as important to address as the physical issues. Martins et al. (2016) also highlight how seeking support and information may protect them from maladaptive responses as does having a partner's support and being able to openly discuss matters.

INFERTILITY AND LOW SPERM COUNT (OLIGOZOOSPERMIA)

Approximately 30% of infertility issues between couples are isolated as male in origin, with 20% being a combination of male and female in origin (Leaver, 2016). Interestingly, 15% of causes remain unknown. In men, the primary issue is low sperm count (**oligozoospermia**) or sperm that have poor motility (**asthenozoospermia**) or abnormalities (**teratozoospermia**). This low sperm count may be secondary to an obstruction in the vas deferens or may be as a result of impaired sperm production. Additionally, men may produce high-quality sperm and semen but may have erectile or ejaculatory dysfunction that results in a physical impairment that prevents effective fertilisation of the female ovum. We will begin this chapter by addressing these core issues, some of which stem from early in life which include:

- Undescended testes (**cryptorchidism**)
- **Hydrocele**
- **Variocele**
- **Hypogonadism**
- **Epididymitis**
- Torsion of the testes

We will then address those issues that can come at any stage in life, which include:

- **Urethral strictures**
- Erectile and ejaculatory dysfunction
- **Benign prostatic hyperplasia**
- **Phimosis** and **paraphimosis**
- Prostate and testicular **cancer**

Undescended testes (cryptorchidism)

Cryptorchidism, or undescended testis, occurs in 1–4% of full-term and up to 30% of preterm male neonates (Goel et al., 2015). This can include failure of one testis to descend (unilateral) or both (bilateral); this has the potential to cause infertility later in life, reducing fertility by one-third and two-thirds respectively, largely as a result of impaired **spermatogenesis**, endocrine dysfunction and increased risk of testicular cancer, particularly if not treated early in life (Goel et al., 2015). Cryptorchidism is therefore often associated with infertility in men. **Azoospermia**, where there is no sperm present in semen, is more likely to occur in bilateral cryptorchidism.

Hydrocele

This is a collection of serous fluid in the **tunica vaginalis** that normally occurs unilaterally (Figure 19.1). The accumulation of fluid is thought to occur as a result of the patency of the **processus vaginalis** (the peritoneal tunnel through which the testes migrate from the retroperitoneum toward the scrotum during embryological development) in infants, permitting peritoneal fluid to pass into the scrotum and surround the testicle (Dagur et al., 2016). When excess fluid cannot drain, the hydrocele forms. It may also form as a result of traumatic injury or epididymitis. The Go Deeper box identifies the classifications of hydroceles, with many types indicating their cause (Dagur et al., 2016).

─────────────── **REVISE: A&P RECAP** ───────────────

Anatomy of the testes

A hydrocele involves the tunica vaginalis. Figure 19.1 shows the anatomy of the testes and the location of the tunica vaginalis.

(Continued)

(Continued)

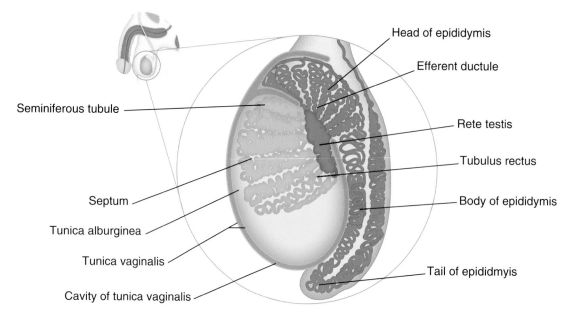

Head of epididymis

Efferent ductule

Seminiferous tubule

Rete testis

Tubulus rectus

Septum

Body of epididymis

Tunica alburginea

Tunica vaginalis

Cavity of tunica vaginalis

Tail of epididmyis

Illustrated by Shaun Mercier © SAGE Publications

Figure 19.1 Tunica vaginalis of the testes

GO DEEPER

Hydrocele

A hydrocele is defined as an accumulation of serous fluid in a body sac.
Eightfold classification of hydroceles (Dagur et al., 2016):

1. Primary
2. Secondary communicating
3. Secondary non-communicating
4. Microbe-induced
5. Inflammatory/iatrogenic
6. Trauma/tumour-induced
7. Canal of Nuck (an abnormal patent pouch of peritoneum) – present in females only
8. **Congenital** and giant

Non-communication hydrocele: when the processus vaginalis is not patent (normal) but fluid collects in the tunica vaginalis.

Communicating hydrocele: when the processus vaginalis remains patent (it normally closes after formation of the tunica vaginalis), this permits fluid in the tunica vaginalis to move into the abdomen.

Hydrocele of the cord: this occurs when fluid collects in a sealed-off section of the spermatic cord (it does not communicate with the tunica vaginalis). It may also be present in the tunica vaginalis.

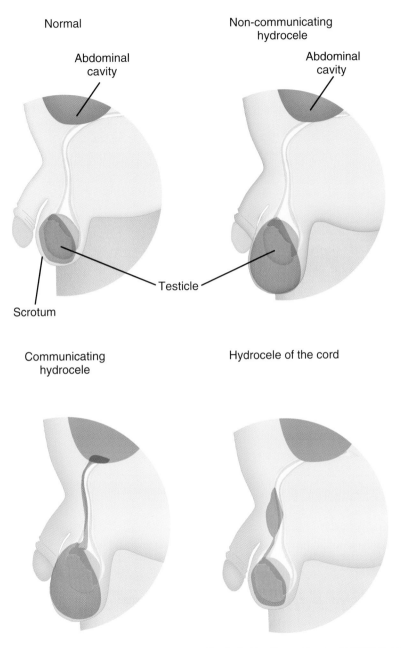

Figure 19.2 Hydrocele in men

Illustrated by Shaun Mercier © SAGE Publications

Varicocele

This is a vascular abnormality of the testicular venous drainage system whereby these veins become abnormally dilated and tortuous (Figure 19.3). It more commonly occurs in the left testicular vein as blood flow is turbulent and results in venous dilation; the left testicular vein (LTV) joins the left renal vein at a right-angle (Sofikitis et al., 2014). In contrast, the right testicular vein merges smoothly into the inferior vena cava and therefore blood flow is more laminar. Ineffective or reduced numbers of valves in the LTV can also contribute to venous dilation and distension, as may **retrograde** blood flow as a result of contraction of the LTV by **catecholamines** from the left adrenal gland; these drain into the left renal vein and may enter the LTV (Sofikitis et al., 2014).

The varicocele can result in impaired male fertility. The pooling of warm, refluxed blood in the veins is thought to raise scrotal temperature which in turn reduces testosterone synthesis by **Leydig cells** and reduces Sertoli cell secretory function (Sofikitis et al., 2014). The result is reduced testosterone production. Varicoceles are also associated with **spermatozoa** DNA damage and impaired testis and spermatozoa maturation (Sofikitis et al., 2014). Other theories have been hypothesised, such as testicular hypoxia and possible effects of adrenal and renal metabolites contained within retrograde blood flow, but are yet to be proven with solid evidence.

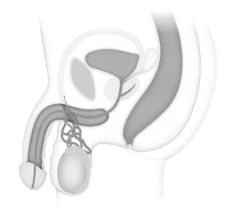 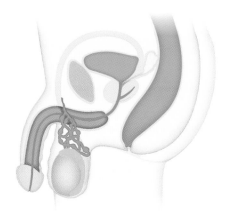

Normal   Varicocele

Illustrated by Shaun Mercier © SAGE Publications

Figure 19.3 Varicocele

Hypogonadism

Congenital hypogonadotropic hypogonadism (CHH) is a heterogeneous **disease** characterised by a failure, or delayed onset, of puberty and infertility secondary to the deficient secretion or action of **gonadotrophin-releasing hormone (GnRH)**; more than two dozen genetic loci have been identified (Dwyer et al., 2016). Timely release of GnRH is critical for the onset of puberty and subsequent sexual maturation. **Follicle-stimulating hormone (FSH)** stimulates rapid reproduction of immature **Sertoli cells** and **spermatogonia** and **luteinising hormone (LH)** stimulates Leydig cells to produce testosterone. It is this intensive stimulation of Sertoli cells and raised intragonadal testosterone levels that initiate spermatogenesis (Boehm et al., 2015). However, in CHH, deficit secretion or the action of GnRH results in insufficient, or absent, production of FSH and LH (via the hypothalamic–pituitary–gonadal axis), leading to impaired gonadal maturation (see Figure 19.4). CHH has two classifications (Dwyer et al., 2016):

1. Normosmic CHH (when the sense of smell is intact) or
2. Kallmann syndrome (KS) when associated with **anosmia**. Anosmia occurs secondary to the absence or hypoplasia of the olfactory bulbs and the lateral olfactory tracts; one of the genes affected in KS is *KAL1* which codes for the glycoprotein anosmin-1; anosmin-1 is necessary to promote neurodevelopment of the olfactory neurons and so its absence will result in suboptimal neuronal branching of the olfactory neurons, affecting the olfactory bulb, tract and cortex (Gillespie, 2013).

CHH can be reversible under certain conditions.

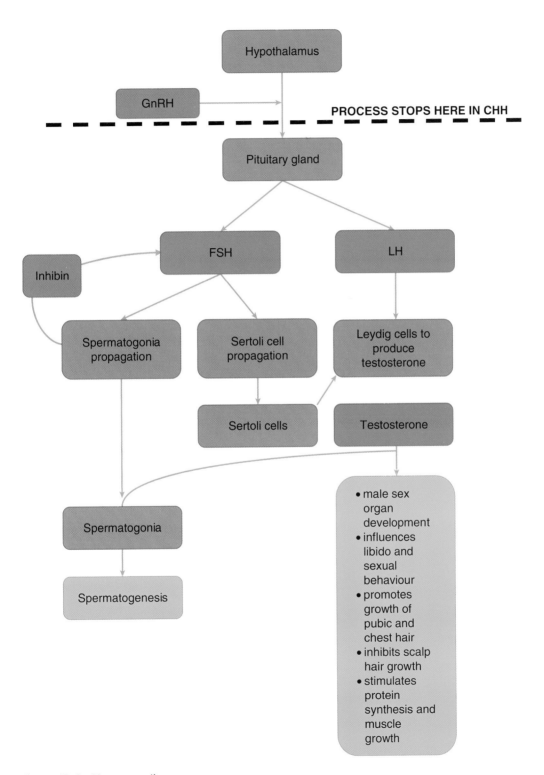

Figure 19.4 Hypogonadism

Epididymitis

Epididymitis is infection or **inflammation** of the epididymis, largely as a result of bacterial infection and normally occurring unilaterally. This has the potential to spread to the testis, in which case it is then known as **epididymo-orchitis**. Common urinary tract pathogens and **sexually transmitted infections** (notably *Chlamydia trachomatis* and *Neisseria gonorrhoea*) are largely the causes of epididymitis. It may also be caused by retrograde flow of urine in older men. The condition may be classified as acute, when there is pain and **oedema**, or more commonly chronic, when there is pain (Çek et al., 2017).

The condition occurs when bacteria ascend the urinary tract, translocating into the vas deferens and making their way to the epididymis. Bacterial colonisation begins at the tail of the epididymis, spreading to its body and head (Garthwaite, 2017), and results in suppurative inflammation with **fibrin** covering. Pus may collect within the epididymal duct, causing it to rupture, creating sperm **granulomas** (Farris and Nielson, 2017). Treatment is largely by antibacterial medication.

Torsion of the testes

Testicular torsion occurs when there is a twisting of the testis on the spermatic cord, obstructing the blood flow to the testis (Karaguzel et al., 2014). It largely occurs as a result of an abnormality in the tunica vaginalis which permits the testis to move, resulting in axial rotation in the spermatic cord above. It occurs more commonly in the second decade of life, but rarely after the age of 30; the incidence under the age of 25 is 3.5 cases per 100,000 (Lee et al., 2014). Disruption in blood flow occurs as the testicular artery (and deferential and cremasteric arteries) are contained within the spermatic cord; any torsion on the spermatic cord will compress these arteries and can lead to cell damage within hours; it is therefore a medical emergency requiring immediate attention. The duration of torsion and degree of obstruction of blood flow determine the extent of the ischaemic-reperfusion injury (Karaguzel et al., 2014).

Urethral strictures

A urethral stricture is a narrowing of the urethral lumen; it may be obstructive or disruptive to flow through the urethra or the person may be asymptomatic. However, men that are symptomatic tend to have a reduced quality of life as a result of obstructive flow and an impact on the bladder storage of urine (Lazzeri et al., 2016); those who have to self-catheterise or perform urethral dilation long term are particularly impacted by pain, discomfort and disruption to daily life (Lubahn et al., 2014). There is no consensus on the incidence of urethral strictures although it is confirmed as a common condition that primarily affects men after the age of 45; younger people with this condition tend to have a **bulbar stricture** and adult men have the stricture elsewhere in the urethra (Lazzeri et al., 2016). The main causes of anterior urethral strictures are identified as:

- Congenital abnormality of the urethral mucosal membrane
- Any condition that may result in urethral scarring from infection or inflammation:
  - **Urethritis** (40%)
  - Blunt perineal trauma
  - Trauma from urethral instrumentation and catheterisation
  - Corrective **surgery** for **hypospadias** (when the urethral opening is on the underside of the penis)
  - Inflammatory disease of the **corpus spongiosum** secondary to lichen sclerosus (an autoimmune skin condition that affects primarily the genitalia)
  - Penile lichen sclerosus
  - Sexually transmitted infections.

The anterior urethral **mucosa** is surrounded by the corpus spongiosum along its length (Figure 19.5). This highly vascular erectile tissue provides the vascular supply to the urethra and there is therefore a direct link between urethral strictures and the health of the corpus spongiosum. When there are fibrotic changes in the corpus spongiosum, this impacts upon the extent and severity of the stricture in the underlying urethra (Gallegos and Santucci, 2016). These fibrotic changes result in scar formation, a progressive process referred to as **spongiofibrosis**. In spongiofibrosis, **spongiosal tissue** (tissue of the corpus spongiosum) is replaced by dense scar tissue that lacks elasticity and contains **fibroblasts**, forming the urethral stricture (Gallegos and Santucci, 2016). The posterior urethra (which stems from the bladder neck to the bulb) is not surrounded by the corpus spongiosum. Therefore, the pathophysiological process that occurs in the anterior urethra is not responsible for strictures here; spongiofibrosis is not the cause but fibrotic changes from trauma and infection remain implicated.

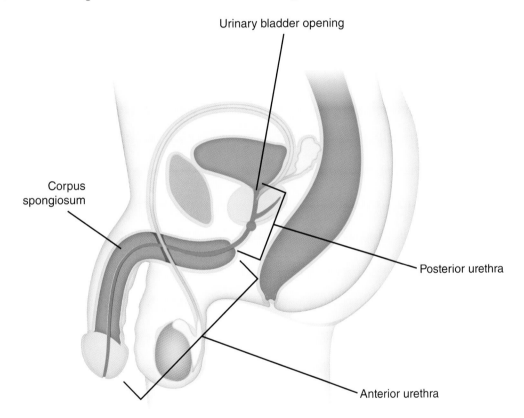

Illustrated by Shaun Mercier © SAGE Publications

Figure 19.5   Urethral strictures

APPLY

Treatment of urethral strictures

The traditional approach to treating urethral strictures was to physically dilate them (urethral dilation) or to undertake a **urethrotomy** (incision of the fibrotic scar tissue in the urethra).

(Continued)

(Continued)

However, while these are the most common forms of treatment, both have the lowest success rate as repeated dilation can cause further traumatic scarring and does not remove scar tissue, and urethrotomy will also result in scar tissue formation. **Urethroplasty** is identified as a more successful approach and is increasingly more commonly used to resolve strictures (Gallegos and Santucci, 2016). Interestingly, tissue-engineered **buccal mucosa** is now being used as an innovative approach to urethroplasty as buccal mucosa has healing properties that largely do not result in the formation of fibrotic scar tissue.

Erectile dysfunction

--------- **REVISE: A&P RECAP** ---------

Before reading this section on erectile dysfunction, it is advisable to refresh your memory on the physiology of sexual arousal and the stages of sexual response in Chapter 16, The Reproductive Systems, in *Essentials of Anatomy and Physiology for Nursing Practice* (Boore et al., 2016).

Erectile dysfunction (ED) is a complex condition that occurs secondary to neural, vascular and/or hormonal dysfunction (Gratzke et al., 2010). However, these are considered as organic origins of ED and psychogenic causes are also identified. These are all discussed below:

Neural: Neural regulation of penile erection involves **neurotransmitter**s and neural structures with both spinal and supraspinal pathways. Neurological disorders affecting these can result in ED. Cavernous nerve injury, which can occur during prostatic surgery for example, is another leading cause of neural ED (Matsui et al., 2015).

Vascular: Efficient blood flow to the corpus cavernosum is essential for an erection to take place. Should any factor impede this blood flow, it may cause the corporo-veno-occlusive mechanism to fail (Gratzke et al., 2010). It is therefore no surprise that the presence of coronary artery disease, peripheral arterial disease and cerebrovascular disease are associated with ED. Additionally, **hypercholesterolaemia** and **hypertension**, both associated with vascular disease, are associated with ED (Gratzke et al., 2010). Indeed, ED can be a predictor of cardiovascular disease, preceding a cardiac event by three years on average (Gandaglia et al., 2014). Diabetes mellitus is also a known factor in ED; changes occur in the arteries and smooth muscle of the corpus cavernosum alongside the impaired endothelium-dependent relaxation of the associated corporeal smooth muscle (Gratzke et al., 2010). Additionally, it is well documented that **nitric oxide (NO)** has a key role in vasodilation necessary for an erection to occur (Matsui et al., 2015). Reduced **bioavailability** of NO can therefore impair the necessary blood flow to achieve an erection.

Hormonal: It is thought that a threshold level of testosterone is necessary for an erection to occur; consequently, **hypogonadism** can lead to ED as a result of insufficient testosterone.

Psychogenic: Psychogenic causes of ED are related to the psychological factors involved in the sexual arousal mechanisms. These can include depression, performance anxiety and low libido. Psychogenic ED is thought to occur secondary to inhibition of the spinal erection centre and/or excessive levels of peripheral catecholamines (Matsui et al., 2015); the latter can inhibit the necessary blood flow to induce an erection.

Ejaculatory dysfunction

Ejaculatory dysfunction is the most common sexual dysfunction that men experience. It can range from ejaculating early (premature ejaculation) to a delay in ejaculation (**delayed ejaculation**) and also includes **retrograde ejaculation**, where the ejaculate is misdirected. Ejaculatory dysfunction can be psychologically stressful but can also be a cause of infertility as it can inhibit the fertilisation of the female ovum.

Premature ejaculation

With a prevalence of up to 20%, premature ejaculation is the most frequent form of ejaculatory dysfunction (Gross et al., 2015). There are two forms of premature ejaculatory dysfunction:

Primary: This form occurs from the first sexual intercourse onwards, whereby early ejaculation occurs within 30-60 seconds in most cases or between 1-2 minutes. This form is also referred to as lifelong. It is thought that men can have a genetic predisposition for lifelong premature ejaculation whereby they are predisposed to the impairment of inhibitory serotonergic pathways that regulate ejaculation (Chung et al., 2015). Additionally, **dopaminergic** and **oxytocinergic** factors are thought to play a role and are the subject of further research in this area.

Secondary: In this form, the man will have had normal ejaculatory experiences and then developed early ejaculation. This form is also termed as **acquired**. It is normally associated with performance or relationship challenges. However, it can have an organic cause and be related to ED, **prostatitis, hyperthyroidism**, or be secondary to weaning from medication (McMahon et al., 2016). The same risk factors for ED also apply to premature ejaculation, such as diabetes, cardiovascular disease and hypertension. In this regard, causes are neuroendocrine as well as psychogenic and relational. Psychological factors are likely to reduce the sympathetic threshold for ejaculation alongside neglecting the signs (**prodromal** sensations) that precede ejaculation due to focusing on performance.

APPLY

Characteristics of premature ejaculation

McMahon et al. (2016) highlight that ejaculatory dysfunction is characterised by:

- Ejaculation occurring prior to or within 1 minute of sexual intercourse (primary) or significant reduction in latency time (< 3 minutes) (secondary).
- An inability to delay ejaculation during intercourse.
- Negative personal experience as a result of premature ejaculation. (Serefoglu et al., 2014)

These characteristics are used in clinical practice to determine the origins of premature ejaculation but may be multifactorial.

Delayed ejaculation

Delayed ejaculation, a delay in orgasmic response and subsequent ejaculation despite sufficient sexual stimulation, is associated with low androgen levels, notably testosterone (McMahon et al., 2016). Testosterone regulates the expression and activity of NO which performs as a local neurotransmitter, triggering relaxation of the intracavernosal **trabeculae**, maximising blood flow and penile **engorgement**

(Sansone et al., 2015). When there are low levels of testosterone, the subsequent reduction in NO can lead to penile flaccidity which can reduce ejaculatory volume but also lead to a loss of psychogenic libido. Additionally, delayed ejaculation may also occur secondary to the threshold for ejaculation not being met or delayed, also exacerbated by a loss of psychogenic libido. Delayed ejaculation can also occur secondary to medication and alcohol use.

Retrograde ejaculation

Retrograde ejaculation is when semen is directed to exit the body through the urethra but is misdirected into the bladder. Normally, the internal urethral **sphincter** contracts at the time of ejaculation, preventing this from occurring and directing semen to leave the body via the urethra. In retrograde ejaculation, this contraction does not occur and the semen enters the bladder as it is the path of least resistance. The cause of the urethral sphincter not contracting is largely related to either neural impairment as a result of surgery or degenerative processes or as a side-effect of medication. The external urethral sphincter can also contract, preventing external urethral outflow (Figure 19.6).

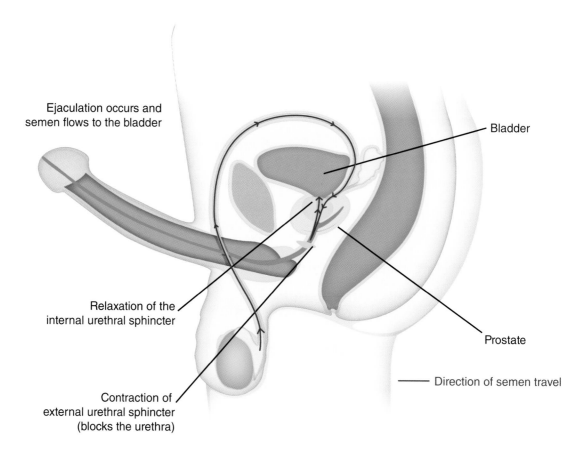

Ejaculation occurs and semen flows to the bladder

Bladder

Relaxation of the internal urethral sphincter

Prostate

Direction of semen travel

Contraction of external urethral sphincter (blocks the urethra)

Illustrated by Shaun Mercier © SAGE Publications

Figure 19.6 Retrograde ejaculation

Benign prostatic hyperplasia

Benign prostatic hyperplasia (BPH) occurs when there is a hyperproliferation of the epithelial and stromal cells in the transitional zone of the prostate gland (Lee and Kuo, 2017). BPH is very prevalent in men; by the age of 60, 50% of men have BPH and by the age of 80, this increases to 90%. The causes of BPH are multifactorial:

Testosterone: Testosterone is converted to dihydrotestosterone in the prostate gland; the latter is known to trigger cell **proliferation** and **differentiation** and so can lead to BPH; when this conversion is blocked with medication (5α-reductase inhibitors), the **progression** to BPH is reduced (Lee and Kuo, 2017).

Inflammation: Inflammation is thought to be a key mechanism by which BPH occurs. It is thought that cytokine release in inflammation may promote the presence of growth factors that trigger cell proliferation in the prostate.

Other factors include **metabolic syndrome**, age and genetics.

Once cell proliferation begins, enlargement of the prostate occurs and can result in intrusion into the lumen of the urethra, contributing to the obstruction of urinary flow. There are two key phases to BPH (Patel and Parsons, 2014):

1. There is an increase in stromal nodules in the periurethral zone.
2. There is a significant increase in size of glandular nodules.

It is thought that chronic inflammation and hormonal changes result in altered prostatic **homeostasis** and tissue damage. The result is hyperplasia and fibrotic changes to prostatic tissue (Schalken, 2015). The goal of treatment is therefore to reduce inflammation and restore homeostatic endocrine control.

APPLY

The personal impact of erectile and ejaculatory dysfunction

Consider the impact that erectile and ejaculatory dysfunction could have on a person. Men with these conditions can have higher levels of personal distress and interpersonal difficulties (Rowland et al., 2007). In a more recent study, this personal burden was found to be threefold:

- The emotional burden
- The health burden
- The relationship burden

Reflect on these three areas and think about how issues would fall under each of these. How would you support a person with erectile or ejaculatory dysfunction from the perspective of being person-centred?

Phimosis

Phimosis is when there is an inability to retract the foreskin over the glans penis (Figure 19.7). It can be congenital or secondary to recurrent **balanitis** (inflammation of the glans penis). Phimosis occurs secondary to **adhesions** between the epithelial layers of the inner prepuce and glans; as the male matures, repeated foreskin retractions and erections normally cause these adhesions to break down, eliminating the phimosis. However, repeated balanitis and forced foreskin retractions result in pathologic phimosis whereby scarring of the **preputial orifice**s occur as a result of trauma and repeated inflammation. Pathological phimosis must be treated early in order to avoid serious complications; if the condition is permitted to remain and worsens over time, it can result in the venous and lymphatic return being impaired, leading to engorgement of the glans, exacerbating the condition. Eventually, the restriction caused by the foreskin, which is now tightly encasing the engorged glans, will result in the reduced and eventual occlusion of arterial blood flow to the glans. The end result can be **infarction** and potential autoamputation of the glans.

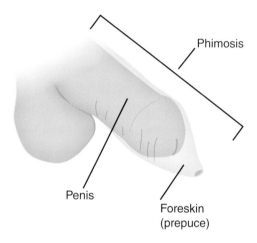

Illustrated by Shaun Mercier © SAGE Publications

Figure 19.7 Phimosis

Paraphimosis

Paraphimosis occurs when the foreskin becomes trapped behind the corona of the glans penis, compromising arterial supply to the gland and preventing venous and lymphatic return (Figure 19.8). **Ischaemia** and **necrosis** can result, similar to that in phimosis. Paraphimosis is largely iatrogenically induced when the foreskin is retracted for personal hygiene measures or urethral catheter insertion.

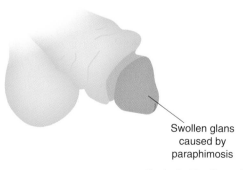

Illustrated by Shaun Mercier © SAGE Publications

Figure 19.8 Paraphimosis

CANCERS OF THE MALE REPRODUCTIVE SYSTEM

Prostate cancer

Prostate cancer (PCa) is a **malignant tumour** of glandular origin in the prostate. It presents most commonly in older men. PCa is graded using the **Gleason score** (the sum of two scales scored 1 to 5 that designates the degree of differentiation of the tumour's predominant cell lines). PCa tends to be multizonal, occurring in different zones of the prostate. However, most (70%) PCa occurs in the peripheral zone (Figure 19.9), with the remaining largely occurring equally in the transitional and anterior zones.

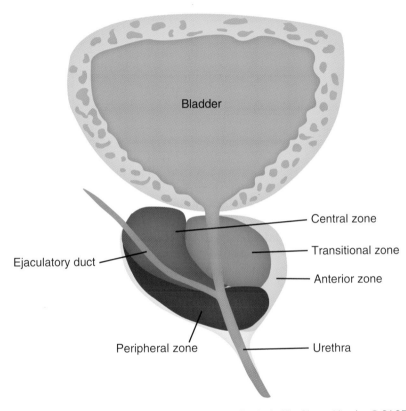

Illustrated by Shaun Mercier © SAGE Publications

Figure 19.9 Zones of the prostate

It was long believed that prostate cancer (PCa) was linked to high levels of testosterone and that low levels protected men against this disease. This was termed the *Androgen Hypothesis*. This hypothesis is not supported by evidence and is now replaced by the *Saturation Model* which reflects the notion that PCa is sensitive to low levels of testosterone but not sensitive to normal and high levels (Khera et al., 2014). In this respect, once a threshold level of testosterone is reached, any rise in testosterone beyond that threshold does not induce any androgen-driven changes in prostate tissue. Prostate tissue also seems to have a saturation point for **androgens**, which may explain this.

PCa occurs when cell division exceeds cell death. Ninety-five per cent of cases are **adenocarcinomas** and 4% occur from prostatic urethral changes. Squamous cell carcinomas make up the final 1% and can be secondary to radiation and/or hormone therapy. There are genetic links with PCa; Table 19.1 shows some implicated **mutations.** Alterations in genes *8p22-23* and *p53* are associated with the progression and severity of PCa (Benedettini et al., 2008). Gene *8q24* is associated with early onset PCa in young African-American men.

Table 19.1   Gene mutations in PCa

Genetic mutation	Influence
8p22-23	Influences progression and severity of PCa
8q24	Associated with early onset of PCa in young African-American men
p53	Failure of tumour suppressor gene that influences metastasis of PCa

Prostate cancer is largely classified as an adenocarcinoma, whereby glandular cells mutate into cancer cells. When it first develops, small collections of cancer cells stay in the glands which are otherwise normal, called prostate intraepithelial neoplasia (PIN) (or carcinoma in situ) (Mustafa et al., 2016). These cancer cells then begin to multiply and invade the surrounding prostatic tissue and result in tumour formation. Over time, this may result in an invasion of the surrounding tissues such as the seminal **vesicles** or rectum, or in travel through circulation around the body to other locations. The prostate gland uses zinc to make citrate which is an important component of semen. This process uses significant amounts of energy. Cancerous prostate cells are found to be devoid of zinc and therefore use the energy not used to generate citrate to proliferate (Mustafa et al., 2016). Introducing zinc into cancerous prostate cells is known to eliminate them as it induces **apoptosis** in abnormal cells. However, this is reliant on a transport protein (ZIP1) to bring zinc into the cell, and the gene to create this transport protein is suppressed in prostate cancer. Additionally, **prostate specific membrane antigen (PSMA)** stimulates the development of PCa through raising intracellular folate levels, enabling the survival of the cancer cells alongside being protected by androgen receptors that prevent apoptosis (Mustafa et al., 2016). Through a variety of complex mechanisms, prostate specific antigen (PSA) is known to promote tumour growth, invasion and metastasis of PCa (Altuwaijri, 2012). These processes include **oxidative stress**, gene mutation and the degradation of extracellular matrix (Altuwaijri, 2012).

APPLY

Gleason score

The Gleason score (or grade/system) is used to grade PCa. The score represents how aggressive the tumour is and its likelihood of metastasising (Drudge-Coates and Turner, 2013). PCa is normally present in more than one area of the prostate – the two areas with the greatest amount of cancer cells are biopsied and graded. The scale of the scoring system is from 1 to 5, where 1 describes the normal prostate tissue and 5 the most abnormal cells. Biopsies from each area are scored and the two scores are added together, with the most common tissue type presented first.

The score denotes how aggressive the tumour is and the likelihood of it spreading and is used alongside additional diagnostic information in determining treatment options. The grade ranges from 3 for cancer cells that look almost normal, to 5 for very abnormal cells, with the primary grade being the most common pattern, and the secondary grade being second. To get a total Gleason score out of 10, the two numbers are added. For example, a Gleason score of 4 + 3 = 7 means that pattern 4 was the most common pattern and pattern 3 the second.

APPLY

PSA screening for prostate cancer

While PSA levels have long been used to support the diagnosis of PCa, this method of screening has been considered controversial in recent years as the evidence base that it reduces mortality and morbidity is somewhat lacking (Ilic et al., 2018). More recently, Ilic et al. (2018) highlight that the US Preventive Services Task Force (USPSTF) has moved away from the position that PSA should not be used as a screening tool and has changed its recommendation to where an individual approach to screening is advocated instead (Fenton et al., 2018). Ilic et al. (2018), in a systematic review and meta-analysis, determine that PSA screening appears to improve the detection of PCa at any stage and has a modest positive impact in reducing prostate cancer-specific mortality. This screening and detection, however, are associated with intervention-associated complications (e.g. sepsis, erectile dysfunction) and it is debated whether, in some cases, no intervention would have led to a high quality of life without a hastening of life. The debate continues, and PSA remains a biochemical marker that can help identify the presence of PCa.

Testicular cancer

Testicular cancer is a rare form of cancer but the most common form of cancer in young men. Risk factors for the condition include:

- Cryptorchidism
- **Orchidopexy** (surgical treatment of undescended testis)
- Testicular torsion
- Mumps

The majority of testicular cancers are germ cell tumours, of which there are two main types:

Seminomas: slower-growing cells that contain only seminomatous elements; there are no **teratoma** cells in the tumour

Non-seminomas: faster-growing cells that are either embryonal carcinoma, yolk sac carcinoma, **choriocarcinoma**, or teratoma.

It is common for both cell types to be present (mixed germ cell tumour).

APPLY

Early detection and treatment

Discussing matters related to sexual health can be challenging for many people. It can also be something that many health care professionals avoid as they do not know how to raise the issue and perhaps feel awkward in doing so. However, this is not an acceptable excuse for health care professionals;

(Continued)

(Continued)

awkwardness does not excuse not raising and discussing something that is fundamental to health; an omission in this regard is negligence and so it is essential that as a health care practitioner you consider how you can meet the needs of someone with sexual dysfunction. There are two models that are very helpful in guiding you: the PLISSIT model (Annon, 1976) and the EX-PLISSIT model (Taylor and Davis, 2007).

Go online and read about both of these models to ensure that you are ready and able to begin discussing these important aspects of someone's health with them. The articles are freely available but if you are using the eBook you can just click on the icons to access them.

Article 1: Plasiano, B. (2017) PLISSIT model: introducing sexual health in clinical care. *Psychiatry Advisor* [online].

Article 2: Taylor, B. and Davis, S. (2007) The extended PLISSIT model for addressing the sexual well-being of individuals with an acquired disability or chronic illness. *Sexuality and Disability*, 25 (3): 135-9.

ARTICLE:
PLISSIT MODEL

ARTICLE:
EX-PLISSIT MODEL

Testicular cancer is associated with specific chromosomal gains at **chromosomes** 7, 8, 12, 21 and X, and by specific chromosomal losses at chromosomes 11, 13 and 18 (Garner et al., 2005). Healthy germ cells express core **pluripotent** transcription factors, namely NANOG, SOX2 and OCT4. However, when these are absent, malignant proliferation occurs from a loss of these germ line-specific inhibitors, enabling pluripotency and self-renewal which cause healthy germ cells to convert to germ line cancer stem cells (Clark, 2007). As a result, **neoplasm**s are derived from **gonocytes** that have failed to differentiate into spermatogonia. However, their ability to invade the surrounding tissues is not activated until puberty when they are triggered by hormonal changes (Hanna and Einhorn, 2014). Seminomas therefore resemble healthy gonocytes but are unable to differentiate correctly. In terms of non-seminomas, embryonal carcinoma cells are undifferentiated stem cells with gene patterns that resemble stem/germ cell neoplasms (Hanna and Einhorn, 2014). Yolk sac carcinomas and choriocarcinomas have **extraembryonic** differentiation, whereas teratomas have **somatic** differentiation (Hanna and Einhorn, 2014). In essence, all testicular cancers arise from gonocytes; low-level **DNA methylation** of germ cell tumours leads to seminomas, and intermediate and high-level DNA methylation of germ cell neoplasms leads to non-seminomas (Hanna and Einhorn, 2014). The proliferation of malignant cells occurs beyond the basement membrane and this can eventually replace healthy testicular parenchyma.

The **tunica albugenia** is a natural barrier to metastatic growth and so can contain the cancer. This is one reason why a needle biopsy is not performed as it can compromise the tunica albugenia and permit metastatic growth. As a result, any testicular growth is largely considered to be malignant.

APPLY

Testicular self-examination

Early detection of testicular cancer is central to optimal outcomes. As a result, men are encouraged to perform testicular self-examination as routine as once monthly to maximise early detection and treatment. The Testicular Cancer Society has been proactive in addressing this issue and has developed a smart application to encourage and support men to undertake this health-protective measure. The app can be located at the URL below and is available at the Apple™ and Android Play™ stores:

www.testicularcancersociety.org/ball-checker.html

Health promotion is central to early detection and treatment.

CHAPTER SUMMARY

In this chapter you will have learned about reproductive health issues that can affect men across the life span. While these problems are largely pathophysiological in origin, they can have a significant impact on health-related quality of life; this is a challenge to someone's personhood and requires person-centred practitioners to engage with the people in their care in an effective and compassionate manner. You must also remember to work with someone's belief system and values in order to consider their care in the context of their culture and wishes. Sexual health problems can extend beyond the person directly affected and impact on the wider family. As person-centred practitioners, we must ensure that we support people during these challenges and intervene to maximise positive outcomes.

KEY POINTS

- Reproductive disorders have the potential to devastate a person's life and impact widely on their wider family circle.

- People can find it challenging to discuss sexual health matters due to the intimate and personal nature of the subject. Being person-centred requires us to be skilled, proactive and compassionate in this regard, remembering that early detection means better care outcomes can be achieved.

- A variety of conditions can occur early in life that can lead to infertility and low sperm count, particularly cryptorchidism, hydrocele, varicocele and hypogonadism.

- Other reproductive health issues can occur across the life span that impact on fertility, with ejaculatory dysfunction being a common reproductive dysfunction affecting men. Others include erectile dysfunction, epididymitis and testicular torsion, the latter being a medical emergency.

- Urethral strictures represent a distressing condition which common practices over the years have not been successful in resolving. Newer therapies have shown more promise and this may lead to improving health-related quality of life for men affected as practices improve.

- Phimosis and paraphimosis are conditions that require urgent treatment in order to prevent significant disfigurement and distress.

REVISE

TEST YOUR KNOWLEDGE

In this chapter you have learned about a variety of disorders of the male reproductive system. Try to answer the following questions to check your knowledge and understanding.

Answers are available online. If you are using the eBook just click on the answers icon below. Alternatively go to **https://study.sagepub.com/essentialpatho/answers**

1 Which form of cryptorchidism is more likely to lead to no sperm production?

2 What causes a hydrocele to occur?

3 What is the theory behind how a varicocele impairs fertility?

4 Why will deficit secretion or action of GnRH lead to hypogonadism?

5 What is the most common cause of epididymitis?

6 What is the most common cause of testicular torsion and what may it lead to?

7 Explain the pathophysiology behind how anterior urethral strictures form.

8 What are the main causes of erectile dysfunction?

9 Describe the three types of ejaculatory dysfunction and how they could impair fertility.

10 What is benign prostatic hyperplasia and how does it occur?

11 Explain the difference between phimosis and paraphimosis.

12 What is the link between zinc and prostate cancer?

13 From what cells does testicular cancer originate?

REVISE

ACE YOUR ASSESSMENT

- Further revision and learning opportunities are available online
- Test yourself away from the book with **Extra multiple choice questions**
- Learn and revise terminology with **Interactive flashcards**

If you are using the eBook access each resource by clicking on the respective icon. Alternatively go to **https://study.sagepub.com/essentialpatho/chapter19**

CHAPTER 19 ANSWERS

EXTRA QUESTIONS

FLASHCARDS

REFERENCES

Altuwaijri, S. (2012) Role of prostate specific antigen (PSA) in pathogenesis of prostate cancer. *Journal of Cancer Therapy, 3* (4): 331.

Annon, J.S. (1976) The PLISSIT model: a proposed conceptual scheme for the behavioral treatment of sexual problems. *Journal of Sex Education and Therapy, 2* (1): 1–15.

Benedettini, E., Nguyen, P. and Loda, M. (2008) The pathogenesis of prostate cancer: from molecular to metabolic alterations. *Diagnostic Histopathology, 14* (5): 195–201.

Boehm, U., Bouloux, P.M., Dattani, M.T., De Roux, N., Dodé, C., Dunkel, L. et al. (2015) Expert consensus document: European Consensus Statement on congenital hypogonadotropic hypogonadism – pathogenesis, diagnosis and treatment. *Nature Reviews Endocrinology, 11* (9): 547–64.

Boore, J., Cook, N. and Shepherd, A. (2016) *Essentials of Anatomy and Physiology for Nursing Practice.* London: Sage.

Çek, M., Sturdza, L. and Pilatz, A. (2017) Acute and chronic epididymitis. *European Urology Supplements, 16* (4): 124–31.

Chung, E., Gilbert, B., Perera, M. and Roberts, M.J. (2015) Premature ejaculation: a clinical review for the general physician. *Australian Family Physician, 44* (10): 737–43.

Clark, A.T. (2007) The stem cell identity of testicular cancer. *Stem Cell Reviews, 3* (1): 49–59.

Dagur, G., Gandhi, J., Suh, Y., Weissbart, S., Sheynkin, Y.R., Smith, N.L. et al. (2016) Classifying hydroceles of the pelvis and groin: an overview of etiology, secondary complications, evaluation, and management. *Current Urology, 10* (1): 1–14.

Drudge-Coates, L. and Turner, B. (2013) Prostate cancer overview. Part 1: non-metastatic disease. *British Journal of Nursing, 21* (9): S23–S28.

Dwyer, A.A., Raivio, T. and Pitteloud, N. (2016) Management of endocrine disease: reversible hypogonadotropic hypogonadism. *European Journal of Endocrinology, 174* (6): R267–R274.

Farris, A.B. and Nielson, G.P. (2017) Genitourinary infectious disease pathology. In R.I. Kradin (ed.), *Diagnostic Pathology of Infectious Disease*, 2nd edn. Philadelphia, PA: Elsevier Saunders. pp. 429–67.

Fenton, J.J., Weyrich, M.S., Durbin, S., Liu, Y., Bang, H. and Melnikow, J. (2018) Prostate-specific antigen-based screening for prostate cancer: evidence report and systematic review for the US Preventive Services Task Force. *JAMA, 319* (18): 1914–31.

Gallegos, M.A. and Santucci, R.A. (2016) Advances in urethral stricture management. *F1000Research, 5*: 2913. http://doi.org/10.12688/f1000research.

Gandaglia, G., Briganti, A., Jackson, G., Kloner, R.A., Montorsi, F., Montorsi, P. et al. (2014) A systematic review of the association between erectile dysfunction and cardiovascular disease. *European Urology, 65* (5): 968–78.

Garner, M.J., Turner, M.C., Ghadirian, P. and Krewski, D. (2005) Epidemiology of testicular cancer: an overview. *International Journal of Cancer, 116* (3): 331–9.

Garthwaite, M. (2017) Inflammation – epididymitis and scrotal abscess. In F.C. Hamdy and I. Eardley (eds), *Oxford Textbook of Urological Surgery*. Oxford: Oxford University Press. pp. 72–5.

Gillespie, D.C. (2013) Sensory organ disorders (retina, auditory, olfactory, gustatory). In J. Rubenstein and P. Rakic (eds), *Neural Circuit Development and Function in the Brain*, 3rd edn. San Diego, CA: Elsevier. pp. 731–59.

Goel, P., Rawat, J.D., Wakhlu, A. and Kureel, S.N. (2015) Undescended testicle: an update on fertility in cryptorchid men. *Indian Journal of Medical Research, 141* (2): 163–71.

Gratzke, C., Angulo, J., Chitaley, K., Dai, Y.T., Kim, N.N., Paick, J.S. et al. (2010) Anatomy, physiology, and pathophysiology of erectile dysfunction. *Journal of Sexual Medicine, 7* (1 pt2): 445–75.

Gross, O., Sulser, T. and Eberli, D. (2015) Erectile and ejaculatory dysfunction. *Praxis, 104* (24): 1337–41.

Hanna, N.H. and Einhorn, L.H. (2014) Testicular cancer: discoveries and updates. *New England Journal of Medicine*, *371* (21): 2005–16.

Ilic, D., Djulbegovic, M., Jung, J.H., Hwang, E.C., Zhou, Q., Cleves, A. et al. (2018) Prostate cancer screening with prostate-specific antigen (PSA) test: a systematic review and meta-analysis. *BMJ*, *362*: k3519.

Karaguzel, E., Kadihasanoglu, M. and Kutlu, O. (2014) Mechanisms of testicular torsion and potential protective agents. *Nature Reviews Urology*, *11* (7): 391–8.

Khera, M., Crawford, D., Morales, A., Salonia, A. and Morgentaler, A. (2014) A new era of testosterone and prostate cancer: from physiology to clinical implications. *European Urology*, *65* (1): 115–23.

Lazzeri, M., Sansalone, S., Guazzoni, G. and Barbagli, G. (2016) Incidence, causes, and complications of urethral stricture disease. *European Urology Supplements*, *15* (1): 2–6.

Leaver, R.B. (2016) Male infertility: an overview of causes and treatment options. *British Journal of Nursing*, *25* (18): S35–S40.

Lee, C.L. and Kuo, H.C. (2017) Pathophysiology of benign prostate enlargement and lower urinary tract symptoms: current concepts. *Tzu-Chi Medical Journal*, *29* (2): 79–83.

Lee, S.M., Huh, J.S., Baek, M., Yoo, K.H., Min, G.E., Lee, H.L. et al. (2014) A nationwide epidemiological study of testicular torsion in Korea. *Journal of Korean Medical Science*, *29* (12): 1684–7.

Lubahn, J.D., Zhao, L.C., Scott, J.F., Hudak, S.J., Chee, J., Terlecki, R. et al. (2014) Poor quality of life in patients with urethral stricture treated with intermittent self-dilation. *Journal of Urology*, *191* (1): 143–7.

Martins, M.V., Basto-Pereira, M., Pedro, J., Peterson, B., Almeida, V., Schmidt, L. et al. (2016) Male psychological adaptation to unsuccessful medically assisted reproduction treatments: a systematic review. *Human Reproduction Update*, *22* (4): 466–78.

Matsui, H., Sopko, N.A., Hannan, J.L. and Bivalacqua, T. (2015) Pathophysiology of erectile dysfunction. *Current Drug Targets*, *16* (5): 411–19.

McMahon, C.G., Jannini, E.A., Serefoglu, E.C. and Hellstrom, W.J. (2016) The pathophysiology of acquired premature ejaculation. *Translational Andrology and Urology*, *5* (4): 434–49.

Mustafa, M., Salih, A.F., Illzam, E.M., Sharifa, A.M., Suleiman, M. and Hussain, S.S. (2016) Prostate cancer: pathophysiology, diagnosis, and prognosis. *IOSR Journal of Dental and Medical Sciences (IOSR-JDMS)*, *15* (6): 4–11.

Patel, N.D. and Parsons, J.K. (2014) Epidemiology and etiology of benign prostatic hyperplasia and bladder outlet obstruction. *Indian Journal of Urology: IJU*, *30* (2): 170–6.

Rowland, D.L., Patrick, D.L., Rothman, M. and Gagnon, D.D. (2007) The psychological burden of premature ejaculation. *Journal of Urology*, *177* (3): 1065–70.

Sansone, A., Romanelli, F., Jannini, E.A. and Lenzi, A. (2015) Hormonal correlations of premature ejaculation. *Endocrine*, *49* (2): 333–8.

Schalken, J.A. (2015) Inflammation in the pathophysiology of benign prostatic hypertrophy. *European Urology Supplements*, *14* (9): e1455–e1458.

Serefoglu, E.C., McMahon, C.G., Waldinger, M.D., Althof, S.E., Shindel, A., Adaikan, G. et al. (2014) An evidence-based unified definition of lifelong and acquired premature ejaculation: Report of the Second International Society for Sexual Medicine Ad Hoc Committee for the Definition of Premature Ejaculation. *Journal of Sexual Medicine*, *11* (6): 1423–41.

Sofikitis, N., Stavrou, S., Skouros, S., Dimitriadis, F., Tsounapi, P. and Takenaka, A. (2014) Mysteries, facts, and fiction in varicocele pathophysiology and treatment. *European Urology Supplements*, *13* (4): 89–99.

Taylor, B. and Davis, S. (2007) The extended PLISSIT model for addressing the sexual wellbeing of individuals with an acquired disability or chronic illness. *Sexuality and Disability*, *25* (3): 135–9.

APPENDIX 1

AMERICAN ENGLISH SPELLING GUIDE

This book is written using UK spelling. If you are using American English, the following guide may be helpful.

Table A.1 UK and American spelling

UK spelling	American spelling	Examples (UK/American)	Variances
-ae-	-e-	aetiology/etiology anaesthetic/anesthetic haemoglobin/hemoglobin leukaemia/leukemia phaeochromocytoma/ pheochromocytoma	aero- words are the same in UK and US spellings, e.g. anaerobic
-oe-	-e-	diarrhoea/diarrhea diethylstilboestrol/ diethylstilbestrol dyspnoea/dyspnea oestrogen/estrogen oesophagus/esophagus oedema/edema	
-re	-er	centre/center fibre/fiber litre/liter metre/meter titre/titer	

(Continued)

Table A.1 (Continued)

UK spelling	American spelling	Examples (UK/American)	Variances
-our	-or	behaviour/behavior colour/color humour/humor tumour/tumor	
-logue	-log	homologue/homolog	
-lyse	-lyze	analyse/analyze catalyse/catalyze haemolyse/hemolyze hydrolyse/hydrolyze	Applies to verbs derived from 'lysis' only
-ical	-ic	biological/biologic serological/serologic	
-ence	-ense	defence/defense	
-lled, -lling, -eller	-led, -ling, -eler	labelled/labeled modelled/modeled modelling/modeling traveller/traveler	
-trophic, -trophin	-tropic, -tropin	adrenocorticotrophic/ adrenocorticotropic gonadotrophin/ gonadotropin thyrotrophin/thyrotropin	When trophic relates to nourishment, UK spelling is always used (e.g. heterotrophic) When tropic refers to directional growth, US spelling is always used (e.g. geotropic)

GLOSSARY

A master set of glossary flashcards is available online: go to **https://study.sagepub.com/essentialpatho**

Abscess   A collection of pus restricted to a specific area in tissue, organs or confined space

Absorption   The process by which one substance absorbs or is absorbed (taken in or assimilated) by another

Acanthosis   Epidermal hyperplasia (thickening of the skin)

Acetylcholinesterase inhibitors   Drugs that inhibit acetylcholinesterase activity (i.e. inhibit the breakdown of acetylcholine)

Achondroplasia   A genetic disorder characterised by an abnormally slow conversion of cartilage to bone during bone development, resulting in short stature (causing disproportionate body structure: normal size trunk, short limbs)

Acidaemia   The state of low blood pH caused by an increase in hydrogen ions

Acidosis   Clinical condition as a result of a low arterial blood pH<7.35. Can be either respiratory or metabolic

Acinar cells   Exocrine cells of the pancreas that secrete pancreatic enzymes

Acini   Plural of acinus

Acinus   A respiratory unit made up of alveoli or a small sac-like cavity in a gland, surrounded by secretory cells (a berry-like cluster of cells)

Acne vulgaris   Chronic inflammatory dermatosis affecting the pilosebaceous unit, leading to inflammatory and non-inflammatory lesions

Acquired   Develops after birth (with reference to a condition/disorder)

Acquired immunodeficiency syndrome (AIDS)   A syndrome associated with HIV that is characterised by immunosuppression and opportunistic infections, malignant tumours, cachexia and central nervous system (CNS) degeneration

Acromegaly   Abnormal, large growth of the hands, feet and face, caused by overproduction of growth hormone by the pituitary gland

Acute   Condition in which signs and symptoms develop suddenly and usually last a short time

Acute cough   A cough that occurs in response to illness that lasts less than three weeks

Acute kidney injury (AKI)   A rapid decline in kidney function occurring over hours to days, resulting in the inability to maintain fluid, electrolyte and acid–base balances, evidenced by a decrease in the glomerular filtration rate and urine output and an increase in nitrogenous waste, leading to azotaemia and uraemia

Acute lung injury (ALI)   An acute lung disease with bilateral pulmonary infiltrate consistent with oedema with no evidence of left atrial hypertension

Acute lymphocytic leukaemia (ALL)   Also known as acute lymphoblastic leukaemia, this form of leukaemia arises from lymphoid stem cells. As abnormal cells accumulate in the bone marrow, they crowd out the bone marrow and this prevents the further production of healthy cells

Acute myeloid leukaemia (AML)   An acute form of leukaemia affecting the myeloid stem cells that results in blast cells that do not differentiate into the types of leucocytes needed to fight off pathogens

Acute myocardial infarction (AMI)   Rupture or erosion of an atherosclerotic plaque with thrombotic occlusion of an epicardial coronary artery and ischaemia across the wall of the heart (myocardium) that leads to infarction (local death of tissue)

Acute on chronic   When a chronic condition has an acute exacerbation, requiring more intensive treatment

Acute pancreatitis   Reversible inflammation of the pancreas that occurs suddenly due to premature activation of pancreatic enzymes that may be caused by gallstones or increased alcohol intake

Acute respiratory distress syndrome (ARDS)   An acute inflammatory lung injury associated with increased pulmonary vascular permeability, increased lung weight and loss of aerated tissue

Acute tubular necrosis (ATN)   Acute kidney injury (AKI) secondary to damage to the renal tubules as a result of ischaemia and the initiation of an inflammatory response that promotes the production of toxic oxygen free radicals, leading to oedema, injury and necrosis. The nephrotoxic form is a result of poison, toxins or medication

Addison's disease   A chronic endocrine disorder in which the adrenal glands do not produce enough steroid hormones due to a progressive destruction of the adrenal cortex

Adenocarcinoma   A tumour formed when glandular cells mutate into cancer cells

Adenoma   A benign tumour formed from glandular structures in epithelial cells

Adenosine deaminase (ADA)   An enzyme eliminates a molecule, called deoxyadenosine, produced when DNA is broken down. ADA converts deoxyadenosine, which is toxic to lymphocytes, to deoxyinosine, which is not toxic

Adenosine triphosphate (ATP)   The energy store of the cell used to power cellular activities

Adenoviruses   Any of a group of DNA viruses discovered in adenoid tissue

Adhesins   Surface molecules that enable bacteria to attach to a host cell

Adhesions   Fibrous bands of scar tissue that form between tissues

Adiadochokinesia   An inability to perform rapid alternating movements

Adipocytes   Fat cells that make up adipose tissue

Adipokines   Cell-signalling proteins from adipose tissues, a form of cytokine

Adiponectin   A protein hormone involved in regulating glucose levels as well as fatty acid breakdown

Adjuvant therapy   Therapy given in addition to the primary/initial therapy to maximise its effectiveness

Adrenal (cortical) insufficiency   A condition in which the adrenal cortex does not produce adequate amounts of steroid hormones

Adrenocorticotropic hormone (ACTH)   A hormone produced by the pituitary gland that stimulates the production and release of cortisol from the adrenal cortex

Adrenogenital syndromes (congenital adrenal hyperplasia)   A group of disorders caused by adrenocortical hyperplasia or malignant tumours, leading to the abnormal secretion of adrenocortical hormones and characterised by masculinisation of women, feminisation of men, or precocious puberty

Aerobic metabolism   Metabolism of glucose in the presence of oxygen

Aetiological epidemiology   Searches for factors (hazardous or beneficial) influencing health status (e.g. toxins, poor diet, pathogenic microorganisms, health-promoting behaviours)

Agonists   Substances/drugs which, through binding with receptors, alter cell activity in some way to modify a specific mechanism within the cell; the substance therefore initiates or activates a physiological response when combined with a receptor or a muscle whose action is opposed by another muscle (antagonist)

Agraphia   An inability to locate the words for writing

Akinesia   An impairment of voluntary movement

Albuminuria   The presence of albumin in the urine

Alexia   Reading difficulties

Alkalosis   Clinical condition as a result of a high arterial blood pH greater than 7.45. Can be either respiratory or metabolic

Alkaptonuria   A genetic disorder that prevents the body fully breaking down two amino acids, tyrosine and phenylalanine, leading to build-up of homogenistic acid which may lead to black urine

Alkylating agents   The shape of DNA is changed through alkyls forming bonds with the DNA (alkylation), thus inducing cell death or slowing the replication of tumour cells

Allele   An alternative form of the same gene located at the corresponding position on homologous chromosomes

Allergen   A substance that can cause an allergic reaction

Allergic reaction   Type 1 hypersensitivity where a person has a hypersensitive immune response to an environmental substance

Alloimmunity   The immune response against the tissue of another individual (e.g. in organ transplantation or blood transfusion)

Alopecia   Hair loss

Alopecia areata   A noncicatricial T-cell-mediated autoimmune process that targets anagen stage hair follicles, disrupting the growth of hair through destruction of the hair follicle

Alternative therapy   When a non-mainstream therapeutic intervention is used instead of conventional (Western) medicine

Alveolar ventilation   The amount of inspired air that reaches the alveoli during a breath

Alzheimer's disease   A neurodegenerative condition characterised by the development of intracellular neurofibrillary tangles and deposits of extracellular amyloidal (beta) protein, leading to plaque formation in the CNS that leads to decreased acetylcholine production

Amenorrhoea   Absence of menstruation

Amniotic fluid embolism   When some amniotic fluid enters the maternal circulation and results in a serious reaction which may result in cardiorespiratory collapse and serious bleeding

Amygdala   Part of the limbic system of the brain that contributes to the storage of emotional experiences as memories and regulates emotional learning

Amylase   An enzyme that digests carbohydrates

Amyloidosis   A build-up of amyloid protein (an abnormal protein) in organs and tissues, impairing their function

Amyotrophic lateral sclerosis (ALS)   *See* Motor neuron disease

Anabolism   The building up or synthesising of large and complex molecules from smaller ones. This process requires energy

Anaemia   A deficiency of erythrocytes or haemoglobin

Anaemic hypoxia   When blood is unable to carry enough oxygen to the tissues

Anaesthesia   The practice of administering medications to block the feeling of pain and other sensations. General anaesthesia also causes unconsciousness

Anaesthetic   A drug/agent that blocks nociception or awareness of pain

Anagen phase   The first phase of hair growth

Analgesia   A drug/agent that diminishes nociception without loss of consciousness

Anaphylactic reaction   A systemic response to a hypersensitivity reaction (type 1), resulting in life-threatening clinical features such as difficulty in breathing due to severe bronchoconstriction, low blood pressure as a result of vasodilation and widespread oedema

Anaphylactic shock   An extreme allergic hypersensitive reaction to an antigen which can be life-threatening

Anaplasia   When cells are poorly differentiated (normally seen in cancer cells)

Androgenic alopecia   Male pattern baldness – polygenetic hair loss in genetically susceptible hair follicles in androgen-dependent areas of the scalp

Androgens   Male sex hormones

Anencephaly   A neural tube defect in which major portions of the brain, skull and scalp fail to develop

Aneuploidy   An abnormal number of chromosomes in a cell (not an exact multiple of the haploid number i.e. 23)

Aneurysm   The ballooning and widening at a specific point of an artery as a result of weakening of the arterial wall

Angina (pectoris)   Angina, meaning pain, and pectoris, meaning chest, is chest pain. This normally refers to pain incurred as a result of myocardial ischaemia and occurs when myocardial oxygen demands are increased (e.g. during exercise)

Angiogenesis   The formation of new blood vessels

Angioplasty   An endovascular procedure to widen narrowed or obstructed blood vessels, often through dilation with a balloon. The procedure enables the placement of a stent

Angiotensin converting enzyme (ACE) inhibitors Drugs that block the conversion of angiotensin I to angiotensin II (the active form) and therefore prevents its effects. Angiotensin II leads to biological responses that increase blood pressure so blocking its production will lower blood pressure

Ankylosis Joint stiffening and immobility due to fusion of the bones

Anomia The inability to name an object

Anomic aphasia Persistent inability to supply words for the things the person wants to say

Anorexia When the normal physiological stimuli that produce hunger remain intact but there is a lack of desire to eat

Anosmia Loss of olfaction (smell)

Anovulation When ovaries do not release an oocyte during a menstrual cycle

Anoxia An extreme form of hypoxia in which there is total depletion of oxygen

Antagonists Substances/drugs which interact with a cell receptor and, by so doing, interfere with or inhibits the physiological action of another substance. This therefore inhibits the action of the other substance. *Also* a muscle that opposes an action of another muscle (agonist)

Anterior cord syndrome Damage to the anterior two-thirds of the spinal cord or the anterior spinal artery, leading to loss of motor function, pain and temperature sensation below the area of injury/damage

Anthracycline A type of drug derived from the bacteria *Streptomyces* used in cancer chemotherapy

Antibodies Glycoprotein immunoglobulins (Igs), produced by lymphocytes, that combine with antigens to inactivate them by changing the antigen's chemical composition, render them immobile or preventing them from penetrating cells

Antidiuretic hormone (ADH) A hormone produced by the hypothalamus and released by the pituitary gland. It results in water reabsorption in the renal tubule to retain/increase water levels in the body

Antigen Any substance foreign to the body that evokes an immune response

Antigen-presenting cells A type of immune cell that enables a T cell to recognise an antigen in order to generate an immune response against the antigen

Antigen–antibody complexes When antibodies bind to either self-antigens or foreign antigens in the circulation and are then deposited in the vessel wall or tissues

Antimetabolites Substances that disrupt metabolic pathways of the cell and interfere with nucleic acid metabolism, thus preventing normal cell division

Antinuclear antibodies (ANA) A type of autoantibody that attacks protein structures within the nucleus of a cell. Also known as antinuclear factor (ANF)

Antiretroviral drugs Drugs that interfere with the viral life cycle and stop its progression

Anti-tumour antibiotics Antibiotics that affect the function of DNA by binding to it and preventing normal cell division and function

Anuria Complete suppression of urine formation, with no or minimal output

Aortic stenosis A narrowing of the aorta that restricts the blood flow leaving the left ventricle

Aphasia Severe difficulty or inability in producing or understanding language and/or speech. Usually due to left-sided brain damage. May be unable to speak. Also refers to a group of language disorders

Aplastic anaemia A form of anaemia where there is a failure in the production of the haematopoietic stem cells in the bone marrow

Apoptosis Programmed cell death

Appendicitis Inflammation with or without infection of the vermiform appendix

Apraxia Lack of awareness of certain body parts and/or surrounding space. Difficulty with motor planning for tasks of movements

Aquaretics A class of drug that promotes aquaresis, excretion of water without loss of electrolytes. *See also* Vaptans

Aqueduct stenosis A congenital narrowing of the channel between the third and fourth ventricles of the brain

Arachnoid villi Small projections of the arachnoid matter of the brain that reabsorb CSF

Arrhythmias Irregular or abnormal heart rhythms; disorders of the cardiac conduction cycle

Arrhythmogenesis The development or onset of arrhythmia

Arrhythmogenic Producing, or a tendency to produce, cardiac arrhythmias

Arteriosclerosis When the arterial walls become thickened and hardened as smooth muscle is replaced by collagen and hyaline cartilage. No lipid material is deposited. The blood vessel becomes less compliant and is associated with raised blood pressure

Arthralgia Joint pain

Arthritis Joint inflammation

Arthus reaction A severe, local immune reaction to the intradermal injection of a vaccine into a sensitised host

Articular cartilage A thin layer of hyaline cartilage that covers the epiphysis of one bone where it forms a joint with another bone

Ascites Accumulation of fluid in the peritoneal cavity

Asepsis The absence of microorganisms

Asthenozoospermia Sperm that have poor motility

Asthma *See* Bronchial asthma

Astrocytes Neuroglia in the CNS that secure neurons to their blood supply, form the blood–brain barrier and regulate the external chemical environment of neurons by removing excess ions and promoting the re-uptake of neurotransmitters released during synaptic transmission

Asynergia Loss of coordination of motor movements

Atelectasis Lack of gas exchange within alveoli, due to alveolar collapse or fluid consolidation

Atheroma A reversible build-up of degenerative material in the inner layer of an artery wall, consisting of macrophages, fats, calcium and fibrous connective tissue

Atheroprone Prone to development of atherosclerosis

Atherosclerosis Chronic inflammatory disease where atheroma builds up in the arteries as plaque is laid down and this in time narrows the arteries and reduces the blood flow

Atopy   The genetic tendency to develop allergic diseases such as allergic rhinitis, asthma and atopic dermatitis (eczema) associated with heightened immune responses to common allergens, especially inhaled and food allergens

Atrial fibrillation (AF)   A disorder with uncoordinated, irregular atrial contractions that result in a deterioration of atrial function

Atrial flutter   Organised atrial rhythm with a rate of typically 250–350 beats per minute

Atrial septal defect   A shunting of blood between the systemic and the pulmonary circulations via a patent foramen ovale, a secundum atrial septal defect or atrial shunting effect at atrial level

Atrioventricular (AV) bundle   A specialised nerve tract that divides into right and left bundle branches which pass down the septum of the heart, dividing out to each ventricle to distribute the impulse

Atrioventricular septal defect (AVSD)   A spectrum of defects where there is incomplete development of the atrioventricular septum alongside atrioventricular (AV) valve abnormalities

Atrophy   When cells decrease in size, resulting in a wasting of part of the organ or structure of the body

Atypia   Cells that appear abnormal but are not malignant

Aura   A subjective sensation including experiences from dreamlike feelings, alterations in smells, hearing, vision or other sensation. This disturbance of perception may represent a focal electrical disturbance

Autism spectrum disorder (ASD)   A group of neurodevelopmental disorders with symptoms that are seen on a continuum ranging from mild to severe. These symptoms include deficits in social reciprocity, communication challenges and repetitive behaviours that may be considered by some as unusual and restrictive

Autoantigens   An antigen that, despite belonging to the host, is the target of a humoral or cell-mediated immune response, e.g. as in autoimmune disease

Autoimmune disease   *See* Autoimmunity

Autoimmunity   When the immune system fails to recognise self-antigens and reacts to them as (foreign) antigens

Autologous immune enhancement therapy (AIET)   When immune cells from the person's own body are extracted and treated to increase their efficacy against cancer

Autonomic dysreflexia   A syndrome whereby the sympathetic nervous system is hyperstimulated (e.g. raising blood pressure excessively) but where there is little or no parasympathetic response to counter-balance this sympathetic reflex activity

Autoregulation   The inherent ability of an organ to maintain a constant blood flow despite changes in perfusion pressure

Autosomal aneuploidy   When individual autosomal chromosomes are missing or an extra one is present

Autosomal inheritance   A pattern of inheritance in which the transmission of traits depends on the presence or absence of particular alleles on the autosomes

Azoospermia   The absence of sperm in semen

Azotaemia   An increased blood serum level of urea, and frequently of creatinine, caused by both renal insufficiency and renal failure

Bacteraemia   Bacteria in the blood

Bacteria   Plural of bacterium – a single-celled spherical, spiral, or rod-shaped microorganism that appears singly or in chains, existing independently or parasitically

Balanitis   Inflammation of the glans penis

Baroreceptors   Sensory receptors that respond to changes in pressure

Basal ganglia/nuclei   Nuclei of grey matter buried within the white matter

Basophils   Granulocytes that assist in the inflammatory response by secreting histamine and heparin which increases blood flow by vasodilation and thinning the blood

Becker muscular dystrophy (BMD)   Similar to Duchenne muscular dystrophy (DMD) but occurs later in childhood with slower, less severe progression

Benign   When neoplasms have well-differentiated cells that are encapsulated, and do not metastasise

Benign cystic teratomas   Germ cell tumours derived from all germ cell layers but mainly ectoderm

Benign prostatic hyperplasia (BPH)   Hyperproliferation of epithelial and stromal cells in the transitional zone of the prostate gland

Beta-blockers   Drugs that are beta-adrenergic blocking agents, preventing other substances from binding with the receptors. This reduces sympathetic nervous system stimulation of the cardiovascular system, lowering blood pressure

Bilirubin   A breakdown product of haemoglobin converted from biliverdin

Binge eating disorder (BED)   A condition in which a person feels compelled to eat in large quantities on a frequent basis, regardless of their state of hunger. This is often followed by feelings of guilt, disgust and low mood

Bioavailability   The amount/proportion of an administered dose of unchanged drug that reaches the systemic circulation and is therefore available to act on its target

Biofilms   Complex multicellular masses consisting of interactive bacterial cells attached to a solid surface or to each other

Bipolar disorder   Enduring mood disorder whereby the person experiences periods of mania and hypomania alternating with periods of depression

Blastocyst   Formed in early pregnancy by the development of a solid ball of cells (the morula) which develops a fluid-filled space and then imbeds into the uterine wall at about day seven of pregnancy

Blood–brain barrier (BBB)   A structural and chemical barrier that strictly regulates substances passing from the circulatory system into the nervous system

Borborygmus   A rumbling sound made by the movement of intestinal fluid/gas

Bradycardia   Slow heart rate, usually less than 60 beats per minute

Bradykinesia   Slowness of movement, possibly with weakness, tremor and rigidity

Bradykinin   An inflammatory mediator that causes the contraction of smooth muscle and the dilation of blood vessels

Bradypnoea   Decreased respiratory rate

Brain tissue oxygenation (PbtO$_2$)   Partial pressure of oxygen in the brain tissue

Broad spectrum antibiotics   Antibiotics that act against both gram-positive and gram-negative bacteria

Broca's aphasia   Non-fluent aphasia – severely reduced speech output as Broca's area of the brain has been affected. Speech is limited mainly to short utterances of less than four words, with limited access to vocabulary. Formation of sounds is laborious and clumsy but the person may understand speech and be able to read, but have limited writing ability

Bronchial asthma   A chronic inflammatory disease, commonly known as asthma, associated with the release of inflammatory mediators from mast cells in the airways, leading to a response clinically manifested as expiratory wheeze, experience of chest tightness, dyspnoea, tachypnoea and cough

Bronchiectasis   The permanent dilation of the bronchi caused by destruction of the bronchial wall and elastic supporting tissue

Bronchiolitis   The most common lower respiratory tract infection in the first year of life; it is caused by a range of viruses

Bronchoconstriction   Constriction of the airways in the lungs as a result of the contraction of surrounding smooth muscle

Bronchospasm   A spasm of bronchial smooth muscle, resulting in a narrowing of the bronchi

Brown–Séquard syndrome (lateral cord syndrome)   Spinal cord injury with ipsilateral (belonging to or occurring on the same side of the body) muscle paralysis (corticospinal tract injury), ipsilateral loss of vibration and position sensation (posterior column injury)

Brudzinski sign   Flexion of the knees and hips when the neck is flexed forward rapidly

B-type natriuretic peptide (BNP)   A polypeptide released by the ventricles of the heart in response to excessive stretching of the heart or heart failure

Buccal mucosa   Mucosa of the buccal cavity (mouth)

Budd–Chiari syndrome   Obstruction of the hepatic vein, draining the liver

Bulbar stricture   Stricture in the bulbar urethra which can reduce urine flow

Bullae   Large air spaces formed from the destruction of alveoli in emphysema

Bullous   Characterised by blisters

Bundle of His   *See* Atrioventricular bundle

Butterfly fracture   A fracture where two oblique fracture lines meet to form a wedge-shaped fracture resembling a butterfly

Cachexia   Weight loss, muscle atrophy, fatigue and weakness caused by the release of inflammatory cytokines, loss of appetite and high metabolic rate. It is characterised by physical wasting

Calibre   Internal diameter

Callus   Bony healing tissue formed around the ends of a fracture

Cancer   A disease of the cell, where abnormal cell growth and division are uncontrolled, leading to altered function of the cells and tissue

Carboxypeptidase   An enzyme that digests proteins

Carcinogenesis   When a normal cell is changed into a malignant cell through changes in its genetic structure

Carcinogenic   Any substance that can induce carcinogenesis

Carcinogens   Substances capable of inducing cancer

Carcinoma   Cancer that originates in the epithelial tissue of the skin or tissue that lines the internal organs

Cardiac output   The volume of blood pumped out of the heart per minute = stroke volume × heart rate

Cardiac tamponade   Fluid in the pericardium compressing the heart

Cardiogenic shock   A type of shock that occurs because the heart is no longer able to pump blood round the body adequately

Cardiomegaly   Abnormal enlargement of the heart

Cardiomyopathies   A group of cardiac disorders that affect the myocardium

Cardiomyopathy   A disease of the heart muscle which affects its size, shape and structure, often including hypertrophy

Cardiovascular disease   Diseases that affect the heart or blood vessels. *See* Coronary artery disease

Catabolism   The breaking down of nutrients to provide energy and raw materials for anabolism

Catagen phase   The second phase of hair growth

Catecholamines   Hormones/neurotransmitters (such as dopamine, noradrenaline [norepinephrine] and adrenaline [epinephrine]) produced by the adrenal glands, the brain and some specialised nerve cells that stimulate alpha-adrenergic and beta-adrenergic receptors

Cauda equina   Nerves resembling a horse's tail that extend from the lower spinal cord down to the sacrum and supply the pelvic organs and lower limbs

Cauda equina syndrome   A syndrome where there is compression of the lumbar, sacral and coccygeal nerve roots, extending from the conus medullaris and affecting innervation of the legs, feet and pelvic organs

Caudal neuropore   A temporary opening at the extreme caudal end of the neural tube

Cell-mediated immunity   The immune response to an antigen involving the activation of phagocytes, antigen-specific cytotoxic T-cells, and the release of cytokines

Central cord syndrome   A spinal cord injury with disproportionately greater motor impairment in the arms than legs and accompanying bladder dysfunction. Anteroposterior compressive forces distribute pressure and damage onto the corticospinal tracts, innervating the arms

Central neurogenic diabetes insipidus (CNDI)   A condition where there is a deficit in the production and secretion of ADH as a result of injury or genetic defect to the neurohypophysis and therefore there are insufficient amounts to stimulate the renal tubule to reabsorb water and concentrate the urine

Central pontine myelinolysis   An irreversible demyelination of neurons in the pons which occurs from too rapid serum sodium level correction

Central precocious puberty   The early activation of the hypothalamic–pituitary–gonadal axis that triggers early puberty

Centriacinar   Refers to the central or proximal parts of the acini

Cerebellar hypoplasia   An incomplete or underdeveloped cerebellum

Cerebral contusions   Bruising to cerebral parenchyma, largely due to blunt trauma to the head causing micro-haemorrhages

Cerebral lacerations   Tears to the brain tissue

Cerebral oedema   An increased accumulation of water in the intracellular and interstitial fluids within the brain

Cerebral palsy   A group of non-progressive disorders of movement, posture and coordination, occurring in early childhood

Cerebral perfusion pressure (CPP)   The net pressure gradient that causes cerebral blood to perfuse the tissues of the brain; CPP = MAP (mean arterial pressure) – ICP (intracranial pressure)

Cerebral salt wasting syndrome (CSWS)   A condition in which there is a loss of both sodium and water from the ECF as a result of a renal loss of sodium which takes water with it. ADH levels are often elevated in an attempt to reabsorb water. However, the primary cause of water depletion is sodium excretion, which is why it is called a salt wasting syndrome

Cerebrospinal fluid (CSF)   Fluid formed in the choroid plexus that protects and nourishes the CNS

Chelation therapy   The use of drugs/infusions that bind iron with a substance that then can be excreted from the body, reducing iron levels in the body

Chemical gastropathy   The injury caused to gastric mucosa from long-term reflux into the stomach of duodenal contents, pancreatic secretions and bile

Chemokine   Signalling cytokine

Chemokine receptor   Cell membrane protein receptors for chemokines

Chemotaxis   The chemical attraction of a cell to a location

Chemotherapy   The use of drugs to treat cancer; it can be used alone or in combination with other therapies and other anticancer drugs. Most chemotherapeutic agents are cytotoxic and act on a specific phase of the cell cycle (cell division)

Chiari malformation   When the cerebellar tonsils descend into the foramen magnum, impairing CSF circulation and affecting cerebellar function

Chitin   A fibrous polysaccharide sugar found in the cell walls of fungi

Chlamydia   Sexually transmitted infection caused by the bacteria *Chlamydia trachomatis*, a gram-negative obligate intracellular pathogen

Cholangitis   Inflammation of the common bile duct

Cholecystitis   Diffuse inflammation of the gall bladder

Choledocholithiasis   Gallstones in the common bile duct

Cholelithiasis   Formation of gallstones through the solidification of substances found in bile, primarily cholesterol and bilirubin

Cholesterol   The most common steroid molecule and the precursor for the steroid hormones

Chondroblast   A cell actively producing the components of the extracellular matrix, which may differentiate into a chondrocyte

Chondrocyte   A mature cartilage cell derived from chondroblasts

Choriocarcinoma   A malignant uterine tumour that originates in the fetal chorion

Chorion   The outermost membrane surrounding an embryo that contributes to the formation of the placenta

Choroid plexus   A network of blood vessels in each ventricle of the brain that produce CSF

Chromosomal abnormality   A disorder that results from a change in the number or structure of chromosomes

Chromosome   Structures in the nucleus composed of DNA tightly coiled many times around proteins. They are responsible for genetic expression

Chronic   Persisting for a long time or constantly recurring

Chronic bronchitis   An inflammatory respiratory condition characterised by a persistent cough and sputum production for at least three months per year for two consecutive years

Chronic cough   A cough that occurs in response to illness and lasts more than eight weeks. May also be referred to as persistent

Chronic illness   One that persists over an extended period of time described in terms of months and years rather than days and weeks, and usually longer than three months. The illness may also be progressive

Chronic kidney disease (CKD)   A slow, progressive and irreversible permanent loss of nephrons, tubular absorptive capacity, decline in renal function and loss of endocrine functions. GFR decreases to less than 60 ml/min per 1.73m^2, albuminuria occurs or both for three or more months

Chronic lymphocytic leukaemia (CLL)   A malignant disorder that originates with lymphoid stem cells and results in immature lymphocytes. It is more common in Western society; the cause is largely unknown and it occurs more commonly in those over 50 years of age

Chronic myeloid leukaemia (CML)   A chronic form of leukaemia affecting myeloid stem cells. CML is associated with an abnormal chromosome known as the Philadelphia chromosome, affecting chromosomes 22 and 9. In this form of leukaemia, there is an overproduction of granulocytes and their precursors

Chronic obstructive pulmonary disease (COPD)   A group of respiratory disorders that are characterised by persistent respiratory symptoms and airflow limitation due to abnormalities caused by exposure to noxious particles or gases

Chronic pancreatitis   The progressive and irreversible fibrotic destruction of the exocrine pancreas that over time leads to the destruction of the endocrine pancreas

Chylomicrons   A type of lipoprotein created in the small intestine to aid absorption

Chylothorax   The presence of lymphatic fluid in the pleural space

Chyme   Partly digested food mixed with digestive enzymes

Chymotrypsin   A digestive enzyme which breaks down proteins in the small intestine

Chymotrypsinogen   A proteolytic enzyme and a precursor of the digestive enzyme chymotrypsin. Formed in the pancreas

Cicatricial   Scarring

Cicatricial alopecia   A form of hair loss where there is progressive and permanent destruction of hair follicles that is followed by replacement with fibrous tissue

Cingulate gyrus/cortex   Part of the limbic system thought to integrate emotion and sensory experiences, plus learning and memory

Circadian rhythm   The inherent biological clock related to biological processes that occur regularly at about 24-hour intervals

Cirrhosis   An irreversible, inflammatory, fibrotic liver disease in which hepatocytes are destroyed faster than they can be regenerated. Liver tissue becomes scarred and destroyed through inflammation and fibrosis

Citrullination   The modification of the amino acid arginine to citrulline, a non-essential amino acid

Clinical epidemiology   Describes the natural course of a disease in patient population and evaluates the effects of diagnostic procedures and treatment

Clinical trial   A study in which one group of people with a particular condition receive a specified treatment and their progress is compared with a second control group who are not receiving the active intervention

Clonic   Phase of a seizure in which there are violent muscular contractions

Clonus   Involuntary rhythmic contractions triggered by stretch of the muscle

Cluster headache   Clusters of episodic headaches occurring 1–8 times daily for weeks or months

Coarctation of the aorta (CoA)   A localised narrowing of the aortic lumen secondary to medial wall thickening and infolding aortic wall tissue

Coeliac disease   A condition in which there is malabsorption in the small intestine with associated inflammation

Cognition   The mental process of acquiring and interpreting knowledge, including perception, intuition and reasoning

Collagen   The primary structural protein in connective tissue

Collagenase   An enzyme that breaks down collagen

Collateral   Secondary or accessory rather than direct or immediate or a small branch, e.g. nerve or blood vessels

Colostrum   The first breast milk produced after delivery of the baby

Colour agnosia   Difficulty identifying colour

Coma   A state of unconsciousness where the person cannot be aroused and there is no detectable behavioural awareness

Combined immunodeficiency   Impairment of T lymphocyte and/or B lymphocyte development

Comminuted fracture   Fracture of a bone into more than two pieces

Communicable disorders/disease   A disease spread by contact, e.g. by pathogens transmitted to people from other people, from animals (zoonoses), or from other reservoirs of infection in the environment

Community trial   A study examining the effect of an intervention on a community as the unit of study, not individuals

Compact bone   Strong, dense bone tissue

Complement proteins   Plasma proteins that facilitate the phagocytosis of bacteria through opsonisation

Complementary and alternative medicine   Therapies outside mainstream medicine (i.e. medical approaches to care which originated in Western civilisation)

Complementary therapy   When a non-mainstream therapeutic intervention is used together with conventional (Western) medicine

Compression fracture   A fracture where two bones are crushed together through compressive forces

Concussion   When the brain is exposed to rapid acceleration, deceleration and rotational forces that stretch and distort neural structures, causing transient neurological dysfunction, e.g. headaches and problems with concentration, memory, balance and coordination

Congenital   Present from birth (with reference to a condition/disorder)

Congenital adrenal hyperplasia   *See* Adrenogenital syndromes

Congenital hypogonadotropic hypogonadism (CHH)   A heterogeneous disease characterised by a lack of puberty and infertility, secondary to the deficient secretion or action of gonadotropin-releasing hormone (GnRH)

Congestive heart failure   *See* Heart failure

Coning   When intracranial pressure reaches the point of irreversible decompensation, the brain will begin to herniate, forcing the brain to displace into any available space, often through the foramen magnum

Conjunctivitis   Inflammation of the conjunctiva of the eye

Connective tissue   Structural tissues that provide structural support for the organs of the body

Consciousness   A state of explicit awareness dependent on both biological arousal in the brain and the processing of experiences (perception)

Consolidation (pulmonary)   When an aerated section of the lung becomes filled with fluid

Constipation   Infrequent or difficult defaecation, usually indicating a decrease in the number of bowel movements per week and hard stools that are difficult to pass

Contrecoup   In head injury, damage on the opposite side of the brain from the impact

Contusion   A bruise resulting from direct trauma whereby the injured tissues undergo a sequence of events including the microscopic rupture of blood vessels, damage to muscle cells, swelling and inflammation

Conus medullaris   A narrowing of the lumbar part of the spinal cord into a conical shape

Conus medullaris syndrome   Trauma to the conus medullaris that leads to radicular pain (down the course of the nerve root), bowel and bladder dysfunction, loss of sensation and lower limb weakness relative to the lumbar and sacral nerve pathways affected

Convalescence   The period of recuperation and recovery from disease

Convulsion   Overt, major motor manifestations of a seizure

Cor pulmonale   Enlargement of the right side of the heart, secondary to lungs or pulmonary blood vessel disease

Corneocytes   Terminally differentiated keratinocytes composing most of the stratum corneum, the outermost part of the epidermis

Coronary artery disease (CAD)   When the major blood vessels that supply the heart with blood, oxygen and nutrients (coronary arteries) become damaged or diseased. Plaque develops over time and reduces myocardial blood flow

Coronary heart disease   *See* Coronary artery disease

Corpus spongiosum   Cylindrical body of erectile tissue in the penis

Corticosteroids   Steroid hormones produced in the adrenal cortex (glucocorticoids and mineralocorticoids) that are involved in metabolism and inflammatory response

Cortisol   A steroid hormone (glucocorticoid class)

Coryzal illness   Inflammation of nasal cavities, mouth and throat, caused by a virus

Cough   Protective reflex that helps clear the airways

Counter anti-inflammatory response syndrome (CARS)   A systemic deactivation of the immune system with the aim of restoring homeostasis from an inflammatory state

Coup   Under the area of impact in head injury. *See also* Contrecoup

Creatinine   A compound molecule generated from creatine during muscle metabolism

Crepitus   Grating, crackling or popping sounds or sensations due to air in the subcutaneous tissue, or in damaged bones or joints

Crohn's disease   A recurrent granulomatous type of inflammatory response that can affect any part of the GIT from the mouth to the anus. It is slowly progressive and can be a life-limiting and disabling disease

Croup   An inflammatory condition that affects the airways of babies and young children aged between 3 months and 3 years

Cryptorchidism   Undescended testis or testes

Crystalloid solution   The most commonly used type of intravenous fluids; a solution in which crystals can or may form but can diffuse across cell membranes

Curettage   The use of a curette (scoop) to remove uterine tissue

Cushing's syndrome (hypercorticalism)   A metabolic disorder caused by the overproduction of corticosteroid hormones by the adrenal cortex

Cyanosis   Bluish discolouration of the skin and/or mucous membranes due to increased levels of deoxygenated blood in the small vessels

Cyclin-dependent kinases   Enzymes that bind with cyclins to monitor and control different stages of the cell cycle, including repair of DNA at the checkpoints

Cyclins   Proteins that control stimulation and progression through the cell cycle

Cystadenomas   A benign tumour that develops from ovarian tissue

Cystic fibrosis (CF)　An autosomal recessive condition that occurs because of mutations in the *CFTR* (cystic fibrosis transmembrane conductance regulator) gene, resulting in disruption in the transport of salt and water across cell membranes in the pancreas, lungs, liver and salivary glands

Cystitis　Infection/inflammation of the lower urinary tract, primarily the bladder

Cystocele　When the support of the bladder base is weakened, the bladder falls below the uterus and the bladder wall causes the anterior vagina wall to bulge. The bladder also herniates into the vagina, particularly when coughing, lifting and defaecating

Cytokines　Small proteins which act to pass signals between cells

Cytotoxic antibiotics　*See* Anti-tumour antibiotics

Cytotoxic T cells/lymphocytes　T lymphocytes that destroy cancer cells, cells infected by viruses or cells that are damaged

Debridement　The removal of dead, damaged or infected tissue to facilitate healing

Decubitus ulcer　A wound that occurs in the upper layers of the skin secondary to sustained, externally applied pressure that causes localised ischaemia and an inflammatory response

Deep vein thrombosis (DVT)　When a thrombus (clot) develops in a deep vein (usually lower leg); it can potentially move and occlude a blood vessel (as an embolus)

Dehydration　A condition that results from the excessive loss of water from body tissues

Delayed ejaculation　A delay in orgasmic response and subsequent ejaculation despite sufficient sexual stimulation

Delayed-type mediated hypersensitivity (DTH)　The activation of CD4+ T-helper cells and the secretion of cytokines that promote an inflammatory reaction in people who are sensitised to an antigen, 24–72 hours after exposure

Demyelination　Loss or destruction of myelin around the axon of neurons

Dendritic cell　Antigen-presenting cells

Dendritic spine　A small membranous protrusion from a neuronal dendrite that receives input from a single axon at the synapse

Denervation　Loss of nerve supply

Depolarisation　Reversal of the resting electrical potential in the neuronal cell membrane when stimulated

Depression　A neurological disorder characterised by low mood, a loss of pleasure or interest, reduced energy and feelings of guilt or low self-worth secondary to pathophysiological changes in the amygdala, hippocampus and prefrontal cortex

Dermatitis　An inflammatory condition of the skin associated with epidermal barrier dysfunction

Descriptive epidemiology　Health and disease and their trends over time in specific populations

Desquamate　To shed surface keratinised cells from the stratum corneum

Detrusor　The main muscle of the bladder formed of smooth muscle fibres in spiral, longitudinal and circular bundles which empties the bladder with contraction

Diabetes insipidus (DI)　A condition where there is insufficient secretion of or a lack of response to ADH (anti-diuretic hormone), resulting in polyuria

Diabetes mellitus (DM) A chronic, life-long condition of glucose metabolism in which the body responds abnormally (insulin resistance) or does not produce enough insulin to control the blood glucose level. There are two main categories of DM:

- Type 1: characterised by the destruction of pancreatic beta cells and can be subdivided into two categories: type 1A (immune-mediated diabetes) and type 1B (idiopathic diabetes). This results in insulin dependence as no or very little insulin is produced
- Type 2: characterised by an inadequate amount of insulin being produced, or insulin resistance

Diabetic autonomic neuropathy A complication associated with diabetes, it is a form of peripheral neuropathy, i.e. damage to either the parasympathetic or sympathetic nerves or both

Diabetic fibrous mastopathy Tough, benign masses that develop in breast tissue; a complication of type 1 diabetes mellitus

Diabetic ketoacidosis (DKA) A complication of type 1 diabetes mellitus when the body begins to break down fat for energy, producing ketones, as it is unable to use glucose because of a lack of insulin

Diaphoresis Excessive perspiration

Diarrhoea The excessive passage of loose, watery stools

Diastolic dysfunction When the myocardium loses elasticity and therefore has reduced filling

Differentiation (cellular) The process by which a less specialised cell becomes more specialised

Diffuse axonal injury (DAI) Neuronal axonal damage from a variety of mechanisms; mechanical breaking/shearage of the axonal cytoskeleton, transport disruption along the axon, inflammation of the neuronal axon, or through secondary pathophysiological changes

Dilated cardiomyopathy Cardiomyopathy in which the heart becomes dilated, which results in the walls of the myocardium thinning with a consequent impaired ability to pump

Direct cell-mediated response When CD8+ cytotoxic T lymphocytes directly kill target cells expressing foreign antigens

Disability-adjusted life years The number of years of possible life lost as a result of premature mortality and the years of productive life lost due to disability/illness

Disease A state of disordered physiological functioning; disordered homeostasis

Dislocation Loss of contact between the articulating surfaces of two bones at a joint

Disseminated intravascular coagulation (DIC) Systemic activation of coagulation whereby fibrin is generated and deposited, causing microvascular thrombi in various organs that can lead to multiple organ dysfunction syndrome (MODS)

Distribution In pharmacokinetics, distribution is the reversible movement of a drug between blood and interstitial and intracellular fluids (extravascular tissues), normally through passive diffusion

Distributive shock A form of shock in which there is a disturbance in the distribution of circulatory volume through bypassing capillaries or pooling in capillary beds

Diverticula (plural diverticulae) Herniations (protrusions) of mucosa and submucosa through muscle layers, occuring primarily in the wall of the sigmoid colon

Diverticulitis Inflammation of the diverticula in the large intestine

DNA methylation An epigenetic mechanism involving the addition of a methyl (CH_3) group to DNA, modifying the function and expression of genes

Dominant inheritance When only one allele is required for the trait to be observed

Dopamine A neurotransmitter of the catecholamine type

Dopaminergic Releasing or involving dopamine

Double-inlet ventricle When more than half of both atria are joined to one dominant ventricle through either two separate atrioventricular (AV) valves or a common AV valve

Duchenne muscular dystrophy (DMD) An X-linked recessive type of muscular dystrophy caused by a mutation in the dystrophin gene that results in a lack of dystrophin, a protein, causing fibres to tear. Free calcium enters the muscle cells, causing degeneration and necrosis, with skeletal muscle fibres being replaced with fat and connective tissue. The muscle increases in size with a subsequent reduction in muscle strength and function

Ductus arteriosus A blood vessel connecting the main pulmonary artery to the proximal descending aorta that permits blood from the right ventricle to bypass the fetal lungs

Dysarthria Difficulty in forming words or speaking them because of a weakness of muscles used in speaking or because of disruption in the neuromotor stimulus patterns required for accuracy and velocity of speech

Dysbiosis Microbial imbalance/maladaptation in the gastrointestinal tract

Dyscalculia Difficulty with mathematics

Dyslipidaemia Distorted lipoprotein cholesterol

Dysmenorrhea Painful menstruation with associated abdominal cramps

Dysmetria An inability to judge distance and when to stop

Dyspareunia Difficult or painful sexual intercourse

Dysphagia Difficulty in swallowing

Dysphasia Language disorder. An inability to speak words which one has in mind or to think of the correct words; or an inability to understand spoken or written words

Dysphonia Difficulty in speaking due to a physical impairment of the mouth, tongue, throat or vocal cords

Dysplasia A condition in which the cells of a particular tissue vary in size and shape, mitosis is increased and large cell nuclei are seen

Dyspnoea Difficulty in breathing

Dysuria Painful or difficult urination

Eburnation Conversion of bone or cartilage through thinning or loss into a hard dense mass with a polished, ivory-like finish

Ecchymotic Discolouration (black/blue) of tissue due to the extravasation of blood, e.g. bruising

Eclampsia A condition whereby a pregnant woman develops neurological disturbances and seizures secondary to hypertension (has pre-eclampsia)

Ectasia Dilation or distention of tubular structures, including blood vessels

Ectopic   In an abnormal place or position

Ectopic pregnancy   Pregnancy in which the fetus develops outside the uterus, usually within a fallopian tube

Eczema   *See* Dermatitis

Ejaculatory dysfunction   Sexual dysfunction of ejaculation in men that includes premature ejaculation, delayed ejaculation and retrograde ejaculation

Ejection fraction   The volume, or percentage, of blood pumped (or ejected) out of the ventricles with each contraction

Elastin   An elastic, fibrous glycoprotein in connective tissue

Electrolyte   A substance that dissociates into ions when dissolved in a solution and attains the ability to conduct electricity

Embolism   (plural emboli) When an embolus occludes a blood vessel

Embolus   A blood clot, air bubble, segment of fatty deposit, or other substance carried in the bloodstream that lodges in and occludes a vessel

Emesis   The forceful expulsion of chyme (stomach and/or intestinal contents) through the mouth (the act of vomiting)

Emphysema   An obstructive airway disease characterised by destructive changes of the alveolar walls and irreversible enlargement of the alveolar sacs with a loss of surface area for gaseous exchange

Empyema   Accumulation of pus in a body cavity

Encephalitis   Inflammation of the brain parenchyma

Endarterectomy   An endovascular procedure to remove atheromatous plaques in the lining of an artery

Endemic   When a condition is generally present in a group or an area

Endometriosis   A condition in which functional endometrial tissue, normally within the uterine cavity, is found in sites outside the uterus, usually the ovaries, fallopian tubes, other organs of the reproductive system, uterosacral ligaments, intestines and pelvic organs

Endometrium   The mucous membrane lining the uterus

Endospore   Highly resistant structures that can remain dormant for many years and are resistant to desiccation, toxic chemicals and UV irradiation. When conditions become favourable, they become active and germinate

Endothelial cells   Cells that line the interior surface of the blood and lymphatic vessels

Endothelium   The tissue formed by a single layer of cells, lining various organs and body cavities

Endotoxin   A toxic substance bound to the wall of gram-negative bacteria

Engorgement   When an organ or tissue is filled with blood or fluid to the point of congestion/capacity

Enteral   Involving or passing through the gastrointestinal tract (e.g. through oral ingestion or tube feeding)

Enterocele   When a portion of the small bowel descends into the space between the posterior surface of the vagina and the anterior surface of the rectum

Enterotoxins   Specific exotoxins that affect the gastrointestinal tract

Eosinophils   Granulocytes that function in allergic responses and in resisting some infections by engulfing antigen–antibody complexes, allergens and inflammatory chemicals. They also weaken or kill parasites by secreting chemical agents

Ependymal cells/tissue   Cells that form the epithelial lining of the ventricles of the brain

Epidemic   Widespread distribution of a condition in a specific area at a specific time

Epidemiology   The scientific study of health and disease in populations to understand the range of factors which influence the distribution of disease through the population and how it spreads between populations

Epidermoid cysts   Dome-shaped lesions of the pilosebaceous follicle, largely formed as a result of infection; they are benign encapsulated, sub-epidermal nodules filled with keratin

Epidermolysis bullosa acquisita (EBA)   A heterogeneous, organ-specific autoimmune disease that occurs when autoantibodies to type VII collagen are induced, causing mucocutaneous blisters

Epididymitis   Infection or inflammation of the epididymis

Epididymo-orchitis   Infection or inflammation of the epididymis and the testes

Epigenetic therapy   The use of drugs that inhibit DNA methylation and histone deacetylation, thereby reversing epigenetic modifications

Epigenetics   The study of changes caused by the modification of gene expression rather than alteration of the genetic code itself

Epilepsy   A distinct, chronic seizure disorder characterised by an imbalance between excitatory and inhibitory neurotransmitter activity in cerebral neuronal ions. A tendency toward recurrent seizures unprovoked by any systemic or acute neurologic insults

Epileptogenesis   A sequence of events that converts a normal neuronal network into a hyperexcitable network that leads to the development of spontaneous recurrent seizures

Epithelium   The covering of the internal and external surfaces of the body, including the lining of vessels and other small cavities

Erectile dysfunction (ED)   A complex condition that occurs secondary to neural, vascular and/or hormonal dysfunction that impairs penile erection

Erythrocytosis   An increase in the number of circulating erythrocytes

Essential hypertension   *See* Primary hypertension

Euploidy   When a cell has any number of complete chromosome sets (an exact multiple of the haploid number)

Evaluative epidemiology   Evaluates preventative interventions and estimates risk of specific diseases for people exposed to hazards

Excitotoxicity   The pathophysiological process whereby neurons are damaged and killed by the overactivation of receptors for excitatory glutamate (neurotransmitter), and intracellular organelles are damaged, leading to death of the neuron

Excretion   A process of eliminating metabolic waste from an organism

Expressive dysphasia   A type of dysphasia where a person has partial or total loss of producing language in different modes (spoken, manual or written); comprehension is usually intact

Extracorporeal life support (ECLS) The use of equipment external to the body to carry out the functions of a non-functioning organ

Extradural (epidural) haematoma A collection of blood between the skull and the dura matter when a force has resulted in periosteal dura mater-bone cleavage

Extraembryonic Referring to outside of the embryo

Fabry disease Deficiency of the enzyme alpha-galactosidase A

Facioscapulohumeral muscular dystrophy (FSHD) An autosomal-dominant inherited form of muscular dystrophy in which the muscles of the limbs, shoulders and face weaken

Faecalith A hard piece of stool/faeces

Failure to thrive Insufficient weight gain or inappropriate weight loss

Farber disease An inherited disorder of lipid metabolism associated with the deficiency of the enzyme ceramidase and accumulation of ceramide in the lysosome

Fascia A band or sheet of subcutaneous tissue that anchors, encloses and separates muscles and other internal organs

Fibrin An insoluble protein formed from fibrinogen during blood clotting that forms a fibrous web in haemostasis

Fibrinogen A glycoprotein involved in blood clotting

Fibrinolytic Processes or substances that result in the disintegration or dissolution of fibrin, usually through enzymatic action

Fibrinopurulent Pus or exudate that contains a relatively large amount of fibrin

Fibroadenomas Benign breast tumours composed of glandular and stromal (connective) tissue

Fibroatheroma A lipid-rich necrotic core encapsulated by collagen-rich fibrous tissue; an advanced lesion of coronary atherosclerosis

Fibroblasts Cells that synthesise the extracellular matrix and collagen

Fibrocystic changes Non-malignant changes in the breasts that include breast pain, cysts and lumpiness

Fibroids *See* Leiomyomas

Fibroma A benign fibrous tumour of connective tissue

Fibromyalgia A chronic syndrome affecting the musculoskeletal system that is characterised by widespread pain, increased sensitivity to touch, fatigue, non-restorative sleep, anxiety and depression

Fibrosis Thickening and scarring of connective tissue, usually as a result of injury

First pass metabolism The metabolism of a proportion of a drug administered before it reaches the systemic circulation (usually due to passage through the liver)

Fissure A groove or cleft (normal or abnormal) on the surface of an organ or bony structure

Flaccid paralysis Weakness and loss of muscle tone secondary to lower motor neuron dysfunction

Follicle stimulating hormone (FSH) A hormone that activates Sertoli cells in men, and stimulates the growth of ovarian follicles in women

Foramen magnum decompression   The removal of sub-occipital bone to increase space and allow CSF to flow

Foramen ovale   An opening in the septum between the two atria of the heart that is normally patent only in the fetus

Fracture   A break or disruption in the continuity of a bone

Fragility fracture   A fracture of a bone from a fall or bump that would not ordinarily have caused a bone to break

Fucosidosis   A lysosomal storage disease

Fundus   Part of a hollow organ (such as the uterus or the gall bladder) that is furthest from the opening. Also refers to the upper part of the stomach

Fungi   Any of a wide variety of single or multi-cell organisms that reproduce by spores, including the mushrooms, moulds, yeasts and mildews

Galactokinase deficiency   A genetic metabolic disorder characterised by an accumulation of galactose and galactitol as a result of decreased conversion of galactose to galactose-1-phosphate by galactokinase

Galactorrhoea   Spontaneous milk secretion

Galactosaemia   An inherited disorder of galactose metabolism that primarily occurs in newborn children

Gamma-aminobutyric acid (GABA)   An inhibitory neurotransmitter that blocks the transmission of nerve impulses in the central nervous system

Gangliosidoses   A group of disorders of the accumulation of lipids known as gangliosides

Gangrene   Tissue death secondary to inadequate blood supply

Gastritis   Inflammation of the gastric mucosa

Gastroesophageal reflux disease (GORD/GERD)   Persistent reflux of stomach contents, i.e. acid, pepsin and bile salts, into the oesophagus, causing oesophagitis

Gaucher disease   A genetic disorder of metabolism where glucocerebroside (a lipid) cannot be adequately broken down

Gene expression   The process by which specific genes are activated to produce a required protein, i.e. the functional gene product

Gene therapy   Using genes to treat or prevent disease by inserting a gene into a patient's cells. *Or* the use of drugs that suppress overactive oncogenes to activate tumour suppressor genes

Germline mosaicism   When some germline cells have a normal chromosomal make-up while others carry a chromosome change

Gestational hypertension   Hypertension that occurs after 20 weeks of gestation but where there are no other signs of pre-eclampsia and it disappears within three months of delivery

Gestational trophoblastic disease   A group of disorders in which tumours grow in the uterus during pregnancy

Ghon complex   The collective term for the primary lung lesion and lymph node granulomas in tuberculosis

Ghon focus   A granulomatous lesion containing tubercle bacilli, modified macrophages and other immune cells

Ghrelin   The 'hunger hormone' produced by cells in the stomach which enhances the sensation of feeling hungry before an expected meal

Gilbert's syndrome   A genetic disorder of bilirubin metabolism

Gleason score   The sum of two scales scored 1 to 5 that designates the degree of differentiation of the tumour of the prostate gland predominant cell lines

Gliadin   A protein that is a component of gluten

Gliosis   A fibrous proliferation of glial cells in injured areas of the CNS, leading to scar tissue formation

Global aphasia   When a person will produce few recognisable words and understand little or no spoken language. They can also neither read nor write

Glomerular filtration rate (GFR)   The rate at which the filtrate is formed in the Bowman's capsule of the kidneys, measured in millilitres per minute

Glomerulonephritis   Inflammation of the renal glomeruli

Glomerulosclerosis   Formation of scar tissue in glomeruli

Glucagon   A peptide hormone that raises the blood glucose level when it falls too low by stimulating conversion of glycogen in the liver into glucose

Glucocorticoids   Any of a group of anti-inflammatory corticosteroids involved in the metabolism of carbohydrates, proteins and fats

Gluconeogenesis   The production of glucose from lactate, amino acids and the glycerol component of fat

Glucosuria   *See* Glycosuria

Glutamate   An excitatory neurotransmitter

Glycogen   Carbohydrate store in the body

Glycogen storage disease type II   An autosomal recessive metabolic disorder whereby there is a deficiency in an enzyme (acid alpha-glucosidase [acid maltase[) needed to break down glycogen, resulting in an accumulation of glycogen in lysosomes

Glycogenolysis   The conversion of glycogen to glucose

Glycoprotein   Proteins which have oligosaccharide chains

Glycosuria   Glucose in the urine

Goblet cells   Cells that produce mucus, found in the respiratory and gastrointestinal tracts

Gonadal dysgenesis   Loss of germ cells; congenital developmental disorder of the reproductive system in the male or female

Gonadotropin-releasing hormone (GnRH)   A hormone secreted by the hypothalamus that triggers the anterior pituitary to release gonadotropins

Gonocytes   Germ cells responsible for spermatogenesis and oogenesis

Gonorrhoea   A sexually transmitted infection caused by *Neisseria gonorrhoeae*, a gram-negative diplococcus bacterium that is spread by direct contact with the mucosa of an infected individual

Gout   A syndrome that results in hyperuricaemia caused by either increased uric acid production or decreased uric acid excretion by the kidneys, leading to uric acid deposition in joints

Granular cell tumour   A tumour (usually benign) that probably originates from Schwann cells of the peripheral nervous system

Granuloma   A mass of granulation tissue that occurs in response to infection, inflammation or the presence of a foreign body

Granulomatous   Of, relating to or characterised by granuloma

Granulomatous hypersensitivity   A chronic type IV reaction where macrophages are activated in response to microbial antigens

Granulysin   A cytokine which is identified as the key mediator of keratinocyte destruction through apoptosis

Graves' disease   An autoimmune condition in which the body's immune system attacks its own tissues which stimulates growth of the thyroid gland and increased thyroid hormone secretion

Guillain-Barré Syndrome (GBS)   An acute inflammatory demyelinating polyneuropathy or an acute motor axonal neuropathy. Rapid-onset muscle weakness is caused by immune system damage of the peripheral nervous system

Gumma   A soft, necrotic, fibrous granuloma resulting from the tertiary stage of syphilis

Haematemesis   The vomiting of blood

Haematocrit   The ratio of the volume of erythrocytes to the total volume of blood

Haematogenous spread   Spread via the bloodstream

Haematoma   A large area of accumulated blood from a local haemorrhage

Haematopoietic   Pertaining to the formation of blood or blood cells

Haematuria   The presence of blood in urine

Haemochromatosis   A genetic disorder whereby there is excess iron absorption

Haemoglobin   A protein composed of globin and haem and containing four globin chains and four haem units, enabling each haemoglobin molecule to carry four oxygen molecules

Haemoglobinopathies   Conditions in which there is an abnormality in structure of (one) of the globin chains of the haemoglobin molecule

Haemoglobinuria   The presence of free haemoglobin in the urine

Haemolytic anaemia   A type of anaemia whereby erythrocytes are prematurely destroyed and eliminated

Haemophilia   An X-linked condition where a deficiency of clotting factors leads to an impaired ability of the blood to clot

Haemoptysis   The coughing up of blood or bloody secretions

Haemorrhagic stroke   A stroke caused by the rupture of a blood vessel in the brain

Haemostasis   The process by which bleeding is stopped

Haemothorax   The presence of blood in the pleural cavity

Hamartoma   A benign uncommon tumour of varying amounts of glandular, adipose and fibrous tissue

Hapten   An incomplete soluble antigen which, when combined with a larger carrier protein, is recognised as an antigen

Haustrum   (plural haustra) A structure resembling a recess or sac formation

Haversian canals   Minute tubes which form a network in bone and contain blood vessels

Health improvement   Interventions to improve the health and well-being of individuals or communities through facilitating the adoption of healthy lifestyle choices and tackling factors that influence health in society (poverty, social housing, education)

Health promotion   The facilitation of people to take positive, autonomous control of their health through a diverse set of approaches that improve health-related quality of life through the prevention of ill-health

Health protection   The area of public health practice concerned with actions to reduce exposure to factors which can impact on the development of ill-health

Health services epidemiology   Describes and analyses the work of the health services

Heart failure   Failure of the heart to effectively pump blood around the body, so that its ability to respond to increased demands for cardiac output is impaired

Helminths   Multi-cellular parasitic worms

Hemiparesis   Weakness down one side of the body

Hepatic encephalopathy   The totality of central nervous system (CNS) manifestations of liver failure, characterised by a variety of neural disturbances

Hepatitis   Inflammation of the liver

Hepatocytes   Liver cells

Hepatomegaly   Abnormal enlargement of the liver

Heterogeneous (genetic)   When there are mutations at two or more genetic loci that yield the same or similar phenotypes

Heteroplasmy   When a cell has some mitochondria that have a mutation in the mitochondrial DNA and some that do not

Heterozygote screening   Genetic testing of a population or sub-population to identify heterozygous carriers of a disease-causing allele who are healthy but have the potential to produce children with the disease

Hiatal hernia   A diaphragmatic protrusion (herniation) of the stomach (upper part) through the diaphragm into the thorax

Hiatus hernia   *See* Hiatal hernia

High-density lipoproteins (HDLs)   A type of lipoprotein that mops up cholesterol in the blood, transporting it to the liver for elimination in bile

High glycaemic index carbohydrates   The index represents the relative ability of a carbohydrate food to increase the level of glucose in the blood. Foods that score highly should be avoided

Hippocampus   Part of the limbic system primarily associated with the formation of memory, and organising sensory and cognitive experiences for storage

Hirsutism   Unwanted, male-pattern hair growth in women

Histamine   An inflammatory agent released by cells in response to an injury/allergy/inflammation that causes dilation of capillaries and contraction of smooth muscle

Histone modification   Epigenetic mechanism post-translational the modifications (the modification of proteins following protein biosynthesis) that regulate gene expression

Histotoxic hypoxia   When cells are unable to use the oxygen reaching them

Homeostasis   Regulation of the internal environment in order that a level of consistency is maintained necessary for the cells and organs of the body to operate optimally

Homocystinuria   A disorder of methionine metabolism, leading to accumulation of homocysteine (an amino acid created during the metabolism of methionine and cysteine) and its metabolites in blood and urine

Hormone antagonist   Substances that act upon the hormone receptors of cells to inhibit the endocrine function

Human chorionic gonadotrophin (hCG)   A placental hormone that maintains the corpus luteum during pregnancy

Human immunodeficiency virus (HIV)   A virus that destroys the CD4+ cells of the immune system and suppresses the immune response. It can cause acquired immunodeficiency syndrome (AIDS)

Human leucocyte antigen (HLA)   The subset of major histocompatibility complex (MHC) genes encoding for cell surface antigen-presenting antigens

Humoral immunity   The immune response mediated by antibodies, complement proteins and certain antimicrobial peptides within the extracellular fluid

Huntington's disease (HD)   An autosomal-dominant, progressive disease of the central nervous system; degeneration of the brain results in uncontrolled movements, emotional problems and cognitive impairment

Hydatidiform mole   Growth of an abnormal fertilised ovum or an overgrowth of placental tissue (during pregnancy)

Hydrocele   A collection of serous fluid in the tunica vaginalis surrounding the testis, normally occurring unilaterally

Hydrocephalus   Enlargement of the CSF containing cavities, the ventricles, within the brain due to impairment of flow or absorption of the CSF

Hydrolytic enzymes   Enzymes that catalyse the hydrolysis of a chemical bond

Hydrosalpinx   A distally occluded Fallopian tube filled with serous or clear fluid

Hydrostatic pressure   The pressure exerted by the blood against the artery wall by the heart pumping blood at force

Hydrothorax   The collection of serous fluid in the pleural cavity caused by increased hydrostatic pressure or decreased osmotic pressure in blood vessels

Hyperactivation   A state of increased activity or agitation

Hyperaemia   An increase in blood supply to an organ

Hyperaldosteronism   An excessive secretion of aldosterone that disrupts electrolyte homeostasis, causing an increase in sodium reabsorption in the renal tubule and promoting the loss of potassium and hydrogen. These are often due to aldosterone-secreting adenomas or hyperplasia

Hypercapnia   Increased levels of carbon dioxide content of the blood

Hypercholesterolaemia   High levels of cholesterol in the blood

Hyperhomocysteinaemia   Elevated levels of homocysteine in the blood

Hyperinsulinaemia   High levels of insulin in the blood

Hypernatraemia   High levels of sodium in the blood

Hyperosmolar hyperglycaemic non-ketotic syndrome (HHNKS)   A complication of type 2 diabetes mellitus in which hyperglycaemia results in high osmolarity without significant ketoacidosis

Hyperosmolarity   The condition of having abnormally high osmolarity

Hyperparathyroidism   An excess amount of parathyroid hormone in the blood

Hyperpituitarism   Increased pituitary secretion

Hyperplasia   When cell division multiplies, resulting in an increasing number of cells in the organ or tissue affected

Hyperpnoea   An increase in the rate and depth of breathing (normal during exercise)

Hypersensitivity   When the immune response to a substance that is normally harmless is altered, causing damage to cells, tissues and organs (e.g. allergy, autoimmunity)

Hypersomnia   A disorder of sleep characterised by excessive daytime sleepiness, excessive sleep periods and/or the absence of feeling refreshed/reenergised after sleep

Hypersynchronisation   When numerous neurons in the brain fire excessively from a large electrical impulse generated in one part of the brain, triggering a seizure

Hypertension   Persistently elevated blood pressure

Hyperthyroidism   When the thyroid gland is overactive and produces too much thyroxine

Hypertonia   High/increased muscle tone

Hypertriglyceridaemia   High blood triglyceride levels

Hypertrophic cardiomyopathy   Cardiomyopathy in which hypertrophic changes of the myocardium occur, including of the ventricular septum, without an obvious cause, resulting in a reduced ability to pump blood effectively

Hypertrophy   When cells grow in size and increase the size of an organ or tissue. The cells have grown bigger rather than increasing the number

Hyperventilation   Ventilation in excess of what is needed for normal elimination of CO_2

Hypervolaemia   Excess volume

Hypo   Low

Hypoglycaemia   Low blood sugar

Hypogonadism   *See* Congenital hypogonadotropic hypogonadism (CHH)

Hypoinsulinaemia   Low levels of insulin in the blood

Hypokalaemia   Low potassium in the blood

Hypomania   When someone is persistently disinhibited and euphoric (but less than with mania)

Hyponatraemia   Low sodium in the blood

Hypophosphataemia   An abnormally low level of phosphate in the blood

Hypopituitarism   Decreased pituitary secretion

Hypoplasia   Underdevelopment or incomplete development of a tissue or organ

Hypoplastic left heart syndrome   A syndrome characterised by the left-sided heart structures being underdeveloped, thereby resulting in a left ventricle that is unable to pump with enough force to meet the needs of the systemic circulation

Hypospadias   When the urethral opening is on the underside of the penis

Hypotension   Low blood pressure

Hypothalamic–pituitary–adrenal (HPA) axis   A complex neuroendocrine network of relay interactions between the hypothalamus, pituitary gland and adrenal glands that modulate stress responses and other homeostatic processes (e.g. digestion, immune response, and energy regulation)

Hypothalamus   Several nuclei and tracts of axons in a small area below the thalamus that control the autonomic nervous system, neuroendocrine system and limbic system and management of many crucial functions

Hypothyroidism   When underactivity of the thyroid gland results in insufficient thyroid hormones to meet the needs of the body, causing reduced anabolism and a fall in metabolic rate

Hypotonia   Low/reduced muscle tone

Hypoventilation   Decreased ventilation; being unable to eliminate adequate amounts of CO_2

Hypovolaemia   Low blood volume

Hypovolaemic shock   Shock induced by a reduction in circulating blood volume

Hypoxaemia   Decreased levels of oxygen in the blood

Hypoxia   A reduction in tissue oxygenation

Hypoxic hypoxia   When inadequate amounts of oxygen enter the lungs

Hysteroscopy   When the cavity of the uterus is viewed directly through a hysteroscope (a fine telescope)

Iatrogenic   Relating to illness or an adverse effect (physical or psychological) caused by health care intervention

Ictal phase   A seizure itself; consists of the paroxysmal firing of cerebral neurons

Ictus phase   *See* Ictal phase

Idiopathic (primary) epilepsy   Epilepsy for which there is no apparent cause

Idiopathic hypertension   *See* Primary hypertension

Idiosyncratic reactions   Serious drug reactions that occur rarely and unpredictably

Immune complexes   *See* Antigen–antibody complexes

Immune tolerance therapies   Therapies that modify the immune system to prevent it attacking its own body cells in autoimmune disease, or foreign cells present in an organ after transplantation

Immunisation   The process of inducing immunity to an infectious organism or agent in an individual or animal through vaccination

Immunodeficiency   A condition in which the body is unable to produce sufficient antibodies or immunologically sensitised T cells in response to antigens

Immunoglobulins   A class of proteins that function as antibodies

Immunoreactive trypsinogen (IRT)   A pancreatic enzyme precursor released by the pancreas and elevated in infants and children with cystic fibrosis

Immunosuppression   Partial or complete suppression of the immune response

Immunotherapy   The use of agents/drugs to modulate the immune response

Impacted fracture   Fracture where fracture fragments wedge together

Impetigo vulgaris   A common infection of the superficial layers of the epidermis, commonly caused by gram-positive bacteria and being highly contagious. It is characterised by erythematous plaques with a yellow crust that may be itchy or painful to touch

Incretins   A group of metabolic hormones released in response to food intake that stimulate a decrease in blood glucose levels by increasing insulin secretion and decreasing glucose production by the liver

Incubation period   The period between the introduction of microbe to host and the onset of symptoms of the illness

Independent prescribers (UK)   Health care professionals able to prescribe medicines on their own initiative from the British National Formulary (includes doctors, dentists and some non-medical health professionals, including nurses, pharmacists and, more recently, registered chiropodists/podiatrists, physiotherapists, optometrists and registered therapeutic radiographers)

Induration   Swelling or hardening of normally soft tissue

Infarction   Tissue death due to inadequate blood supply

Infectious enterocolitis   Inflammation of both the small and large intestine due to infection

Infiltration   The diffusion, entry or accumulation of a substance in a tissue or cell

Inflammation   When there is an increased blood supply to a site of injury that triggers an inflammatory response to prevent infection. The second stage of wound healing

Inflammatory bowel disease (IBD)   A group of idiopathic chronic inflammatory disorders of the gastrointestinal tract that includes two major phenotypes, Crohn's disease and ulcerative colitis

Influenza   A viral infection caused by viruses that belong to the Orthomyxoviridae family that can affect both the upper and lower respiratory tract

Inotropes   Drugs that increase the contractile force of the heart

Insulin   An anabolic hormone which promotes the synthesis of proteins, carbohydrates and nucleic acids, reduces blood glucose levels and facilitates entry into the cells of glucose, potassium (K^+) magnesium (Mg^{2+}) and phosphate (PO_4^{3-}). It binds to and activates the appropriate cell membrane receptors, causing glucose transporters to promote glucose uptake followed by diverse metabolic events through the body

Insulin shock   A physiological state characterised by excess insulin in the blood, low blood glucose, weakness and potentially loss of consciousness

Interferons   Proteins that prevent viruses replicating

Interleukins   A group of cytokines expressed by leucocytes which promote the development and differentiation of T and B lymphocytes and haematopoietic cells

Internal cervical os   The opening of the cervix into the uterus

Interphase   Stage of cell cycle when growth and preparation for division occur, including duplication of proteins and organelles

Interstitial lung disease (ILD)   A group of diffuse parenchymal lung disorders associated with substantial morbidity and mortality

Interstitium   An interstitial space within a tissue or an organ

Intestinal obstruction   Impaired movement of chyme through the intestinal lumen

Intima   The innermost layer of an artery or vein

Intracerebral haemorrhage/haematoma (ICH)   A subset of stroke in which a rupture occurs in a cerebral blood vessel (typically arteries/arterioles), resulting in haemorrhage and haematoma formation in the cerebral parenchyma which can extend into the subarachnoid space

Intracranial hypertension   Raised intracranial pressure

Intrinsic AKI   Acute kidney injury (AKI) as a result of abnormalities within the kidney (including damage to the blood vessels, glomeruli and tubules)

Irritable bowel syndrome (IBS)   A gastrointestinal disorder associated with recurrent abdominal pain and altered bowel habits and can be either diarrhoea prevalent or constipation prevalent

Ischaemia   A reduction in blood supply to tissue that results in the the supply being insufficient

Ischaemic heart disease   *See* Coronary artery disease

Ischaemic hypoxia   When blood supply to the tissue is inadequate

Ischaemic stroke   A type of stroke (85% of strokes) secondary to inadequate blood flow to the brain as a result of a partial or complete occlusion of an artery. It can be caused by a thrombus or embolus

Isovaleric acidaemia   An autosomal recessive metabolic disorder in which there is impairment of the normal metabolism of the amino acid leucine that leads to acidaemia

Isthmus   A final section of the aortic arch (the connection between the ascending and descending aorta)

Jaundice   Yellow discolouration of the skin and whites of the eyes due to high bilirubin levels

Joint effusion   The presence of increased intra-articular fluid

Kaposi sarcoma (KS)   A malignancy of the endothelial cells of blood and lymphatic vessels that initially manifests as a lesion on the skin and mucosal membrane of the mouth

Karyotype   The number and appearance of chromosomes in the nucleus

Keratinocytes   Cells that produce keratin

Kernig sign   Resistance to knee extension in the supine position with the hips and knees flexed against the body

Ketones   Any of a class of organic compounds characterised by a carbonyl group attached to two carbon atoms. They are byproducts of the breakdown of fatty acids

Ketonuria   The excretion of large amounts of ketone bodies in the urine

Krabbe disease   A lysosomal storage disease whereby an enzyme deficiency leads to a lack of myelin and neurodegeneration

Kussmaul respirations   Laboured, deep breathing often associated with severe metabolic acidosis

Kyphosis   Excessive convex curvature of the spine

Lactate   An ester or salt of lactic acid, the final byproduct of anaerobic glycolysis

Lactiferous duct   Ducts that converge to create a network connecting the nipple to the lobules of the mammary gland and that carry breast milk

Lactose intolerance   The inability to digest lactose

Legionnaires' disease   A type of pneumonia caused by *Legionella pneumophila* (gram-negative bacteria) that thrives in warm, moist environments

Leiomyomas   Benign growths derived from smooth muscle and the commonest type of female reproductive tumours, known as fibroids

Leptin   The 'satiety hormone' which regulates how much fat is stored in the body by adjusting the sensation of hunger and the amount of energy expended

Lesion   An area of abnormal tissue change

Leucocytes   White blood cells that provide protection against pathogens. They are mostly found in connective and lymphatic tissue, normally only circulating in the blood for a number of hours

Leucocytosis   An increase in the number of leucocytes in the blood

Leukaemias   Malignant disorders of haemopoietic (blood forming) tissue within the bone marrow or peripheral blood supply

Leukopenias   Conditions in which there is a reduction in the number of leucocytes

Leukotrienes   Inflammatory mediators released by mast cells; they are primarily responsible for bronchoconstriction in an asthma attack

Leydig cells   Cells outside the seminiferous tubules that produce testosterone

Lichen sclerosus/Lichen sclerosis   An autoimmune condition in which the vulva is inflamed with areas of very thin epithelium with superficial ulcers due to scratching because of itching

Lipase   An enzyme that digests fats

Lipolysis   The breakdown of fats/lipids into fatty acids and glycerol

Lipoma   A benign tumour composed of mature fat cells

Lipophagy   The breakdown and elimination of lipids from cells

Lipopolysaccharides   A molecule consisting of combined lipid and polysaccharide

Lipoproteins   Large molecules which play a central role in the absorption of lipids, and of transporting cholesterol, triglycerides and fat-soluble vitamins through body fluids to and from peripheral tissues and the liver

Locked in syndrome   A loss of voluntary control of movement, usually from some form of brain stem damage/disorder, but arousability and awareness are retained, that is, the person remains conscious

Low-density lipoproteins (LDLs)   A type of lipoprotein largely composed of cholesterol – cells use enzymes to break them down to release the cholesterol

Lumpectomy   Surgical removal of a lump of tissue

Lupus   *See* Systemic lupus erythematosus (SLE)

Luteinising hormone (LH)   A hormone that stimulates Leydig cells to secrete testosterone in men, and ovulation and development of the corpus luteum in women

Lymphadenopathy   Abnormal enlargement of the lymph nodes

Lymphocytes   Agranulocytes that can destroy cancer cells, cells with a viral infection and foreign cells. There are three types of lymphocytes: B cells, T cells and natural killer (NK) cells

Lymphocytopenia   An abnormal reduction in the amount of lymphocytes

Lymphoedema   Oedema caused by the impaired lymphatic drainage of extracellular fluid

Lymphomas   Cancer of the lymphoid tissue

Lymphopenia   *See* Lymphocytopenia

Lysis   Deconstruction of a cell by rupture of the cell membrane

Lysosomal enzymes   Enzymes that break down macromolecules and bacteria

Lytic enzymes   Enzymes that cause lysis

Macrocephaly   When the circumference of the head is larger than expected parameters

Macrocytic   When a substance is larger in size than normal

Macrophage   A form of phagocyte which has a role in both non-specific (innate) and specific (adaptive) defence mechanisms in the body – a mature monocyte

Maculopapular rash   A skin rash characterised by a flat, red area covered with small confluent bumps

Major histocompatibility complex (MHC)   Proteins that are recognised as 'self', which in humans are known as the HLA (human leucocyte antigen)

Malabsorption   The inability of the intestinal mucosa to absorb digested nutrients

Malabsorption syndromes   Disorders that interfere with intestinal absorptive processes

Malaise   A feeling of general discomfort, uneasiness or pain

Malignant   When neoplasms have poorly differentiated, rapid growing cells that are not encapsulated and have the ability to break loose, migrate and form secondary tumours

Malignant hypertension   A rapid, extreme form of hypertension that can lead to organ damage

Malnutrition   A lack of nourishment due to inadequate/inappropriate amounts of calories, macro-nutrients (fat, protein and carbohydrates) and micronutrients (vitamins and minerals). Malnutrition includes undernutrition and overnutrition (excess consumption of nutrients)

Mammary duct ectasia   When the lactiferous duct becomes dilated as the duct becomes blocked or clogged and chronic inflammation develops in the surrounding tissues

Maple syrup urine disease   A genetic metabolic disorder affecting the ability to process certain branched-chain amino acids (valine, leucine, isoleucine)

Marfan syndrome   A connective tissue disorder that results in elongated bones, leading to individuals who are tall and thin, with long extremities and digits

Mast cells   Cells that contain basophil granules that release histamine and other inflammatory agents during inflammation and allergic reactions

Mastectomy   Surgical removal of a breast, including breast tissue, skin and nipple

Mastitis   Breast inflammation

Megakaryocyte   A large bone marrow cell responsible for the production of thrombocytes

Memory cells   Lymphocytes that have previously encountered specific antigens that on re-exposure to the same antigen rapidly initiate the immune response (memory T cells) or proliferate and produce large amounts of specific antibodies (memory B cells)

Meninges   Three layers of connective tissue that surround the brain and spinal cord

Meningitis   Infection and inflammation of the membranes (meninges) and fluid (cerebrospinal fluid) surrounding the brain and spinal cord

Meningocele   A protrusion of the meninges through a gap in the spine due to a congenital defect – it contains no neural tissue

Menorrhagia   Excessive menstrual flow

Messenger RNA (mRNA)   A molecule that carries codes from DNA in the cell nucleus to sites of protein synthesis in ribosomes in cytoplasm. Acts as a template for the polypeptide chain forming a protein

Metabolic acidosis   An acidosis secondary to the metabolic production of acid in greater quantities than can be buffered

Metabolic bone disease   Disorders of bone metabolism resulting in structural effects on the skeleton

Metabolic syndrome   A complex syndrome of several pathophysiological conditions marked by obesity, cardiovascular changes and significant insulin resistance

Metabolism   All of the organic and chemical reactions in the body, using all of the nutrients that the body takes in to create molecules for structure, chemical reactions and energy

Metachromatic leukodystrophy (MLD)   A lysosomal storage disease

Metaplasia   When one type of mature cell becomes converted into another which is better able to deal with the conditions causing the change

Metastasis   (verb metastasise) The process whereby cancer cells spread from their original site and proliferate in distant sites

Metastatic spread   *See* Metastasis

Microbiome   The ecological community of commensal, symbiotic and pathogenic microorganisms that coexist within and on the body

Microcephaly   When the circumference of the head is smaller than expected parameters

Microcytic   When a substance is smaller in size than normal

Microvesiculation   Extracellular vesicles associated with pathophysiological processes

Migraine   A severe intermittent disturbance of sensory processing in the CNS that results in a failure in full inhibitory pain control with an associated reduction in attentional functional capacity: moderate or severe headache, often felt as a throbbing pain on one side of the head

Minimally conscious state (MCS)   A disorder of consciousness where a person has a shifting awareness of others and their environment, sometimes responding to some stimuli. Responses are inconsistent but reproducible and indicate that the person is interacting with their environment to some degree

Minute volume   The volume of air/gas inhaled (inhaled minute volume) or exhaled (exhaled minute volume) from a person's lungs in one minute

Mitochondria   The plural of mitochondrion – a cellular organelle known as the 'power house'. ATP is created for storage of energy, which is released when required

Mitosis phase   The stage of the cell cycle when nuclear division occurs

Mixed urinary incontinence   When stress incontinence and urge incontinence co-exist

Monoclonal antibodies   Antibodies made in the laboratory to target a specific antigen and numerous copies are produced

Monoploidy   Where one member of the chromosome pair is missing

Monosomy   When there is only one copy of a specific chromosome instead of the normal two

Morbidity   The incidence or prevalence of disease

Morula   A small bunch of embryonic cells when they enter the uterus (at about three days after fertilisation)

Mosaicism   The presence of two or more populations of cells with different complements of chromosomes in the same individual

Motor neuron disease (MND)   A selective and progressive functional loss in upper and lower motor neurons, resulting in impairment or loss of motor function

Movement agnosia   An inability to recognise movement of an object

Mucociliary clearance/escalatory/function   The propelling of mucus by cilia from the distal to the proximal lung airways

Mucosa   The mucous membrane or a lining of a part of the body that secretes mucus

Mucus   A viscous slippery secretion produced by mucous membranes. Being rich in mucins, its function is to moisten and protect

Multifactorial inheritance   The inheritance of a trait as a result of more than one factor, including gene combinations and environmental factors

Multigenic   Refers to an inherited characteristic specified by a combination of multiple genes

Multiparity   Having given birth two or more times or having given birth to more than one offspring at a time

Multiple organ dysfunction syndrome (MODS)   When two or more organ systems fail due to the overwhelming uncontrolled inflammatory response

Multiple sclerosis (MS)   A chronic, progressive autoimmune disease with multifocal areas of neuronal demyelination, disrupting the ability of the nerve to conduct action potentials. It is characterised by chronic inflammation, demyelination and gliosis (scarring) in the CNS

Muscular dystrophies   A group of genetic disorders that lead to a progressive loss of muscle fibres, resulting in a weakness of the voluntary muscles (mostly but not exclusively)

Mutagen   A chemical or physical agent capable of causing a change in form, quality or other characteristic in a gene, thereby causing a mutation

Mutation   When changes in DNA affect the functioning of a gene

Myalgia   Muscle pain

Myasthenia gravis   An autoimmune disorder with an antibody-mediated reaction at the postsynaptic neuromuscular synapse, causing muscle weakness

Mycobacterium   Non-motile aerobic bacteria that include numerous saprophytes (microorganisms that live on dead/decaying organic matter) and are the pathogens that cause tuberculosis and leprosy

Mycoplasmas   A microscopic, bacteria-like organism that lacks a cell wall around its cell membrane

Mycoses   Infection/disease caused by a fungus

Myelomeningocele   Neural tissue exposure, resembling a fluid sac adhered to the back. Due to a defect of the spine and spinal cord when the spine and spinal canal do not close properly. A myelomeningocele is the most serious form of spina bifida

Myenteric plexus   The major nerve supply to the gastrointestinal tract

Myocardial infarction   Infarction of the myocardium, normally as a result of occlusion of one or more coronary arteries

Myocarditis   Inflammation of the myocardium

Myocardium   The middle layer of the heart muscle, consisting of thin filaments of actin and thick filaments of myosin

Myoclonus   Brief, sudden, involuntary twitching/jerking of a muscle or a group of muscles

Myocyte   A contractile cell found in muscle tissue

Myofibrils   Small threadlike structures that are the contractile organelles of the skeletal muscle

Myoglobin   Oxygen-transmitting pigment of the muscle, consisting of one haem molecule with one iron molecule attached to a single globin (protein) chain

Myoglobinuria   The presence of myoglobin in the urine

Myometrium   The smooth muscle tissue forming the middle layer of the uterus

Myotonic muscular dystrophy (MMD)   A multisystem disease, caused by genetic mutation, affecting the brain, smooth muscle, skeletal muscle, heart and endocrine systems. It presents with distal muscle weakness, learning difficulties or intellectual disability or both

Myxoedema   Oedema of the skin and underlying tissues, thickening of the tongue and mucous membranes caused by hypothyroidism, resulting in a waxy appearance and dysarthria

Narrow complex tachycardia   Tachycardias that originate in the atria

Natriuretic peptide   A peptide that causes natriuresis (renal loss of sodium)

Natural killer (NK) cells   Cytotoxic lymphocyte

Nausea   A feeling of sickness and unease with an inclination to vomit

Necrosis   Death of one or more cells as a result of injury from external stimuli

Neoplasia   The plural of neoplasm

Neoplasm   'New growth' of cells that is no longer responding to the body's normal regulatory controls and can be benign or malignant

Nephrogenic diabetes insipidus (NDI)   A condition when the renal tubule fails to respond to the presence of ADH and is unable to concentrate urine as a result of failure to reabsorb water back into the intravascular space

Nephropathy   Chronic loss of kidney function

Nephrosclerosis   Development of sclerotic lesions in the renal arterioles and glomerular capillaries, causing them to become thickened and narrowed

Neuralgia   Severe, acute experiences of neuropathic pain that are often repetitive

Neurogenesis   The process of generating new neurons

Neurogenic bladder   Bladder dysfunction secondary to impaired nervous control

Neurogenic bowel   Colon dysfunction secondary to impaired nervous control

Neurogenic shock   A type of shock secondary to disruption of the autonomic pathways within the spinal cord that results in a triad of hypotension, bradycardia and hypothermia

Neuroglia   Non-neuronal cells that support and protect neurons

Neuron   A specialised cell of the nervous system that transmits nervous impulses (action potentials)

Neuronal plasticity/neuroplasticity   The ability of the nervous system to create and reorganise synaptic connections in response to early development, learning, experience, or following injury

Neuropathy   Disease or dysfunction of one or more peripheral nerves, typically causing numbness or weakness

Neurotoxins   Endotoxins that inhibit the release of neurotransmitters

Neurotransmitter   A chemical messenger that transmits nerve signals across a synapse

Neutropenia   A fall in production or an increase in loss from the blood of neutrophils

Neutrophils   Granulocytes that engulf bacteria and cellular debris or use chemical agents (lysozyme and peroxidase) to destroy foreign bodies

Niemann–Pick disease   A genetic disease that affects lipid metabolism

Nitric oxide (NO)   A gas that causes and maintains vasodilation and contributes to increased vascular permeability

NMDA receptor antagonists   A class of anaesthetics that work to antagonise/inhibit the action of the N-Methyl-D-aspartate receptor (NMDAR)

Noncicatricial   Non-scarring

Non-communicable disorders/disease   Disease not contracted by contact but occurring as a result of a range of risk factors or occurrences (e.g. trauma, poor diet)

Non-neoplastic epithelial disorders   Refers to a number of disorders that can affect the vulval epithelium

Normocytic   When a substance is the size expected

N-terminal pro b-type natriuretic peptide (NT-proBNP)   A polypeptide released by the ventricles of the heart in response to excessive stretching of the heart. Can be used to diagnose heart failure

Nuchal   Relating to the nape of the neck

Nutrition   Food or nourishment. Also the branch of science that deals with nutrients and nutrition; the scientific foundation for dietetics

Nystagmus   Rapid involuntary movements of the eyes

Obesity   Abnormal or excessive fat accumulation that may impair health

Oblique fracture   A fracture at an angle through the bone

Obstructive shock   A form of shock that occurs as a result of an obstruction in blood circulation

Oedema   The observable accumulation of excess interstitial fluid secondary to an imbalance between capillary filtration and lymph drainage

Oesophageal varices   Dilated sub-mucosal veins in the lower oesophagus secondary to portal hypertension

Oestrogen   One of several steroid hormones, largely secreted by ovaries and placenta

Oestrogens   Refers to the group of oestrogenic hormones (e.g. oestradiol and oestrogen), classically referred to as female sex hormones although some are present in men in lesser amounts. They are associated with the development of secondary sexual characteristics, growth and maturation of long bones, sexual function and menstruation

Oligoclonal bands   Bands of immunoglobulins suggesting inflammation of the central nervous system due to infection or another disease

Oligodendrocytes   A type of neuroglial cell that produces myelin in the central nervous system

Oligohydramnios   Reduced amniotic fluid

Oligomenorrhea   Infrequent or very light menstruation

Oligozoospermia   Low sperm count

Oliguria   Urine output that is less than 1 ml/kg/h in infants, less than 0.5 ml/kg/h in children, and less than 400 ml or 500 ml per 24 h in adults

Omentum   A fold of visceral peritoneal tissue that hangs from the stomach

Oncogene   A mutated gene that may cause the growth of cancer cells

Oogenesis   The process of female gamete formation

Ophthalmoplegia Paralysis or weakness of the eye muscles

Opsonisation The process by which a pathogen is marked for destruction by phagocytosis

Orchidopexy Surgical treatment of undescended testis

Organomegaly Abnormal enlargement of an organ

Orthopnoea Difficulty in breathing when lying flat

Oscillation Regular fluctuation or vibration about a central point

Osmolality The concentration of osmotically active particles per 1000ml of fluid

Osmolarity The concentration of osmotically active particles per 1000 ml of solution

Osmotic diuresis Excess urine production as a result of osmotic particles being excreted by the kidney, carrying water with them

Osmotic pressure The pressure exerted by plasma proteins and some electrolytes in the plasma inside the capillaries, pulling water and small molecules towards them. Includes the pressure exerted in pulling water across a semipermeable membrane

Ossification Formation of bone

Osteitis deformans See Paget disease of bone (PDB)

Osteoarthritis Joint disease characterised by the loss of and damage to articular cartilage, inflammation, osteophytosis (formation of bone spurs) and thickening of the subchondral bone

Osteoblasts Bone-building cells that synthesise and secrete collagen fibres and other organic components and also initiate the calcification of bone matrix

Osteoclasts Bone cells formed from fused monocytes that secrete powerful lysosomal enzymes and acids for dissolving the protein and mineral matrix

Osteogenesis (ossification) Formation of bone

Osteogenic Bone producing

Osteomalacia A softening of bones due to the inadequate and slowed mineralisation of osteoid in mature bone

Osteomyelitis Infection of bone

Osteopenia/Osteopaenia A reduction in bone density greater than would be expected for age

Osteophytosis New bone formation of joint margins, leading to osteophytes (bone spurs)

Osteoporosis A complex, chronic, progressive metabolic bone disease, multifactorial in nature, characterised by a decrease in bone mineral density (BMD), leading to an increased risk of fractures

Otalgia Ear pain

Otitis media Inflammation of the middle ear

Overactive bladder syndrome A syndrome characterised by increased urinary frequency, nocturia and urgency with or without urge incontinence in the absence of infection

Overflow incontinence The involuntary loss of urine due to bladder distension in the absence of detrusor muscle activity

Overweight   *See* Obesity

Oxidative phosphorylation   The synthesis of ATP by phosphorylation of ADP

Oxidative stress   An imbalance between the production of free radicals and the ability of the body to counteract or detoxify their harmful effects through neutralisation by antioxidants

Oxytocinergic   Releasing or involving oxytocin

Paget disease of bone (PDB)   A progressive bone disease where there is an increased rate of metabolic activity in the bone, leading to localised, abnormal and excessive remodelling of the bone

Panacinar   Involves the acini at the terminal alveoli

Pancreatic exocrine insufficiency   The inability to produce pancreatic enzymes

Pancreatitis   Inflammation of the pancreas

Pandemic   A condition which spreads across a large region or worldwide

Pannus   A thickened layer of fibrovascular tissue or granulation tissue

Papanicolaou (Pap) smear (test)   A procedure in which cells are retrieved from the cervix using a spatula in order to examine them for changes that may indicate cancer or other disease processes

Papilloedema   Oedema of the optic disc

Papules   A solid elevation of skin with distinct margins and no visible fluid

Paracellularly   Refers to the movement/transport of substances between cells

Paraesthesia   Abnormal sensations such as numbness, tingling or burning

Paraneoplastic syndromes   Disorders that are triggered by an altered immune system response to a neoplasm

Paraphimosis   When the foreskin becomes trapped behind the corona of the glans penis, compromising arterial supply to the gland and preventing venous and lymphatic return

Paraplegia   Injury to the thoracic, lumbar or sacral regions of the spinal cord, including the cauda equina and conus medullaris, resulting in loss of function of the lower body

Parasite   An organism which lives in or on another organism (known as the host) and benefits by deriving nutrients from the host but provides no benefit to the host

Parenteral   Referring to a route of entry of a substance other than through the enteral route

Parkinson's/Parkinson's disease   A progressive neurodegenerative disorder associated with decreased dopamine in parts of the brain, largely due to destruction of the nigrostriatal neurons (in the basal ganglia) that results in loss of smooth, coordinated movement

Patent ductus arteriosus (PDA)   When the fetal ductus arteriosus remains patent after birth

Pathogen   An agent causing disease or illness to its host

Pathogenesis   The biological processes that lead to development of a disease

Pelvic inflammatory disease (PID)   Infection of the upper female genital tract, including the uterus, ovaries, fallopian tubes and cervix

Penetrance   The extent that the trait carried in the abnormal gene presents the disorder

Penumbra   An area of ischaemic tissue in which infarction is evolving but is reversible if circulation/perfusion is restored

Pepsinogen   A proenzyme produced by chief cells in the stomach and converted to its active form, pepsin, for the digestion of protein

Peptic ulcer disease   Ulceration that occurs in the gastric or intestinal mucosal lining

Perforation   When erosion, infection or other factors produce a weak point in an organ or structure that can rupture as a result of internal pressure

Perfusion   The delivery of blood to the capillary bed in systemic circulation. Also refers to the amount of blood perfusing the capillaries around the alveoli

Peripartum cardiomyopathy   Cardiomyopathy that develops in the last month of pregnancy or up to five months after delivery

Peripheral artery disease   A circulatory disorder caused by the build-up of plaque in the major arteries that supply the legs, arms and pelvis

Peripheral nerve disorders   Disorders involving motor and/or sensory neurons of the peripheral nervous system, resulting in muscle weakness and/or atrophy and possibly sensory changes

Peristalsis   The ripple-like waves created by the relaxation and contraction of muscle in a tubular structure that results in the movement of material along its length

Pernicious anaemia   Deficiency in the production of erythrocytes through a lack of vitamin B_{12}

Perseveration   Persistence of a single thought

Petechial rash   Pinpoint, round spots on the skin secondary to microhaemorrhages

Phaeochromocytoma   A neuroendocrine tumour of the adrenal medulla that secretes high amounts of catecholamines

Phagocytosis   (verb phagocytose) Process by which a cell (e.g. white blood cell) engulfs a pathogen, other cells, cell debris or foreign particles

Pharmacodynamics   The study of how drugs affect the body

Pharmacokinetics   The study of the physiological absorption, distribution, metabolism and excretion of drugs within the body

Pharmacology   The study of drugs including their origin, composition, pharmacokinetics, therapeutic use and toxicology

Pharyngitis   Inflammation of the pharynx

Phenylalanine   An essential amino acid that is metabolised to tyrosine

Phenylketonuria   A genetic disorder whereby the amino acid phenylalanine builds up in the body as a result of a defect in the gene that helps create the enzyme needed to break it down. Can cause intellectual disability, seizures, behavioural problems and mental disorders

Phimosis   An inability to retract the foreskin over the glans penis

Phlebitis   Inflammation of the walls of a vein

Photosensitivity   Sensitivity to light or ultraviolet radiation

Pilli   Structures on the surface of bacteria that enable them to attach to a host cell

Piloerection   Involuntary erection of hairs on the skin due to a sympathetic reflex

Placenta abruptio/placental abruption   When the placenta comes away from the lining of the uterus before delivery of the baby occurs, most commonly at around 25 weeks of gestation

Placenta praevia   When the placenta has implanted in the lower part of the uterus or over the cervix

Plaque   An accumulation of semi-solid substances on the surface of tissue (e.g. within an artery or on the surface of a tooth)

Plasmids   Pieces of DNA that replicate independently from the host's chromosomal DNA

Platelet-activating factor (PAF)   A pro-inflammatory lipid molecule that activates neutrophils through chemotaxis and causes platelet aggregation and degranulation, inflammation and anaphylaxis

Pleural effusion   An abnormal collection of fluid in the pleural cavity

Plicae   A fold or ridge of tissue

Pluripotent   The ability of a cell to differentiate into any type of cell or tissue but not a complete organism

Pneumonia   An inflammatory condition of the lungs, primarily alveoli and bronchioles

Pneumothorax   The presence of air in the pleural cavity caused by rupture of either the parietal or visceral pleura

Polycystic ovary syndrome (PCOS)   A disorder involving infrequent, irregular or prolonged menstrual periods, anovulation and often excessive androgen levels

Polycythaemia   A condition in which there is a raised level of red blood cells (erythrocytes) or haemoglobin

Polycythaemia vera   A malignant disorder of haematopoietic stem cells, leading to raised amounts of erythrocytes

Polydipsia   Excessive thirst

Polygenic inheritance   The inheritance of a single trait (phenotype) that is controlled by two or more different genes

Polyhydramnios   Increased amniotic fluid

Polymicrobial   Polymicrobial diseases are caused by combinations of viruses, bacteria, fungi and parasites which together cause more severe diseases

Polymorphic   Occurring in more than one form

Polymorphism   The manifestation of two or more genetically determined phenotypes in a certain population

Polyphagia   Excessive hunger

Polyploidy   When a cell contains more than two paired (homologous) sets of chromosomes

Polyuria   An excessive amount of urine production

Porphyria   A genetic disorder where there is impairment in the ability to produce haem, resulting in the increased formation and excretion of chemicals called porphyrins

Portal hypertension   High pressure in the hepatic portal vein

Posterior cord syndrome   Damage to the posterior third of the spinal cord or the posterior spinal artery, leading to a loss of light touch, vibration, and proprioception sensations

Post-ictal phase   The period after a seizure with temporary neurological dysfunction

Postpartum haemorrhage (PPH)   The loss of 500 ml of blood within 24 hours of delivery

Postrenal AKI   Acute kidney injury secondary to an obstruction in the urinary collection system

Post-traumatic epilepsy (PTE)   A recurrent seizure disorder occurring due to traumatic brain injury

Pre-eclampsia   A disorder of pregnancy characterised by the onset of hypertension and (often) proteinuria

Prefrontal cortex   An area of grey matter in the anterior frontal lobe involved in the complex regulation of cognition, emotion and behavioural function

Preputial orifice   The opening of the foreskin

Pressure ulcers   *See* Decubitus ulcer

Priapism   A prolonged erection of the penis that is non-sexual

Primary adrenal cortical insufficiency   When there is insufficient production of the hormone cortisol from the adrenal cortex. There may also be insufficient aldosterone production

Primary encephalitis   When a pathogen directly infects the brain and spinal cord

Primary hypertension   When blood pressure is elevated without evidence of another disease causing it

Primary immunodeficiency   A disorder as a result of a single gene mutation that results in immune dysregulation, autoimmunity and recurrent infection

Primary injury (neurological)   Referring to damage that occurs at the time of trauma, i.e. the physical effect of mechanical forces on the brain or spinal cord

Primary polydipsia   An excessive intake of water that suppresses the secretion of ADH

Procallus   Granulation tissue formed at the site of fracture

Procarboxypeptidase   The inactive precursor of carboxypeptidase

Processus vaginalis   The peritoneal tunnel through which the testes migrate from the retroperitoneum toward the scrotum during embryological development

Prodromal   The phase that precedes a seizure involving symptoms and signs including insomnia, headache, reduced tolerance threshold, increased agitation, low mood and emotional lability. Also refers to the short time of generalised/mild symptoms (malaise, muscle aches) that precede illness

Progression   Developing or moving gradually towards a more advanced state. For example, when a mutant dividing cell begins to exhibit malignant properties

Prokaryotes   A single-celled organism without a distinct nucleus with a membrane and specialised organelles

Proliferation   Rapid reproduction of a cell, part or organism

Proliferation (cellular)   The process when cells increase in number through mitotic division

Promotion   The proliferation of a cell with a mutation

Prosopagnosia Difficulty in recognising faces

Prostaglandins A group of lipid compounds with hormone-like effects

Prostate cancer (PCa) A malignant tumour of glandular origin in the prostate

Prostate-specific antigen (PSA) A serum protein produced by the prostate gland; raised levels may indicate prostate cancer or benign prostatic hyperplasia

Prostate-specific membrane antigen (PSMA) An antigen that facilitates the development of prostate cancer through raising intracellular folate levels. Levels in plasma correlate with the severity of cancer and are used as indicators

Prostatitis Inflammation of the prostate gland

Protease An enzyme that breaks down proteins

Proteasome Protein complexes which break down proteins by proteolysis

Proteinuria The presence of protein in urine

Proteolysis The breakdown of proteins

Proteolytic enzymes Enzymes that break down proteins into peptides and amino acids

Proto-oncogene A gene that codes for proteins that stimulate cell growth (growth factors) and differentiation

Proton pump inhibitors Drugs that inhibit the activity of pumps transporting hydrogen ions across cell membranes; their main use is to reduce the amount of stomach acid produced

Protozoa A diverse group of mostly motile unicellular eukaryotic organisms (including amoebas, flagellates, ciliates and sporozoans (e.g. *Plasmodium falciparum*, which causes malaria)) that mostly live parasitically

Pruritus Diffuse itching of the skin

Pseudoangiomatous stromal hyperplasia This is a rare and benign breast lesion, one of a group of such lesions, which includes nodular fasciitis. It is a benign proliferation of myofibrils in the stroma

Pseudopolyps Tongue-like projections that resemble polyps

Psoriasis vulgaris A T-lymphocyte mediated autoimmune skin disorder characterised by the focal formation of inflamed, raised skin plaques that constantly desquamate scales as a result of excessive epithelial cell growth

Psoriatic arthritis (PsA) A chronic inflammatory joint disease that is primarily preceded by psoriasis

Puerperal Related to the period after childbirth

Puerperal fever Any form of bacterial infection of the female reproductive tract following childbirth or miscarriage

Pulmonary embolism (PE) When a blood-borne substance lodges in a branch of the pulmonary artery, occluding pulmonary vasculature

Pulmonary hypertension High blood pressure in the arterial supply to the lungs; an increase in mean pulmonary arterial pressure (PAPm) greater than 25 mmHg at rest as assessed by right-sided heart catheterisation

Pulmonary oedema   Fluid accumulation in the tissues and alveoli of the lungs

Pulmonary stenosis   When there is a narrowing at one or more points between the right ventricle and the pulmonary artery

Pulse pressure   The difference between the systolic and diastolic blood pressure that represents the contractile force of the heart

Purpura   Purple spots on the skin secondary to haemorrhage from small blood vessels

Purulent   Producing or containing pus

Pyelonephritis   Infection/inflammation of the upper urinary tract, i.e. affecting the renal parenchyma, i.e. renal pelvis and medulla (tubules and interstitial tissue)

Pyogenes   Gram-positive bacteria of the genus *Streptococcus*

Quadriplegia   *See* Tetraplegia

Radicular pain   Pain that radiates into a lower extremity directly along the course of a spinal nerve root

Radiotherapy (radiation therapy)   The use of ionising radiation to damage the DNA of cancer cells to delay cell cycle progression and result in apoptosis

Reactive oxygen species (ROS)   Oxygen-containing molecules formed as a by-product of normal oxygen metabolism and which play important roles in cell signalling and homeostasis

Receptive dysphasia   A type of dysphasia when people have difficulty understanding written and spoken language

Recessive inheritance   When a trait is expressed only when an organism has two recessive alleles (one from each parent) for a gene

Rectocele   A prolapse of the wall between the rectum and the vagina

Reelin   A glycoprotein that signals migrating neurons and their position in the developing brain

Refeeding syndrome (RFS)   A syndrome that consists of metabolic disturbances following the reinstitution of nutrition to people who are severely malnourished, starved or metabolically stressed due to severe illness

Remission   A period of time when a disease process is inactive or less severe

Renal calculi   Kidney stones – polycrystalline aggregates composed of materials that the kidney normally excretes

Renal cortex   The outer section of the kidney between the renal capsule and the renal medulla

Renal failure   Significant loss of renal function

Renal insufficiency   A decline to about 25% of normal renal function

Renal tubular acidosis (RTA)   A condition where there is impaired renal hydrogen ion excretion (type 1), impaired bicarbonate reabsorption (type 2), or abnormal aldosterone production or response (type 4). Type 3 is no longer included in classifications

Renin   A hormone from the afferent arteriole of the nephron that converts angiotensinogen in to angiotensin I

Renin–angiotensin–aldosterone system (RAAS)   A hormonal system that regulates blood volume and systemic vascular resistance

Repolarisation   Restoration of the polarised state of a neuronal cell membrane

Respiratory failure   Failure of the respiratory system to adequately oxygenate the body or to eliminate carbon dioxide from the body

Respiratory tract infections (RTIs)   An infectious disease that can affect any part of the respiratory tract

Restrictive cardiomyopathy   Cardiomyopathy in which the ventricular walls become rigid and inflexible, leading to restricted ventricular filling

Retching   The muscular (retroperistalsis) event that occurs in vomiting but no stomach contents are expelled

Reticular activating system (RAS)   An area of the brain composed of a number of nuclei that connect throughout the forebrain, midbrain and hindbrain and controls arousal mechanisms used in maintaining consciousness and awake states essential for selective attention and purposeful responses

Reticular formation   A core of nerve cell bodies which extend from the spinal cord up through the medulla, pons and mid-brain to the hypothalamus and thalamus and with connections to the cerebral cortex involved in regulating skeletal muscle tone, autonomic control of the cardiovascular and respiratory systems, and somatic and visceral sensations. It plays a central role in states of consciousness like alertness and sleep

Retinopathy   A disease of the retina that results in impaired vision and blindness

Retrograde (flow)   Reverse/backward

Retrograde ejaculation   When semen is directed to exit the body through the urethra but is misdirected into the bladder

Retrovirus   A virus whose RNA is used inside a host cell to form DNA by means of the enzyme reverse transcriptase

Reverse transcriptase   An enzyme that converts two identical strands of RNA into double-stranded DNA once inside the host cell

Rheumatoid arthritis (RA)   A chronic, progressive, systemic autoimmune disease with periods of remission and exacerbation characterised by tenderness and swelling which eventually destroys the synovial joint, resulting in disability

Rheumatoid factors   Autoantibodies involved in rheumatoid arthritis

Rhinitis   Inflammation of the mucous membranes of the nose

Rhinorrhoea   Excessive nasal mucous secretion

Sacral sparing   Preserved movement or sensation in the sacrum due to an incomplete spinal cord injury

Salpingitis   An inflammatory condition of the Fallopian tubes

Salpingo-oophorectomy   Removal of the Fallopian tube and ovary from one or both sides of the uterus. Can be combined with hysterectomy, when the uterus is also removed

Sarcoidosis   A systemic granulomatous disease process that may impact on any organ (in particular the lung) and can mimic other disease processes, especially malignancy or infection

Sarcomere   A compartment that is the functional unit of myofibril

Schizophrenia   A syndrome characterised by signs of psychosis that include paranoid delusions and auditory hallucinations. It can occur at any age, but tends to occur in late adolescence

Scoliosis   Abnormal lateral curvature of the spine

Secondary (post-infectious) encephalitis   When a pathogen first infects another part of the body and secondarily enters the brain

Secondary hypertension   When another disorder causes blood pressure to rise

Secondary injury (neurological)   Referring to further damage occurring at cellular level as a result of a primary injury. This can occur over hours or days after the primary injury and includes ischaemia, hypoxia, infection and raised intracranial pressure

Segmental fracture   When at least two fracture lines isolate a segment of bone

Seizure   A single episode of electrical neuronal dysfunction, abnormal and excessive excitation and synchronisation of a population of cortical neurons in the brain, resulting in an acute, temporary change in neurological functioning

Seizure disorders   Any abnormality generating an electrochemical differential across cell membranes and depolarisation, i.e. an abnormality in an action potential, creating uncontrolled neuronal activity

Self-antigens   An antigen that induces antibody formation in another organism but of which the parent organism is tolerant

Self-tolerance   The ability of the immune system to differentiate between self and foreign antigens

Seminomas   Germ cell tumours that are slow growing and contain only seminomatous elements

Sensitisation   A state or condition in which the response to a second or later stimulus is greater than the response to the original. In an immune response, this can lead to hypersensitivity

Sepsis   A life-threatening organ dysfunction caused by a dysregulated host response to infection

Septic shock   A subset of sepsis in which profound circulatory, cellular and metabolic abnormalities are associated with a greater risk of mortality than with sepsis alone

Septum primum   When there is tissue growth down in the single atrium of the developing heart in the human embryo. This growth will result in the single atrium being divided into two atria

Septum secundum   A tissue growth that descends from the upper wall of the right atrium. After birth, it closes the foramen ovale by fusing with the septum primum

Serotonin and norepinephrine reuptake inhibitors   A type of antidepressant that is believed to increase availability of the neurotransmitters serotonin and norepinephrine in the synaptic cleft by limiting their reabsorption (reuptake) into the presynaptic cell. More serotonin and norepinephrine are said to be available to bind to the postsynaptic receptor

Serotonin selective reuptake inhibitors (SSRIs)   A type of antidepressant that is believed to increase availability of the neurotransmitter serotonin in the synaptic cleft by limiting its reabsorption (reuptake) into the presynaptic cell. More serotonin is said to be available to bind to the postsynaptic receptor

Serotype   The category of microorganism as characterised by serologic typing

Sertoli cells   Cells that produce anti-Müllerian hormone and act as the 'nurse' cells for the germ cells in spermatogenesis

Serum amyloid   A protein capable of starting an immune response and triggering cytokine release

Serum sickness   A systemic allergic reaction to an injection of serum

Service improvement   The component of public health concerned with the provision of a range of services that contribute to health in different ways (e.g. practice development, service planning, clinical governance)

Sex-linked inheritance   The inheritance of a trait (phenotype) that is determined by a gene located on one of the sex chromosomes (usually the X chromosome)

Sexually transmitted infections (STIs)   A range of pathogens that can be acquired through sexual contact

Sheehan syndrome   Hypopituitarism caused by ischemic necrosis secondary to blood loss and hypo-volaemic shock during and after childbirth

Sinus arrhythmias   Arrhythmias that occur as a result of disordered sympathetic stimulation and other homeostatic alterations in temperature, oxygen availability and metabolic changes

Sinus bradycardia   A heart rhythm where the PQRST complex is normal but the ventricular rate is slow (<60 beats per minute)

Sinus tachycardia   A heart rhythm where the PQRST complex is normal but the ventricular rate is fast (>100 beats per minute)

Sinusitis   Inflammation/infection of the paranasal sinuses

Sodium–potassium pump   A process of active transport that moves potassium ions into, and sodium ions out of, a cell

Somatic   Refers to the cells of the body, excluding germ cells. Any non-reproductive cell

Somatic cell   Any non-reproductive cell

Spasms   Involuntary movements that often involve multiple muscle groups and joints

Spastic dystonia   Tonic muscle overactivity in the absence of any stimulus

Spasticity   Increased, involuntary, velocity-dependent muscle tone that causes resistance to movement

Spermatocyte   An immature male germ cell, developed from a spermatogonium

Spermatogenesis   The process of male gamete formation involving creation of a spermatocyte from a spermatogonium, meiotic division of the spermatocyte to create four spermatids that are transformed into spermatozoa

Spermatogonia   Germ cells for sperm formation

Spermatozoa   The plural of spermatozoon – sperm, the male gamete

Sphincter   A circular ring of muscle surrounding an opening or a tube that can open or close it

Spina bifida   An open neural tube defect (the incomplete closing of backbone and membranes around the spinal cord) and neuro-developmental disorder that originates during embryogenesis, in the first 30 days after fertilisation

Spinal shock   A transient physiological (rather than anatomical) reflex depression of cord function below the level of injury with an associated loss of all sensorimotor functions

Spiral (torsion) fracture   Fracture that has occurred as a result of rotating force applied along the axis

Spongiofibrosis   When spongiosal tissue is replaced by dense scar tissue that lacks elasticity and contains fibroblasts, forming a urethral stricture

Spongiol tissue   Tissue of the corpus spongiosum

Spongy bone   Softer, honeycomb-like bone tissue on the inside of bones with spaces containing red and yellow bone marrow and blood vessels

Spontaneous abortion (miscarriage)   The spontaneous loss of a pregnancy before 20 weeks of gestation with the fetus not normally judged as viable

Spontaneous bacterial peritonitis (SBP)   Bacterial infection in the peritoneum, resulting in peritonitis

Spontaneous pneumothorax   When an air-filled bleb or blister on the surface of the lung ruptures and air enters the pleural cavity

Sprain   Ligament damage

Squamous cell hyperplasia   A thickened plaque with an irregular surface in the vulva, resulting from pruritus leading to rubbing or scratching

Staging (of tumours)   The process of classifying a cancer by its location, growth and spread

Starvation   A decrease in energy intake below the level needed to maintain homeostasis

Statins   Drugs that lower LDL (low-density lipoprotein) levels by blocking the liver enzymes responsible for making cholesterol

Status asthmaticus   A condition where bronchospasm that occurs in asthma has not responded to bronchodilators and or anti-inflammatory drugs

Steatohepatitis   An inflammatory condition of the liver where there is an accumulation of fat

Steatorrhoea   Fatty, yellow-grey coloured foul-smelling stools

Steatosis   Abnormal retention of lipids within hepatocytes

Stenosis   Abnormal narrowing of a structure

Stent   A tubular structure placed into a blood vessel to maintain its patency

Stevens–Johnson Syndrome (SJS)   A rare range of mucocutaneous diseases usually attributable to severe adverse drug reactions. There is widespread inflammation of the epidermis that results in necrosis and sloughing of tissue

Strain (microbiological)   A genetic variant or subtype of a microorganism (e.g. a virus or bacterium)

Strain (musculoskeletal)   Tendon damage

Stress   The biological and psychological response to any adverse stimulus (physical or emotional) that disrupts homeostasis

Stress incontinence   The involuntary passage of urine on effort, physical exertion, coughing or sneezing

Stricture   The abnormal narrowing of the lumen of a duct, canal or other passage. May be temporary or permanent

Stroke   Gradual or rapid, non-convulsive onset of neurological deficits that fit a known vascular territory and that last for 24 hours or more. There are two types: ischaemic (thromboembolic) and haemorrhagic

Stroke volume   The volume of blood pumped out of each ventricle per heartbeat

Stroma   The supportive connective tissue of an epithelial organ/tissue/growth

Stromal lesions   Lesions of connective tissues

Sub-acute   Refers to conditions which fall between acute and chronic in nature

Subarachnoid haemorrhage   When there is an arterial rupture and blood flows into the subarachnoid space (and sometimes into the ventricles of the brain). A subarachnoid haemorrhage is usually from the rupture of a cerebral aneurysm

Subarachnoid space   The space between the arachnoid and pia mater through which CSF circulates and within which delicate trabeculae (partitions) of connective tissue extend

Subdural haematoma   A collection of blood below the dura above the arachnoid membranes of the brain

Sudden arrhythmic death syndrome (SADS)   The sudden, untimely death of a young, apparently fit and healthy person due to a cardiac arrhythmia

Sudden cardiac death   When death from SADS is thought to be as a direct result of cardiac disease

Superoxide dismutase (SOD1)   An enzyme antioxidant, produced by astrocytes, needed to prevent oxidative stress in a neighbouring motor neuron

Supersaturation of urine   The increased presence in urine of stone components, e.g. calcium salts, uric acid, magnesium ammonium phosphate and cystine

Supplementary prescribers (UK)   Health care professionals permitted to prescribe within the limits of a clinical management plan agreed for a specific group of people by the supplementary prescriber, doctor (independent prescriber) and recipient

Suppurate   Formation of pus

Supraventricular   Relating to the origin of cardiac impulse being above the ventricles

Surgery   When an operative approach, using special techniques manually or with instruments, is used to treat disease, injury or deformity and/or to investigate an illness or improve bodily function or appearance

Symptomatic (secondary) epilepsy   Epilepsy for which there is a known cause

Synaptogenesis   The creation of synapses between neurons in the nervous system

Syncetium   Fusion of several cells to form one cell with several nuclei

Syncope   Partial or complete loss of consciousness with interruption of awareness of oneself and one's surroundings

Syndrome   A set of signs and symptoms which occur together and sometimes indicate a specific condition

Syndrome of inappropriate ADH secretion (SIADH)   A condition in which people develop high levels of, or continuously secrete, ADH; the negative feedback loop that normally controls the amount of ADH secretion fails. As a result, there is increased renal reabsorption of water, resulting in a hypervolaemic, haemodilutional state

Synovial cells   Cells that produce synovial fluid into the capsules of synovial joints

Synovial membrane   A membrane that produces synovial fluid

Synovium   *See* Synovial membrane

Syphilis   A sexually transmitted infection caused by the bacterium *Treponema pallidum,* an aerobic spirochete bacterium

Syringobulbia   A syrinx in the brain stem

Syringomyelia   A syrinx in the upper spinal cord

Syrinx   A CSF filled sac in either the brainstem or the upper spinal cord

Systemic inflammatory response syndrome (SIRS)   Systemic activation of the innate immune response regardless of the cause

Systemic lupus erythematous (SLE) (lupus)   An antibody-mediated autoimmune disease characterised by chronic inflammation of the tissues of the skin, kidney, blood vessels and other tissues

T-helper cells   A type of T cell (lymphocyte) involved in the adaptive immune system that supports the activity of other immune cells by releasing cytokines, helping to regulate the immune response

Tachycardia   Raised heart rate (usually greater than 100 beats per minute)

Tachypnoea   Increased respiratory rate

Tay–Sachs disease   An inherited metabolic disorder caused by deficiency of the enzyme hexosaminidase A that causes a failure to process GM2 ganglioside (a lipid) that accumulates in the brain and other tissues, causing damage

Telogen phase   The final phase of hair growth

Telomere   A short length of specific DNA which acts as a buffer against damage and shortening of the chromosome end

Teniae coli   Three separate longitudinal bands of muscle in the colonic wall

Tenosynovitis   Inflammation and swelling of the fluid filled sheath (synovium) that surrounds a tendon. Can be infectious or non-infectious

Tension pneumothorax   When intrapleural air accumulates under pressure and exceeds atmospheric pressure

Tension type headache (TTH)   The commonest type of headache, episodic or chronic. Some overlap in symptoms with migraine, but are rarely disabling or associated with any significant autonomic phenomena

Teratogenic   Relating to any substance that can disrupt the healthy development of an embryo or fetus

Teratoma   A germ cell tumour composed of different types of tissues

Teratozoospermia   Sperm with abnormalities

Testicular torsion   When there is twisting of the testis on the spermatic cord, obstructing the blood flow to the testis

Tetraplegia   Injury to the cervical spinal cord with an associated loss of motor and/or sensory function in all four extremities

Thalamus   The relay centre for nervous impulses moving to and from the cerebrum

Thalassaemia   A group of conditions in which the rate of formation of haemoglobin is reduced but the structure is normal

Thrombocythaemia   A disorder in which excess thrombocytes are produced

Thrombocytopenia   Low blood platelet count

Thrombocytopenia   When there is a reduced number of thrombocytes being formed, resulting in a low level of platelets in the blood

Thrombolysis   When a thrombus is dissolved using medication

Thrombosis   Formation/presence of a blood clot in a blood vessel

Thyroid storm   *See* Thyrotoxic crisis

Thyrotoxic crisis   An acute, life-threatening hypermetabolic state secondary to excessive levels of thyroid hormone in people with thyrotoxicosis

Thyrotoxicosis   The clinical effects experienced due to an excess of thyroid hormones in the bloodstream (hyperthyroidism)

Tonic   The phase of a seizure in which there is increased tone of voluntary muscle

Tonsillitis   Inflammation of the tonsils

Tophi   Hard, white nodules formed of deposits of crystalline uric acid and other substances

Topical   Relating to the application of medicinal products directly to a part of the body (e.g. to the skin)

Toxic epidermal necrolysis (TEN)   *See* Stevens–Johnson syndrome (SJS)

Trabeculae   Supporting columns of connective tissue within an organ/structure

Transcellularly   Referring to penetration of a cell and travelling through it

Transient ischaemic attack (TIA)   A temporary focal loss of neurological function (less than 24 hours) caused by ischaemia

Translocation   The movement of something from one place to another, e.g. bacteria from the gastro-intestinal tract into the circulation

Transmural   Occurring across the entire wall of an organ/structure

Transposition of the great arteries   When the aorta arises from the right ventricle and the pulmonary artery from the left ventricle, i.e. the opposite to the normal location of these vessels

Transverse fracture   A fracture in which the fracture line is perpendicular to the shaft of the bone

Traumatic subarachnoid haemorrhage   When rotational, stretching and tearing forces cause arteries to rupture with haemorrhage in the subarachnoid space

Trichomoniasis   An STI caused by the protozoan *Trichomonas vaginalis*, an anaerobic flagellated protozoan

Trigeminal neuralgia (TN)   A form of neuralgia that occurs largely from compression of the trigeminal nerve or from another structural abnormality that triggers the nerve

Triglycerides   A type of fat composed of one molecule of glycerol joined with three fatty acid molecules

Trisomy   When there are three copies of a specific chromosome instead of the normal two

Trophoblasts   Cells form the outer layer of the blastocyst

Trypsin   A digestive enzyme which breaks down proteins in the small intestine

Trypsinogen   The inactive precursor of trypsin

Tuberculosis   A highly contagious infection caused by *Mycobacterium tuberculosis* (MTB) (an acid-fast bacillus), usually affecting the lungs but may invade other body systems

Tumour necrosis factor (TNF)   A cytokine, secreted by macrophages, that induces cell death of mutated cells

Tumour   A swelling which can result from various conditions including inflammation and trauma

Tumour markers   Biochemical substances produced by some cancer cells

Tumour nodes metastasis (TNM) system   An international cancer classification system

Tumour suppressor genes (TSG)   Genes that control growth inhibitory signals

Tunica albugenia   A fibrous envelope covering the penile corpora cavernosa that creates partitions between seminiferous tubules

Tunica vaginalis   The serous membrane that covers the anterior and lateral surfaces of the testes

Tyrosinaemia   A genetic disorder characterised by impairment in the process of breaking down the amino acid tyrosine, a building block of most proteins. This results in high levels of tyrosine in the blood

Ubiquitin   A small protein found in all cells of the body which affects proteins in many ways

Ubiquitination   When a protein has ubiquitin attached to it, signalling that the protein is to be transported to a proteasome for degradation, affects their activity, and promotes or prevents protein interactions

Ulcer   An open sore on an external or internal surface of the body (organ or tissue), resulting from necrosis that accompanies inflammatory, infectious or malignant processes

Ulcerative colitis (UC)   A nonspecific inflammatory condition of the colon and rectum

Undernutrition   A nutritional state characterised by being underweight for one's age, having stunted growth and tissue wasting, and being deficient in micronutrients

Unresponsive wakefulness syndrome (UWS)   *See* Vegetative state (VS)

Unstable angina   Chest pain secondary to reduced blood flow to the coronary arteries caused by unstable plaques that rupture or erode, exposing the plaque core to blood flow. In unstable angina, the person will experience pain at rest as a result of myocardial ischaemia secondary to insufficient oxygen to meet myocardial tissue demands

Uraemia   High blood urea

Uraemic syndrome   A syndrome characterised by increased blood serum levels of urea and creatinine alongside neurological changes, nausea, vomiting, anorexia and fatigue

Urethral stricture   A narrowing of the urethral lumen; it may be obstructive or disruptive to flow through the urethra or the person may be asymptomatic

Urethritis   Inflammation of the urethra

Urethrocele   When part of the vaginal wall fused to the urethra descends and causes disruption of continence

Urethroplasty   Repair of a damaged urethra

Urethrotomy   Incision of the fibrotic scar tissue in the urethra

Urge incontinence   The involuntary loss of urine accompanied by, or immediately preceded by, urgency

Urinary incontinence   The loss of voluntary control of the bladder, resulting in involuntary leakage of urine

Urinary oxalates   Chemicals in the urine which can form kidney stones

Urticaria   A skin reaction characterised by fluid-filled blisters known as wheals and surrounded by an area of redness known as flares

Uterine prolapse   When the main supportive ligaments for the uterus are stretched and the uterus bulges down into the vagina

Uveitis   Inflammation of the uvea, the middle layer of the eye between the sclera and the retina

Vaccination   The administration of a vaccine (antigenic material) – a biological preparation that stimulates an individual's immune system to develop adaptive immunity to a specific infectious disease

Vacuolating toxin   A toxin involved in *Helicobacter pylori* pathogenesis

Vaginitis   Inflammation of the vagina with discharge, itching, burning, redness and swelling

Vaptans   Oral vasopressin antagonists

Variable expression   The extent to which a phenotype is expressed to different degrees among individuals with the same genotype

Varicocele   A vascular abnormality of the testicular venous drainage system whereby these veins become abnormally dilated and tortuous

Vascular endothelial growth factor (VEGF)   A signal protein that stimulates the proliferation of vascular endothelial cells, contributing to blood vessel development

Vasculitis   Inflammation of a blood vessel(s)

Vasoconstriction   A narrowing of the lumen of blood vessels through contraction of the smooth muscle within the vessel walls

Vasodilation   A widening of the lumen of blood vessels through relaxation of the smooth muscle within the vessel walls

Vasopressors   Drugs/agents that cause vasoconstriction

Vasospasm   An arterial spasm that leads to vasoconstriction

Vegetative state (VS)   A disorder of consciousness where a person appears awake but displays no behavioural signs of awareness; a sleep–wake cycle is present and there may be reflexive and spontaneous behaviours but not in response to stimuli

Ventilation   The amount of air that enters the alveoli

Ventilation/Perfusion (V/Q) mismatch   Abnormal ventilation/perfusion ratio, e.g. when areas of the lungs are better perfused by blood than they are ventilated (e.g. a lack of alveoli), or better ventilated than perfused with blood (e.g. a lack of blood supply to a well-ventilated lung with sufficient alveoli)

Ventricular fibrillation (VF)   A disorder with uncoordinated ventricular activation that results in the deterioration of ventricular function; the ventricles fibrillate (i.e. quivering movement – uncoordinated contraction) and therefore do not contract sufficiently to produce cardiac output

Ventricular septal defects (VSDs)   Openings in the ventricular septum, enabling blood to shunt from one side to the other

Ventricular tachycardia (VT)   When the cardiac impulse is generated from increased automaticity at a single point in either the left or the right ventricle that leads to a fast, organised rhythm

Very-low-density lipoproteins (VLDLs)   Precursors to LDLs, these lipoproteins have their triglycerides removed in adipocytes and become LDLs

Vesicle   A cellular organelle comprised of fluid enclosed by a lipid bilayer membrane, within which substances can be stored for secretion

Vesiculation   Blistering

Viron   The extracellular infective form of a complete virus particle consisting of a single or double strand of RNA or DNA surrounded by a protein coat

Virus   Any of a wide variety of mostly pathogenic microorganisms consisting of a single nucleic acid chain surrounded by a protein coat, capable of replication only within another living cell

Viscosity   The thickness of a fluid; a measure of its resistance to flow

Vitamin D   A lipophilic vitamin and hormone synthesised in the skin by the conversion of 7-dehydrocholesterol to Vitamin D by ultraviolet radiation from the sun

Vitiligo   A skin depigmentation condition where patches of skin progressively lose pigmentation, characterised by white skin with sharp, distinct margins

Volume-responsive (prerenal) AKI   Acute kidney injury as a result of decreased blood supply to the kidneys (glomeruli and renal tubule undamaged)

Vomiting   *See* Emesis

Vulvodynia   Vulval pain or a burning sensation without visible lesions

Waterhouse–Friderichsen syndrome   Adrenal gland failure due to haemorrhage into the adrenal glands, commonly caused by severe bacterial infection

Wernicke's aphasia   Fluent aphasia – impairment of the ability to grasp the meaning of spoken words. The person can usually produce correct speech but sentences often do not connect well. Reading and writing are usually severely impaired

Wolman disease   A severe type of lysosomal acid lipase deficiency that results in the impaired metabolism of lipids

X-linked   Mode of inheritance. *See* Sex-linked inheritance

Zona fasciculata   A layer of the adrenal gland that secretes glucocorticoid hormones, including cortisol

Zona glomerulosa   A layer of the adrenal gland that secretes aldosterone

Zona reticularis   A layer of the adrenal gland that produces androgens

INDEX

Abscess 199, 231, 316, 355, 356, 357, 358, 491, 493, 509, 559, 580

Absorption 11, 14, 88–92, 93, 95, 96–97, 107, 119, 205, 212, 282, 283, 308, 309, 310, 311, 319, 322, 323, 336, 338, 340, 352, 353, 356, 359, 362, 390, 391, 395, 397, 405, 424, 425, 433, 455, 469, 485, 493, 538

Acanthosis 261

Acetylcholinesterase Inhibitors 512

Achondroplasia 64, 108, 538

Acidaemia 120, 373

Acidosis 115, 191, 196, 291, 306, 310, 311, 318, 323, 325, 326, 338, 350, 358, 373, 377, 379, 380, 393, 413, 426, 428, 439, 487, 546, 574

Acinar cells 364, 365, 392

Acini 419, 431, 581

Acne vulgaris 266–268
  Acne and self-esteem 267
  Processes involved in acnegenesis 268
  Types of acne lesions 267

Acquired Immunodeficiency Syndrome (AIDS) 8, 9, 11, 151, 164, 166, 169, 204, 340, 341, 546

Acromegaly, *see* Growth hormone

Acute illness 7, 166, 378

Acute kidney injury (AKI) 272, 320, 321–324, 361, 365
  Acute tubular necrosis (ATN) 322
  Causes 322
  Classification 323
  Diagnosis and treatment 323–324
  Intrinsic 322
  Nephrotoxic ATN 322
  Oliguria 322
  Postrenal 322
  Relationship between AKD, AKI and CKD 321
  RIFLE criteria and kidney disease 321
  Volume-responsive (prerenal) 322

Acute liver disease 400–401

Acute lung injury (ALI) 438–439

Acute lymphocytic leukaemia (ALL), *see* Leukaemias

Acute myeloid leukaemia (AML), *see* Leukaemias

Acute myocardial infarction (AMI) 7, 215–217, 466
  Biochemical markers 217
  ECG changes 216
  Factors 216
  Lived experience of 217
  Signs and symptoms 216
  Thrombolytic therapy in 217

Acute on Chronic 9, 403

Acute respiratory distress syndrome (ARDS) 60, 365, 425, 438

Acute respiratory failure 438, 439
  Type I 439
  Type II 439

Acute Tubular Necrosis (ATN) 322

Addison's disease 547
  Characteristics 547
  Signs and symptoms 548

Adenocarcinoma 233, 251, 347, 561, 564, 609, 610

Adenosine deaminase (ADA) 162

Adenosine triphosphate (ATP) 114, 191, 193, 196, 218, 229, 230, 231, 341, 372, 373, 403, 414, 487

Adenoviruses 417, 422

Adhesins 172

Adhesions 178, 358, 509, 558, 562, 566, 607, 608

Adiadochokinesia 490

Adipocytes 232, 342, 389, 395, 580

Adipokines 342, 389

Adiponectin 341, 342, 388, 389

Adjuvant therapy 54, 59, 565

Adrenal cortical insufficiency 546–547
  Addison's disease 547
  Causes 546
  Primary adrenal cortical insufficiency 546
  Secondary adrenal cortical insufficiency 547

Adrenal medulla 12, 450, 543
  Disorders of 547–549
  Excessive mineralocorticoid/catecholamine secretion 547

Adrenocortical hyperfunction 543–546
  Adrenogenital syndromes (congenital adrenal hyperplasia) 545–546
  Cushing's syndrome (hypercorticalism) 543–544
  Hyperaldosteronism 544–545
  Adrenocorticotropic Hormone (ACTH) 242, 243, 536, 537, 543, 544, 546, 547

Adrenogenital syndromes (congenital adrenal hyperplasia) 545–546

Adverse drug events 96–100
Allergic reaction 99
Altered drug activity 96
Anaphylactic shock 99
Carcinogenic 99
Drug development 98
Fetal abnormalities 99
Idiosyncratic reactions 99
Immunological reactions 99
Known effect of drug 99
Preventable adverse events 98
Preventing adverse effects 98
Stages in drug development 98
Teratogenic 100
Unrelated to known action of drug 99_
Aerobic metabolism 191, 487
Ageing 15–16
Clinical implications 16
Reactive oxygen species 15
Agonists 87, 392
Akinesia 514
Albuminuria 324, 325
Alexia 489
Alkalosis 358, 413, 426
Alkaptonuria 373
Alkylating agents 245
Allele 105, 159, 235, 263, 289, 352
Allergen 60, 104, 152, 153, 154, 155, 156, 262, 417,
425, 427, 428
Allergic reaction 57, 99, 152, 153, 154, 586
Allergies, see Type I immediate hypersensitivity
disorders
Alloimmunity 151, 168, 206
Blood transfusion 168
Direct pathway 168
Indirect pathway 168
Transplant rejection 168
Alopecia 269–271
Alopecia areata 269
Androgenic alopecia 270
Cicatricial alopecia 270
Personal impact of 271
Alternative therapy(ies) 47, 49, 50, 294
Alveolar ventilation 413, 439
Alzheimer's Disease 8, 92, 113, 114, 132, 389, 483,
485, 493, 511–512
Acetylcholinesterase inhibitors 512
Formation of Beta-Amyloid Plaques in
Alzheimer's Disease 512_
Amenorrhoea 377, 534, 536
Amino acid disorders 399
Amniotic fluid embolism, see Postpartum disturbances
Amygdala 132, 133, 134, 140
Amylase 351, 352, 364
Amyloidosis 546
Amyotrophic lateral sclerosis (ALS), see Motor
neuron disease
Anabolism 372, 373, 376
Anaemia 6, 11, 56, 108, 155, 159, 160, 174,
203–207, 239, 241, 242, 291, 306, 325, 347,
353, 356, 357, 405, 432, 563

Abnormal haemoglobin formation 205
Blood loss 206
Bone marrow dysfunction 205
Extrinsic causes of haemolysis 206
Haemolytic 155, 361, 380
Impaired red cell formation 205
Increased red cell destruction 205
Iron deficiency anaemia 205, 230, 351
Macrocytic anaemias 205
Management of 207
Nutritional deficiencies 205
Pernicious 347
Types of 204
Vitamin B_{12} deficiency 205
Anaemic hypoxia 206, 414
Anaesthesia 52, 53, 91, 565
Anaesthetics 53, 425
Anagen phase 269, 270
Analgesia 53, 63, 293
Anaphylactic reaction 154
Anaphylactic shock 11, 99, 154, 199–200
Anaplasia 229
Androgenic Alopecia 270
Androgens 268, 283, 543, 545, 555, 568, 609
Anencephaly 113, 522
Aneuploidy 109, 111
Aneurysm 176, 195, 197, 212, 424, 485
Angina (pectoris) 206, 213, 215–216, 438
Angiogenesis 232, 237, 252, 261, 289, 569
Angioplasty 195, 217
Angiotensin Converting Enzyme (ACE)
inhibitors 195
Ankylosis 291
Anomia 489
Anomic aphasia 214
Anorexia 13, 206, 240, 291, 320, 338, 346, 356,
360, 363, 365, 404, 414, 421, 435
Anorexia nervosa 11, 67, 341
Anosmia 417, 600
Anovulation 568
Anoxia 197, 350
Antagonists 87, 162, 246, 309, 328, 350, 389
Anterior Cord Syndrome 500
Anthracyclines 58
Antibodies 59, 151, 152, 155, 156, 159, 160, 162,
163, 166, 168, 169, 171, 176, 206, 242, 246,
262, 289, 315, 347, 352, 419, 426, 427, 429,
515, 520, 521, 522, 539
Antidiuretic hormone (ADH) 306, 307, 308, 309,
310, 312, 451, 535, 537
Antigen 16, 17, 57, 59, 60, 151, 152, 155, 156, 157,
158, 159, 165, 168, 199, 238, 239, 242, 243,
246, 261, 269, 289, 348, 352, 353, 354, 383,
384, 419, 420, 426, 427, 435, 575, 610
Antigen presenting cells 159, 168
Antigen-antibody complexes 156
Antimetabolites 246
Antimicrobial resistance 181–182, 317
Antibiotic resistance 182, 317
Mechanism of bacterial resistance to drugs 181
Antinuclear antibodies (ANA) 159, 160

Antiretroviral drugs 167
Anti-tumour antibiotics 246
Anthracyclines 58
Anuria 323
Aortic stenosis 467
Aphasia 66, 214–215, 393, 495
    Anomic aphasia 214
    Aphasia etiquette 215
    Broca's aphasia ('non-fluent aphasia') 214
    Global Aphasia 214
    Mixed non-fluent aphasia 214
    Primary progressive aphasia 215
    Wernicke's aphasia ('fluent aphasia') 214, 489
Aplastic anaemia 204, 205
Apoptosis 15, 137, 139, 159, 226, 227, 230, 231,
    234, 237, 245, 263, 272, 349, 383, 384, 392,
    487, 509, 514, 569, 610
Appendicitis 358
Apraxia 489
Aquaretics 309
Aqueduct stenosis 493
Arrhythmias 61, 200, 306, 377, 459–467, 469, 521
    Arrhythmogenesis 459–460
    Atrial disturbances 461–464
    Atrial fibrillation (AF) 16, 461, 463
    Atrial flutter 463
    Causes 460
    Narrow complex tachycardia 463
    Sinus arrhythmias 465, 466
    Surviving cardiac arrest 467
    Ventricular fibrillation (VF) 464, 465
    Ventricular tachycardia (VT) 464, 465
Arteriosclerosis 192
Arthralgia 159, 542
Arthritis 8, 9, 64, 159, 160, 292, 542, 558
Arthus reaction 156
Articular cartilage 286, 287, 288, 289, 291
Ascites 404, 405, 456, 569, 570
Asepsis 52, 54, 579
Asthenozoospermia 597
Asthma 9, 60, 104, 151, 153, 154, 344, 389, 411,
    414, 422, 423, 424, 425–429, 538
Asynergia 490
Atelectasis 359, 413, 414, 422, 423, 424,
    Types of 424, 425
Atheroma 192–194
    Development of atheroma 193
    Stages of atheroma development 194
Atheroprone 193
Atherosclerosis 24–25, 58, 113, 192–195, 212, 218,
    230, 395, 448, 454, 455, 542
    Atheroma 192–194
    Complications of 194
    Ischaemic heart disease 24–25
    Management of 195
    Pathophysiological changes 192
Atopy 25, 104
Atrial fibrillation (AF) 16, 461–463
    Electrical Pathways 462
    Management 463
    Sinus Rhythm Versus Atrial Fibrillation 463

Sub classifications 461
Atrial flutter, see Arrhythmias
Atrial septal defect 469
    Patent foramen ovale 469
    Secundum atrial septal defect 469
Atrial tachycardia (AT), see Narrow complex
    tachycardia
Atrioventricular nodal reentrant tachycardia
    (AVNRT), see Narrow complex tachycardia
Atrioventricular reciprocating tachycardia (AVRT),
    see Narrow complex tachycardia
Atrioventricular septal defect (AVSD) 469–470
    Types of Shunting in AVSD 470
Atrophy 14, 16, 108, 133, 135, 228, 285, 316, 324,
    340, 346, 347, 353, 380, 484, 502, 518, 564
Atypia 581
Aura 507, 517
Autism spectrum disorder (ASD) 113, 132,
    137–138, 140–141
    Gene expression 140
    Macrocephaly 140
    Proinflammatory cytokines 139
    Reelin 138
    Social reciprocity 138
Autoantigens 383, 384
Autoimmune disorders 11, 60, 150, 156, 158–162
    Antigen-presenting cells 159
    Rheumatoid arthritis (RA) 160–162
    Self-tolerance 159
    Systemic lupus erythematous (SLE) 159–160
Autologous immune enhancement therapy (AIET) 58
Autonomic dysreflexia, see Spinal cord injury
Autosomal Aneuploidy 109–111
Azoospermia 597
Azotaemia 320, 321, 325

Bacteraemia 179, 198, 558, 588
Bacterial infection, see Infection
Balanitis 607, 608
Becker Muscular Dystrophy (BMD) 295
Benign cystic teratomas 569
Benign prostatic hyperplasia (BPH) 595, 597, 607
Beta-blockers 195, 377
Bilirubin 361, 362, 363, 400
Bioavailability 88, 604
Biofilms 172–173
Bipolar disorder 8, 64, 113, 132, 136–137, 213
    Apoptosis 137
    Classification 136
    Dendritic spine loss 137
    Depression 136
    Exercise 137
    Hypomania 136
    Mania 136
    Mitochondria 137
    Signs and symptoms 137
Blastocyst 571, 575
Blood Brain Barrier (BBB) 91, 92, 177, 178, 310,
    509, 515
Blood flow 63, 95, 96, 156, 190–196, 230, 232, 322,
    329, 349, 350, 358, 363, 404, 405, 436, 437,

438, 468, 469, 471, 484, 486, 487, 490, 493, 571, 576, 578, 599, 600, 602, 604, 606, 608 (also *see* Shock)
Arterial disturbances 192
Effects of reduced blood flow 190–192
Metabolic changes 191
Organ damage 210
Bone disorders 121,
Metabolic bone disease 281–285
Borborygmus 352, 358
Bradycardia 200, 345, 378, 414, 465–466, 499, 574
Bradykinesia 514
Bradykinin 14
Bradypnoea 413
Brain tissue oxygenation (PbtO$_2$) 488–489
Breast
Benign disorders of 579
Cancer of (also *see* Breast Cancer) 582
Developmental abnormalities 579
Disorders of 579–586
Fat necrosis 580
Fibrocystic changes 580
Inflammatory disorders of 580
Mammary duct ectasia 580
Mastitis 580
Neoplasms 582
Nonproliferative lesions 581
Proliferative lesions 581
Stromal lesions 581
Breast cancer 34, 58, 109, 112, 118, 225, 234, 235, 246, 247, 254, 459, 570, 580, 582–586
Histological grading of 582
Lymphoedema 585
Main types 582
Risk factors 584
Treatment 583
Types of Invasive Carcinoma 583
Broad spectrum antibiotics 181, 199, 361
Broca's aphasia 214
Bronchial asthma 154, 425–429,
Allergic (atopic) asthma 425–426
Asthma and long- term treatment 429
Bronchial tube in asthma 428
Living with asthma 425
Non-allergic (non-atopic) asthma 426
Pathophysiology 427
Signs and symptoms 428
Treatment 429
Bronchiectasis 107, 432–433
Finger clubbing 433
Bronchiolitis 422
Bronchoconstriction 153, 154, 426
Bronchospasm 99, 199, 422, 425, 426, 427, 428
Brown-Séquard Syndrome (Lateral Cord Syndrome) 500
Brudzinski sign 178
B-type natriuretic peptide (BNP) 310, 458
Budd-Chiari syndrome 400, 401
Bulbar stricture 602
Bullae 432
Bullous 263, 264

Burns 11, 61, 171, 173, 197, 230, 265, 270–272, 322, 350
Counter anti-inflammatory response syndrome (CARS) 272
Systemic impact 272
Systemic inflammatory response syndrome (SIRS) 272
Zones of injury 271
Butterfly fracture, *see* Fracture

Cachexia 164, 166, 239, 240, 241, 242, 340
Calibre 194
Callus 281
Cancer 8, 9, 11, 25, 50, 54, 55–59, 69, 100, 104, 108, 109, 118, 162, 163, 164, 176, 178, 204, 208, 224, 225, 229, 230, 232–254, 337, 338, 340, 342, 352, 355, 358, 378, 400, 402, 403, 404, 420, 459, 561, 562–565, 568, 569, 570, 580, 582–586, 597, 609–613
Aetiology 249
Alcohol consumption 251
Anaemia 241
Angiogenesis 237
Blood tests 242
Cachexia 240
Chemotherapeutic agents and mechanism of action 245–246
Chemotherapy 245
Classification of tumours 244
Development and progression of malignant cells 236
Diagnosis 242
DNA methylation 236
Epidemiology 247
Epigenetic therapy 246
Epigenetics 235, 236
Evasion of body's immune system 238
Fatigue 241
Gene and molecular therapy 247
Genetic mechanisms 234
Global impact 247
Grading 243
Histone modification 236
Immunotherapy 239
Immunotherapy 246
Infections and inflammation 251
Initiation 237
Living with familial bowel cancer 244
Mechanism by which tumour cells evade the immune system 238
Metastasis 237
Nutrition, obesity and physical activity 251
Oncogenes 234
Pain 240
Paraneoplastic syndromes 242
Prevention 253
Progression 237
Promotion 237
Radiation 253
Radiation therapy 245
RN-induced 236

Screening 254
Side-effects of chemotherapy 246
Staging 243
Stem cell transplantation 247
Surgery 245
Terminology and characteristics 232
TNM system 244
Tobacco 250
Treatment 244
Tumour markers 242
Tumour suppressor genes 234
Tumour tissue biopsy 243
Vaccination 253
Carcinogenesis 98, 99–100, 234
Carcinogenic 100
Carcinogens 225, 237, 250, 251
Cardiac tamponade
Cardiogenic shock 200–201
    Management of 201
Cardiomyopathies 467–468
    Dilated 468
    Hypertrophic 466, 468
    Inherited 466
    Pathophysiology of Primary
        Cardiomyopathies 468
    Peripartum 468
    Primary and Secondary Cardiomyopathies 467
    Restrictive 468
Cardiovascular disease 8, 11, 34, 40, 69, 104, 108,
    326, 342, 374, 389, 391, 395, 448, 449, 453,
    454, 475, 568, 604, 605
Carotid artery disease 211
Catagen phase 270
Catecholamines 12, 142, 201, 272, 293, 449, 499,
    547, 600, 604
Cauda Equina Syndrome 501
Caudal neuropore 522
Cell adaptation 223, 224, 227–229
    Anaplasia 229
    Atrophy 228
    Dysplasia 229
    Hyperplasia 229
    Hypertrophy 228–229
    Metaplasia 229
    Neoplasm 229
Cell cycle 223, 225–227, 234, 245
    Cyclins 226
    Cell growth and division 224, 225–232, 254, 583
Cell injury 163, 172, 230–232, 455, 493
    Apoptosis 231
    Causes 230
    Mechanisms 230
    Necrosis 231–232
Cell-mediated immunity 383, 403
Central Cord Syndrome 500
Central neurogenic diabetes insipidus (CNDI), see
    Diabetes insipidus
Central pontine myelinolysis 309, 310
Central precocious puberty 541
Cerebellar hypoplasia 524
Cerebral contusions 486

Cerebral herniation 491–492
    Primary types 492
Cerebral infarction, see Intracranial hypertension
Cerebral ischaemia, see Intracranial hypertension
Cerebral lacerations 486
Cerebral oedema 211, 212, 308, 310, 486, 487, 491,
    492–493, 576
    Cytotoxic 493
    Interstitial 493
    Vasogenic 493
Cerebral palsy 64, 345, 524
Cerebral perfusion pressure (CPP) 488
    Formula 488
Cerebral salt wasting syndrome (CSWS) 307, 310
Cervix 59, 175, 176, 229, 249, 556, 556, 557, 558,
    560, 561, 564, 572, 575, 576, 586, 588
    Premalignant and cancerous lesions of 560–561
Chelation therapy 205
Chemical gastropathy 346
Chemokine 164, 419
Chemokine receptor 164
Chemotaxis 432
Chemotherapy 47, 54, 55–59, 163, 178, 209,
    245–247, 341, 565, 577, 585, 586
    Antracyclines 58
    Immune checkpoint inhibitors 59
    Monoclonal antibodies 59, 586
Chiari malformation 522–524
    Types 523–524
Chitin 173
Chlamydia, see Sexually transmitted infections
Cholangitis 362, 363, 400
Cholecystitis 362, 363
    Signs and symptoms 363
Choledocholithiasis 363
Cholelithiasis 362–363, 364
    Cholesterol and Pigment Gallstones 362
    Factors contributing to gallstone
        formation 362
    Signs and symptoms 363
Cholesterol 14, 24, 28, 40, 86, 97, 108, 113, 192,
    193, 195, 361, 362, 373, 374, 376, 388, 389,
    395, 397, 398, 400, 403, 516, 543
Chondroblast 281
Choriocarcinoma, see Gestational trophoblastic
    disease
Chorion 571, 573
Chromosomal abnormality 105
Chronic bronchitis, see Chronic obstructive
    pulmonary disease
Chronic illness 9, 69, 113, 164, 538, 612
Chronic kidney disease (CKD) 9, 218, 292, 303,
    316, 320, 324–326
    Classification 325
    Diagnosis and treatment 326
    ESRD/ESKD and renal replacement therapy
        (RRT) 326
    Signs and symptoms 325
    Stages 325
Chronic liver disease 403
    Alcohol-related liver disease 403

Cirrhosis 404–405
　Complications 405
　Non-alcoholic fatty liver disease (NAFLD) 404
Chronic lymphocytic leukaemia (CLL), *see*
　Leukaemias
Chronic myeloid leukaemia (CML), *see* Leukaemias
Chronic obstructive pulmonary disease (COPD) 62,
　340, 411, 429–433, 437, 464
　Bronchiectasis 107, 432–433
　Characteristics of Emphysema and Chronic
　　Bronchitis 430
　Chronic bronchitis 8, 9, 107, 419, 424, 429, 430
　Emphysema 349, 424, 429, 430, 431–432
Chronic Pancreatitis 341, 352, 365
Chylothorax 424
Chyme 338, 339, 357, 364, 502
Cicatricial Alopecia 269, 270
Cingulate gyrus/cortex 133, 134, 517
Circadian rhythm 15, 518, 535, 544
Cirrhosis (of liver) 11, 371, 379, 400, 402, 403,
　404–405
　Personal stories 405
　Symptoms 404
Citrullination 162
Clonus 503, 506
Cluster headache, *see* Headache
Coarctation of the aorta (CoA) 452, 469
Coeliac disease 67, 335, 352–353, 385
　Living with coeliac disease 352
Cognition 106, 133, 142, 306, 488, 511
Colostrum 580
Colour agnosia 490
Coma 197, 203, 373, 377, 378, 379, 383, 393, 405,
　414, 483, 495, 575, 576
Combined immunodeficiency 162
Comminuted fracture, *see* Fracture
Common cold, *see* Upper respiratory tract infections
Communicable disorders/disease 10, 35
Complement (proteins) 99, 151, 155, 156, 159, 162,
　163, 179, 180, 292, 325, 384, 419, 520, 521
Complementary and alternative medicine (CAMs)
　48, 49, 70–72
　Acupuncture 71,
　Aromatherapy 72
　Chiropractic 70, 71
　Osteopathy 70, 71
Complementary therapies 49, 50, 70, 71–72, 73
Compression fracture, *see* Fracture
Concussion 486
Congenital adrenal hyperplasia, *see* Adrenogenital
　syndromes
Congenital hypogonadotropic hypogonadism
　(CHH), *see* Hypogonadism
Congestive heart failure 454, 548
Coning 491
Conjunctivitis 153, 175
Consciousness 178, 196, 203, 211, 306, 378, 424,
　483, 494, 503, 505, 506, 537
　Coma 495
　Disorders of 494

Minimally conscious state (MCS) 496
　Physiology of 495
　Prolonged disorders of 496
　Vegetative state (VS) 495
Consolidation (pulmonary) 413, 418, 419, 430
Constipation 13, 16, 56, 206, 306, 329, 336–337,
　353, 357, 365, 375, 378, 414, 502, 547, 548, 563
　Indicators 337,
　Normal transit constipation 337
　Pelvic floor/outlet dysfunction 337
　Slow transit constipation 337
Contrecoup 486
Contusion(s) 274, 486
Conus medullaris 497, 501, 502
Conus Medullaris Syndrome 501
Convalescence 174
Convulsion 9, 405, 504, 506, 575, 576
Cor pulmonale 432, 434, 435
Corneocytes 262
Coronary artery disease (CAD) 160, 215, 394, 447,
　448, 449, 454, 458, 466, 467, 604
Coronary heart disease 35, 215, 449,
　Acute myocardial infarction (AMI) 215–217
　Angina 215
　Unstable angina 215
Corpus spongiosum 602, 603
Corticosteroids 13, 14, 160, 162, 246, 543, 545,
　546, 576
Cortisol 12, 18, 201, 272, 283, 536, 543, 544,
　546, 547
Coryzal illness 422
Cough 16, 66, 155, 166, 171, 177, 216, 239, 295,
　344, 413, 415, 416, 418, 419, 421, 422, 423,
　424, 425, 428, 430, 432, 433, 434, 435, 438,
　457, 498, 503
　Acute cough 413
　Chronic cough 413
Counter Anti-inflammatory Response Syndrome
　(CARS) 272
Coup 486
Creatinine 199, 306, 320, 323, 324, 325, 326, 576
Crepitus 280
Crohn's disease 204, 286, 354–355, 358
　Signs and symptoms 355
Croup, *see* Upper respiratory tract infections
Cryptorchidism, *see* Infertility
Curettage 565, 576
Cushing's syndrome 18, 242, 389, 538, 543–545
　Endogenous Causes 543
　Lived experience of 544
　Signs and symptoms 544, 545
Cushing's Syndrome (Hypercorticalism) 18, 242,
　389, 538, 543–545
Cyanosis 192, 197, 199, 413, 414, 424, 430,
　435, 456
Cyclin-dependent kinases 226
Cyclins 226–227
Cystadenomas 569
Cystic fibrosis (CF) 341, 352, 364, 406, 411, 423,
　432, 433–434

Cystitis 313–315, 555
 Diagnosis and treatment 313–314
 Signs and symptoms 313
 Urinalysis 314
Cystocele 565
Cytokines 59, 134, 139, 152, 153, 156, 157, 158,
 160, 161, 162, 165, 166, 168, 172, 179, 180,
 198, 240, 246, 261, 262, 263, 268, 272, 287,
 289, 290, 323, 340, 342, 349, 364, 365, 383,
 384, 389, 417, 419, 434, 439, 511, 515, 524
Cytotoxic antibiotics 246
Cytotoxic T cells 238, 384

Debridement 232, 233
Decubitus ulcers, *see* Pressure ulcers
Deep vein thrombosis (DVT), *see* venous thrombosis
Dehydration 16, 190, 262, 305, 306, 308, 310, 357,
 358, 359, 360, 385, 393, 426, 433, 546
Delayed ejaculation, *see* Ejaculatory dysfunction
Delayed-type mediated hypersensitivity (DTH), *see*
 Type IV cell-mediated hypersensitivity disorders
Demyelination 309, 514, 515, 518, 519, 520, 521
Denervation 228, 358, 502
Depression, *see* unipolar depression
Dermatitis 25, 104, 157, 262
Detrusor 327, 328, 329, 502
Diabetes insipidus (DI) 197, 307–308
 Central neurogenic diabetes insipidus (CNDI) 308
 Nephrogenic diabetes insipidus (NDI) 307–308
Diabetes mellitus 4, 8, 11, 13, 16, 26, 28, 34, 67,
 190, 195, 307, 311, 312, 324, 337, 341, 342,
 364, 365, 380, 382–394, 455, 538, 539, 542,
 544, 564, 571, 604
 Classification 382
 Complications 392–394
 Lived experiences of 392
 Managing diabetes 394
Diabetes mellitus (DM) type 1 347, 376, 380,
 381, 581
 Autoimmunity 384
 Diabetic ketoacidosis (DKA) 393
 Pathogenesis 384
 Signs and symptoms 385
 Treatment 386
 Type 1A – immune-mediated DM 383
 Type 1B – idiopathic DM 385
Diabetes mellitus (DM) type 2 58, 68, 372, 374,
 380, 404
Diabetic autonomic neuropathy 337
Diabetic Fibrous Mastopathy 581
Diabetic ketoacidosis (DKA) 377, 393
Diaphoresis 197, 339, 358, 414, 435, 499, 521
Diarrhoea 13, 56, 93, 155, 169, 172, 197, 246, 306,
 337–338, 347, 351, 352, 353, 355, 356, 357,
 360, 361, 375, 377, 380, 547, 548, 586, 617
 Characteristics 338
 Motility diarrhoea 338
 Osmotic diarrhoea 337
 Secretory diarrhoea 338
Diastolic dysfunction 455, 457, 458

Diffuse axonal injury (DAI) 485, 495
Dilated cardiomyopathy 467–468
Direct cell-mediated response 156, 157
Disability 5, 8, 18, 52, 69, 110, 111, 112, 119, 120,
 141, 260, 286, 289, 295, 399, 483, 485, 515, 612
Disability-adjusted life years (DALYs) 132, 482
Disease 6–18
 Aetiology 10
 Communicable 10
 Diagnosis 17
 Non-communicable 8, 10, 27, 39, 40
 Presentations 6
 Syndromes 18
Disease presentations 4, 6–10
 Acute 7
 Acute on chronic 9
 Chronic 8
 Sub-acute 10
Dislocations, *see* Soft tissue injury
Disseminated Intravascular Coagulation (DIC) 40,
 180, 198, 439, 547
Distributive shock 198–200
 Anaphylactic shock 11, 99, 154, 199–200
 Septic shock 172, 179, 180, 197, 198–199, 272
Diuretics 197, 292, 308, 309, 311, 341, 405
Diverticula(e) 357, 358
Diverticular disease 357
 Signs and symptoms 357
Diverticulitis 357
DNA 55, 57, 58, 87, 88, 98, 99, 105, 106, 108, 114,
 115, 118, 122, 125, 159, 162, 164, 165, 170,
 171, 173, 176, 181, 205, 224, 226, 227, 228,
 230, 234, 235, 236, 237, 245, 246, 250, 251,
 252, 253, 402, 513, 562, 576, 600, 612
 Damage 55, 58, 108, 252, 253
 Methylation 236, 251, 612
 Mutation 58, 99, 104, 106, 107, 114, 250
DNA Methylation *see* DNA
Dominant inheritance 105
Double Uterus (uterus didelphys) 557
Double-inlet ventricle 470
Down syndrome 64, 65, 110, 121, 469, 471, 538
Drug administration 90–96
 Adverse drug events 96
 Adverse drug reaction profile 95
 Drug therapy through the life span 95
 Enteral 90,
 Essentials of 94
 First pass metabolism 90
 Intervals 90
 Parenteral 91
 Patient safety 93–94
 Rectal 91
 Sublingual 91
 Topical 91
Drug classification 84–85
Duchene Muscular Dystrophy (DMD) 64, 108,
 294–295
Ductus arteriosus 469, 472, 473
Duodenal ulcer, *see* Peptic ulcer disease

Dysarthria 66
Dysbiosis 353
Dyscalculia 489
Dyslipidaemia 195, 397
Dysmenorrhoea 562
Dysmetria 490
Dyspareunia 558, 560, 561
Dysphagia 66, 489
Dysphasia 66
Dysphonia 490
Dysplasia 121, 229, 254
Dyspnoea 166, 199, 202, 306, 345, 377, 413, 419, 421, 422, 423, 424, 425, 428, 430, 432, 433, 435, 437, 438, 456, 457
Dysuria 175, 176, 313, 316, 558

Ecchymotic 274,
Eclampsia, *see* Hypertension
Ectasia 261, 580
Ectopic pregnancy 197, 558, 559, 566,571–572, 576
Sites of 572
Eczema, *see* Dermatitis
Ejaculatory dysfunction 596, 597, 605–606, 607
Delayed ejaculation 605–606
Premature ejaculation 605
Retrograde ejaculation 606
Ejection fraction 455, 458
Elastin 432
Embolism 196, 200, 202, 240, 241, 436, 578
Embolus/emboli 196, 202, 211, 212, 213, 414, 437, 461
Emesis, *see* vomiting
Emphysema 349, 424, 429, 430, 431–432.
Centriacinar 431
Panacinar 431
Structural alveolar changes in emphysema 431
Empyema 424
Encephalitis 9, 508–509,
Pathogenic causes 508
Primary 508
Secondary 508
Treatment 509
Encephalitis 9, 508–509
Endarterectomy
Endometrial cancer 246, 563–565, 568
Diagnosis and treatment 564
Types of 564
Endometriosis 195
Endospore 172
Endothelial cells / endothelium 152, 166, 169, 179, 193, 194, 237, 291, 349, 361, 439, 493, 452, 515, 561, 604
Endothelin 438, 452
Endotoxin 172, 179, 198, 230, 358, 403
Engorgement 419, 581, 605, 608
Enterocele 565
Enterotoxins 172, 360
Eosinophils 151, 153, 154, 155, 417, 426, 427
Ependymal cells/tissue 493
Epidemic 8, 27, 39, 164, 177, 360, 374, 416

Epidemiology 5, 23, 24–30, 159, 164, 224, 247
Analytical studies 28
Cardiovascular morbidity 27
Case-control studies 28
Cholera 27
Clinical trials 30
Cohort studies 29
Community trials 30
Contribution of 30
Cross sectional studies 28
Descriptive 26
Ecological studies 28
Experimental studies 30
Intervention studies 30
Prospective 29
Retrospective 29
Epidermoid cysts 269
Classification 269
Epidermolysis bullosa acquisita (EBA) 263–264
Inflammatory 263–264
Mechanobullous 263–264
Epididymitis 175, 597, 602, 613
Epididymo-orchitis 602
Epigenetic therapy 246
Epigenetics 58, 112, 113, 118, 234, 236, 246, 353
Epilepsy 8, 9, 100, 114, 493, 504–507, 568
Categories 504
Causes 505
Epilepsy and genetics 504
Pharmacological treatment 507
Post traumatic 493
Seizures versus epilepsy and convulsions 504
Epileptogenesis 493, 494
Epithelial hyperplasia 581
Erectile dysfunction 400, 542, 604, 611
Hormonal 604
Neural 604
Psychogenic 604
Vascular 604
Erectile dysfunction (ED) 400, 542, 604, 611
Erythrocytosis 207, 306
Essential hypertension 576
Euploidy 109
Excitotoxicity 140, 513
Extracorporeal life support (ECLS) 60, 201
Extradural (epidural) haematoma 485–486
Extraembryonic 612

Fabry disease 395, 396
Facioscapulohumeral (FSH) Muscular Dystrophy 295
Faecalith 358
Failure to thrive 162, 307
Fallopian tube 118, 175, 555, 557, 558, 559, 566, 567, 569, 571, 586, 587,
Disorders of 566
Farber disease 397
Fascia 273, 274
Fibroadenomas 579
Fibroatheroma 194
Fibrocystic changes, *see* Breast

Fibroids 562, 563, 586, 587
Fibroma 233, 569
Fibromyalgia 9, 293–294
  Education and treatment 293
  Signs and symptoms 293
Fibrosis 194, 291, 324, 325, 357, 365, 403, 404,
    430, 431, 434, 435, 438, 460, 468, 502, 581
First pass metabolism 90–92, 95, 386
Fissure 355, 357
Flaccid paralysis 499, 521
Fluid imbalance 305–307
Follicle Stimulating Hormone (FSH) 536, 537, 600, 601
Foramen magnum decompression 523
Foramen ovale 469
Fractures 16, 51, 177, 230, 273, 276–281, 282,
    285, 286, 287, 288, 351, 437, 484, 496,
    534, 544, 555
  Bone repair 281
  Butterfly fracture 278
  Classification 277–279
  Comminuted fracture 277
  Compression fracture 277
  Impacted fracture 278
  Oblique 279
  Segmental fracture 278
  Signs and symptoms 280
  Spiral (torsion) fracture 279
  Transverse 279
Fragility fracture 282, 285
Fucosidosis 396
Fundus (of the stomach) 343, 344, 347, 348, 350
Fungal infection, *see* Infection

Galactokinase deficiency 373, 380
Galactorrhoea 536
Galactosaemia 373, 380
Gamma-Aminobutyric Acid (GABA) 504
Gangliosidoses 396
Gangrene 11, 195, 199, 218, 232, 358, 363
Gastric ulcer, *see* Peptic ulcer disease
Gastritis 346–347, 349
  Acute 346
    Signs and symptoms 346
  Chronic 346
    Chemical gastrophy 347
    Chronic autoimmune gastritis 347
    H. pylori gastritis 347
    Signs and symptoms 346
    Types 347

Gastroesophageal reflux disease (GORD/GERD)
    344–345
  In children 345
    Signs and symptoms 345
  Lifestyle changes and drugs 345
  Predisposing factors 344
  Signs and symptoms 344
Gene expression 107–108, 138, 140, 236, 392
Gene therapy 125, 247, 396
Genetic disorders 26, 104, 105–125, 294, 376, 580

Autosomal aneuploidy 109–110
Autosomal dominant 106
Autosomal recessive 106–107
Chromosomal alterations 109
Diagnosis 116
Ethics 120–121
Family history 116–117
Gene expression 107
Genetic counselling 123
Genogram 117
Germline mosaicism 107
Heel prick test 120
Heteroplasmy 114
Heterozygote screening 122
Karyotype 109
Management of 124–125
Mitochondrial diseases 114
Monosomy 110
Mosaicism 110
Penetrance 107
Polygenic and multifactorial diseases 112
Polygenic inheritance 113
Polyploidy 109
Postnatal screening 119–120
Pregnancy screening 122
Prenatal diagnosis 120
Pre-symptomatic screening 118–119
Principles of inheritance 105
Risk assessment 117–118
Sex chromosome aneuploidy 111–112
Single gene disorders 106, 108
TP53 mutations 108–109
Trisomy 110
Variable expression 107
X-linked 107
Genital herpes, *see* Sexually transmitted
    infections
Germline Mosaicism 107
Gestational disorders 570–571
  Ectopic pregnancy 571
  Spontaneous abortion (miscarriage) 571
Gestational hypertension, *see* Hypertension
Gestational trophoblastic disease 576–577
  Choriocarcinoma 576–577
  Hydatidiform mole 576
Ghon complex 421
Ghon focus 420, 421
Ghrelin 340, 341, 342, 388
Gilbert's syndrome 400
Glasgow Coma Scale 203, 483
Gleason score, *see* Prostate cancer
Gliadin 352
Gliosis 515
Global aphasia 214
Glomerulonephritis 156, 303, 324, 325
Glomerulosclerosis 324
Glucocorticoids 12, 13, 60,134, 283, 543, 548
Gluconeogenesis 13, 180, 340, 380, 383,
    384, 388
Glucosuria 307, 311, 312

Glutamate 134, 138, 140, 487, 504, 513, 514, 517
Glycogen 340, 341, 372, 373, 380, 400
Glycogen storage disease type II 400
Glycogenolysis 340, 383, 384, 388
Glycoprotein 138, 164, 165, 363, 416, 600
Glycosuria 13, 311, 380, 385, 393
Goblet cells 356, 430
Gonadal dysgenesis 569
Gonadotropin-Releasing Hormone (GnRH)
    600, 601
Gonocytes 612
Gonorrhoea, *see* Sexually transmitted infections
Gout 292–293, 318, 401
    Primary 292
    Secondary 292
    Signs and symptoms 293
    Tophi 292
Granular cell tumour 582
Granuloma 158, 232, 421, 435, 580, 602
Granulomatous hypersensitivity, *see* Type IV cell-
    mediated hypersensitivity disorders
Granulysin 263
Graves' disease 151, 156, 376
Growth disorders 537–542
    Short stature in children 537
Growth hormone (GH) 15, 111, 283, 534, 536, 537,
    538–542, 577
    Acromegaly 540
    Deficiency 538
    Deficiency in adults 538
    Excess in adults 542
    Excess in children 540
    Gigantism 540–541
    Marfan syndrome 539
    Precocious puberty 541
Guillain-Barré syndrome (GBS) 439, 519–521
    Axonal degeneration 519–521
    Demyelination 519–521
Gummas 176

Haematemesis 345, 346
Haematocrit 306, 309
Haematoma 10, 274, 275, 281, 484–486, 491,
    493, 575
Haematuria 119, 160, 313, 325
Haemochromatosis 119, 400, 546
Haemoglobin 6, 192, 203–207, 322, 326, 380,
    381, 414
Haemoglobinopathies, *see* anaemia and abnormal
    haemoglobin formation
Haemoglobinuria 322
Haemolytic anaemia 155, 204, 205, 361, 380
Haemophilia 107, 108, 190, 286
Haemoptysis 166, 413, 421, 432, 437
Haemorrhagic shock, *see* Shock
Haemorrhagic stroke 212
Haemostasis 52, 53
Haemothorax 424
Hamartoma 582
Hapten 157

Haustra 357
Haversian canals 283
Headache 13, 18, 71, 72, 166, 176, 178, 203, 263,
    285, 293, 375, 378, 391, 393, 414, 415, 416,
    417, 419, 507, 510, 516–518, 536, 537, 540,
    542, 548, 555, 575, 578
    Cluster headache 517–518
    Lived experience of cluster headaches 518
    Migraine 517
    Primary headache disorder 516
    Secondary headache disorder 516
    Stress and headaches 517
    Tension type headache (TTH) 517
Health improvement 32, 33–34, 40
Health promotion 5, 28, 35, 36, 40, 253, 613
Heart Failure 25, 61, 88, 115, 195, 196, 202, 246,
    350, 375, 377, 430, 432, 438, 454–458, 459,
    460, 461, 464, 468, 473, 541, 548
    Assessment 458
    Failure in compensation 455
    Symptoms 457–458
    Systolic and diastolic dysfunction 455, 457
Heel prick test 120, 399
Helminths 170, 171, 174
Hemiparesis 393
Hepatic encephalopathy 405, 491
Hepatitis 7, 8, 9, 11, 58, 173, 251, 253, 326, 400,
    401, 402–403, 404
Hepatomegaly 373, 380
Hepatotoxicity 99, 401–402
    Paracetamol overdose 402
    Related drugs 401
Heterogeneous (genetics) 98, 141, 263, 600
Heteroplasmy 114
Heterozygote screening 122–123
Hiatal hernia 342–345
    Gastroesophageal reflux disease (GORD/GERD)
        344–345
    Types 342–344
High Density Lipoproteins (HDLs) 395
High glycaemic index carbohydrates 386
Hippocampus 132, 133, 134, 135, 137, 140,
    494, 508
Hirsutism 544, 545, 546, 555, 568
Histamine 14, 99, 152, 153, 154, 349, 350, 417,
    426, 518
Histone modification 235, 236
Histotoxic hypoxia 414
HIV and acquired immune deficiency syndrome
    (AIDS) 8, 164–167
    Clinical features 166
    Diagnosis and testing 166
    Epidemiology 164
    Opportunistic infections and
        co-morbidities 166
    Pathogenesis 164–165
    Risk factors 166
    Testing and counselling 164
    Transmission of HIV infection 165
    Treatment and prevention 167

Homeostasis xii, xxii, 11, 15, 16, 51, 60, 108, 132, 134, 150, 182, 190, 191, 199, 224, 228, 272, 283, 304, 305, 307, 309, 311, 312, 336, 376, 412, 448, 475, 482, 493, 537, 607

Homocystinuria 120, 399

Hormone antagonist 246

Human Chorionic Gonadotrophin (hCG) 243

Human Immunodeficiency Virus (HIV) 8, 11, 92, 163–167, 169, 171, 204, 420, 421, 508, 561

Human Leucocyte Antigen (HLA) 113, 159, 162, 168, 169, 263, 265, 269, 289, 352, 354, 384, 385, 435

Human papilloma virus (HPV), *See* Sexually transmitted infections

Humoral immunity 383, 384, 418, 419

Huntington's Disease (HD) 10, 106

Hydatidiform mole, *see* Gestational trophoblastic disease

Hydrocele 597–599
  Classification of 598
  In men 599

Hydrocephalus 178, 212, 485, 491, 493–494, 509, 510, 524, 536
  Communicating/Non-obstructive 493
  Non-communicating/Obstructive 493

Hydrolytic enzymes 291

Hydrosalpinx, *see* Salpingitis

Hydrostatic pressure 272, 405, 424, 454, 458, 459, 493

Hydrothorax 424

Hyperaemia 269, 271

Hyperaldosteronism, *see* Adrenocortical hyperfunction

Hypercapnia 60, 413, 414, 422, 426, 428, 430, 438, 439
  Effects on the body 414

Hypercholesterolaemia 24, 28, 108, 389, 404, 604

Hypercorticalism, *see* Cushing's syndrome

Hyperhomocysteinaemia 482

Hyperinsulinaemia 388, 389

Hyperosmolar Hyperglycaemic Non-Ketotic Syndrome (HHNKS) 393

Hyperosmolarity 393

Hyperpituitarism 535–536
  Pituitary adenomas 535–536

Hyperplasia 229, 261, 291, 342, 426, 432, 521, 535, 543, 544, 545, 546, 555, 560, 564, 569, 581, 597, 607

Hyperpnoea 413

Hypersensitivity 150, 151–158, 199, 268, 353
  Classification 151
  Type I immediate hypersensitivity disorders (allergy) 152, 199, 425
  Type II antibody-mediated disorders 155
  Type III immune complex-mediated disorders 156, 159
  Type IV cell-mediated hypersensitivity disorders 156, 168, 169

Hypersomnia 134

Hypersynchronisation 494

Hypertension 8, 12, 18, 28, 67, 69, 113, 119, 194, 195, 212, 229, 311, 316, 323, 324, 325, 326, 365, 374, 389, 437, 447, 449–454, 455, 459, 461, 467, 469, 485, 499, 544, 547, 548, 563, 571, 572, 574, 575, 576, 604, 605
  Blood pressure control 449–450
  Chronic hypertension (in pregnancy) 576
  Classification 450–452
  Definition 449
  Diagnosis 452–453
  During pregnancy 574
  Eclampsia 575
  Gestational hypertension 574
  Living with 454
  Malignant 452
  Pre-eclampsia 575
  Primary 450
  Renal disease in pregnancy 576
  Secondary 452
  Stage 1 453
  Stage 2 453
  Treatment 453

Hyperthyroidism 156, 282, 337, 374, 375, 376–377, 536, 605
  Living with 377
  Signs and symptoms 376–377
  Treatment 377

Hypertonia 502, 503

Hypertriglyceridaemia 389

Hypertrophic cardiomyopathy 467–468

Hypertrophy 134, 228, 229, 291, 312, 324, 342, 438, 451, 455, 458, 468, 471, 473, 545, 555

Hyperventilation 413, 426

Hypervolaemia 207, 307, 329

Hypervolaemic 305, 309

Hypoglycaemia 373, 377, 379, 380, 391, 392, 393, 505, 538

Hypogonadism 595, 597, 600–601, 604
  Classification of Congenital hypogonadotropic hypogonadism (CHH) 600

Hypoinsulinaemia 383, 384, 388

Hypokalaemia 311, 312, 338, 341, 358, 544

Hypomania 136

Hyponatraemia 307, 309, 310, 312, 329, 546, 547

Hypophosphataemia 341

Hypopituitarism 535, 537, 538

Hypoplasia 228, 524, 546, 600

Hypoplastic left heart syndrome 471

Hypospadias 602

Hypotension 16, 99, 179, 180, 198, 200, 201, 206, 306, 308, 322, 357, 358, 360, 365, 393, 414, 423, 487, 499, 521, 546

Hypothalamic-pituitary-adrenal axis 134, 544

Hypothyroidism 25, 104, 120, 201, 237, 347, 374, 375, 377–379, 534, 538,
  Living with 379
  Myxoedema 378

Hypotonia 373, 490

Hypoventilation 413, 414, 426, 439

Hypovolaemia 181, 272, 307, 311, 322

Hypovolaemic shock, *see* Shock
Hypoxaemia 60, 413, 414, 419, 422, 424, 426, 428,
    430, 434, 437, 438, 439, 487
Hypoxia 108, 174, 180, 206, 207, 212, 231, 232,
    237, 251, 291, 349, 358, 393, 413, 414, 423,
    432, 438, 439, 455, 484, 495, 505, 524, 537,
    546, 571, 576, 600
    Effects on the body 414
    Types 414
Hypoxic hypoxia 414
Hysteroscopy 565

Iatrogenic 99, 164, 543, 544, 598
Ictal phase 507
Ictus phase *see* Ictal phase
Idiopathic (primary) epilepsy 504
Idiopathic hypertension 452
Idiopathic pulmonary fibrosis 434–435
    Clinical features 434
    Living with 435
Idiosyncratic reactions 99
Immune checkpoint inhibitors 59
Immune complexes 151, 155, 159, 162, 163, 289
Immune tolerance 60, 272, 383
Immune tolerance therapies 60
Immunisation 35, 59, 156, 163, 253, 326, 402, 511
Immunodeficiency disorders 162–169, 421
    Alloimmunity 168
    Primary (congenital) immunodeficiencies 162
    Secondary (acquired) immunodeficiencies 163
Immunoglobulins 108, 163, 243, 289, 418,
    515, 521
Immunosuppression 14, 60, 163, 164, 265,
    272, 558
Immunotherapy 47, 56–60, 155, 239, 245, 246
    Activation immunotherapy 57
    Adjuvant therapy 59
    Allergen immunotherapy 60
    Allergies 60, 155
    Autologous immune enhancement therapy 58
    Cancer 239
    Immune checkpoint inhibitors 59
    Immune tolerance therapies 60
    Microbial therapy and 56–57
    Vaccination 59
Impacted fracture, *see* Fracture
Impetigo vulgaris 259, 264–265
    Bullous 264
    Non-bullous 264
Incretins 388, 389, 391, 392
Incubation period 174, 176, 177, 360, 361
Independent prescribers 85, 86
Induration 273
Infarction 4, 7, 9, 33, 46, 113, 178, 192, 194, 195,
    200, 207, 212, 215, 216, 217, 448, 455, 460,
    465, 466, 467, 493, 537, 548, 571, 608
Infection 5, 7, 8, 9, 10, 11, 14, 16, 26, 31, 39, 52,
    53, 54, 56, 57, 59, 108, 113, 137, 138, 139,
    140, 151, 159, 162, 163, 164, 169–174, 178,
    179, 180, 181, 198, 199, 204, 205, 207, 208,

209, 210, 216, 228, 229, 231, 232, 237, 239,
    240, 242, 250, 251, 252, 253, 254, 264, 265,
    269, 270, 272, 273, 276, 285, 293, 295, 306,
    312, 323, 324, 327, 329, 347, 349, 357, 358,
    360, 361, 363, 364, 376, 377, 378, 383, 385,
    390, 396, 400, 402, 403, 415, 461, 482, 484,
    493, 495, 504, 505, 508, 509, 510, 511, 516,
    521, 524, 537, 541, 546, 547, 554, 555, 557,
    574, 580, 586, 602, 603,
    Bacterial infection 171
    Biofilms 172
    Convalescence 174
    Direct contact 170
    Dissemination within the body 171
    Fungal infection 173
    General characteristics of microorganisms that
        cause disease 169
    Incubation period 174
    Indirect contact 171
    Inflammation 251
    Microbiome 56, 169
    Mycoses 173
    Of female reproductive tract 557
    Parasitic infection 173–174
    Penetration of the skin 171
    Placental 574
    Portal of entry 170
    Respiratory tract 415
    Transmission 171
    Urinary tract 312
    Viral infection 173
Infectious disease 26, 32, 33, 35, 39, 40, 59, 69,
    123, 169, 174, 415,
    Meningitis 177
    Sexually transmitted infections (STIs) 174
Infectious enterocolitis 360–361
    Clostridium difficile and antibiotic therapy 361
    Pathogens 360–361
Infertility 55, 56, 174, 534, 536, 540, 553, 554,
    537, 558, 562, 567, 568, 569, 586–588,
    596–601, 605
    Assisted conception 588
    Hypogonadism 600–601
    Identified Causes of Female Infertility 586
    Low sperm count (oligozoospermia) 596
    Medication 587
    Surgery 587
    Undescended testes (cryptorchidism) 597
Inflammatory Bowel Disease (IBD) 335, 337,
    354–357
    Crohn's disease 354–355
    Ulcerative colitis 354–357
Influenza, *see* Upper respiratory tract infections
Inheritance 104–105, 106, 107, 112, 113, 117,
    118–119, 123, 153, 159, 162, 294, 379, 395,
    396–397
    Laws 105
    Modes 105, 107, 113, 117,
    Patterns of inheritance 104, 106, 153,
        162, 294

Inotropes 201
Insulin-like growth factor 1 (IGF-1) deficiency, *see* Growth hormone (GH) deficiency
Integrated healthcare 45
Interferons 59
Interleukins 59, 153, 180, 292, 417, 426
Internal cervical os 572
Interphase 226
Interstitial lung disease (ILD) 434
Intestinal obstruction 357–360, 558
    Appendicitis 358
    Classification 358
    Consequences 359
    Functional 357
    Mechanical 357
    Signs and symptoms 358
Intracerebral haemorrhage/ haematoma (ICH) 212, 485–486, 495
Intracranial hypertension 380, 488, 490–494
    Cerebral herniation 492
    Cerebral ischaemia and infarction 493
    Cerebral oedema 492–493
    Hydrocephalus 493–494
    Intracerebral and Extracerebral Causes 491
    Intracranial volume-pressure relationship 491
Intraductal papillomas 581
Intrinsic AKI 322, 323, 324
Irritable bowel syndrome (IBS) 67, 337, 338, 353
    Presentation 353
Ischaemia 194, 215, 216, 232, 242, 272, 273, 322, 323, 349, 350, 358, 363, 364, 393, 460, 484, 493, 575, 608
Ischaemic heart disease 25, 195, 461
Ischaemic hypoxia 414
Ischaemic stroke, *see* Stroke
Isovaleric acidaemia 120, 373

Jaundice 363, 373, 402, 403, 404
Joint disorders 286–293
    Gout 292–293
    Osteoarthritis 286–288
    Rheumatoid arthritis 160–162, 289–291
Joint effusion 262

Kaposi Sarcoma (KS) 166, 251
Kernig sign 178
Ketonuria 14, 385
Kidney dysfunction 320
Klinefelter syndrome 111–112
Krabbe disease 397
Kussmaul respirations 373
Kyphosis 288, 542, 555

Labour 524, 554, 558, 575, 576, 577
    Fetal problems during 577–578
    Problems related to labour and delivery 577–578
    Timing of 577
Lactate 137, 181, 191, 196, 199, 340, 358, 487
Lactiferous duct 580, 581

Lactose intolerance 67, 337, 352
Larvae therapy 233
Legionnaires' disease 419
Leiomyomas 562–563, 571
Leptin 341, 342, 388, 389
Lesion 166, 175, 176, 194, 420, 421, 483, 500, 502, 561, 567, 579, 582
Leucocytosis 179, 208, 313, 357, 358, 360, 365
Leukaemias 208–209, 233
    Acute lymphocytic leukaemia (ALL) 208
    Acute myeloid leukaemia (AML) 208
    Chronic lymphocytic leukaemia (CLL) 209
    Chronic myeloid leukaemia (CML) 208
    Treatment of 209
Leukopenias 208, 209–210
    Lymphocytopenia (lymphopenia) 209
    Neutropenia 209
    Treatment of 210
Leydig cells 600, 601
Lichen sclerosus 560, 602
    Treatment of 560
Lipase 351, 352, 364, 390, 397
Lipid-storage disorders 395–398
    Drug therapy 397
    Statins 397–398
Lipolysis 340, 342
Lipoma 233, 582
Lipophagy 376
Lipopolysaccharides 172, 198
Lipoproteins 395
Locked in syndrome 496
Low Density Lipoproteins (LDLs) 194, 395
Lower respiratory tract infections (LRTIs) 169, 415, 418–422
    Bronchiolitis 422
    Pneumonia 418–419
    Tuberculosis 419–422
Lumpectomy 584
Lupus 159–160, 324
Luteinising Hormone (LH) 536, 537, 600, 601
Lymphadenopathy 176, 291
Lymphocytopenia (lymphopenia), *see* Leukopenias
Lymphoedema 111, 459, 585
Lymphomas 166, 208–209, 233, 246
    Treatment of 209
Lymphopenia 209
Lysis 165, 173, 177, 292, 618
Lysosomal enzymes 156, 292
Lytic enzymes 420

Macrocephaly 140
Maculopapular rash 176
Major Histocompatibility Complex (MHC) 113, 162, 168, 238, 269, 289, 352, 354, 384, 385, 435
Malabsorption 282, 283, 337, 351, 352, 356, 358, 362, 365, 405, 433, 538
Malabsorption syndromes 351
    Signs and symptoms 351
Malaise 8, 178, 316, 356, 360, 416, 419, 558

Malformations of the Uterus 556, 571
Malignant 54, 55, 57, 58, 59, 108, 164, 169, 207, 208, 209, 225, 227, 228, 229, 232–254, 424, 452, 535, 536, 537, 545, 547, 554, 559, 560, 561, 567, 576, 579, 581, 582, 584, 585, 586, 609, 612
    Disorders 232–254
Malignant hypertension, *see* Hypertension
Malnutrition 92, 163, 164, 265, 273, 306, 340, 341, 403, 404, 430, 459
Mammary duct ectasia, *see* Breast
Mantoux test 158
Maple syrup urine disease 120, 373, 399
Marfan syndrome, *see* Growth hormone
Mast cells 99, 151–154, 156, 194, 417, 419, 425, 426
Mastectomy 118, 585
Mastitis 580
    Acute 580
    Granulomatous mastitis 580
Medical interventions 22, 47, 51–61
    Chemotherapy 55–56
    Immunotherapy 56–60
    Microbial therapy 56–57
    Organ support and transplantation 60–61
    Radiotherapy 54–55
    Surgery 51–54
Megakaryocyte 432
Memory cells 59, 157, 261
Meningitis 163, 166, 177–178, 483, 504, 508, 509–511, 537, 558
    Acute pyogenic 177
    Aseptic 178
    Bacterial 177–178, 509
    Cerebrospinal fluid changes in meningitis 510
    Chronic 178, 510
    Fungal 511
    Prevention 511
    Signs and symptoms 510
    Viral 178, 509–510
Meningocele 522
Menopause 86, 225, 250, 260, 282, 534, 554, 555, 561, 563, 564, 579, 584, 586
Menorrhagia 563
Metabolic acidosis 291, 310, 325, 338, 358, 373, 380, 393
Metabolic bone disease 281–286
    Osteomalacia 283–285
    Osteomyelitis 285–286
    Osteopenia 281
    Osteoporosis 282–283
    Paget disease of bone (osteitis deformans) 285
Metabolic syndrome 342, 373, 374, 376, 382, 404, 539, 568, 607
Metachromatic leukodystrophy (MLD) 397
Metaplasia 229, 347
Metastasis 163, 228, 237, 241, 243, 244, 610
Microbial therapy 47, 56–57
    Allergies 57
    Faecal microbial therapy 57

Microbiome 39, 56, 58, 169, 232, 266, 268, 338, 361, 365, 383, 432
Microcephaly 139
Microcytic 204, 205
Microvesiculation 269
Migraine, *see* Headache
Minimally Conscious State (MCS) 495–496
Minute volume 413
Miscarriage, *see* gestational disorders
Mitochondrial disease(s) 114–116, 513
Mitochondrial disorder 114, 115, 125
Mitochondrial replacement therapy 115–116
Mitosis phase 226
Mixed urinary incontinence 327
Monoclonal antibodies 59, 246, 429, 586
Monoploidy 109
Monosomy 110, 111
Mood Disorders 132, 133–137, 140
    Bipolar disorder 136–137
    Unipolar depression 133–135
Morbidity 8, 27, 28, 34, 69, 164, 178, 213, 224, 247, 317, 341, 353, 361, 429, 434, 438, 448, 449, 485, 570, 611
Mosaicism 107, 110
Motor neuron disease (MND) 511, 512–513, 519
    Variants 513
Movement Agnosia 490
Mucociliary clearance 430
Mucociliary escalator 415, 418
Mucociliary function 154
Multifactorial inheritance 105
Multiparity 572
Multiple Organ Dysfunction Syndrome (MODS) 180, 199
Multiple Sclerosis (MS) 8, 9, 62, 64, 92, 156, 158, 327, 337, 385, 502, 511, 514–516, 518
    Influencing factors 516
    Types 515
Muscle disorders 293–295
    Fibromyalgia 293–294
    Muscular dystrophies 294–295
Muscular dystrophies 294–295
    Becker muscular dystrophy (BMD) 295
    Duchenne muscular dystrophy (DMD) 294
    Facioscapulohumeral muscular dystrophy (FSHD) 295
    Myotonic muscular dystrophy (MMD) 295
Mutagenesis 98
Mutation 58, 99, 104, 106–109, 114, 115, 119, 162, 181, 205, 210, 228, 230, 234–238, 250, 252, 253, 285, 294, 295, 307, 311, 433, 434, 437, 466, 504, 513, 514, 524, 540, 541, 547, 564, 569, 570, 583, 609, 610
Myalgia 416, 419, 435
Myasthenia gravis 521–522
    Blocking of nicotinic receptors 522
Mycobacterium 157, 158, 177, 178, 231, 419
Mycoplasmas 422
Mycoses 173
Myelomeningocele 522

Myenteric plexus 502
Myocardial infarction (MI) 4, 7, 9, 33, 46, 62, 113, 192, 194, 195, 200, 207, 215–217, 448, 455, 460, 465, 466, 467, 548
Myocarditis 200
Myoclonus 373
Myocyte 217, 455
Myofibrils 581
Myoglobinuria 322
Myometrium 560, 564
Myotonic Muscular Dystrophy (MMD) 295
Myxoedema 378

Narrow complex tachycardia 463–464
    Atrial tachycardia (AT) 463–464
    Atrioventricular nodal reentrant tachycardia (AVNRT) 463–464
    Atrioventricular reciprocating tachycardia (AVRT) 463–464
Natriuretic peptide 310, 458
Natural Killer (NK) cells 58, 162, 169, 209, 238, 263
Nausea 56, 169, 178, 209, 216, 240, 246, 306, 316, 319, 320, 338, 346, 347, 357, 358, 359, 360, 363, 365, 379, 391, 402, 404, 438, 489, 536, 547, 548
Necrosis 40, 156, 159, 168, 176, 194, 230, 231–232, 242, 263, 269, 273, 294, 322, 358, 368, 361, 364, 402, 419, 421, 422, 435, 464, 537, 580, 608
Neoplasm 229, 233, 240, 516, 535, 544, 545, 546, 547, 563, 582, 612
Nephrogenic diabetes insipidus (NDI), see Diabetes insipidus
Nephropathy 324, 393
Nephrosclerosis 324
Neuralgia 288, 518
Neurogenesis 135, 137, 139
Neurogenic bladder 312, 315, 327, 502
Neurogenic bowel 337, 502
Neurogenic shock, see Shock
Neuromuscular junction disorders 521
    Myasthenia gravis 521
Neuronal plasticity 139 (see neuroplasticity also)
Neuropathy 114, 286, 337, 393, 397, 508, 519, 520
Neuroplasticity 494
Neurotoxins 172
Neutropenia, see Leukopenias
Neutrophilia 208
Niemann-Pick disease 396
Nitric Oxide (NO) 179, 180, 438, 452, 604, 606
NMDA receptor antagonists 135
Noncicatricial 269
Non-communicable disorders/disease 10, 27, 39–40
Non-medical practitioners 61–70
    Chaplain 70
    Dietetics 66–68
    Health psychologist 69–70
    Nutrition 66–68
    Occupational therapy 63–64
    Pharmacist/Pharmacy 68–69
    Physiotherapy 61–63
    Social work 68
    Speech and language therapy 64–66
Non-neoplastic epithelial disorders 560
    Lichen sclerosus (sclerosis) 560
    Squamous cell hyperplasia 560
Non-neoplastic Epithelial Disorders 560
Normocytic 204
N-terminal pro b-type natriuretic peptide (NT-proBNP) 458
Nutrition 5, 6, 24, 35, 39, 48, 61, 66, 67, 68, 108, 113, 204, 205, 228, 230, 237, 251, 323, 335, 336, 338, 340, 341, 356, 379, 394, 538, 570, 579
Nystagmus 490

Obesity 11, 18, 28, 29, 34, 40, 58, 67, 69, 113, 192, 194, 196, 230, 250, 251, 286, 341–342, 344, 349, 362, 364, 373, 374, 382, 385–390, 404, 430, 437, 538, 544, 554, 563, 564, 568, 575, 584
Oblique fracture 276
Obstructive lung disorders 424–433
    Asthma/bronchial asthma 425–429
    Chronic obstructive pulmonary disease (COPD) 429–433
Obstructive shock 202
    Cardiac Tamponade 202
    Pulmonary embolism 202
    Tension pneumothorax 202
Oedema 14, 153, 154, 155, 157, 177, 179, 180, 195, 199, 200, 212, 230, 261, 262, 269, 272, 273, 274, 275, 287, 291, 306, 313, 316, 322, 323, 349, 351, 355, 357, 358, 359, 364, 365, 374, 376, 380, 402, 404, 414, 418, 419, 422, 425, 426, 427, 430, 432, 438, 454, 456, 458–459, 490, 503, 508, 574, 575, 579, 602
    Causes 459
Oesophageal varices 197, 405
Oligoclonal bands 515
Oligodendrocytes 134, 135, 515
Oligohydramnios 577
Oligomenorrhea 545
Oligozoospermia, see Infertility
Oliguria 322–323
Omentum 344
Oncogene 108, 208, 234, 236, 237, 247, 252, 253
Ophthalmoplegia 115, 373
Opsonisation 151, 155, 163
Orchidopexy 611
Organ support 47, 60
Organ transplantation 60
Organomegaly 373, 396
Orthopnoea 413, 456, 457
Osmolality 385, 393
Osmolarity 307–310, 323, 324, 393, 426
Osmotic diuresis 311, 385, 393
Osmotic pressure 385, 405, 424, 459
Ossification 281–283
Osteitis deformans 285
Osteoarthritis 16, 286–288, 342

Disease process 287
Living with 288
Risk factors 286
Signs and symptoms 287
Osteogenesis *see* Ossification
Osteomalacia 282, 283–285, 380
Signs and symptoms 285
Osteomyelitis 273, 285–286
Chronic non-bacterial osteomyelitis / chronic recurrent multifocal osteomyelitis 286
Contiguous 285
Haematogenous 285
Osteopenia 281–282
Osteophytosis 286–287
Osteoporosis 8, 14, 16, 260, 276, 282–283, 285, 353, 375, 399, 534, 544, 555,
Primary 282
Secondary 282
Otalgia 345, 417
Otitis media, *see* Upper respiratory tract infections
Ovarian cancer 118, 569–570
Adult granulosa cell tumour 569
Epithelial cell tumours 569
Germ cell tumours 569
Gonadal stromal cell tumours (ovarian granulosa cell tumours) 569
Juvenile granulosa cell tumour 569
Risk factors 570
Treatment 570
Ovarian disorders 567–570
Benign ovarian tumours and cysts 567
Cystic ovaries 567
Ovarian cancer 569–570
Ovarian tumours (benign) 569
Polycystic ovary syndrome (PCOS) 568–569
Overflow incontinence, *see* Urinary incontinence
Overweight and obesity 341–342
Oxidative phosphorylation 373
Oxidative stress 15, 58, 134, 137, 401, 403, 513, 514, 524, 610
Oxytocinergic 605

Paget disease of bone (osteitis deformans) 285
Signs and symptoms 285
Panacinar 431
Pancreatic exocrine insufficiency 352
Pancreatitis 306, 341, 352, 363, 364–365, 439
Acute pancreatitis 306, 364–365
Signs and symptoms 365
Chronic pancreatitis 341, 352, 365
Signs and symptoms 365
Risk factors
Pandemic 39, 40, 418
Pandemic spread 39
Pannus 160–161, 289–291
Papilloedema 452
Papules 263, 266, 435, 558
Paracellularly 509
Paraesthesia 347, 385, 390, 517, 521, 542, 544
Paraneoplastic syndromes 242

Paraphimosis 597, 608
Paraplegia 497–498
Parasitic infection, *see* Infection
Parkinson's Disease 62, 64, 327, 337, 481, 483, 511, 513–514
Reducing the risk 514
Patent ductus arteriosus (PDA) 469, 472–473
Pathophysiology xi, xiii, xxi–xxiii
Pelvic inflammatory disease (PID) 174, 558, 566, 586
Penetrance 107, 108
Age-related 107
Reduced 107
Penumbra 493
Pepsinogen 347, 349
Peptic ulcer disease 347–351
Duodenal ulcer 349–350
Gastric ulcer 349–350
Risk factors 348
Stress ulcers 350
Treatment 350–351
Peptidoglycan 172
Perforation 357–359, 363, 417
Perfusion 16, 96, 97, 180, 181, 196, 198, 199, 200, 201, 202, 216, 271, 272, 273, 323, 324, 359, 413, 414, 426, 430, 432, 454, 455, 459, 464, 488, 493, 506, 575, 602
Peripheral artery disease
Peripheral nerve disorders 518–521
Guillain-Barré syndrome 520–521
Types 519
Peripheral vascular disease 217–218
Peristalsis 95, 155, 339, 358, 361, 502
Pernicious anaemia 11, 204, 205, 347
Perseveration 489
Person-centred Nursing xxi, 4, 15, 18, 46, 47, 55, 74, 260, 271, 336, 412, 534
Interprofessional collaboration 72
Mental ill-health 141
Person-Centred Nursing Framework xxii
Petechial rash 178, 510
Phaeochromocytoma 119, 547–549
Phagocytosis 14, 151, 155, 156, 163, 292, 580
Pharmaceutical regulations 84, 85–86
General Sales List (GSL) 85
Independent prescribers 85
Nurse prescribers 86
Over The Counter (OTC) 85
Pharmacy medicines 85
Prescribers 85
Prescription Only Medicines (POMs) 85
Supplementary prescribers 85
Pharmacodynamics 84, 87–88, 92, 96
Agonists 87
Antagonists 87
Drug receptors 87–88
Pharmacokinetics 84, 88–93, 95, 96
Absorption 88–91, 96–97
Absorption processes 92
Binding 97

Bioavailability 88
Distribution 89, 92, 97
Excretion 89, 93, 97
Factors influencing 93
First pass metabolism 90–91
Metabolism 89, 92–93, 97
Pharmacokinetic mechanisms 89
Plasma concentration 90
Pharmacology 51, 84, 507 (*see* also Chapter 4)
Pharyngitis 175
Phenylalanine 398–399
Phenylketonuria 108, 120, 373, 398, 399
Heel prick test 120, 399
Phimosis 597, 607–608
Phlebitis 178
Photosensitivity 159–160
Pilli 172
Piloerection 499
Pituitary adenomas 243, 535–536
Prolactinomas 536
Signs and symptoms 536
Placenta abruptio, *see* Placental disorder
Placenta praevia, *see* Placental disorder
Placental disorder 571–574
Placenta abruptio 572, 574
Placenta praevia 572
Placental infections 574
Twin pregnancy 571, 573
Placental infections, *see* Placental disorder
Plasmids 171, 181
Platelet-Activating Factor (PAF) 179, 349, 364
Pleural effusion 422, 424
Chylothorax 424
Empyema 424
Haemothorax 424
Hydrothorax 424
Pleural effusion 422, 424
Plicae 559
Pluripotent 612
Pneumonia 11, 163, 164, 173, 177, 179, 181, 312, 344, 414, 416, 417, 418–419, 424, 432, 509
Atypical pneumonia 419
Classifications 418
Typical pneumonia (acute bacterial) 419
Pneumothorax 411, 422–423
Primary spontaneous 423
Secondary spontaneous 423
Signs and symptoms 423
Spontaneous 422
Tension pneumothorax 202, 423
Traumatic 423
Polycystic ovary syndrome (PCOS) 389, 568–569, 586, 587
Androgen-related symptoms 568–569
Polycystic ovary 568
Polycythaemia 207, 430
Polycythaemia vera 207
Secondary polycythaemia 207
Polydipsia 306–308, 312, 385, 390, 393, 394
Polygenic inheritance 105, 112–113

Polyhydramnios 571
Polymicrobe 175
Polymorphic 466–467
Polymorphism 162, 262
Polyphagia 385
Polyploidy 109
Polyuria 307, 308, 316, 325, 380, 385, 390, 393, 394
Porphyria 373, 519
Portal hypertension 61, 404–405
Posterior cord syndrome 501
Post-ictal phase 507
Post-natal depression, *see* Postpartum disturbances
Postpartum disturbances 578–579
Amniotic fluid embolism 578
Post-natal depression 578
Postpartum haemorrhage 577, 578
Puerperal fever 578–579
Uterine damage 578
Postpartum haemorrhage, *see* Postpartum disturbances
Postrenal AKI 322
Post-traumatic epilepsy (PTE), *see* Traumatic brain injury
Precocious puberty, *see* Growth hormone
Pre-eclampsia 572, 574, 575, 576
Phases 575
Premature ejaculation 605
Characteristics of 605
Primary 605
Secondary 605
Preputial orifice 608
Pressure ulcers (decubitus ulcers) 171, 273
Grades 273
Priapism 499
Primary (congenital) immunodeficiencies 162–163
Antibody deficiencies 163
Combined 162–163
Complement deficiencies 163
Failure to thrive 162
Single gene mutation 162
Primary adrenal cortical insufficiency, *see* Adrenal cortical insufficiency
Primary Brain Injury 484–486, 487, 489
Focal Primary Brain Injuries 486
Primary Brain Injuries and their Pathophysiology 484–486
Primary encephalitis, *see* Encephalitis
Primary hypertension, *see* Hypertension
Primary immunodeficiency 162
Primary injury, *see* Primary brain injury
Primary polydipsia 308
Procallus 281
Procarboxypeptidase 352
Processus vaginalis 597–598
Prodromal 139, 507, 605
Progression 8, 9, 29, 162, 167, 174, 208, 226, 232, 236, 237, 239, 240, 246, 252, 295, 326, 347, 430, 435, 438, 607, 609, 610
Prokaryotes 170–171

Prolactinomas, *see* Pituitary adenomas
Proliferation (cellular) 108, 225, 227, 234, 237, 240, 241, 266, 268, 269, 291, 432, 509, 515, 569, 581, 607, 612
Proliferative disorders 207–209
Promotion 237, 240, 252
Prosopagnosia 489
Prostaglandins 268, 270, 349, 417, 426
Prostate cancer 118, 235, 239, 243, 247, 584, 609–611
  Gene mutations in 610
  Gleason score 610
  PSA screening 611
  Zones of the prostate 609
Prostate Specific Antigen (PSA) 243, 610
Prostate Specific Membrane Antigen (PSMA) 610
Prostatitis 175, 605
Protease 167, 172, 239, 261, 287, 349, 417, 432, 433, 439
Proteasome 513
Proteinuria 160, 316, 325, 326, 575, 576
Proteolysis 340
Proteolytic enzymes 153, 160, 194, 364, 431
Protozoa 169, 170, 171, 173, 174, 177, 558, 571
Protozoan infection, *see* Sexually transmitted infections
Pruritus 264, 402, 404, 558, 560
Pseudoangiomatous stromal hyperplasia 581
Pseudopolyps 356
Psoriasis 259, 261–262, 286,
  Cellular changes in 261
  Lived experience of 262
Psoriatic Arthritis (PsA) 262
Public health 23, 24, 25, 26, 30–40, 50, 66, 67, 152, 181, 324, 341, 416
  Agriculture and livestock 39
  Challenges 38–39
  Governance 36
  Health disorders 39–40
  Health improvement 33–34
  Health literacy 36
  Health promotion 35
  Health protection 32–33, 36
  Inequalities 38
  Infrastructure 38
  Population growth 38
  Service improvement 34
  Value of 35
Puerperal fever, *see* Postpartum disturbances
Pulmonary disorders 91, 424–436, 458
  Atelectasis 424–425
  Obstructive lung disorders 424–436
Pulmonary embolism (PE) 200, 202, 377, 436–437, 461,
  Risk factors 437
Pulmonary fibrosis, *see* Idiopathic pulmonary fibrosis
Pulmonary hypertension 414, 430, 432, 434, 436, 437–438, 439
  Classification 438

Pulmonary oedema 199, 272, 310, 414, 439, 454, 456–459, 473
Pulmonary stenosis 473
Pulse pressure 196
Purpura 178, 210, 361
Pyelonephritis 11, 312, 313, 315–317, 324
  Acute pyelonephritis 315–316
    Diagnosis and treatment 316
    Signs and symptoms 316
  Antibiotic resistance 317
  Antibiotic stewardship (AS) 317
  Chronic pyelonephritis 316–317
    Diagnosis and treatment 317
    Signs and symptoms 316
Pyogenes 546

Quadriplegia 498

Radicular pain 501
Radiotherapy (radiation therapy) 47, 54–55, 209, 245, 541, 561, 565, 582, 584, 585
Raised intracranial pressure, *see* Intracranial hypertension
Reactive oxygen species 15, 272, 349, 439, 509, 514
  Apoptosis 15
  Mitochondria 15
Recessive inheritance 395
Rectocele 565
Reelin 138
Refeeding syndrome (RFS) 340–341
Regulation 46–51, 84
  Advanced Nurse Practitioner 48
  British Acupuncture Council 50
  Complementary and Natural Healthcare Council 50
  Genetic Counsellor Registration Board 50
  Nursing and Midwifery Council (NMC) 48
  Pharmaceutical 50, 84
  Statutory 48
  UK Public Health Register 50
Remission 139, 160, 244, 289, 348, 350, 355, 436, 515
Renal calculi (kidney stones) (urolithiasis) 315, 318–320, 544
  Diagnosis and treatment 319–320
  Signs and symptoms 319
  Types 318
Renal failure 7, 8, 61, 67, 119, 195, 197, 306, 320, 321, 324, 325, 393
Renal insufficiency 320, 393
Renal tubular acidosis (RTA) 311–312, 379
Renin 310, 451
Renin-Angiotensin Aldosterone System (RAAS) 304, 310, 311, 449, 450, 451, 452, 455
Respiratory disease 8, 173, 400, 415, 425, 429, 432, 433
  Phases of 415
Respiratory failure 415, 434, 438, 439
Respiratory tract infections (RTIs) 154, 169, 412, 415–422

Lower respiratory tract infections (LRTIs) 418–422
Upper respiratory tract infections (URTIs) 415–418
Restrictive Cardiomyopathy 467–468
Retching 338–339
Reticular Activating System (RAS) 495
Reticular formation 495, 502
Retinopathy 393
Retrograde ejaculation, *see* Ejaculatory dysfunction
Retrovirus 164
Reverse transcriptase 164, 167
Rheumatoid arthritis (RA) 8, 9, 55, 151, 156, 158, 159, 160–162, 204, 209, 276, 289–291, 349, 385
   Citrullination 162
   Clinical features 162
   Disease process 290
   Environmental risk factors 289
   Lived experience of 291
   Pannus formation 161
   Rheumatoid factors 162
   Signs and symptoms 291
Rheumatoid factors 162, 289, 290
Rhinitis, *see* Upper respiratory tract infections
Rhinorrhoea 415–417, 426
Rickets 35, 283, 285, 399

Sacral sparing 499
Salpingitis 559
   Acute suppurative salpingitis 559
   Chronic salpingitis 559
   Hydrosalpinx 559
   Tubo-ovarian abscesses 559
Salpingo-oophorectomy 565
Sarcoidosis 423, 434, 435–436, 537, 546
Schizophrenia 64, 113, 132, 137–140
   Amygdala 140
   Excitotoxicity 140
   Hippocampus 140
   Microcephaly 139
   Prefrontal cortex 140
   Proinflammatory cytokines 139
   Psychosis 138, 140
   Reelin 138
   Signs and symptoms 140
   Stages 139
Sclerosing adenosis 581
Scoliosis 119, 295, 439
Secondary (acquired) immunodeficiencies 163–167
   Causes 163
   HIV and acquired immune deficiency syndrome (AIDS) 164–167
   Protein-calorie malnutrition 164
Secondary (post-infectious) encephalitis 508
Secondary adrenal cortical insufficiency, *see* Adrenal cortical insufficiency
Secondary Brain injury 483, 484, 485, 487–503
   Cellular effect of 487
Secondary hypertension, *see* Hypertension

Secondary injury (neurological) 484, 487
Segmental fracture, *see* Fracture
Seizures 51, 119, 178, 309, 373, 379, 393, 396, 397, 493, 494, 503, 504–507, 536, 538
   Classification of seizures 505–506
   Phases of 507
   Types of seizures 505
Seizure disorders 482, 503–507
Self-antigens 151, 156, 158, 159, 289
Self-tolerance 59, 159, 162, 516
Seminomas 611–612
Sensitisation 57, 152, 425
Sepsis 52, 177, 178–181, 197, 198, 272, 306, 322, 340, 350, 363, 365, 401, 436, 439, 459, 579, 611
   Mediators 180
   Pathophysiology 179
   Septic shock 179
   Systemic inflammatory response syndrome (SIRS) 179
   Treatment 180
Septic shock, *see* Distributive shock
Septum primum 469
Septum secundum 469
Serotype 360, 416
Sertoli cells 600–601
Serum amyloid 435
Serum sickness 156
Sex-linked inheritance 105, 106
Sexually transmitted infections (STIs) 170, 174–177, 602
   Chlamydia 175
   Genital herpes 176
   Gonorrhoea 175
   Human papilloma virus (HPV) 176–177
   Pathogens 174
   Protozoan infection 177
   Syphilis 175–176
Sheehan syndrome 537
Shock 154, 178, 179, 195, 196–203, 218, 272, 350, 359, 365
   Anaphylactic 11, 99, 154, 199–200
   Cardiogenic shock 200–201, 378
   Distributive shock 198–200
   Haemorrhagic shock 197
   Hypovolaemic shock 197–198, 206
   Key facts 196
   Management of 202–203
   Neurogenic shock 200, 499
   Obstructive shock 202
   Pathophysiology 196–197
   Septic 172, 179, 180, 197, 198–199, 272
   Spinal shock 499
Short stature in children 537–538
   Causes 538
Sinus arrhythmias 465–466
   Bradycardia in healthy people 466
   Sinus bradycardia 465–466
   Sinus tachycardia 466
Sinus bradycardia, *see* Sinus arrhythmias

Sinus tachycardia, *see* Sinus arrhythmias
Sinusitis, *see* Upper respiratory tract infections
Skin Disorders 16, 261–274
  Acne vulgaris 266–268
  Alopecia 269–271
  Burns (thermal injury) 270–272
  Dermatitis/Eczema 262
  Epidermoid cysts 269
  Epidermolysis bullosa acquisita (EBA) 263–264
  Impetigo vulgaris 264–265
  Pressure ulcers (decubitus ulcers) 273–274
  Psoriasis 261–362
  Stevens–Johnson Syndrome/toxic epidermal
    necrolysis 262–263
  Vitiligo 265–266
Soft Tissue Injury 274–276
  Contusion 274
  Dislocations 276
  Haematoma 274
  Muscle tears 276
  Strains/sprains 275
  Treatment 275
Somatic cell 235
Spasms 306, 503, 505
Spastic dystonia 503
Spasticity 63, 87, 502–503
  Benefits of mild spasticity 503
  Effects in the limbs 503
Spermatogenesis 597, 600, 601
Spermatogonia 600–601, 612
Spermatozoa 107, 600
Spina bifida 64, 113, 121, 521–522
Spinal cord injury 327, 439, 484, 496–503
  Autonomic dysreflexia 499
  Classification 497
  Incomplete Spinal Injury Syndromes 500–501
  Levels of Injuries and Associated Impairments 498
  Neurogenic bowel and bladder 502
  Neurogenic shock 499
  Spasticity 502–503
  Spinal shock 499
  Vulnerable injury points on the spine 497
Spinal shock, *see* Spinal cord injury
Spiral (torsion) fracture, *see* Fracture
Spongiofibrosis 603
Spontaneous abortion (miscarriage), *see* gestational
    disorders
Spontaneous Bacterial Peritonitis (SBP) 405
Spontaneous pneumothorax 423
Sprain 273–275, 286
Squamous cell hyperplasia, *see* Non-neoplastic
    epithelial disorders
Stages of puberty 554
Starvation 230, 340, 362, 385
Statins 24, 25, 86, 97, 195, 397–398
Steatohepatitis 403–404
Steatorrhoea 351–352, 365
Steatosis 403–404
Stem cell transplantation, *see* cancer
Stenosis 194, 215, 468, 473, 493, 501

Stent 195
Stevens–Johnson Syndrome 262–263
  Common drug causes 263
Strain
  Muscular/tissue 11, 275, 577
  Pathogenic 317, 417, 420
Stress 5, 10, 12–15, 53, 69, 113, 132, 133, 134, 135,
    137, 139, 142, 176, 180, 209, 231, 276, 293,
    306, 338, 341, 349, 353, 354, 517, 534, 535,
    546, 548
  Alarm reaction 13
  Catecholamines 12
  Circadian rhythm 15
  Cognition 142
  Diabetes 14
  Glucocorticoids 12, 13–14
  Headaches 517
  Hypothalamus 12
  Response 12, 133, 535
Stress incontinence, *see* urinary incontinence
Stricture 315, 365, 602–603
Stroke 11, 35, 62, 64, 65, 92, 113, 114, 192, 194,
    195, 200, 207, 211–215, 315, 327, 337, 373,
    394, 395, 400, 461, 463, 482, 485, 502, 504,
    505, 524, 548
  Anticoagulant treatment 212
  Communication loss 214–215
  Effect on each side of the brain 213
  Embolic 212
  Haemorrhagic stroke 212
  Identification 212–213
  Ischaemic stroke 211–212
  Life after stroke 211
  Physiological changes in 211
  Thrombolysis 212
  Thrombotic 211
  Transient ischaemic attack (TIA) 213–214
Stromal lesions, *see* Breast
Subarachnoid haemorrhage 212, 309, 310, 485,
    495, 537
Subdural haematoma 10, 484–486
Sudden arrhythmic death syndrome (SADS)
    18, 466
Sudden cardiac death 466
Superoxide Dismutase (SOD1) 513
Supersaturation of urine 319
Supplementary prescribers 85–86
Suppurate 313
Supraventricular 356
Surgery 6, 26, 51–54, 55, 60, 64, 69, 93, 107,
    118, 177, 195–197, 202, 217, 231, 245, 322,
    327, 340, 350, 377, 424, 437, 459, 537, 541,
    561–562, 565–566, 569, 577–580, 584–587,
    602, 604, 606
Symptomatic (secondary) epilepsy, *see* Epilepsy
Synaptogenesis 134
Syncetium 583
Syncope 437, 438, 466, 506
Syndrome of inappropriate secretion of ADH
    (SIADH) 309–310

Syphilis 174, 175–176
  Stages of 176
Syringobulbia 523
Syringomyelia 523
Syrinx 523
Systemic inflammatory response syndrome (SIRS) 179, 272, 365, 401
  Diagnosis 179
Systemic lupus erythematous (SLE) 159–160
  Antinuclear antibodies (ANA) 159
  Clinical signs and symptoms 159–160
  Epidemiology 159

T helper cells 156, 160, 383, 384, 430
Tachycardia 13, 179, 180, 198, 308, 339, 356, 358, 373, 377, 393, 414, 419, 423, 424, 460, 463, 464, 465, 466, 548, 574
Tachypnoea 179, 339, 365, 413, 419, 422, 424, 425, 428, 433
Tay-Sachs disease 122–123, 396
Telogen phase 269–270
Teniae coli 357
Tenosynovitis 262
Tension pneumothorax 202
Tension type headache, see Headache
Teratogenic 100, 522
Teratoma 611
Teratozoospermia 597
Testicular cancer 7, 25, 225, 596, 597, 611–613
  Early detection and treatment 611–612
  Risk factors 611
  Testicular self-examination 612–613
  Types 611
Testicular torsion 595, 602, 611
Tetraplegia 497–498
Thalassaemia 6, 204
Thermal injury, see Burns
Thrombocythaemia 210
Thrombocytopenia 160, 361, 405
Thrombolysis 212
Thrombosis 46, 156, 178, 194–196, 207, 210, 212, 215, 230, 271, 358, 436
Thyroid storm 377
Thyrotoxic crisis 377
Thyrotoxicosis, see hyperthyroidism
Tonsillitis 175
Tophi 292
Torsion of the testes, see Testicular torsion
Toxic epidermal necrolysis, see skin disorders (Stevens–Johnson Syndrome)
Transient ischaemic attack (TIA) 195, 211, 213–214
  ABCD^2 tool 213–214
Translocation 365, 403, 418
Transmural 355
Transposition of the great arteries (TGA) 474–475
Transverse fracture, see Fracture
Traumatic brain injury (TBI) 308, 310, 483–496, 502, 537, 538
  Classification of severity 483
  Disorders of consciousness 494–496

Glasgow Coma Scale 483
Intracranial hypertension (raised intracranial pressure) 490–491
Living with a brain injury 488
Lobal Effects of Brain Injury 489–490
Post-traumatic epilepsy (PTE) 493–494
Primary Brain Injury 484–486
Secondary Brain injury 487–488
Traumatic subarachnoid haemorrhage 485
Trichomoniasis 174, 177
Trigeminal neuralgia 518
  Divisions of the trigeminal nerve 519
Trisomy 110–111
Trophoblast 575
Tuberculosis (TB) 35, 123, 157, 158, 166, 177, 178, 232, 401, 419–422, 423, 432, 510, 546
  Primary TB 421
  Risk factors 420
  Secondary TB 421–422
Tumour 54, 55, 59, 108, 119, 136, 198, 227, 229, 232–240, 242–247, 253, 292, 308, 357, 358, 376, 401, 425, 501, 504, 505, 535, 536, 538, 540–543, 564, 569, 582, 584, 585, 598, 609, 610, 611, 618
Tumour markers 242–243
Tumour Necrosis Factor (TNF) 153, 160, 162, 179, 180, 198, 263, 271, 286, 287, 289, 364, 384, 419, 426, 432, 515, 618
Tumour Nodes Metastasis (TNM) system 243
Tumour suppressor genes (TSG) 234–237, 247, 253
Tumours 54, 55, 57, 109, 119, 164, 227, 228, 229, 233, 243, 244–246, 254, 358, 424, 436, 491, 493, 535, 536, 537, 541, 543, 547, 560, 611, 612
  Characteristics of 227–228
  Nomenclature of benign and malignant tumours 233
  Staging and grading of 243–244
Tunica albugenia 612
Tunica vaginalis 597–598, 602
Twin pregnancy 571
  Types of Placentae with Twin Pregnancies 573
Type 2 diabetes mellitus 4, 58, 68, 372, 374, 380, 382, 386–393, 404
  Causes and risk factors 387
  Hyperosmolar hyperglycaemic non-ketotic syndrome (HHNKS) 393
  Incretins 392
  Insulin deficiency 390
  Insulin resistance 398–390
  Insulin sensitisers 390
  Obesity 389
  Pathogenesis of insulin resistance 388
  Signs and symptoms 390
  Treatment 390–392
Type I immediate hypersensitivity disorders (allergy) 152–155
  Allergen 152
  Allergic reaction 152
  Allergic Rhinitis 154–155

Anaphylactic reactions 154
Antibodies 152
Asthma 153
Bronchial Asthma 154
Cytokines 152
Food allergies 155
Genetic susceptibility 153
Histamine 152
Immunotherapy 155
Inflammation 153
Late/delayed response 153
Mast cells 152
Primary/immediate response 153
T-helper lymphocytes 152
Tumour necrosis factor (TNF) 153
Urticaria 153
Type II antibody-mediated disorders 155–156
    Antibodies 155
    Complement 156
    Graves' Disease 156
    Immune complexes 155
    Opsonisation 155
Type III immune complex-mediated disorders 156
    Antigen–antibody complexes 156
    Complement 156
Type IV cell-mediated hypersensitivity disorders
        156–158
    Delayed-type mediated hypersensitivity
        (DTH) 156
    Direct cell-mediated response 156
    Granulomatous hypersensitivity 158
    Latex allergy 158
    Mantoux test 158
    Reactions 156, 157
Tyrosinaemia 373, 399

Ubiquitin 513
Ubiquitination 512
Ulcerative colitis 8, 354–355, 356–357
    Signs and symptoms 356
Unipolar depression 132, 133–135
    Altered synaptogenesis 134
    Amygdala 133
    Antidepressant therapy 135
    Atrophy 133
    Basal ganglia 133
    Cingulate cortex 133
    Cognition 133
    Cytokines 134
    Elements 134
    Glucocorticoids 134
    Glutamate 134
    Hippocampus 133
    Hypothalamic–pituitary–adrenal (HPA) axis 134
    Limbic system 134
    Living with depression 141
    Low mood 133
    Neurogenesis 135
    Neuronal hypertrophy 134
    Neurotransmitters 134–135

Oxidative stress 134
    Prefrontal cortex 133
    Pyramidal neurons 133
    Signs and symptoms 135
Unresponsive Wakefulness Syndrome (UWS) 495
Unstable angina 215
Upper respiratory tract infections (URTIs) 415–418
    Common cold 416
    Croup 417–418
    Influenza 416–417
    Otitis media 417
    Rhinitis 417
    Sinusitis 417
Uraemia 320–321, 323, 325
Uraemic syndrome 320, 361
Urethral strictures 602–604
    Treatment of 603–604
Urethritis 175, 602
Urethrocele 565
Urethroplasty 604
Urethrotomy 603–604
Urge incontinence, see urinary incontinence
Urinary incontinence 327–329
    Age 329
    Diagnosis and treatment 328
    Overflow incontinence 327
    Stress incontinence 327
    Urge incontinence 327
Urinary oxalates 561
Urinary tract infection (UTI) 7, 174, 303, 312–317,
        319, 555
    Aetiological factors 312
    Cystitis 313–314
    Pyelonephritis 315–317
    Types 313
Urticaria 153
Uterine prolapse 327, 565–567
    Stages of 565, 567
Uterosacral ligaments 560, 562, 565–567
    Disorders of 565
    Effects of 566
Uterus didelphys, see Double Uterus
Uveitis 436

Vaccination 35, 59, 150, 169, 177, 253, 402
Vacuolating toxin 349
Vaginal disorders 561
    Cancer of the vagina 561
    Vaginitis 561
Vaginitis, see Vaginal disorders
Vaptans 309
Variation 4–6
    Behavioural 5
    Physical 5
Varicocele 599–600
Vascular Endothelial Growth Factor (VEGF)
        237, 432
Vasculitis 156, 162
Vasoconstriction 178, 201, 206, 230, 322, 323, 325,
        414, 438, 449, 451, 499, 575

Vasodilation 13, 152, 153, 154, 179, 180, 310, 365, 376, 401, 414, 426, 427, 491, 499, 517, 604
Vasopressors 180, 201
Vasospasm 485, 576
Vegetative state (VS) 495
Venous thrombosis 195–196, 207, 210
   Deep vein thrombosis (DVT) 196
   Pulmonary embolism 196
Ventilation 13, 199, 202, 412, 413, 418, 425, 426, 428, 439, 498
Ventilation/Perfusion (V/Q) mismatch 16, 413, 414, 426, 430, 432, 436
Ventricular fibrillation (VF), *see* Arrhythmias
Ventricular septal defects (VSDs) 471–472
   Shunting in ventricular septal defect 472
Ventricular tachycardia (VT), *see* Arrhythmias
Very Low Density Lipoproteins (VLDLs) 395
Vesiculation 520
Viral infection, *see* Infection
Vitamin D 6, 14, 16, 251, 283, 306, 318, 351, 516
Vitiligo 265–266, 548
   Living with 266
   Non-segmental 265
   Psychological burden of 266
   Segmental 265
   Types of vitiligo presentation 265
Volume-Responsive (prerenal) AKI 322–324
Vomiting 13, 56, 93, 154, 155, 172, 178, 197, 216, 240, 246, 306, 316, 319, 320, 335, 338, 339–340, 346, 350, 353, 357, 358, 359, 360, 363, 365, 373, 379, 380, 397, 402, 404, 438, 536, 546, 547, 548
   Vomiting reflex 339
Vulvodynia 561

Waterhouse-Friderichsen Syndrome 547
Wernicke's aphasia 214, 489
Wolman disease 397

Zona fasciculata 543
Zona glomerulosa 543
Zona reticularis 543